Handbook
of
Multiple
Sclerosis

NEUROLOGICAL DISEASE AND THERAPY

Advisory Board

Additional Volumes in Preparation

Handbook
of
Multiple
Sclerosis

Third Edition

edited by
Stuart D. Cook

University of Medicine and Dentistry of New Jersey
and New Jersey Medical School
Newark, New Jersey

MARCEL DEKKER, INC.   NEW YORK • BASEL

ISBN: 0-8247-0485-1

This book is printed on acid-free paper.

Headquarters
Marcel Dekker, Inc.
270 Madison Avenue, New York, NY 10016
tel: 212-696-9000; fax: 212-685-4540

Eastern Hemisphere Distribution
Marcel Dekker AG
Hutgasse 4, Postfach 812, CH-4001 Basel, Switzerland
tel: 41-61-261-8482; fax: 41-61-261-8896

World Wide Web
http://www.dekker.com

The publisher offers discounts on this book when ordered in bulk quantities. For more information, write to Special Sales/Professional Marketing at the headquarters address above.

Series Introduction

Multiple sclerosis (MS) is a common disease of the central nervous system, affecting young women in particular. This disease can devastate the professional and social life of those affected. There has been a recent explosion in knowledge about how to diagnose MS and understand its pathophysiological mechanisms as well as provide efficacious treatment. The third edition of the *Handbook of Multiple Sclerosis* has documented the impressive and dramatic advances that have occurred. In particular, the immunopathology of the disease is now well established. MS at one time was considered an untreatable disease; however, now there are many therapeutic approaches. As Dr. Cook states, these advances have led to a reduction in disability and a dramatic increase in the quality of life for patients suffering with this potentially disabling disease.

This edition of the *Handbook of Multiple Sclerosis* provides clinicians with informative and detailed information regarding almost every aspect of MS. For health care professionals working with MS patients, this book provides an invaluable resource. Treatment modalities are thoroughly discussed and comments are given about the ongoing research in MS, which will lead to better understanding and treatment in the future.

William C. Koller

Preface

Only ten years have passed since publication of the first edition of the *Handbook of Multiple Sclerosis*, and impressive advances have been made in our understanding of multiple sclerosis (MS), particularly with regard to its natural history, immunopathology, lesion evolution based on imaging techniques, and therapy. Physicians are now in a much better position to prescribe medications that can modify disease course, decrease lesion burden, and alleviate symptoms. Many patients can look forward to fewer exacerbations, a slower rate of deterioration, and a better quality of life. Although current treatments are only palliative, the exciting prospect of medications that can prevent further disability, and even promote recovery from fixed neurological deficits, no longer seems so remote.

Increased funding for MS research from a variety of sources, including federal funding agencies, the pharmaceutical industry, and national MS societies worldwide, has led to more scientists and clinicians partaking in basic and clinical studies directed toward finding the cause and cure of this enigmatic disorder. Patients are much better informed about cutting-edge treatments and ongoing clinical trials through information available on the Internet.

Over the next few years, we can expect further advances in our knowledge about genetic susceptibility and environmental factors causing MS, and about the interaction between those factors and the immune response that results in lesion pathogenesis. This should lead to better-focused research and more rapid development of effective therapies.

This edition of the *Handbook of Multiple Sclerosis* will provide the reader with the most up-to-date and detailed information currently available about all aspects of MS. It should provide a valuable resource to anyone interested in this disease, be it patient, student, clinician, or scientist. I am very grateful to the contributors, who are world leaders in MS research and treatment. This book is dedicated to those individuals who bravely cope with MS on a daily basis, their devoted friends and family members, and their caring physicians.

Stuart D. Cook

Contents

Contents

Contributors

Khurram Bashir, M.D.   Department of Neurology, University of Alabama at Birmingham, Birmingham, Alabama

Etty N. Benveniste, Ph.D.   Department of Cell Biology, University of Alabama at Birmingham, Birmingham, Alabama

Suprabha Bhat, M.D.   Department of Neurology, The University of Texas—Houston, Health Science Center, Houston, Texas

Carl Bjartmar, M.D., Ph.D.   Department of Neurosciences, Lerner Research Institute, Cleveland Clinic Foundation, Cleveland, Ohio

Peter Calabresi   University of Maryland Medical Center, Baltimore, Maryland

Christian Confavreux, M.D.   Service de Neurologie A, Hôpital Neurologique, Lyon, France

Stuart D. Cook, M.D.   University of Medicine and Dentistry of New Jersey and New Jersey Medical School, Newark, New Jersey

Fiona Costello, M.D.   Memorial University of Newfoundland, St. John's, Newfoundland, Canada

Anne H. Cross, M.D.   Department of Neurology and Neurosurgery, Washington University School of Medicine, St. Louis, Missouri

Gary Cutter, Ph.D.   AMC Cancer Institute, Denver, Colorado

Mauro C. Dal Canto, M.D.   Departments of Pathology (Neuropathology) and Neurology, Northwestern University Medical School, Chicago, Illinois

Jill S. Fischer, Ph.D.　Mellen Center for Multiple Sclerosis Treatment and Research, Cleveland Clinic Foundation, Cleveland, Ohio

Donald E. Goodkin, M.D.　Department of Neurology, UCSF/Mt. Zion MS Center, San Francisco, California

Jan Hillert, M.D., Ph.D.　Karolinska Institutet at Huddinge University Hospital, Huddinge, Sweden

Lawrence Jacobs, M.D.　Department of Neurology, School of Medicine and Biomedical Sciences, State University of New York at Buffalo, Buffalo, New York

Kenneth P. Johnson, M.D.　Department of Neurology, University of Maryland Medical Center, Baltimore, Maryland

Orhun H. Kantarci, M.D.　Department of Neurology, Mayo Clinic and Foundation, Rochester, Minnesota

Mariko Kita, M.D.　Department of Neurology, UCSF/Mt. Zion MS Center, San Francisco, California

Fred D. Lublin, M.D.　Corinne Goldsmith Dickinson Center for Multiple Sclerosis, Mount Sinai School of Medicine, New York, New York

Jeri-Anne Lyons, Ph.D.　Department of Neurology and Neurosurgery, Washington University School of Medicine, St. Louis, Missouri

Thomas Masterman, B.A., B.S.　Karolinska Institutet at Huddinge University Hospital, Huddinge, Sweden

W. I. McDonald, Ph.D., FRCP　Royal College of Physicians, London, England

Henry F. McFarland, M.D.　Neuroimmunology Branch, National Institute of Neurological Disorders and Stroke, National Institutes of Health, Bethesda, Maryland

Aaron E. Miller, M.D.　Maimonides Medical Center and State University of New York Health Science Center at Brooklyn, Brooklyn, New York

Marc R. Nuwer, M.D., Ph.D.　Department of Neurology, UCLA School of Medicine, and Department of Clinical Neurophysiology, UCLA Medical Center, Los Angeles, California

Hillel Panitch, M.D.　Department of Neurology, University of Maryland School of Medicine, Baltimore, Maryland

John W. Prineas, M.D., FRCP　Veterans Administration Medical Center, East Orange, New Jersey, and Institute of Clinical Neurosciences, Department of Medicine, The University of Sydney, Sydney, Australia

William Pryse-Phillips, M.D., FRCP, FRCP(C)   Memorial University of Newfoundland, St. John's, Newfoundland, Canada

George P. A. Rice, M.D., FRCPC   The Multiple Sclerosis Clinic, London, Ontario, Canada

Nancy Richert, M.D., Ph.D.   Laboratory of Diagnostic Radiology Research, Clinical Center, National Institutes of Health, Bethesda, Maryland

Christine Rohowsky-Kochan, Ph.D.   University of Medicine and Dentistry of New Jersey and New Jersey Medical School, Newark, New Jersey

Peter Rudge, FRCP   The National Hospital for Neurology and Neurosurgery, London, England

Richard Rudick, M.D.   Mellen Center for Multiple Sclerosis Treatment and Research, Cleveland Clinic Foundation, Cleveland, Ohio

Randall T. Schapiro, M.D.   Fairview MS Center and University of Minnesota, Minneapolis, Minnesota

Labe Scheinberg, M.D.   Professor Emeritus, Department of Neurology, Albert Einstein College of Medicine, New York, New York

Charles R. Smith, M.D.   Multiple Sclerosis Comprehensive Care Center, St. Agnes Hospital, White Plains, New York

Lael A. Stone, M.D.   Mellen Center for Multiple Sclerosis Treatment and Research, Cleveland Clinic Foundation, Cleveland, Ohio

Bruce D. Trapp, Ph.D.   Department of Neurosciences, Lerner Research Institute, Cleveland Clinic Foundation, Cleveland, Ohio

Ute Traugott, M.D.   New York Medical College, Valhalla, St. Agnes Hospital, White Plains, and Bronx Lebanon Hospital, Bronx, New York

Raymond Troiano, M.D.   University of Medicine and Dentistry of New Jersey and New Jersey Medical School, Newark, New Jersey

John L. Trotter, M.D.   Department of Neurology and Neurosurgery, Washington University School of Medicine, St. Louis, Missouri

Sandra Vukusic, M.D.   Service de Neurologie A, Hôpital Neurologique, Lyon, France

Stephen G. Waxman, M.D., Ph.D.   Department of Neurology and PVA/EPVA Neuroscience Research Center, Yale University School of Medicine, New Haven, and Rehabilitation Research Center, VA Connecticut, West Haven, Connecticut

Brian G. Weinshenker, M.D.   Department of Neurology, Mayo Clinic and Foundation, Rochester, Minnesota

John N. Whitaker, M.D.   Department of Neurology, University of Alabama at Birmingham and The Neurology and Research Services of the Birmingham Veterans Medical Center, Birmingham, Alabama

Jerry S. Wolinsky, M.D.   Department of Neurology, The University of Texas–Houston, Health Science Center, Houston, Texas

Handbook
of
Multiple
Sclerosis

1

The History of Multiple Sclerosis

W. I. MCDONALD

Royal College of Physicians, London, England

I. INTRODUCTION: THE EARLY HISTORY OF MULTIPLE SCLEROSIS

The first depiction of the central nervous system in what we now recognize as multiple sclerosis was published by Carswell (1) in 1838. As Compston (2) has established, Cruveil-hier's pictures soon followed (3). To them were attached the first brief clinical descriptions. Valentiner (4) in 1856, working in the Department of Frerichs (who had also described cases of multiple sclerosis), reported exacerbations and remissions, and—it is interesting to note—mental changes as well. In 1864 Fromann (5) described and illustrated demyelination.

Thus the main clinical and pathological characteristics of multiple sclerosis were already recognized by the mid-1860s. It was Charcot (6), however, who in 1868 drew the threads together, adding new observations and making prescient pathophysiological interpretations in his magisterial lectures.

Babinski (7,8) described further important histological details, illustrating, for example, macrophages containing debris alongside axons denuded of myelin. The term *segmental demyelination* could not be used of central demyelination at that time, since—on the authority of Ranvier (9)—nodes were held not to exist on central nerve fibers. (It is interesting to note, in passing, that Babinski's drawings of normal central fibers show short gaps in the myelin that surely must be nodes, though he does not label them as such. He had, in his thesis, already disagreed with Charcot on a point of detail; perhaps he did not wish to contradict explicitly another great contemporary figure of the Parisian scientific world.)

II. THE TWENTIETH CENTURY

The history of the growth of understanding of multiple sclerosis in the twentieth century is one of growing complexity, since disciplines as various as particle physics, molecular biology, and population genetics have provided techniques and approaches that have helped to elucidate different aspects of the disease. It is convenient to consider the evolution of our knowledge under a number of headings.

A. Pathology

Marburg (10), early in the new century, described acute, rapidly fatal multiple sclerosis and emphasized the importance of axonal degeneration in many lesions. But it was Dawson (11) who, in 1916 provided the definitive histological account of the disease in his huge monograph. Little was then added until the introduction of the electron microscope to human neuropathology in the 1960s, followed by the application of the techniques of histochemistry and immunohistochemistry in the past three decades. The occurrence of remyelination was established and the patterns of myelin breakdown were documented (12–16). A rich variety of immunopathological changes in the lesions (and in the normal-appearing white matter) has been documented (see reviews in Refs. 17 and 18), though a coherent scheme for the initiation and evolution of the lesion making sense of both the immunopathology and the neuropathology, including that of the glia, has still to be established (see below).

B. Neurobiology

The importance of an understanding of the development and maintenance of neurons and their supporting structures is crucial to an understanding of the pathogenesis of multiple sclerosis and of repair mechanisms that compensate for the damage and are so strikingly effective in the early stages of the disease. The recognition by Raff and colleagues (19,20) of the different elements in the glial cell lineage in rodents was an important advance, as was the demonstration that similar cells exist in the central nervous system of adult human beings (21). Growing numbers of factors that influence cell division, differentiation, and migration are being recognized (see reviews in Refs. 22 and 23). How they interact in the normal and diseased nervous system is a major area of current investigation.

C. Pathophysiology

Charcot (6) was explicit that the areas of demyelination cause the symptoms of multiple sclerosis, and it is implicit in his account that loss of function was due to block of electrical conduction. Holmes (24) deduced from a postmortem study of spinal cord compression that demyelination must lead to conduction block. The first demonstration that this is so came, however, only during the Second World War, when Denny-Brown and Brenner (25), who were investigating the mechanisms of nerve injury, showed experimentally that chronic compression of a motor nerve could produce focal demyelination and that stimulation distal to such a lesion resulted in muscular contraction, whereas stimulation proximal to it did not.

The late 1940s saw a rapid development in the understanding of conduction in normal nerve; in particular, Huxley and Stämpfli (26) proved the existence of saltatory conduction in myelinated fibers. It then became of physiological interest to define the details of the consequences of demyelination. In the early 1960s, conduction block was demonstrated directly by recording from the lesion itself and the adjacent histologically normal fibers, and a new phenomenon, slowing of conduction, was demonstrated in single fibers (27–29) as well as in compound action potentials (30,31). Similar properties were soon identified in demyelinated central nerve fibers (32). The latter single-fiber study revealed intermittent conduction block, which resulted in irregular transmission of impulses, thus providing evidence for a speculation of Charco (6) a century earlier. In the 1970s the marked thermolability of fibers traversing a demyelinating lesion was demonstrated (33,34), and it was found that demyelinated axons can acquire the ability to conduct continuously, as in unmyelinated fibers (35). Restoration of conduction was shown to depend on the development of large numbers of sodium channels in the denuded internodal axon (36,37). It was later shown that a similar increase in the number of sodium channels occurs in surviving demyelinated axons in multiple sclerosis lesions (38). It is reasonable to conclude that this is a crucial element in remission.

Remyelination in the central nervous system was convincingly demonstrated experimentally by Bunge et al. (39) in 1961 and was later shown to restore secure conduction (40). As already mentioned, remyelination occurs in multiple sclerosis. Recent evidence suggests that under certain circumstances it may be extensive, though in many lesions at postmortem it is scanty and confined to the edges of lesions (12,41). The role of remyelination in different lesions at different ages and perhaps in different individuals (is it, for example, more extensive in benign multiple sclerosis?) has still to be defined.

What of the mechanism of the irrecoverable deficit that develops in most patients after the initial relapsing and remitting phase, in which recovery from individual relapses is often virtually complete? The use of magnetic resonance imaging (MRI) and magnetic resonance spectroscopy (MRS) techniques sensitive to neuronal and axonal loss has in the past 5 years provided evidence that the degenerative element in the pathological process (known since Charcot (6) and repeatedly reaffirmed; see review in Ref. 42) plays an important part (44–47) (see review in Ref. 48). It is nevertheless likely that failure of the early recovery mechanisms with the reappearance of conduction block in chronically demyelinated fibers also contributes (49).

D. Diagnosis

A practical consequence of the demonstration of slowing of conduction in demyelinated fibers was the introduction of the evoked potential method as a diagnostic technique. In the 1960s there had been a rapid development of nerve conduction studies as an aid to pathological diagnosis in peripheral neuropathy: demyelinating neuropathies were associated with marked slowing of conduction, while degenerative neuropathies were not. Recording of cerebral evoked potentials after peripheral stimulation had become feasible with the introduction of averaging techniques by Dawson (50). They were being increasingly used in the 1960s in the physiological investigation of cerebral function and had been studied in neuronal diseases affecting the cerebral cortex (51). Martin Halliday and I therefore decided to see whether evoked potentials could be used diagnostically in a way analogous to nerve conduction studies—given that, as in the peripheral nervous system, experimental degenerative lesions were not associated with slowing of conduction, whereas demyelinating lesions were (52). We started with the visual evoked potentials (VEP) in optic neuritis. Its potential value was at once clear: substantial delays were seen in more than 90% of cases (53). Exploitation of the somatosensory and brainstem auditory evoked potentials along similar lines quickly followed (see review in Ref. 54). The technique quickly became established as an invaluable noninvasive diagnostic procedure in the assessment of patients suspected of having multiple sclerosis (55). Overall abnormalities were found in 70% of patients with clinically definite multiple sclerosis, although the changes were not specific. From the point of view of pathophysiology, the evoked potential techniques have provided invaluable confirmation of mechanisms of symptom production predicted from animal studies (56,57).

Cerebrospinal Fluid Analysis.

Lumbar puncture was introduced by Quinke (58) and Wynter (59) in the late nineteenth century, and by 1925 it was well established that multiple sclerosis was associated with a particular abnormality known as the ''paretic colloidal gold curve'' (from its association with syphilitic general paralysis of the insane) (60). This abnormality is now known to be due to the presence of oligoclonal IgG. The demonstration of the latter depended on the application of electrophoresis to cerebrospinal fluid, first by Kabat et al. (61) in 1942. Later the introduction of polyacrylamide gels and isoelectric focusing increased the sensitivity to over 90%, though the specificity remains as poor as it was in the 1920s. Interpretation of the meaning of the observed abnormalities—as in evoked potentials and MRI— still depends on the clinical and other investigative contexts.

Magnetic Resonance Imaging

The demonstration in 1981 that MRI reveals abnormalities in multiple sclerosis represents a landmark in the history of our understanding of the disease (62). That these abnormalities correspond with plaques at postmortem was soon shown, and it became clear that MRI abnormalities are found in more than 95% of patients with clinically definite disease (63–65). As the following section recounts, the exploitation of MRI and MRS has also led to new insights into the pathogenesis of the disease.

E. Pathogenesis

While there was general agreement in the nineteenth century on the pathological changes in the nervous system in multiple sclerosis, there was a sharp division of opinion between Rindfleisch (66) and Charcot (6) on the mechanisms that lead to their development. Rindfleisch concluded that the primary change was inflammation. Charcot, on the other hand, took the view that the initial change was hyperplasia of the glia. The inflammatory hypothesis gradually gained support in the latter part of the twentieth century because of the similarity in the histology of multiple sclerosis and the T cell–mediated demyelinating disease experimental allergic encephalomyelitis, especially in its chronic relapsing form (13). Support also came from the similarities between the acute form of experimental disease and acute disseminated encephalomyelitis, and especially from fatal cases of encephalomyelitis following antirabies inoculation (67) in the 1970s. But it was the development of MRI and MRS in the 1980s and 1990s that provided compelling evidence for the role of inflammation in the evolution of the new lesion.

It has already been mentioned that the abnormalities on standard MRI correspond with lesions at postmortem. In the 1980s it was found that some lesions exhibit enhancement after the injection of gadolinium-DTPA, while some do not (68,69). Experimental, postmortem, and biopsy correlations provided good evidence that in this context enhancement indicates an increase in the permeability of the blood-brain barrier in association with inflammation (70). Serial studies at intervals as short as 1 week showed that enhancement (signaling inflammation) is the earliest event detectable by MRI in most lesions in relapsing/remitting and secondary progressive multiple sclerosis (71). It seems, however, that a few lesions in these forms of the disease (72,73) and the majority of the lesions in primary progressive multiple sclerosis (74) do not show evidence of inflammation *by these methods*. The situation is a complex one, since, at postmortem, inflammatory cells are present in primary progressive multiple sclerosis, though in smaller numbers than in secondary progressive multiple sclerosis (75).

MRS revealed that myelin breakdown occurs early in the inflammatory phase of the lesion (76). It is generally assumed that it is a consequence of the immune-mediated inflammation. However, Lassmann and colleagues (18,77), on the basis of biopsy and postmortem studies, have recently suggested that inflammation and demyelination may occur independently of each other and have proposed that several distinct pathogenetic mechanisms may exist in different clinical subgroups of patients with multiple sclerosis.

F. Etiology

What initiates the pathogenetic processes that lead to the pathology we see at postmortem and lead to the symptomatology we see during life? Charcot (6) confessed that it was not possible to have a clear idea of the cause of multiple sclerosis at the time that he lectured. By the last decade of the nineteenth century, however, the discovery that certain acute illnesses were caused by bacteria led to Marie's conviction (without evidence) that infection would be found to be the cause of multiple sclerosis (78). Some not very convincing evidence for infection (by spirochetes or the "spherula insularis") was adduced in the first part of the twentieth century but did not survive close examination (see review in Ref. 79). The conviction that a viral infection is the direct cause of multiple sclerosis has from time to time been held equally vehemently and with equally little objective support. And so it remains: though spontaneously occurring demyelinating diseases due to viral infection in animals are well recognized, repeated efforts to demonstrate persistent viral infection in multiple sclerosis have failed. That, however, does not exclude the possibility that infection—perhaps viral—might play a role in initiating the disease or in precipitating relapse. Indeed there is evidence that the latter is the case (80). What of the former? This brings us to a consideration of the epidemiology of multiple sclerosis.

G. Epidemiology

The earliest recognition (81) that there are differences in the frequency of multiple sclerosis in different populations came in 1903. Further evidence emerged from the consideration of the morbidity in ex-servicemen in the United States after the First World War (82). After the Second World War, Dean (83) observed an unexpectedly low prevalence of multiple sclerosis in South Africa. This observation was quickly followed by extensive epidemiological studies in many parts of the world (see review in Ref. 84). It soon became clear that there were real differences in the frequency of multiple sclerosis in different populations: it is an order of magnitude less prevalent among Orientals than among individuals of northern European origin. Among the latter the frequency varies with place of birth, residence, and age at migration (when this has taken place). These observations have been interpreted as indicating the existence of an environmental factor or factors in the cause of multiple sclerosis, and apparent spatiotemporal clusters of cases have been taken to support this view (85). What these factors might be, however, remains uncertain.

Genetic Factors

The epidemiological data and, in particular, the relative rarity of multiple sclerosis among Orientals suggested the operation of genetic factors influencing susceptibility. The familial occurrence of multiple sclerosis has been recognized since early in the twentieth century. Families usually share environments, but three sets of observations indicated that genetic factors are important: there is a higher concordance rate among monozygotic (about 30%) than dizygotic (about 2%) twins (86,87); adoptees living with the parent or a sibling with multiple sclerosis do not have an increased risk of developing the disease (88); and half siblings have a significantly lower risk of developing multiple sclerosis than full siblings, there being no difference in risk for those reared together and those reared apart (89). But given that about 70% even of monozygotic twins are not concordant and not all twin studies have yielded the same results, it is clear that genetic factors play only a part in the etiology of the disease.

How might the genetic factors operate? The observation of an association between the HLA system and multiple sclerosis was a promising start, but the recent results of large international collaborative investigations have made it clear that there is not a single major susceptibility locus and that a number of genetic factors other than those related to the HLA region are involved (90–94) (see review in Ref. 95). The mechanism of susceptibility thus remains elusive.

H. Treatment

Physicians, of course, must try to help their patients whether or not the mechanism of the disease is fully understood. In the nineteenth century as now, treatments were designed partly to relieve symptoms and partly to modify the course of the disease. The treatments used for Augustus D'Este in the 1830s and 1840s [and recorded in meticulous detail by him (96)] had a basis rational enough to his physicians but are wholly without basis from our perspective (79).

Treatments Based on Theories of Etiology

Marie's (78) advocacy of infection as the cause of multiple sclerosis was accompanied by his recommendation that mercury should be used for its "disinfective properties." Because of their effectiveness in syphilis, organic arsenical compounds were recommended when a spirochete was thought to be the cause (97). In 1924 the fashion changed to malarial treatment (with the same rationale) (98). But malaria was not readily available for transmission in northern Europe; therefore, intramuscular injections of typhoid vaccine or sterile milk three times weekly were used instead to induce the supposedly beneficial fever. But as Denny-Brown (who had experience of administering these treatments when he was a resident at Queen Square) later commented (99), they were "seldom beneficial and sometimes disastrous." Although the spirochetal theory was largely abandoned by 1929, arsenic continued to be used for another 30 years. McAlpine still had an arsenic clinic in the Middlesex Hospital in the 1950s. Marie's idea of chronic bacterial infection still lingered until that time, and tonsillectomy to eradicate it was still recommended (100).

Treatments Based on Theories of Pathogenesis

Marie (78) in the late nineteenth century had also recommended iodide to modify the sclerosis which Charcot (6) believed was the primary disease mechanism. Putnam (101), in the 1930s, noting the perivenular arrangement of the plaques at postmortem, concluded that the pathogenesis was ischemic and used anticoagulants to prevent thrombosis in the venules he thought he saw that but others before and after did not. The ischemic theory was revived in the 1980s (though the pathology had not changed) and led to the widespread use of hyperbaric oxygen, which, as expected, was not shown to be of benefit. Swank (102) and later Baker et al. (103) advocated a metabolic pathogenesis on the basis of epidemiological and postmortem biochemical studies. The resulting use of polyunsaturated fatty acid regimes did not, however, confer convincing benefit (104).

By far the most influential pathogenetic theory has been that of autoimmunity. Although the initiating event must necessarily be different, it was logical to try to modify the immune response. In principle three approaches are possible. The first to be employed was immunosuppression: nonspecific methods (using, for instance, cyclophosphamide, azathioprine, cyclosporine, or total lymphoid irradiation) have not proved convincingly effective, though a metanalysis of azathioprine has suggested that a further trial, probably in combination with other treatments such as beta interferon, may be worthwhile (105). Mitoxantrone, another nonspecific immunosuppressant, depresses MRI evidence of disease activity over a 6-month period, though whether this is translated into clinical benefit remains to be seen (106). Turning to more specific forms of immunotherapy, anti-CD4 antibodies have proved ineffective (107), though the humanized monoclonal antibody Campath-1H has a dramatic effect on MRI activity (108,109). Whether clinical benefit justifying the not inconsiderable risk of side effects will follow is currently under investigation.

Historically, the second approach to be used was induction of tolerance, though two decades elapsed before convincing benefit was shown. Glatairimer acetate has now been shown to reduce the relapse rate by about one-quarter and possibly to slow progression, though the latter claim requires confirmation (110).

The third approach was immune modulation using the interferons, though they were originally employed for their antiviral properties. Interferon beta-1b (111) and beta-1a (112,113) reduce the relapse rate by about one-third. It has been reported that in secondary progressive multiple sclerosis, interferon beta-1b slows progression of disability (114). These issues are discussed in detail elsewhere in this volume.

The results of these recent trials—showing a modest effect in changing the course of the disease—are encouraging, not least because they reflect the power of clinical trials utilizing improved design and greater rigor of conduct of therapeutic investigations. The process of refinement of trial design and methods of analysis is still continuing. It is interesting to review how the present position was reached. Undoubtedly the most important step forward was the introduction of statistics, the methods of which grew out of the concerns of physicians, physiologists, anthropologists, and what we would now call social scientists in the nineteenth century to deal with data derived from populations [see review by Matthews (115)]. The great debates in Paris in the 1830s and 1840s, in Germany in the 1880s, and in London at the turn of the century gradually led to an agreed methodology. The next crucial contributions were Fisher's (116) *The Design of Experiments* in 1935 and then the introduction of the principle of randomization by Bradford Hill; the triumphant vindication of this approach in a chronic disease came in 1948, with the trial of streptomycin in tuberculosis (117).

Coming specifically to multiple sclerosis, the first important step was the introduction by Kurtzke (118) in 1955 of a scale that provided a way of measuring the physical impact of the disease on the patient. He pointed out its limitations, and they are widely agreed on. Modifications have been introduced, but the Kurtzke scale remains central to clinical trials. Criteria for diagnosis were accepted at a meeting of the New York Academy of Sciences (119) in 1965; in 1983, they were refined to include the results of investigations (120). In the same year the National Multiple Sclerosis Society of the United States (the founding of which by Sylvia Lawry in 1946 must itself be counted as a major step in the history of multiple sclerosis) held a meeting of great significance for the design of clinical trials for therapeutic agents in multiple sclerosis (121). The necessity for the double-blind placebo-controlled trial was agreed on.

In the 1990s, three significant developments have taken place. First, there has been the realization of just how large clinical trials must be if valid conclusions about therapeutic effectiveness are to be drawn. The natural history data of Weinshenker et al. (122,123) have been exploited to good effect. Second, MRI has been introduced as a method for monitoring treatment. It is at its best in screening putative therapies for an effect on "disease activity." However, the methods so far used—as the interferon beta trials so clearly show—relate but weakly to an effect on progression of disability. The prospect for improving the relationship between MRI and clinical data is, however, good (124).

The very success of the recent clinical trials has paradoxically created a major problem for the future. Given that we now have treatments that modify (albeit modestly) the course of multiple sclerosis, it is no longer ethically justifiable to carry out such large, prolonged, double-blind placebo-controlled trials as were needed to demonstrate the effectiveness of the recently licensed products. A new approach is needed, and as the twenty-first century begins, an international group of investigators is working under the auspices of the International Federation of Multiple Sclerosis Societies to do just that.

III. CONCLUSION

This short account of the history of demyelinating disease has been written from the standpoint of the medical scientist. But as physicians our concern is equally with individuals and their suffering. It is important that we know what it is like to experience multiple sclerosis. A number of accounts have appeared in writing, in the cinema, and on television. None is more effective than the first, by Augustus D'Este (an illegitimate grandson of King George III of England), who kept a diary of his illness, which began 16 years before Carswell's (1) depiction of the pathology and ended fatally 20 years before Charcot's (6) account. It was published, with a commentary, after the Second World War (96). It is still worth reading today.

ACKNOWLEDGMENT

This chapter is based on a paper on the history of demyelinating disease published in *Affection demyelinisantes—collection traite de neurologie*. Rueil Malmaison: Groupe Liaison S.A., 1998.

REFERENCES

1. Carswell R. Pathological Anatomy: Illustrations of the Elementary Forms of Disease. London: Longmans, 1838.
2. Compston DAS. The 150th anniversary of the first depiction of the lesions of multiple sclerosis. J Neurol Neurosurg Psychiatry 1988; 51:806–813.
3. Cruveilhier J. Anatomie pathologique du corps humain: descriptions avec figures lithographiées et coloriées; des diverses alterations morbides dont le corps humain est susceptible. Paris: Ballière, 1835–1842.

4. Valentiner W. Ueber die Sclerose des Gehirns und Ruckenmarks. Dtsch Klin 1856; 8:147–151.

5. Fromann C. Untersuchungen uber die normale und pathologische Amatomie des Ruckenmarks, zweiter Theil. Jena: Frommann, 1864, pp. 128

6. Charcot J-M. Histologie de la sclérose en plaques. Gaz Hôpitaux Paris 1868; 141:554–555, 557–558

7. Babinski J. Etude anatomique et clinique sur la sclérose en plaques. Paris: Masson, 1885.

8. Babinski J. Recherches sur l'anatomie pathologique de la sclérose en plaques et étude comparative des diverses variétés de scléroses de la moelle. Arch Physiol 1885; 5:186–202.

9. Ranvier LA. Lecons sur l'histologie du système nerveux, Paris, Librarie F. Savy, 1878.

10. Marburg O. Die sogenannte "akute Multiple Sklerose" (Encephalomyelitis periaxialis scleroticans). Jahrb Psychiatr Neurol (Leipzig) 1906; 27:213–312.

11. Dawson JW. The histology of disseminated sclerosis. Proc R Soc Edinb 1916; 17:229–416.

12. Prineas JW, Connell F. Remyelination in multiple sclerosis. Ann Neurol 1979; 5:22–31.

13. Lassmann H. Comparative Neuropathology of Chronic Experimental Allergic Encephalomyelitis and Multiple Sclerosis. Berlin, Springer, 1983.

14. Princeas JW, Kwon EE, Cho E-S, Sharer LR. Continual breakdown and regeneration of myelin in progressive multiple sclerosis plaques. In: Scheinberg L, Raine CS, eds. Multiple Sclerosis: Experimental and Clinical Aspects, vol. 436. New York: Annals of the New York Academy of Sciences, 1984, pp. 11–32.

15. Ghatak NR, Leshner RT, Price AC, Felton WL. Remyelination in the human central nervous system. J Neuropathol Exp Neurol 1989; 48:507–518.

16. Prineas JW, Barnard RO, Revesz T, Kwon EE, Sharer L, Cho E-S. Multiple Sclerosis: Pathology of Recurrent Lesions. Brain 1993; 116:681–693.

17. Raine CS. The Dale E McFarlin memorial lecture: The immunology of the multiple sclerosis lesion. Ann Neurol 1994; 36:S61–S72.

18. Lassmann H. Pathology of multiple sclerosis. In: Compston A, Ebers G, Lassmann H, McDonald I, Matthews B, Wekerle H, eds. McAlpine's Multiple Sclerosis, 3rd ed. London: Harcourt Brace, 1998; pp. 323–358.

19. Raff MC, Miller RH, Noble M. A glial progenitor that develops in vitro into an astrocyte or an oligodendrocyte depending on culture medium. Nature 1983; 303:390–396.

20. Raff MC. Glial cell diversification in the rat optic nerve. Science 1989; 243:1450–1455.

21. Scolding NJ, Rayner PJ, Sussman J, Short C, Compston DAS. A proliferative adult human oligodendrocyte progenitor. Neuroreport 1995; 6:441–445.

22. Compston A, Zajicek J, Sussman J, Webb A, Hall G, Muir D, Shaw C, Wood A, Scolding N. Glial lineages and myelination in the central nervous system. J Anat 1997; 190:161–200.

23. Compston A. Neurobiology of multiple sclerosis. In: Compston A, Ebers G, Lassmann H, McDonald I, Matthews B, Wekerle H, eds. McAlpine's Multiple Sclerosis, 3rd ed. London: Harcourt Brace, 1998, pp. 283–322.

24. Holmes G. On the relation between loss of function and structural change in focal lesions of the central nervous system, with special reference to secondary degeneration. Brain 1906; 29:514–523.

25. Denny-Brown D, Brenner C. Lesion in peripheral nerve resulting from compression by spring clip. Arch Neurol Psychiatry 1944; 52:1–19.

26. Huxley AF, Stämpfli R. Evidence for saltatory conduction in peripheral myelinated nerve fibres. J Physiol 1949; 108:315–339.

27. McDonald WI. Conduction in muscle afferent fibres during experimental demyelination in cat nerve. Acta Neuropathol 1962; 1:425–432.

28. McDonald WI. The effects of experimental demyelination on conduction in peripheral nerve: a histological and electrophysiological study. II. Electrophysiological observations. Brain 1963; 86:501–524.

29. Hall JI. Studies in demyelinating peripheral nerves in guinea pigs with experimental allergic

neuritis: a histological and electrophysiological study. Part 2: Electrophysiological observations. Brain 1967; 90:313–332.

30. Kaeser HE, Lambert H. Nerve function studies in experimental polyneuritis: Electroencephalogr Clin Neurophysiol 1962; 29(suppl):29–35.

31. Cragg BG, Thomas PK. Changes in nerve conduction in experimental allergic neuritis. J Neurol Neurosurg Psychiatry 1964; 27:106–115.

32. McDonald WI, Sears TA. The effects of experimental demyelination on conduction in the central nervous system. Brain 1970; 93:583–598.

33. Davis FA, Jacobson S. Altered thermal sensitivity in injured and demyelinated nerve: A possible model of temperature effects in multiple sclerosis. J Neurol Neurosurg Psychiatry 1971; 34:551–561.

34. Rasminsky M. The effect of temperature on conduction and demyelinated single nerve fibres. Arch Neurol 1973; 28:287–292.

35. Bostock H, Sears TA. The internodal axon membrane: Electrical excitability and continuous conduction in segmental demyelination. J Physiol (Lond) 1978; 280:273–301.

36. Waxman SG, Ritchie JM. Organisation of ion channels in the myelinated nerve fibre. Science 1985; 228:1502–1507.

37. Black JA, Felts P, Smith KJ, Kocsis JD, Waxman SG. Distribution of sodium channels in chronically demyelinated spinal cord axons: Immuno-ultrastructural localization and electrophysiological observations. Brain Res 1991; 544:59–70.

38. Moll C, Mourre C, Lazdunsky M, Ulrich J. Increase of sodium channels in demyelinated lesions of multiple sclerosis. Brain Res 1991; 556:311–316.

39. Bunge MB, Bunge RP, Ris H. Ultrastructural study of remyelination in an experimental lesion in adult cat spinal cord. J Biophy Biochem Cytol 1961; 10:67–94.

40. Smith KJ, Blakemore WF, McDonald WI. The restoration of conduction by central remyelination. Brain 1981; 104:383–404.

41. Prineas JW, McDonald WI. Demyelinating diseases. In: Graham DI, Lantos PL, eds. Greenfield's Neuropathology. 6th ed., vol. I. Sevenoaks, UK: Edward Arnold 1997, pp. 813–896.

42. Kornek B, Lassmann H. Axonal pathology in multiple sclerosis: A historical note. Brain Pathol 1999; 9:651–656.

43. Perry VH, Anthony DC. Axon damage and repair in multiple sclerosis. Phil Trans R Soc Lond B 1999; 354:1641–1647.

44. Davie CA, Barker GJ, Webb S, Tofts PS, Thompson AJ, Harding AE, McDonald WI, Miller DH. Persistent functional deficit in multiple sclerosis and autosomal dominant cerebellar ataxia is associated with axon loss. Brain 1995; 118:1583–1592.

45. Losseff NA, Webb SL, O'Rioradan JI, Page R, Wang L, Barker GJ, Tofts PS, McDonald WI, Miller DH, Thompson AJ. Spinal cord atrophy and disability in multiple sclerosis: A new reproducible and sensitive MRI method with potential to monitor disease progression. Brain 1996; 119:701–708.

46. Truyen L, van Waesberghe JHTM, van Walderveen MAA, et al. Accumulation of hypointense lesions ("black holes") on T1 spin-echo MRI correlates with disease progression in multiple sclerosis. Neurology 1996; 47:1469–1476.

47. Van Walderveen MAA, Kamphorst W, Scheltens P, et al. Histopathologic correlate of hypointense lesions T1-weight spin-echo MRI in multiple sclerosis. Neurology 1998; 50:1282–1288.

48. Barkhof F, van Walderven M. Characterisation of tissue damage in multiple sclerosis by nuclear magnetic resonance. Phil Trans R Soc Lond B 1999; 354:1675–1686.

49. Smith KJ, McDonald WI. The pathophysiology of multiple sclerosis: Mechanisms underlying the production of symptoms and the natural history of the disease. Phil Trans R Soc Lond B 1999; 354:1649–1673.

50. Dawson GD. A summation technique for the detection of small evoked potentials. Electroencephalogr Clin Neurophysiol 1954; 6:65–84.

51. Halliday AM. The electrophysiological study of myoclonus in man. Brain 1967; 90:241–284.

52. McDonald WI, Robertson MAH. Changes in conduction during nerve fibre degeneration in the spinal cord. Brain 1972; 95:151–162.

53. Halliday AM, McDonald WI, Mushin J. Delayed visual evoked response in optic neuritis. Lancet 1972; 1:982–985.

54. Halliday AM, ed. In: Evoked Potentials in Clinical Testing. Edinburgh: Churchill Livingstone, 1993.

55. Halliday AM, McDonald WI, Mushin J. Visual evoked response in diagnosis of multiple sclerosis. BMJ 1973; 4:661–664.

56. Persson HE, Sachs C. Visual evoked potentials are listed by pattern reversal during provoked visual impairment in multiple sclerosis. Brain 1981; 104:369–382.

57. Youl BD, Turano G, Miller DH, Towell AD, MacManus DG, Moore SG, Jones SJ, Barrett G, Kendall BE, Moseley IF, Tofts PS, Halliday AM, McDonald WI. The pathophysiology of acute optic neuritis: an association of gadolinium leakage with clinical and electrophysiological deficits. Brain 1991; 114:2437–2450.

58. Quincke H. Die Lumbar punktion des Hydrocephalus. Klin Wochenschr 20:929–933, 1891.

59. Wynter WE. Four cases of tubercular meningitis in which paracentesis of the theca vertebralis was performed for the relief of fluid pressure. Lancet 1891; 1:981–982.

60. Greenfield JG, Carmichael EA. The Cerebro-Spinal Fluid in Clinical Diagnosis. London: MacMillan, 1925, p. 272.

61. Kabat EA, Moore DH, Landow H. An electrophoretic study of the protein components in cerebrospinal fluid and their relationship to the serum proteins. J Clin Invest 1942; 21:571–577.

62. Young IR, Hall AS, Pallis CA, Legg NJ, Bydder GM, Steiner RE. Nuclear magnetic resonance imaging of the brain in multiple sclerosis. Lancet 1981; 2:1063–1066.

63. Lukes SA, Crooks LE, Aminoff MJ, Kaufman L, Panitch HS, Mills C, Norman D. Nuclear magnetic resonance imaging in multiple sclerosis. Ann Neurol 1983; 13:592–601.

64. Stewart WA, Hall LD, Berry K, Paty DW. Correlation between NMR scan and brain slice data in multiple sclerosis. Lancet 1984; 2:412.

65. Ormerod IEC, Miller DH, McDonald WI, du Boulay EPGH, Rudge P, Kendall BE, Moseley IF, Johnson G, Tofts PS, Halliday AM, Bronstein AM, Scaravilli F, Harding AE, Barnes D, Zilkha KJ. The role of NMR imaging in the assessment of multiple sclerosis and isolated neurological lesions: A quantitative study. Brain 1987; 110:1579–1616.

66. Rindfleisch E. Histologisches Detail zu der grauen Degeneration von Gehirn und Ruckenmark. (Zugleich ein Beitrag zu der Lehre von der Entstehung und Verwandlung der Zelle.) Arch Pathol Anat Physiol Klin 1863; 26:474–483.

67. Shiraki H. Aetiopathogenesis of multiple sclerosis mainly from the neuropathological viewpoint. In: Multiple Sclerosis in Asia. Tokyo: University of Tokyo Press, 1976, pp. 161–192.

68. Grossman RE, Gonzales-Scarano F, Atlas SW, Galetta S, Silberberg DH. Multiple sclerosis: Gadolinium enhancement in MR imaging. Radiology 1986; 161:721–725.

69. Miller DH, Rudge P, Johnson G, et al. Serial gadolinium enhanced magnetic resonance imaging in multiple sclerosis. Brain 1988; 111:927–939.

70. Katz D, Taubenberger JK, Cannella B, McFarlin DE, Raine CS, McFarland H. Correlation between MRI findings and lesion development in chronic active multiple sclerosis. Ann Neurol 1993; 34:661–669.

71. Kermode AG, Thompson AJ, Tofts PS, MacManus DG, Kendall BE, Kingsley DPE, Moseley IF, Rudge P, McDonald WI. Breakdown of the blood-brain barrier precedes symptoms and other MRI signs of new lesions in multiple sclerosis: Pathogenic and clinical implications. Brain 1990; 113:1477–1489.

72. Filippi M, Yousry T, Campi A, et al. Comparison of triple dose versus standard dose gadolin-

ium-DTPA for detection of MRI enhancing lesions in patients with MS. Neurology 1996; 46:379–384.

73. Silver NC, Good CD, Barker GJ, et al. Sensitivity of contrast enhanced MRI in multiple sclerosis: Effects of gadolinium dose, magnetisation transfer contrast and delayed imaging. Brain 1997; 120:1149–1161.

74. Thompson AJ, Kermode AG, Wicks D, et al. Major differences in the dynamics of primary and secondary progressive multiple sclerosis. Ann Neurol 1991; 29:53–62.

75. Revesz T, Kidd D, Thompson AJ, Barnard RO, McDonald WI. A comparison of the pathology of primary and secondary progressive multiple sclerosis. Brain 1994; 117:759–765.

76. Davie CA, Hawkins CP, Barker GJ, Brennan A, Tofts PS, Miller DH, McDonald WI. Serial proton magnetic resonance spectroscopy in acute multiple sclerosis. Brain 1994; 117:49–58.

77. Lucchinetti CF, Bruck W, Rodriguez M, Lassmann H. Distinct patterns of multiple sclerosis pathology indicate heterogeneity in pathogenesis. Brain Pathol 1996; 6:259–274.

78. Marie P. Lectures on the Diseases of the Spinal Cord. Trans. Lubbock M. London: New Sydenham Society, 1895, pp. 134–136, 153.

79. McDonald WI. Attitudes to the treatment of multiple sclerosis. Arch Neurol 1983; 40:667–670.

80. Sibley WA, Bamford CR, Clark K. Clinical viral infections and multiple sclerosis. Lancet 1985; 1:1313–1315.

81. Bramwell B. On the relative frequency of disseminated sclerosis in this country (Scotland and the North of England) and in America. Rev Neurol Psychiatry (Edinb) 1903; 1:12–17.

82. Davenport CD. Multiple sclerosis from the standpoint of geographic distribution and race. Arch Neurol Psychiatry 1922; 8:51–58.

83. Dean G. Disseminated sclerosis in South Africa. BMJ 1949; 1:842–845.

84. Kurtzke JF. Epidemiologic contributions to multiple sclerosis: An overview. Neurology (Minneapolis) 1980; 30(7 pt 2):61–79.

85. Kurtzke JF, Hyllested K. Multiple sclerosis in the Faroe Islands: 1. Clinical and epidemiological features. Ann Neurol 1979; 5:6–21.

86. Ebers GC, Bulman DE, Sadovnik AD, Paty DW, Warren S, Hader W, Murray TJ, Seland P, Duquette P, Grey T, Nelson R, Nicolle M, Bruenet D. Population-based studies of multiple sclerosis in twins. N Engl J Med 1986; 315:1638–1642.

87. Mumford CJ, Wood NW, Kellar-Wood H, Thorpe JW, Miller DH, Compston DAS. The British Isles survey of multiple sclerosis in twins. Neurology 1994; 44:11–15.

88. Ebers GC, Sadovnick AD, Risch NJ. A genetic basis for familial aggregation in multiple sclerosis. Nature 1995; 377:150–151.

89. Sadovnick AD, Ebers GC, Dyment DA, Risch N. The Canadian Collaborative Study Group: Evidence for genetic basis of multiple sclerosis. Lancet 1996; 347:1728–1730.

90. Bell JI, Lathrop GM. Multiple loci for multiple sclerosis. Nature Genet 1996; 13:377–378.

91. Ebers GC, Kukay K, Bulman DE, Sadovnick AD, Rice G, Anderson C, Armstrong H, Cousin K, Bell RB, Hader W, Paty DW, Hashimoto S, Oger J, Duquette P, Warren S, Gray T, O'Connor P, Nath A, Auty A, Nelson R, Freedman M, Brunet D, Bouchard JP, Hinds D, Risch N. A full genome search in multiple sclerosis. Nature Genet 1996; 13:472–476.

92. Sawcer S, Jones HB, Feakes R, Gray J, Smaldon N, Chataway J, Robertson N, Clayton D, Goodfellow PN, Compston A. A genome screen in multiple sclerosis reveals susceptibility loci on chromosome 6P21 and 17Q22. Nature Genet 1996; 13:464–468.

93. Haines JL, Terminassian M, Bazyk A, Gusella JF, Kim DJ, Terwedow H, Pericakvance MA, Rimmler JB, Haynes CS, Roses AD, Reyes C, Ribierre F, Gyapay G, Weissenbach J, Hauser SL, Goodkin DE, Lincoln R, Usuku K, Garciamerino A, Gatto N, Young S, Oksenberg JR. A complete genomic screen for multiple sclerosis underscores a role for the major histocompatibility complex. Nature Genet 1996; 13:464–468.

94. Kuokkanen S, Sundvall M, Terwilliger JD, Tienari PJ, Wikstrom J, Holmdahl R, Pettersson

U, Peltonen L. A putative vulnerability locus to multiple sclerosis maps to 5p14-p12 in a region syntenic to the murine locus Eae2. Nature Genet 1996; 13:477–480.

95. Compston A. The genetic epidemiology of multiple sclerosis. Phil Trans R Soc Lond B 1999; 354:1623–1634.

96. Firth D. The case of Augustus d'Este. Cambridge, UK: Cambridge University Press, 1948.

97. Buzzard EF. The treatment of disseminated sclerosis: A suggestion. Lancet 1911; 1:98.

98. Grosz K. Malaria-behundlung der multiplen Sclerose. Jahrbuch Psychiatr Neurol 1924; 43: 198–214.

99. Denny-Brown D. Multiple sclerosis: The clinical problem. Am J Med 1952; 12:501–509.

100. McAlpine D, Compston ND, Lumsden CE. Multiple Sclerosis. Edinburgh: E & S Livingstone 1955; p. 191.

101. Putnam TJ. Evidence of vascular occlusion in multiple sclerosis and "encephalomyelitis." Arch Neurol Psychiatry 1937; 37:1298–1321.

102. Swank RL. Multiple sclerosis: A correlation of its incidence with dietary fat. Am J Med Sci 1950; 220:441–450.

103. Baker RWR, Thompson RHS, Zilkha KJ. Fatty acid composition of brain lecithins in multiple sclerosis. Lancet 1963; 1:26–27.

104. Paty DW, Cousin HW, Read S, Adlakh AK. Linoleic acid in multiple sclerosis: Failure to show any therapeutic benefit. Acta Neurol Scand 1978; 58:53–58.

105. Yudkin PL, Ellison GW, Ghezzi A, Goodkin DE, Hughes RAC, McPherson K, Mertin J, Milanese C. Overview of azathioprine treatment in multiple sclerosis. Lancet 1991; 338: 1051–1055.

106. Edan G, Miller D, Clanet M, Confavreux C, Lyon-Caen O, Lubetzki C, Brochet B, Berry I, Rolland Y, Froment J-C, Dousset V, Cabanis E, Iba-Zizen M-T, Gandon J-M, Lai HM, Moseley I, Sabouraud O. Therapeutic effect of mitoxantrone combined with methylprednisolone in multiple sclerosis: A randomised multicentre study of active disease using MRI and clinical criteria. J Neurol Neurosurg Psychiatry 1997; 62:112–118.

107. Llewellyn-Smith N, Lai M, Miller DH, Rudge P, Thompson AJ, Cuzner ML. Effects of anti-CD4 antibody treatment on lymphocyte subsets and stimulated tumor necrosis factor alpha production: A study of 29 multiple sclerosis patients entered into a clinical trial of cM-T412. Neurology 1997; 48:810–816.

108. Moreau Th, Coles A, Wing M, Thorpe J, Miller D, Moseley I, Issacs J, Hale G, Clayton D, Scolding N, Waldmann H, Compston A. Campath-1H in multiple sclerosis. Mult Scler 1996; 1:357–365.

109. Coles A, Paolili A, Molyneux P, Wing MG, Hale G, Miller D, Waldman H, Compston A. Monoclonal antibody treatment exposes three mechanisms underlying the clinical course of multiple sclerosis. Ann Neurol 1999; 46:296–304.

110. Johnson KP, Brooks BR, Cohen JA, Ford CC, Goldstein J, Lisak RP, Myers LW, Panitch HS, Rose JW, Schiffer RB, Vollmer T, Weiner LP, Wolinsky JS, and the Copolymer 1 Multiple Sclerosis Study Group. Copolymer 1 reduces relapse rate and improves disability in relapsing-remitting multiple sclerosis: Results of a phase III multicenter, double-blind, placebo-controlled trial. Neurology 1995; 45:1268–1276.

111. The IFNB Multiple Sclerosis Study Group. Interferon beta-1b is effective in relapsing-remitting multiple sclerosis: I. Clinical results of a multicenter, randomized, double-blind, placebo-controlled trial. Neurology 1993; 43:655–661.

112. Jacobs LD, Cookfair DL, Rudick RA, Herndon RM, Richert JR, Salazar AM, Fischer JS, Goodkin DE, Granger CV, Simon JH, Alam JJ, Bartoszak DM, Bourdette DN, Braiman J, Brownscheidle CM, Coats ME, Cohan SL, Doughterty DS, Kinkel RP, Mass MK, Munschauer FE III, Priore RL, Pullicino PM, Scherokman BJ, Weinstock-Guttman B, Whithma RH, and the Multiple Sclerosis Collaborative Research Group (MSCRG). Intramuscular interferon beta-1a for disease progression in relapsing multiple sclerosis. Ann Neurol 1996; 39:285–294.

113. Ebers GC and PRISM (prevention of relapses and disability by interferon beta-1a subcutane-
     ously in multiple sclerosis): Randomised double-blind placebo-controlled study of interferon
     beta-1a in relapsing/remitting multiple sclerosis. Lancet 1998; 352:1498–1504.
114. Kappos L and European Study Group on Interferon-beta in Secondary Progressive MS.
     Placebo-controlled-center randomised trial of interferon beta-1b in treatment of secondary
     progressive multiple sclerosis. Lancet 1998; 352:1491–1497.
115. Matthews JR. Quantification and the Quest for Medical Certainty. Princeton, NJ: Princeton
     University Press, 1995, p. 195.
116. Fisher RA. The design of Experiments. Edinburgh: Oliver and Boyd, 1935.
117. Tuberculosis Trials Committee. Streptomycin treatment of pulmonary tuberculosis: A Medi-
     cal Research Council investigation. BMJ 1948; 2:769–782.
118. Kurtzke J. A new scale for evaluating disability in multiple sclerosis. Neurology 1955; 5:
     580–583.
119. Schumaker GA, Beebe G, Kibler RF, Kurland LT, Kurtzke JR, McDowell F, Nagler B,
     Sibley WA, Tourtellotte WW, Willmon TL. Problems of experimental trials of therapy in
     multiple sclerosis: Report by the panel on the evaluation of experimental trials of therapy
     in multiple sclerosis. Ann NY Acad Sci 1965; 122:552–568.
120. Poser CM, Paty DW, Scheinberg L, McDonald WI, Davis FA, Ebers GC, Johnson KP, Sibley
     WA, Silberberg DH, Tourtellotte WW. New diagnostic criteria for multiple sclerosis: guide-
     lines for research protocols. Ann Neurol 1983; 13:227–231.
121. Multiple sclerosis. Arch Neurol 1983; 40:683–710.
122. Weinshenker BG, Rice GPA, Noseworthy JH, Carriere W, Baskerville J, Ebers GC. The
     natural history of multiple sclerosis: A geographically based study. 3. Multivariate analysis
     of predictive factors and models of outcome. Brain 1991; 114:1045–1056.
123. Weinshenker BG, Rice GPA, Noseworthy JH, Carriere W, Baskerville J, Ebers GC. The
     natural history of multiple sclerosis: A geographically based study. 4. Applications to plan-
     ning and interpretation of clinical therapeutic trials. Brain 1991; 114:1057–1067.
124. Miller DH, Grossman RI, Reingold SC, McFarland HF. The role of magnetic resonance
     techniques in understanding and managing multiple sclerosis. Brain 1998; 121:3–24.

2

The Epidemiology of Multiple Sclerosis

WILLIAM PRYSE-PHILLIPS and FIONA COSTELLO

Memorial University of Newfoundland, St. John's, Newfoundland, Canada

I. INTRODUCTION

Although there is agreement that exogenous factors are very relevant in the pathogenesis of multiple sclerosis (MS), the genetic aspects have been studied more since the second edition of this book was published in 1996. The compelling data from twin studies leave no doubt that there is a strong familial factor in MS, with a concordance rate for monozygotic twins of nearly 40% (although this necessarily means that there is more than a 60% discordance)—a figure increasing with duration of follow-up. The rates in fraternal twins and nontwin siblings are similar at about 3%, translating into a prevalence of 2000 per 100,000. This high rate, if only partly the product of genetic influences, must spring largely from environmental effects if it is supposed that fraternal twins are frequently in each other's company. Studies of large enough numbers of twins separated from an early age will soon be available, and the ongoing Canadian Collaborative Study on Genetic Susceptibility to MS has shown that among the adopted siblings of MS patients, the prevalence of MS is much the same as in the general population (1). Hence, one persists in examining the epidemiology of the disease in order to draw inferences about its possible causes. In the 4 years since the second edition of this book, some new data have been produced; these are examined here, the overall format being maintained.

II. MORTALITY STUDIES

The mortality rate for MS is the number of deaths attributable to MS in a specified time period, as recorded on death certificates; but although these figures are readily available, the cause of death may be actually quite unrelated to MS. Apparent inconsistencies in

15

rates may also be due to differences in recording practices (2). Such survival data are important in assessing the prognosis for individual patients and are of interest in considering the long-term effects of MS on the budgets of paying agencies, but they tell little or nothing about the etiology of MS. Figures from the unusually complete Danish MS registry (3) indicate that the course of the disease is generally worse than neurologists care to think, let alone to mention. The mean survival time after the diagnosis of MS is made is reduced by about 14 years compared with that of healthy controls—particularly for those with later onset of disease or with early cerebellar signs and in men. In Switzerland, increased prevalence rates between the 1950s and 1986 were considered to be due to the increased life span of the affected subjects; similarly, increased longevity was reported from Italy. Life tables indicate that the overall life expectancy for MS is only about 6 or 7 years less than for the insured population without MS (4).

Severe MS disability, as measured by an Extended Disability Status Scale (EDSS) score of 7.5 or higher, is a major risk factor for death. The case fatality ratios for patients in this group approach four times the rate for controls, while the ratios for those with mild or moderate disability (EDSS ≥ 7) are about 1.5 times that of age- and sex-matched comparison groups.

III. PREVALENCE RATIOS AND INCIDENCE RATES

Most epidemiology studies report incidence and/or prevalence ratios in defined geographical regions over a specified time period. Many have attested to the nonrandom distribution of the disease; the reviews of Sadovnick and Ebers (5), Poser (6), Weinshenker (7), and Rosati (8) are comprehensive. Further studies continue to be published, but although these data are of interest, simple prevalence studies still have not incriminated any single external Inciting cause for MS, which was the object of the research in the first place. Unfortunately, the prevalence ratios reported in most studies are subject to so many contaminating factors that interpretation is difficult (7,9). Further confounding the issue, demographic peculiarities can skew prevalence data, and the diagnostic criteria used in the published studies have varied, some being more and some less inclusive. Thus the 1954 diagnostic criteria of Allison and Miller have been considered to lack specificity and to overestimate the true rate (10). The paucity of published confidence intervals, lack of an agreed standard population, variability of diagnostic criteria, and discrepancies in survival times may also be responsible for variations in reported rates when actually none may exist.

It should be repeated that the differential diagnosis of MS is seldom considered in retrospective studies; Poser (6) has listed some of the other conditions in which clinical or laboratory findings may suggest the diagnosis of MS, including granulomatous, idiopathic, infectious, and autoimmune diseases. Diagnostic errors involving such conditions are likely to be of relevance in studies performed in many parts of the world. The problems of isolated optic neuritis and of primary progressive multiple sclerosis (PPMS) are examples, for it is still uncertain whether these are the same as typical MS or different disorders. The proportion of subjects with optic neuritis going on to develop features of MS varies with the length of follow-up, and certain clinical and laboratory features suggest that PPMS may be a different form of the disease (11,12) and unusually hard to diagnose even with magnetic resonance imaging (MRI) studies of the spinal cord. Many cases may thus be missing or, alternatively, cases of PPMS may have been inappropriately included.

A. Racial Factors

The proportion of North American MS patients with an affected family member is about 6% (2 to 16%); but in Asia and Chile, the figure is substantially lower (13). Multiple sclerosis is very rare among black Africans and postmortem confirmation of the diagnosis has not been obtained in any case. In one study, half of the black patients reported (14) were blind because of optic neuritis, indicating a real difference in the phenotype of the disease in this population. Other resistant isolates include the Inuit, Japanese, Amerindians, Maoris, Lapps, and Hungarian Gypsies (15). In Kuwait, the prevalence of MS among Palestinians is more than double that among the native Kuwaitis (16). The Palestinians and Kuwaitis had differences in eye color, blood group distribution, and HLA-DR or HLA-DQ epitope frequency, so the discrepancy in disease susceptibility might be attributable to genetic/racial differences among Arabs originating from the eastern Mediterranean basin. Again, in Jordan, MS was twice as common among Palestinians than among Jordanians (17). Thus, some studies have demonstrated that two racially different populations sharing the same environment can have different risks of developing MS, others that the same can be true for two racially similar populations sharing the same environment.

B. Prevalence and Incidence Studies

The more recent prevalence ratios for MS in over 80 sites within more than 45 countries have been listed (5,18). The prevalence rate for clinically definite/probable MS in London, Ontario, Canada, in 1984 was 94 per 100,000, and the estimated annual incidence rate for this population in 1974–1983 was 3.4 per 100,000, with a female-to-male sex ratio of 2.5 to 1. A family history of MS was recorded in 14.4% of close relatives (17% when distant relatives were included) (19). In Denmark, the prevalence rate was 112 per 100,000 in 1990 (20). These figures may be regarded as typical for central Canada and for northern Europe at those times, but they may be higher now, either as a result of better ascertainment or because of a real increase in the occurrence of the disease.

The existence of a latitudinal gradient, with incidence and prevalence rates increasing as one moves farther from the equator, is evident, although there has been discussion of the responsibility of genetics for at least part of this trend, since it was largely northern Europoid people that colonized those areas of the world in which MS prevalence is now high. North-south gradients exist independently of genetic or racial factors, but major differences occur in MS prevalence at the same latitude (as do west-east gradients in the United States), such that prevalence rates among people of the same ethnic background tend to differ in separated areas. The association between latitude and risk of MS in the United States was corroborated in the two Nurses' Health Studies, which are of particular interest, since the first (studying older women) strongly supported the existence of a north-south gradient in the United States, while this gradient vanished in the case of younger women studied later (21). This finding could provide new clues to identifying environmental causes of the disease, possibly met with as an effect of increasing travel.

An exception to the north-south rule is found in Japan, which is northerly but has low rates, and the gradient is now less easily defined in Europe as a result of numerous studies showing that the average annual incidence there correlates poorly with latitude (8). Prevalence rates are much higher in Sardinia than on the Italian mainland (22) but similar throughout England (23), though lower there than in Scotland, where Rothwell (24) documented crude annual incidence rates of probable or definite MS of up to 12.2

per 100,000 (95%; CI 10.8–13.7) and standardized prevalence rates of up to 219 per 100,000 (95%; CI 191–251). Some confusion arises, however, from the larger numbers of people with "Mc" or "Mac" as a prefix to their name, and thus presumably of Celtic origin, living in the northern British Isles. Searches in large databases for England and Wales suggest a standardized prevalence rate of 115 (95%; CI 112–120). There is thus confirmed the existence of a north-south gradient in the United Kingdom, the main island portion of which extends over about 1000 km.

The varying prevalence ratios described in eastern Europe, the Middle East, the Mediterranean (25), Norway (26), Russia, India, and possibly the United States have been taken as evidence of the influence of genetic rather than of environmental factors. For example, an inexplicable and possibly chance finding has been an excess of female patients with probable or definite MS in Jersey, compared with the (somewhat low) numbers in the adjacent island of Guernsey (27). On the other hand, a logistic regression analysis of veterans (28) showed that variations in MS risk in the United States are associated most strongly with latitude and population ancestry group; in particular, subjects of Swedish or French ancestry had higher risks of MS. In general, the authors concluded that an individual's ethnicity seems to be of less relative importance in determining MS risk than is population ancestry, suggesting that MS is a disease of *place* as long as the meaning of the word is expanded to include not only attributes of the locale (e.g., latitude) but also of its populace (e.g., ancestry).

Future studies will best be undertaken on genetically homogeneous populations living in a country with varying geographic conditions, such as Chile (over 4000 km long north to south), bearing in mind that in the eastern Australian states, a real south-north gradient has indeed been demonstrated (29) within such a homogeneous population. In Chile (13) neither overall prevalence ratios nor the north-south demographic figures are available, but they are for Australia, where there is a significant increase in prevalence with increasing southern latitude. This discrepancy occurs in the absence of differences between the genetic constitution of the populations, as judged by the frequency of HLA-DR2 antigen and by the names starting with "Mac" and "Mc" in telephone books. It was also notable that there was no excess of people with presumed Scottish ancestry in increasingly southern latitudes of Australia, suggesting that if the Scots are unusually susceptible to MS, this appears to be so only while they still live in Scotland. The results of a carefully performed study (29) represent important evidence for of the role of environmental factors in the pathogenesis of MS.

Poser and colleagues (30) have suggested that the best prevalence indicator is one referring retrospectively to all patients whose symptoms eventually lead to the diagnosis of MS, even if the diagnosis may not have been established on an earlier prevalence day, and that only those patients of the same ethnic background who have spent their prepubertal years in the geographic area in the study should be included. They called the measure they advocate the *onset-adjusted prevalence rate*. To date, no others have recalculated their figures in accordance with these suggestions.

A north-south gradient might be a methodological artifact, resulting from better ascertainment; but when prevalence figures for MS in the southern United Kingdom were adjusted to account for unobserved cases, the difference persisted. The prevalence of MS in the northern part of the United Kingdom appeared to be at least 180 per 100,000, whereas the maximum prevalence in the southern part of the United Kingdom was less than 160 per 100,000. Thus the distribution of MS in the United Kingdom is not uniform and is consistent with the hypothesis that populations with a high prevalence of MS may be genetically predisposed to the disease (31). The geographic distributions of cancer of the colon, dental caries, Parkinson's disease, and prostatic cancer also show a geographic gradient (32), but interpretation of the meaning of these observations is less mature.

C. Stability of Incidence Rates

Proof of a cyclic variation in the incidence rates of MS in a defined geographic region would be important evidence of an environmental cause and possibly of its nature. This has been described in Newfoundland (33) and eastern Norway (34), and it might be discerned in the figures from Iceland between 1910 and 1990 (36) and elsewhere (35). The dangers of overinterpretation have, however, been stressed by Giger and others, who have shown, using stochastic mathematical models, that fluctuation rates of up to 20% could be due merely to chance (36).

The figures published for incidence (and for prevalence) are difficult to interpret because of confounding factors, such as the uncertainty of the precise date of onset, improving documentation and diagnostic tools, variability in case-finding methods and diagnostic criteria, and increasing physician and population awareness. Another problem is that many studies have recorded the date of diagnosis rather than the date of onset of the first symptoms; but the latter is more likely to yield information of value in the determination of etiology, although itself flawed because of the frequent failure of recollection of minor symptoms and by virtue of the unknown latency between exposure to a putative environmental agent and the onset of clinical symptoms.

In almost all areas that have been sampled more than once, an increase in the number of detected cases has been found; this is true in various parts of Europe but especially in Norway, the United Kingdom, and Newfoundland (33), probably in Minnesota, and (as discussed in previous editions of this book) in the Orkney and Shetland islands. Crude prevalence rates have also increased in almost every state surveyed in Australia (29). The possible reasons for this are mentioned in the foregoing. Retrospective analyses of onset times, however, indicate that the incidence rates in the North Atlantic islands were relatively stable at least until 1969, whereas in the Orkneys there has been a steady reduction in incidence since 1964. Whether these changes in incidence are biological or sociological is not yet certain, although the former seems more likely. As a result of the changes recently reported, the stable or decreasing rates in the northern United Kingdom and Sardinia (75) and the increasing rates in some southern countries are leading to a reduction in the magnitude of the gradient with latitude, although it is still clearly present.

Any increase in MS among the Japanese could be ascribable to an increased awareness of the disease in Japan, to the profusion there of magnetic resonance imaging (MRI) scanners, or to a real increase in occurrence. However, the availability of MRI had less impact on the epidemiology of MS than expected in one study (37), in which only 3 of 69 patients diagnosed in Germany would have been missed without MRI. In 18 of 50 patients, however, the diagnostic classification did change, mostly from ''possible'' to ''probable'' MS.

In Westlock, Alberta, Canada, a steadily increasing incidence rate was recorded over the four decades starting in the 1950s (1.91, 2.85, 3.82, and 7.26 per 100,000) (38). The local prevalence rate in the current decade is 200 per 100,000, but in a population of less than 12,000, every case identified changes the figure by about 17 per 100,000. In western Norway, MS incidence rates doubled over the 20 years ending in 1987, whereas a decline followed by an increase in onset age supported the concept of real time–space fluctuations in MS incidence in this period. The nature of the factors contributing to this increase in incidence is undetermined. In Gothenburg, Sweden, however, the incidence rate fell; although the authors expressed caution about the adequacy of case ascertainment (39).

D. Point Source Outbreaks and Clustering

Clusters are geographically bounded occurrences of a trait that are of sufficient size and concentration to make them unlikely to have occurred by chance. A high prevalence of MS within a defined region excites interest because of the possibility that the finding might indicate the nature of an external, inciting cause. Sadly, despite numerous such reports, no single cause has been found or, if suggested, has proven relevant. Familial clustering, random accumulations occurring by chance, out-migration of the healthy with resultant condensation of the affected, less mobile patients in the area surveyed, and the wide confidence intervals for mean values in different areas all reduce the strength of the observation. In-migration is another confounding factor. Since more factors influence prevalence than incidence rates (for example, the size of the area surveyed), perhaps it is incidence rather than prevalence that should be emphasized in the future. Large, validated registries of MS patients have been compiled in Canada and in Europe (40), leading to the hope that enough reliable data could be obtained to obviate the necessity for such laborious and expensive studies elsewhere. However, unless some attempt is also made within these data banks to document both temporal and geographic factors, allowing the determination of space-time clusters, this hope is likely to be futile.

The factors that have determined the uneven prevalence of MS in various parts of the Canadian province of Alberta (38,41–42) have not been determined, but these were often in defined, rather small prairie regions. The crude prevalence rate is high at up to 216 per 100,000 (97), but too few data on incidence and familial linkages have been reported to allow confident interpretation of these figures, and the etiological significance of these observations remains undetermined. In Sweden, similarly high rates in a small community (253 per 100,000) were noted (44), but 22 of the 33 affected subjects were related to each other, and incidence rates were not reported. The appropriate geographic unit for prevalence studies has not yet been defined; the rate in the household of one MS patient living alone is, after all, 100,000 per 100,000, which is meaningless. Small numbers are also a problem, as with the cluster of 30 cases reported in Key West, Florida, between 1970 and 1986 (45), in which avian viruses have been implicated (46) without serological proof. A cluster of MS incidence among women in a defined census area of central New-foundland in the early 1970s has been detected (Guy and Pryse-Phillips, 1998; unpublished data). But although reports of such clusters continue to be published, one can make nothing meaningful of such anecdotes, although their occurrence demands explanation (47).

IV. MIGRATION STUDIES

It is not certain that immigrants are truly characteristic of the country from whence they come, nor that they settle randomly in their new country (5). Consequently, the interpretation of the following figures is not as easy as it first appears. However, MS is uncommonly recorded among the Japanese; in ethnic Asians on the Indian subcontinent; among Asians and Africans resident in African countries within the Commonwealth and in the

West Indies; and in those who have migrated from those countries to England after the age of about 15 years. The low rate of MS susceptibility associated with birth in many of these countries appears to be retained if the subject moves to high-risk areas after that age. Children born to such immigrants who came to the United Kingdom after World War II are now entering the age range within which MS has its greatest incidence, and the MS rate among them is comparable with that of the remainder of the population in South London. Thus the protective factor, whatever it is, does not extend to the second generation. The potential biases of the study in either direction include incomplete ascertainment, incorrect estimation of local population rates, certainty of diagnosis, imperfect demographic calculations, and—to a smaller extent (since confidence intervals were quoted)—the effects of small numbers. However, the conclusion that those who migrate from an area of low to one of high risk take with them the low risk only if they emigrate *after* about the age of 15 years still stands (48), and confidence in the role of some (still unidentified) environmental factor is further augmented by the results of studies of Britons and other Europoids in Africa, Japanese in Hawaii, Indian and Pakistani immigrants to England, and of (French) Algerians in France, indicating some robustness of these conclusions based on migration data. Caribbean immigrants who have a higher MS prevalence in their native land than do Asian immigrants did not show this difference (49). This study supports others showing that the environment during childhood is a major factor in determining the risk of developing MS. The study of North African migrants to France is of interest, since the incidence rate for the immigrants was substantially higher than that of the native French population, leading Kurtzke and his colleagues (50) to the conclusions that MS is primarily an environmental disease acquired after childhood, that acquisition requires prolonged or repeated exposure (here 3 years for these medium-to-high MS-risk migrants) followed by a prolonged latent or incubation period between acquisition and symptom onset (here 10 years), and that MS is most likely a widespread but unknown persistent infection which results in clinical MS in only a small proportion of those affected.

In the attempt to determine whether migration studies support the genetic or the environmental hypotheses, a study from Israel (51) is of interest in that it led to the conclusions that native-born Israelis whose fathers were born in Europe or America had MS incidence and prevalence rates at least as high as those of immigrants in previous studies, whereas those whose fathers were born in Asia or Africa had significantly higher rates than those of immigrants from those countries. Both the genetic and the environmental hypotheses are thus supported. Nevertheless, in Israel the MS prevalence rates differ between those of Sephardic stock (low) and those of Ashkenazi origin (high) (35).

Despite the overall strong impression of the importance of migration studies, caution must be used in interpreting the results. Among 246 MS patients who migrated to France from North Africa, 11% had had their first symptoms before migration. No differences were found between the mean age of MS onset in this group of patients and in those matched for sex and age who had been born in France. Hence it is likely that MS was acquired by the same age in migrants as in French-born patients (50). These findings may constitute indirect support for the hypothesis that the (unknown) causative factors of MS are equally frequent whatever the latitude of origin. Martyn (25) has suggested that these data might indicate the existence of a protective factor operating in childhood in countries where MS has low prevalence rates, referencing older studies showing that the age of infection with some of the commoner communicable diseases of childhood tends to be greater in subjects with MS than in controls.

V. OTHER FACTORS EXAMINED

Too often, results have been published as a result of the detection of statistical significance, while biological implausibility has been ignored.

A. Birth Month

The report of an association between the occurrence of MS and the birth month of the subject (52) smacks somewhat of astrology, but this finding was not replicated in British Columbia, Canada (53).

B. Trauma

Substantial, indeed forceful, disagreement about the role of physical trauma in precipitating the onset or exacerbation of MS has been shown in the publications of the last few years. Those considering that the relation is strong have the intrinsic advantage that comes from not having to prove a negative, but two studies (54–55) have shown no significant association between cranial or other trauma and the occurrence of the disease. These conclusions were challenged by Poser (56) on the grounds that the initial event in MS is likely to be a breach of the blood-brain barrier, which is exactly what happens with (at least severe) craniocerebral trauma. Despite this, the lack of statistical association now appears watertight, and few dispassionate physicians (or judges) support the position taken by any MS patient that worsening of symptoms following trauma is compensable (57).

C. Diet

The role of vitamin B_{12} in MS remains speculative. That a deficiency of the vitamin is common among MS patients is acknowledged, but its replacement does not seem to have any effect on the subsequent course of the disease. Arguments for the benefit of a diet high in vegetable fats have been reviewed by Granieri (35), but benefit is not confirmed, although one retrospective study has claimed a protective role for dietary fruit, vegetables, and grains, while an increased risk was found with high energy and animal food intake (58). A statistically significant association between the consumption of liquid cow's milk (as opposed to cheese) and MS prevalence has been reported (59–60), though the interpretation of this is unclear. Fresh milk may be a cofactor or may reflect association with another factor. The authors considered that there was significant correlation between MS prevalence and milk production per inhabitant, national bovine density per inhabitant, and local bovine geographic density. Although this may be true worldwide, the high rates of MS in Newfoundland and the northern Canadian tundra (more eschewed than chewed by the cows, so that almost all the milk has to be brought in from other provinces) suggest that this is, at best, an imperfect association.

  The range of dietary factors incriminated in the causation of MS in numerous studies encompasses a huge variety of foodstuffs, ranging from bread and butter through chocolate, oats, and beer to smoked meats. Following his comprehensive reviews, Lauer (61,62) commented that despite a great number of analytical studies, the possible aetiologic role of deleterious or protective dietary factors in MS remains a matter of debate. This represents fair comment on studies in which significance and meaningfulness are at odds.

D. Socioeconomic Factors

Granieri (15) also reviewed reports of a higher risk of MS in higher social classes but noted that the findings are inconsistent. The MS case-control ratios by state originating from the postwar studies of Kurtzke in the United State were compared with a large number of sociogeographic variables by Lauer (63). Latitude was the variable by far most closely associated with MS in univariate testing, whereas factor-analytic studies revealed two independent factors, the first characterized by indicators of higher affluence, better nutrition, and a higher sanitary level and the second comprising characteristics of a colder climate along with such dietary variables as a diet low in fish and high in dairy products. The author considered that the findings suggested a possible interaction of both socioeconomic and geoclimatic factors in the etiology of MS. Similar conclusions were drawn from a more recent study in Israel (64). The finding from Australia (65) that MS is associated with later age of leaving school and with higher educational levels (replicated in some studies from the United Kingdom and the United States but not from others from Spain, the United States, and Germany) remains inexplicable.

E. Toxins and Occupational Exposures

Case-control studies have shown no consistent statistically significant differences between MS patients and controls relative to exposure to organic solvents, welding, or other chemical compounds (66–68). In a Spanish case-controlled study, contact with dogs (but also with cloth) was considered to be significantly associated with MS occurrence (69). Electromagnetic influences appear not to be relevant (20). A cluster of cases among workers at an upstate New York zinc-processing plant was recorded in the last edition of this handbook; the number of patients with confirmed MS is now increased by nine, all with onset in the 1980s, but they did not differ in family histories of MS or in HLA-DR antigenic haplotypes from other MS sufferers. Mercury poisoning (from dental fillings) was popularly considered relevant in this last decade, leading many subjects to demand their replacement. However, the association between MS and dental caries seems to be stronger than that between MS and body mercury levels (70).

F. Other Diseases

According to prospective population-based studies, apart from Hashimoto thyroiditis (71), no diseases appear to occur significantly more often in patients with MS than in those without.

G. Pregnancy

Although received wisdom indicates that MS relapses are especially common in the first few months after pregnancy, Sadovnick, in a prospective study (72), found a reduction in the relapse rate only during the third trimester, with no subsequent increase, concluding that neither pregnancy nor the following 6 months appeared to be risk factors for MS relapses or for pregnancy outcome. In Runmarker's study (73), pregnancy was associated with a lower risk of onset of MS and a better prognosis, while Stenager (74) concluded that pregnancy and childbirth were unlikely to have any influence on the long-term prognosis for MS. However, a recent study of women with definite or probable MS found a decrease of about 70% in the rate of relapse during the third trimester of pregnancy, followed by an increase of about 70% over the prepregnancy rate in the first 3 months postpartum, without long-term effect on the progression of MS (75).

H. Climate

In a preliminary paper, it was suggested (76) that the latitude gradient could be explained by the amount of ambient sunlight acting as an immunosuppressant in youth. Further prospective studies should not be difficult to undertake in order to confirm or refute this theory.

VI. GENETIC AND FAMILY STUDIES

Studies of familial MS previously reviewed have indicated a concordance rate of up to 38% in monozygotic (MZ) twin pairs, dropping to 4% in dizygotic (DZ) pairs and in nontwin siblings; but in a large population-based MS sample within which 54 twin pairs (17 monozygotic) were available for study, concordance rates did not differ significantly for MZ and DZ twin pairs (77). Overall numbers were too small and confidence limits too wide, however, to exclude a type II error.

As Ebers and Sadovnick (78) remarked, "It remains undetermined whether or not genes exist which are truly necessary for the development of the disease," but there is little doubt that at least two genes, and probably more, will be found to influence susceptibility. One of these may well be the class II major histocompatibility complex (MHC); others await identification. Until the Canadian Collaborative Project on Genetic Susceptibility to Multiple Sclerosis (79) has been completed, the relative roles of genetic and environmental factors in the causation of MS will remain speculative.

A. Genetics

This subject is considered in the following chapter, but one point may be made here. Most demographic studies of MS, and of many other autoimmune diseases, have shown a female preponderance. This question was addressed by Duquette et al. (80), who noted that female preponderance is most obvious among cases with early onset and who reviewed the "rules" applicable to multifactorial diseases: early-onset cases are more likely to have a first-degree relative affected; early onset is associated with greater severity of the disease; early onset, severity, and increased familial occurrence should characterize cases of the less affected gender; late cases are milder and more responsive to treatment (none correct for MS); and concordant twin pairs are more likely to have a positive family history (correct for MS). As the authors comment, either the rules are wrong or MS is not multifactorial.

B. Genetic Geography

The suggestion that the prevalence of MS in the United Kingdom correlates with the regional population frequency of the MS-associated HLA-DR2 antigen remains unchallenged but may be of less relevance in view of the Australian (29,47) and other data that cast doubt on the closeness of association of that antigen and the disease.

MS rarely occurs in Gypsies, despite the high frequency of DR2 in that population, among whom it is rather DQw6 which correlates with MS susceptibility. Observations such as these are of limited value when reported in isolation and need confirmation in other populations before they are accorded true etiological significance. The overall prevalence of MS in British Columbia at 64.7 per 100,000 is between four and five times higher than the rate in non-Europoids, such as Asians. MS was not encountered at all in pure-blooded native Amerindians at the Vancouver, B.C., MS clinic.

VII. INFECTIOUS CAUSES

Granieri and Casetta (35) have reviewed this subject noting that a higher proportion of children show positive titers to many viral diseases early in life in areas where MS is rare, as opposed to those where MS is common, suggesting a protective effect. . . . [so that] MS could be an age-dependent response to common viral infections in childhood, considering also that age dependent central nervous system diseases caused by common viruses are well known. Unfortunately, although in some studies the age of, for example, measles or rubella affection was higher in patients than controls, significant differences in the age at which infectious diseases were suffered were only reported in 10 of the 24 studies that they reviewed.

More directly, evidence for the occurrence of repetitive outbreaks of MS in the Faroe Islands after the 1940s was presented by Kurtzke, who considered that four successive epidemics, beginning in 1943, can be discerned and attributed to a primary MS affection (PMSA) brought into the islands by British troops, then spreading to and from successive cohorts of Faroese people (82,83). He considered MS to be a single widespread systemic infectious disease that only seldom goes on to clinical MS and is characterized by a need for prolonged exposure, limited age of susceptibility, and prolonged incubation, with an unidentified retrovirus as the most likely agent. In Iceland, however, previous reports of an "epidemic" of MS following the arrival of Allied troops in the early 1940s have been contradicted by Benedikz et al. (84), who report that onset-adjusted prevalence appears to have increased almost linearly since 1920. This is considered by them to reflect increased longevity and improved case detection in a country that has now one neurologist for every 22,000 people. The reduction of the lag time between first symptom and diagnosis over the last 70 years indirectly confirms the likely influence of improved ascertainment. Although it is easy, in prevalence studies, to correct for the immigration of people who came to a region with preexisting MS symptoms, it is nearly impossible to ascertain how many other people with symptoms had left the region to reside elsewhere; this thus introduces a bias of unknown magnitude into onset-adjusted prevalence figures, which means that the reduction of published rates may be inappropriate.

Unlike the situation with trauma, there is a clinical perception that infections do precipitate exacerbations of MS. Viral upper respiratory infections (URTIs) stimulate the secretion of cytokines, such as interferon gamma, which may explain a seasonal variation in relapse rates. Anecdotal reports as well as clinical experience suggest a strong correlation between the infections and relapses of MS, but the Uhthoff effect (fever-induced conduction block) may be relevant here. One might speculate that if the organisms causing URTIs can precipitate subsequent MS attacks, might they not also be responsible for the first attack? But it is difficult to know which agent should be inculpated, because MS patients tend to have high antibody levels to many of them (85) and the identity of the culprit(s) may actually be irrelevant.

A. Paramyxoviruses

The hypothesis that an environmental agent is involved in the genesis of MS has led to the search for viruses as putative causes; morbilliviruses have been the most studied, as a result of the observation of the similarities between the brain lesions in MS and those of encephalitis caused by measles virus. Antibodies to measles and the serologically near-identical canine distemper virus (CDV) have been found in the blood and/or cerebrospinal fluid (CSF) of MS patients in titers greater than in controls (85), but despite intriguing evidence linking MS with exposure to dogs or to CDV (reviewed in previous editions of this book), the relationships between any of these agents and MS do not fulfill Koch's postulates.

B. Other Infections

No definite cause for the Key West cluster of cases reported by Sheremata (45) has been determined, and Poser has considered the cluster to represent a chance occurrence (6). Human herpesvirus 6 (86,87) and *Chlamydia pneumoniae* have also been incriminated in the genesis of MS (as well as for many other diseases), but no casual association has been proved. A relationship between early infection with herpes zoster virus and the later development of MS has been discerned by Ross (88–92), but until his findings are confirmed, the role of this (as of all the other agents mentioned) in the genesis of MS remains provocatively uncertain.

Epstein-Barr virus (EBV) infection has been suggested as inciting an age-dependent host response of pathogenetic relevance, perhaps especially when linked to retroviral infection (93–95). A Danish cohort study showed a threefold increase in risk of MS in subjects who had serologically confirmed late EBV infection (25,96). The specter of neurotoxicity from hepatitis B infection has been raised (97), but there is no proven causal relationship between MS and hepatitis vaccination, which probably provides more benefit than risk (98). MS-associated retrovirus, a member of the endogenous retrovirus-9 family, is a retroviral sequence that has been isolated from MS material. In addition, special interest has been taken in human T-cell lymphotrophic virus 1 (HTLV-1) because of its role in the genesis of tropical spastic paraparesis, yet the association between the expression of these agents and MS remains tentative (99). No causal association has yet been confirmed between rubella, *Mycoplasma pneumoniae*, vaccinia, adenovirus, varicella, influenza, etc., and the subsequent development of MS or of perinatal infections, according to van Buuren (100).

VIII. CONCLUSION

Epidemiology is inferential; its role is to provide etiologic clues, but it cannot be used to prove or to refute causality. MS is a complex trait that appears to be determined both by genetic and environmental factors. It exhibits a changing incidence over time in an uneven geographic distribution through several areas of the world. The evidence of these spatial and temporal trends and the data from migrant studies affirm the etiological relevance of environmental factors, although their nature remains mysterious and is undoubtedly complex. As Sadovnick and Ebers (5) point out, susceptibility of mice to autoimmune diseases is inherited in a polygenic manner, and "penetrance proved to be very strongly influenced by early life, cleanliness of environment and viral contamination of breeding colonies," a fact that must be relevant to the occurrence of MS.

Risk factors for the development of MS include female gender, age, familial background, ethnic origin, DR2 positivity (7), and probably geography. One might proffer a best-summarizing guess at the disease's causality by supposing that all MS patients possess one of a range of genotypes that confer susceptibility, that different genotypes are associated with different phenotypes, and that about one-third of those susceptible will develop the disease while the remaining two-thirds will not—either because they possess inhibitory or protective genes or because they do not come into contact with the necessary triggering factors in their internal or external environments. The task for classic, inferential epidemiology is still to standardize case finding, diagnostic criteria, and other methodological considerations to discover what those factors might be.

REFERENCES

1. Ebers G, Sadovnick AD, and Risch NJ. The Canadian Collaborative Study Group. A genetic basis for familial aggregation in multiple sclerosis. Nature 1995; 377:150–151.
2. Hibberd PL. Use and misuse of statistics for epidemiological studies of multiple sclerosis. Ann Neurol 1994; 36(suppl 2):S218–S230.
3. Bronnum-Hansen H. Survival in disseminated sclerosis in Denmark. A nation-wide study of the period 1948–1986. Ugeskr Laeger 1995; 15751:7131–7135.
4. Sadovnick AD, Ebers GC, Wilson RW, Paty DW. Life expectancy in patients attending multiple sclerosis clinics. Neurology 1992; 425:991–994.
5. Sadovnick AD and Ebers G. Epidemiology of multiple sclerosis: A critical overview. Can J Neurol Sci 1993; 20:17–29.
6. Poser CM. The epidemiology of multiple sclerosis: A general overview. Ann Neurol 1994; 36(suppl 2):S180–S193.
7. Weinshenker BG. Epidemiologic strategies to detect an exogenous cause of MS. Acta Neurol Scand Suppl 1995; 161:93–99.
8. Rosati G. Descriptive epidemiology of multiple sclerosis in Europe in the 1980s: A critical overview. Ann Neurol 1994; 36(suppl 2):S164–S174.
9. Kahana E, Zilber N. Pitfalls in multiple sclerosis epidemiology: The Israel experience [editorial]. Neuroepidemiology 1996; 155:229–238.
10. Rice-Oxley M. A prevalence survey of multiple sclerosis in Sussex. J Neurol Neurosurg Psychiatry 1995; 581:27–30.
11. Cottrell DA. The natural history of multiple sclerosis: A geographically based study. 6. Applications to planning and interpretation of clinical therapeutic trials in primary progressive multiple sclerosis. Brain 1999; 122(4):641–647.
12. Cottrell DA. The natural history of multiple sclerosis: A geographically based study. 5. The clinical features and natural history of primary progressive multiple sclerosis. Brain 1999, 122(4):625–639.
13. Alvarez G, Castillo JL, Ruiz F, et al. Multiple sclerosis in Chile. Acta Neurol Scand 1992; 851:1–4.
14. Dean G, Bhigjee AI, Bill PL, et al. Multiple sclerosis in black South Africans and Zimbabweans. J Neurol Neurosurg Psychiatry 1994; 579:1064–1069.
15. Granieri E. Multiple sclerosis in Italy. A reappraisal of incidence and prevalence in Ferrara. Arch Neurol 1996; 538:793–798.
16. al Din AS, Khogali M, Poser CM, et al. Epidemiology of multiple sclerosis in Arabs in Kuwait: A comparative study between Kuwaitis and Palestinians. J Neurol Sci 1990; 1001–1002:137–141.
17. al Din AS. Multiple sclerosis in Arabs in Jordan. J Neurol Sci 1995; 1312:144–149.
18. Ebers G, Sadovnick AD. Epidemiology. In Paty DW, Ebers G, eds. Multiple Sclerosis. Philadelphia: Davis, 1998, pp 5–28.
19. Hader WJ, Elliot M, Ebers GC. Epidemiology of multiple sclerosis in London and Middlesex County, Ontario, Canada. Neurology 1988; 384:617–621.
20. Johansen C, Koch-Henriksen N, Rasmussen S, Olsen JH. Multiple sclerosis among utility workers. Neurology 1999; 52:1279–1282.

21. Hernan MA, Olek MJ, Ascherio A. Geographic variation of MS incidence in two prospective studies of US women. Neurology 1999; 538:1711–1718.
22. Rosati G, Aiello I, Pirastru MI, et al. Epidemiology of multiple sclerosis in Northwestern Sardinia: Further evidence for higher frequency in Sardinians compared to other Italians. Neuroepidemiology 1996; 151:10–19.
23. Ford HL, Gerry E, Airey CM, et al. The prevalence of multiple sclerosis in the Leeds Health Authority. J Neurol Neurosurg Psychiatry 1998; 645:605–610.
24. Rothwell PM, Charlton D. High incidence and prevalence of multiple sclerosis in south east Scotland: evidence of a genetic predisposition. J Neurol Neurosurg Psychiatry 1998; 646:730–735.
25. Martyn CN. The epidemiology of multiple sclerosis. Acta Neurol Scand Suppl 1997; 169:3–7.
26. Koch-Henriksen N. Multiple sclerosis in Scandinavia and Finland. Acta Neurol Scand. 1995; (suppl 161):55–59.
27. Sharpe G. Multiple sclerosis in island populations: prevalence in the Bailiwicks of Guernsey and Jersey. J Neurol Neurosurg Psychiatry 1995; 581:22–26.
28. Page WF, Mack TM, Kurtzke JF, et al. Epidemiology of multiple sclerosis in US veterans. 6. Population ancestry and surname ethnicity as risk factors for multiple sclerosis. Neuroepidemiology 1995; 146:286–296.
29. McLeod JG, Hammond SR, Hallpike JF. Epidemiology of multiple sclerosis in Australia. With NSW and SA survey results. Med J Aust 1994; 1603:117–122.
30. Posner CM, Benedikz J, Hibberd PL. The epidemiology of multiple sclerosis: The Iceland model. Onset-adjusted prevalence rate and other methodological considerations. J Neurol Sci 1992; 1112:143–152.
31. Forbes RB, Swingler RJ. Estimating the prevalence of multiple sclerosis in the United Kingdom by using capture-recapture methodology. Am J Epidemiol 1999; 149:1016–1024.
32. Schwartz GG. Multiple sclerosis and prostate cancer: What do their similar geographies suggest? Neuroepidemiology 1992; 114–116:244–254.
33. Pryse-Phillips WEM. The incidence and prevalence of multiple sclerosis in Newfoundland and Labrador, 1960–1985. Ann Neurol 1986; 20:323–328.
34. Edland A. Epidemiology of multiple sclerosis in the county of Vestfold, eastern Norway: Incidence and prevalence calculations. Acta Neurol Scand 1996; 932–933:104–109.
35. Granieri E, Casetta I, Tola MR, et al. Multiple sclerosis: Does epidemiology contribute to providing etiological clues? J Neurol Sci 1993; 115(suppl):S16–S23.
36. Giger A, Wuthrich RJ. Research in epidemiology and causality: The example of the Basel Multiple Sclerosis Study, 1980 to 1986. Schweiz Rundsch Med Prax 1993; 821:18–24.
37. Poser S, Scheidt P, Kitze B, et al. Impact of magnetic resonance imaging MRI on the epidemiology of MS. Acta Neurol Scand 1991; 833:172–175.
38. Warren S, Warren KG. Prevalence, incidence, and characteristics of multiple sclerosis in Westlock County, Alberta, Canada. Neurology 1993; 439:1760–1763.
39. Svenningsson A, Runmarker B, Lycke J, et al. Incidence of MS during two fifteen-year periods in the Gothenberg region of Sweden. Acta Neurol Scand 1992; 82:161–168.
40. Confavreux C. Establishment and use of multiple sclerosis registers—EDMUS. Ann Neurol 1994; 36:S136–S139.
41. Warren S, Warren KG. Prevalence of multiple sclerosis in Barrhead County, Alberta, Canada. Can J Neurol Sci 1992; 171:72–75.
42. Klein GM, Rose MS, Seland TP. A prevalence study of multiple sclerosis in the Crowsnest Pass region of southern Alberta. Can J Neurol Sci 1994; 213:262–265.
43. Svenson LW, Woodhead SE, Platt GH. Regional variations in the prevalence rates of multiple sclerosis in the province of Alberta, Canada. Neuroepidemiology 1994; 131–132:8–13.
44. Binzer M, Forsgren L, Holmgren G, et al. Familial clustering of multiple sclerosis in a northern Swedish rural district. J Neurol Neurosurg Psychiatr 1994; 57:497–499.

45. Sheremata WA, Poskanzer DC, Withum DG. Unusual occurrence on a tropical island of multiple sclerosis [letter]. Lancet 1985; 2:618.

46. McHatters GR, Scham RG. Bird viruses in multiple sclerosis: Combination of viruses or Marek's alone? Neurosci Lett 1995; 1882:75–76.

47. Miller DH, Hammond SR, McLeod JG, et al. Multiple sclerosis in Australia and New Zealand: Are the determinants genetic or environmental? J Neurol Neurosurg Psychiatry 1990; 53:903–905.

48. Gale CR. Migrant studies in multiple sclerosis. Prog Neurobiol 1995; 474–475:425–448.

49. Dean G, Elian M. Age at immigration to England of Asian and Caribbean immigrants and the risk of developing multiple sclerosis. J Neurol Neurosurg Psychiatry 1997; 635:565–568.

50. Kurtzke JF, Delasnerie-Laupretre N, Wallin MT. Multiple sclerosis in North African migrants to France. Acta Neurol Scand 1998; 985:302–309.

51. Kahana E, Zilber N, Abramson JH, et al. Multiple sclerosis: Genetic versus environmental aetiology: Epidemiology in Israel updated. J Neurol 1994; 2415:341–346.

52. Templer DI, Trent NH, Spencer DA, et al. Season of birth in multiple sclerosis. Acta Neurol Scand 1992; 852:107–109.

53. Sadovnick AD, Yee IM. Season of birth in multiple sclerosis. Acta Neurol Scand 1994; 893: 190–191.

54. Siva A, Radhakrishnan K, Kurland LT, et al. Trauma and multiple sclerosis: A population-based cohort study from Olmsted County, Minnesota. Neurology 1993; 43:1878–1882.

55. Sibley, WA. Physical trauma and multiple sclerosis. Neurology 1993; 43:871–1874.

56. Poser CM. Physical trauma and multiple sclerosis. Neurology 1994; 47:1360–1362.

57. Goddin DS, Ebers GC, Johnson KP, et al. The relationship of MS to physical trauma and psychological stress: Report of the Therapeutics and Technology Assessment Subcommittee of the American Academy of Neurology. Neurology 1999; 52:1737–1745.

58. Ghadirian P, Jain M, Ducic S, et al. Nutritional factors in the aetiology of multiple sclerosis: A case-control study in Montreal, Canada. Int J Epidemiol 1998; 275:845–852.

59. Malosse D, Perron H, Sasco A, Seigneurin JM. Correlation between milk and dairy product consumption and multiple sclerosis prevalence: A worldwide study. Neuroepidemiology 1992; 114–116:304–312.

60. Malosse D, Perron H. Correlation analysis between bovine populations, other farm animals, house pets, and multiple sclerosis prevalence. Neuroepidemiology 1993; 121:15–27.

61. Lauer K. Ecologic studies of multiple sclerosis. Neurology 1997; 492(suppl 2):S18–S26.

62. Lauer K. Diet and multiple sclerosis. Neurology 1997; 492(suppl 2):S55–S61.

63. Lauer K. The risk of multiple sclerosis in the USA in relation to sociogeographic features: A factor analytic study. J Clin Epidemiol 1994; 47:43–48.

64. Zilber N. Risk factors for multiple sclerosis: A case-control study in Israel. Acta Neurol Scand 1996; 946:395–403.

65. Hammond SR. Multiple sclerosis in Australia: Socioeconomic factors. J Neurol Neurosurg Psychiatry 1996; 613:311–331.

66. Gronning M, Albrektsen G, Kvale G, et al. Organic solvents and multiple sclerosis: A case-control study. Acta Neurol Scand 1993; 88:47–250.

67. Mortensen JT, Bronnum-Hansen H, Rasmussen K. Multiple sclerosis and organic solvents. Epidemiology 1998; 92:168–171.

68. Landtblom AM. Exposure to organic solvents and multiple sclerosis. Neurology 1997; 492(suppl 2):S70–S74.

69. Beltran I, Molto-Jorda JM, Diaz-Marin C, et al. Analytical epidemiological study of multiple sclerosis in Alcoi. Revista de Neurologia 1998; 26:67–69.

70. McGrother CW, Dugmore C, Phillips MJ, et al. Multiple sclerosis, dental caries and fillings: A case-control study. Br Dent J 1999; 1875:261–264.

71. Karni A, Abramsky O. Association of MS with thyroid disorders. Neurology 1999; 534: 883–885.

72. Sadovnick AD, Eisen K, Hashimoto SA, et al. Pregnancy and multiple sclerosis. Arch Neurol 1994; 51:1120–1124.

73. Runmarker B, Andersen O. Pregnancy is associated with a lower risk of onset and a better prognosis in multiple sclerosis. Brain 1995; 118:253–261.

74. Stenager E. Acute and chronic pain syndromes in multiple sclerosis. A 5-year follow-up study. Ital J Neurol Sci 1995; 169:629–632.

75. Confavreux C, Hutchinson M, Hours MM, et al. Rate of pregnancy-related relapse in multiple sclerosis. Pregnancy in Multiple Sclerosis Group. N Engl J Med 1998; 3395:285–291.

76. Hutter CD, Laing P. Multiple sclerosis: Sunlight, diet, immunology and aetiology. Med Hypotheses 1996; 492:67–74.

77. Multiple sclerosis in 54 twinships: concordance rate is independent of zygosity. French Research Group on Multiple Sclerosis. Ann Neurol 1992; 326:724–727.

78. Ebers GC, Sadovnick AD. The role of genetic factors in multiple sclerosis susceptibility. J Neuroimmunol 1994; 541–542:1–17.

79. Sadovnick AD. Canadian collaborative project on genetic susceptibility to MS, phase 2: rationale and method. Canadian Collaborative Study Group. Can J Neurol Sci 1998; 253: 216–221.

80. Duquette P, Pleines J, Girard M, et al. The increased susceptibility of women to multiple sclerosis. Can J Neurol Sci 1992; 19:466–471.

81. Granieri E. Selected reviews common childhood and adolescent infections and multiple sclerosis. Neurology 1997; 492(suppl 2):S42–S54.

82. Kurtzke JF. MS epidemiology world wide. One view of current status. Acta Neurol Scand Suppl 1995; 161:23–33.

83. Kurtzke JF, Hyllested K, Heltberg A, Olsen A. Multiple sclerosis in the Faroe Islands. 5. The occurrence of the fourth epidemic as validation of transmission. Acta Neurol Scand 1993; 883:161–173.

84. Benedikz J, Magnusson H, Gudmundsson G. Multiple sclerosis in Iceland, with observations on the alleged epidemic in the Faroe Islands. Ann Neurol 1994; 36(suppl 2):S175–S179.

85. Cook SD, Rohowsky-Kochan C, Bansil S, Dowling PC. Evidence for multiple sclerosis as an infectious disease. Acta Neurol Scand Suppl 1995; 161:34–42.

86. Campadelli-Fiume G, Mirandola P, Menotti L. Human herpesvirus 6: An emerging pathogen. Emerg Infect Dis 1999; 53:353–366.

87. Kimberlin DW, Whitley RJ. Human herpesvirus-6: Neurologic implications of a newly-described viral pathogen. J Neurovirol 1998; 45:474–485.

88. Ross RT. The varicella-zoster virus and multiple sclerosis. J Clin Epidemiol 1998; 517:533–553.

89. Ross RT. Varicella zoster antibodies after herpes zoster, varicella and multiple sclerosis. Can J Neurol Sci 1997; 242:137–139.

90. Ross RT. Common infectious diseases in a population with low multiple sclerosis and varicella occurrence. J Clin Epidemiol 1997; 503:337–339.

91. Ross RT. Varicella zoster virus and multiple sclerosis in a Hutterite population. J Clin Epidemiol 1995; 4811:1319–1324.

92. Ross RT, Cheang M, Landry G, et al. Herpes zoster and multiple sclerosis. Can J Neurol Sci 1999; 261:29–32.

93. Haahr S, Koch-Henriksen N, Moller-Larsen A, et al. Increased risk of multiple sclerosis after late Epstein-Barr virus infection: A historical prospective study. Mult Scler 1995; 12:73–77.

94. Haahr S, Sommerlund M, Moller-Larsen A, et al. Is multiple sclerosis caused by a dual infection with retrovirus and Epstein-Barr virus? Neuroepidemiology 1992; 114–116:299–303.

95. MacGregor HS, Latiwonk QI. Complex role of gamma-herpesviruses in multiple sclerosis and infectious mononucleosis. Neurol Res 1993; 156:391–394.

96. Haahr S. Cluster of multiple sclerosis patients from Danish community. Lancet 1997; 3496: 923.

97. Pirmohamed M, Winstanley P. Hepatitis B vaccine and neurotoxicity. Postgrad Med J 1997; 73:462–463.

98. Tosti ME, Traversa G, Bianco E, Mele A. Multiple sclerosis and vaccination against hepatitis B: Analysis of risk benefit profile. Ital J Gastroenterol Hepatol 1999; 315:388–391.

99. Monteyne P, Bureau JF, Brahic M. Viruses and multiple sclerosis. Curr Opin Neurol 1998; 114:287–291.

100. van Buuren S, Zaadstra BM, Zwanikken CP, et al. Space-time clustering of multiple sclerosis cases around birth. Acta Neurol Scand 1998; 976:351–358.

3

The Genetics of Multiple Sclerosis

JAN HILLERT and **THOMAS MASTERMAN**

Karolinska Institutet at Huddinge University Hospital, Huddinge, Sweden

I. INTRODUCTION

A. Background

Theories concerning the etiology and pathogenesis of multiple sclerosis (MS) have changed from time to time, following the evolution of biomedicine. Thus, it is only to be expected that, during the current period of heavy progress in molecular genetics, MS should be widely looked upon as a genetically determined disorder. However, although there is irrefutable evidence that genetic factors do play a role in MS, it is much too early to tell whether the genetic perspective will provide us with information of relevance for the management of MS patients.

The prevailing hypothesis at the beginning of the twenty-first century is that MS is a polygenic disease—i.e., that several different genes jointly confer susceptibility to the disorder—which, of course, does not rule out the possibility of contributing environmental factors. So far, only one genetic factor of confirmed importance has been identified; it is located in the human leukocyte antigen (HLA) class II region on the short arm of chromosome 6. This fact has in essence been known for close to 30 years, and one could argue that little progress has been made since its discovery. However, the last few years have seen tremendous progress in our knowledge of MS genetics, and today we know of a number of additional candidate genes and chromosomal regions of probable importance.

In this chapter we will first outline the existing evidence implicating genetic factors in MS and then briefly review methodological aspects of genetic analysis and review what is known about HLA class II genes and other specific candidate genes in MS. In addition, attention will be focused on data from the published genomic screen studies, which have provided valuable clues about where in the genome to look for MS genes.

B.   MS Genetics: Summary of Present Knowledge

Genetic epidemiology has provided firm evidence for the importance of genes in determining the risk for MS. The existence of familial aggregation can be translated into an increased risk for MS among relatives of MS patients. The high concordance rate of 30% in monozygotic twins, which decreases to 2 to 5% in other full siblings and is still considerably higher in half siblings (1.1 to 1.4%) than in relatives by adoption (0.1%) or the general population (0.1%), underscores the influence inherited genetic factors, believed to be at least a half-dozen in number, exert on predisposition to MS (1–4).

Many studies have confirmed that a genetic factor in the HLA class II region confers an increased risk for MS. More precisely, carrying the HLA-DR-DQ haplotype HLA-DRBI*1501,DRB5*0101,DQA1*0102,DQB1*0602 increases the risk for MS three to four times in western and northern Europeans (for a review, see Ref. 5).

Genome-wide mapping studies have indicated the absence of any single gene with a very high impact in MS and confirmed the importance of the HLA gene complex; moreover, a handful of additional loci have been singled out as being of probable importance (6–9). For a few of these loci, subsequent studies have supported the initial genome-screen findings. In particular, loci on the short arms of chromosomes 2, 3, 5, and 7 and on the long arms of chromosomes 2, 17, and 19 are likely to contain relevant genes (see Table 3). Interestingly, there are indications that some of these regions may also harbor genes predisposing to other autoimmune disorders as well as to experimental animal models of human autoimmune disease (10).

A large number of genetic studies have focused on candidate genes chosen on the grounds of hypotheses about MS pathogenesis. For most of these, existing data are negative or conflicting. The T cell–receptor α- and β-chain genes and the immunoglobulin genes have thus far received the most attention. Although early reports of allelic associations have been difficult to confirm, available linkage data also seem to support the importance of these genes. More recent studies suggest that the gene encoding CTLA-4 may influence susceptibility to MS and that other genes, in particular those of the interleukin-1 cluster, may influence the course of the disease. These claims, however, await confirmation in independent studies.

II.   BASIS OF MS GENETIC STUDIES

A.   A Brief History of MS Genetics

The field of MS genetics is over a century old. Eichorst proposed as early as 1896 that hereditary factors were involved in MS. Pratt reviewed the tendency toward familial aggregation in 1951 and concluded that more than a single gene was required to explain the pattern of inheritance. After the identification of an HLA-associated susceptibility factor in 1972, the search for genetic factors in MS has accelerated steadily, with numerous studies focusing on HLA and non-HLA candidate genes. At present, several major efforts are under way with regard both to the recruitment of MS families and to laboratory-intensive molecular-genetic analysis.

B.   Why Look for Genes in MS?

The reason to identify genes influencing the risk of developing MS is to understand the pathogenesis of the disorder, which could serve as a basis for new therapeutic approaches.

Even in identical twin pairs in which one twin has MS, there is a 70% chance that the other twin will remain unaffected (3). Thus, we should not expect that even a full understanding of MS genetics would allow prenatal diagnosis or serve as a basis for detailed genetic counseling.

C. Genetic Epidemiology: Evidence for Genetics in MS

Family Studies

As outlined in the previous chapter, MS prevalence rates in many areas in the western world are approximately 1 in 1000, which can be translated roughly into a lifetime risk of 1 in 500. Since 20% of patients have a family history of at least one additional case of MS (4,11), there is no doubt that there is familial aggregation in MS. This is clearly not by itself evidence for genetics, however, since family members also share environment and lifestyle.

A number of population-based twin studies have been performed, and three of them have reported very similar results. Concordance rates in these reports were 21.1%, 30.8%, and 25.0% in monozygotic (MZ) twins and 3.6%, 4.7%, and 3.3% in dizygotic (DZ) twins (1,3,12). Of these reports, the one by Sadovnik et al. includes twin pairs with a mean age of more than 50 years and may therefore most accurately reflect the lifetime concordance rates.

The inheritance pattern in MS does not resemble patterns seen in typical genetic diseases, which classically display dominant, recessive, or X-linked modes of inheritance with high penetrance; rather, when MS occurs in families, it appears in an irregular fashion. Further, the number of affected individuals in each family is small, usually only two, with three being unusual and four or more rare. This means that the statistical lifetime risk for MS in a relative to an MS patient is low and, except for MZ twins, always below 5%. In summary, the lifetime risk for MS in first-degree relatives (children, parents, siblings) to MS patients is 3 to 5%; in second- (niece/nephews) and third-degree relatives (first cousins), it is 1.5 to 2.5% (2,13).

Recently, Sadovnik et al. (14) reported the recurrence risk for MS in half-siblings, a highly interesting set of relatives because they are often reared apart. The chief finding in this study—that there was no significant difference in concordance between half-sibs reared together (1.2%) and half-sibs reared apart (1.5%)—indicates that the increased risk is mediated by genes rather than by shared environment. In addition, it made no difference whether half-siblings had a common father or common mother, indicating that mitochondrial or X-linked susceptibility is not a common feature of familial MS.

As stated above, a commonly reported prevalence rate for MS is 1 in 1000. Ebers et al. (15) shown in a large adoptee study that, among 1201 first-degree relatives by adoption to MS patients, only 1 had MS—i.e., a prevalence nearly exactly equal to the expected rate. This also indicates that when MS occurs more than once in a nuclear family, it is most likely due to shared genes.

Recurrence rates in relatives of varying degrees of kinship have been used to rule out different specific patterns of inheritance in MS and to support the notion of polygenicity. Apart from being poorly compatible with the effect of a single autosomal dominant gene, MS familial recurrence data—which show that parents and children to cases have approximately the same risk as siblings—are also incompatible with the effect of a single recessive gene. Further, neither dominant X-linked, recessive X-linked, or mitochondrial inheritance can explain the observed data (2).

Thus, it seems likely that MS is a polygenic disease. Familial recurrence rates may also be used to estimate the number of genes involved in MS. Since family members obviously differ to some degree with regard to environment, twin data are generally more amenable to such calculations, based on the assumption that twins more or less share the same environment. The concordance ratio of 6 to 7 seen in MS between MZ and DZ twins can be interpreted as evidence for the effect of several genes. With an increasing numbers of interacting genes, the ratio should become increasingly higher. On the other hand, the overall concordance rate of MZ twins is in itself not an argument for the involvement of genetic factors. Risch (16) has reported techniques using concordance rates in different degrees of kinship for use in the segregation analysis of polygenic disease. Phillips (17) applied these methods to MS and came up with an estimation of the existence of 5 to 10 susceptibility genes.

Ethnic Comparisons

There are well-known examples of ethnic groups that seem more or less resistant to MS, despite living in the same geographic area as medium- or high-prevalence populations: for instance, Maoris in New Zealand (18), Lapps in Norway (19), Gypsies in Hungary (20), and American blacks (21). Although there may also be environmental reasons for the different frequencies, both in Hungarian Gypsies and American blacks the frequency of the HLA-DR15,DQ6,Dw2 haplotype is strikingly lower than in the ethnically predominant surrounding population (22,23), which supports the view that genes are likely to contribute to these different prevalence figures.

HLA-DR15,DQ6,Dw2

As will be discussed in detail in a later section, this common HLA class II haplotype occurs in 20 to 30% of healthy controls in northern and western Europe and, typically, in 50 to 70% of MS patients in populations from these areas. This association has been observed in a large number of independent studies in many different populations, making it unlikely that it is an effect of sampling bias, a problem often afflicting association studies.

D. Criticisms of Genetic and Polygenic Models

Although the arguments for a polygenic model outlined above are striking, they should perhaps be interpreted with some care. For instance, poliomyelitis, in spite of its apparent infectious cause, displays MZ and DZ concordance rates very similar to those for MS (24). Further, it is possible that the differences in fetal environment between MZ and DZ twins could be of importance for disease later in life (25). Thus, it is possible that twin studies do not really tell us what we think they do. In addition, the confidence intervals of the twin, half-sib, and adoptee studies in MS are wide enough to allow for less confident conclusions regarding the domination of nature over nurture. As for familial aggregation, the lifetime risk for MS is about 1 in 500 in the general population, and the occurrence in first-, second-, or third-degree relatives may be as high as 4 to 5%, which leaves a relative risk of only 4 to 5 to be explained by genes and environment together.

III. METHODOLOGICAL ASPECTS

In principle, there are two different ways of investigating genes in a complex disease such as MS: the candidate gene approach and the more recently developed random genomic screen method.

A. Investigation of Candidate Disease Genes

This method is based on intelligent guesses concerning which genes could theoretically be expected to be important. Examples of this approach include the studies of the insulin gene in diabetes (IDDM), of the myelin basic protein (MBP) gene in MS, and of HLA genes in putatively autoimmune disorders. Traditionally, this method has been used for genes that are known to be polymorphic, allowing the distribution of alleles between patients and healthy controls to be compared for statistical significance. Such association studies can be performed quickly, since unrelated patients are abundant; but they are also fraught with several pitfalls, frequently resulting in positive reports that are never confirmed. A major problem is controlling for ethnicity between patients and the control group. For instance, if MS, as is sometimes argued, is due to a "Scandinavian gene" (26), studies of MS patients in North America would run an increased risk of finding false associations with any allele typical to persons of Scandinavian descent—unless the control group was of the same ethnic background—regardless of whether the particular gene is of any real importance. To overcome this problem, the strategy of using intrafamilial controls has been increasingly practiced. Here, the frequency of transmission of a particular allele from a heterozygote parent to an affected offspring is compared to what would be expected by chance alone.

A different approach to studying candidate genes is to study linkage between genes and disease within families in which more than one person is affected. Linkage analysis is a powerful tool in diseases for which large pedigrees are found; but, as mentioned above, this is not the case in MS. For diseases such as MS, a large number of families are instead required, due to the small number of affected persons within each family. Linkage analysis is most powerful when genetic data are tested against a specific model that is likely to be true—e.g., in the presence of a clearly dominant or recessive pattern of inheritance. Such parametric analyses also include variables such as disease frequency as a function of age ("liability"), disease prevalence in the general population, and the postulated distance between the gene itself and the marker used. However, since several of these variables are unknown in polygenic diseases such as MS, the results of parametric linkage analysis can only be approximate at best and may very well be misleading.

Therefore, several nonparametric methods for linkage analysis have been developed. Here, assumptions of a true model are not required. The most commonly used strategy recently has been to study affected sibling pairs and to compare how often they share marker alleles in relation to what would be seen by chance. If siblings with MS are found to inherit the same parental chromosomal segment more often than expected by chance, it may be due to the presence of an MS gene in that region. One drawback with this method is its lack of statistical power; a large number of affected sibling pairs need to be investigated to attain significant results.

A major disadvantage of the candidate gene approach is that the investigator is limited by what is currently known about the pathogenesis of the disease in focus. For MS, the number of genes of possible importance on theoretical grounds is very high (genes of importance in autoimmunity, genes encoding myelin components, etc.). Thus, in recent years there has been a tendency to look for an alternative strategy.

B. The Genomic Screen Approach

In this approach, no assumptions are necessary concerning which genes could be of importance; rather, the whole genome is surveyed without preformed hypotheses about pathogenesis. Large sets of polymorphic markers, dispersed throughout the genome, are now available. So far, the most commonly used markers are microsatellites—highly polymorphic sequences of two, three, or four nucleotides repeated tandemly a variable number of times. These markers can be studied in a semiautomated fashion based on DNA fragment analysis after fluorescent polymerase chain reaction (PCR) amplification (27). In a genomic screen of a polygenic disease such as MS, usually 300 to 400 markers are studied in at least 100 families. The end result of a genomic screen is the identification of a chromosomal region of considerable size, usually 10 to 20 million base pairs. The task then becomes to identify the exact gene responsible for the positive linkage data. Since a chromosomal region of such size may contain hundreds of genes, many of which will be unknown or uncharacterized, the identification of the disease-predisposing gene is a major undertaking. How this is most efficiently achieved is still not very well known, but it is likely that the completion of the Human Genome Project, which will provide information on the location of all genes, will make it more feasible.

Data from genomic screens, based typically on microsatellite analysis of hundreds of affected siblings, are now available for MS as well as for many other polygenic diseases. The common experience, however, has been one of confusion. Only a few chromosomal regions have been identified with linkage scores strong enough to be formally significant, and results between studies have been inconsistent. The reason for this may be that the number of genes involved in polygenic disorders is large and that each gene only contributes a minor part of the genetic risk. Thus, the number of families required may be much higher than originally anticipated. Therefore, because the linkage strategy has proven difficult, there is a need, yet again, for alternative methods.

Progress in DNA technology, allowing rapid, high-throughput laboratory analysis, has opened up new possibilities, bringing back association analysis as an attractive alternative.

IV. CANDIDATE GENES IN MS: HLA CLASS II

A. Summary

We do know that HLA class II genes play a role in determining susceptibility to MS, although many details are unclear and the mechanisms largely unknown. The present knowledge can be summarized in the following way:

1. MS is associated with the HLA-DR-DQ haplotype DR15,DQ6,Dw2 (HLA-Dw2, for short), which is equivalent to DRB1*1501,DRB5*0101,DQA1*0102,DQB1*0602 in genomic terminology.
2. The HLA-Dw2 association is strongest in Europe and North America but can be seen in most ethnic groups.
3. The Dw2 haplotype is identical in MS patients and controls and confers a four-fold increased risk for MS, but it is not clear what importance it has compared with other possible genetic factors.
4. Among other HLA haplotypes, DR3,DQ2 is positively associated with MS, albeit to a lesser degree than Dw2.
5. HLA-A alleles seem to play a role in MS independent of their proximity to class II haplotypes and appear to interact with Dw2 in determining the risk for MS.

B. HLA Molecules, Genes, and Function

In experiments with skin grafting and transplantation of tumors between different strains of experimental animals in the 1930s, it became clear that genetic factors influence the ability of an animal to accept or reject a transplanted tissue. Later, it became clear that the most important of these genes were inherited closely together in a complex termed the major histocompatibility complex (MHC). In humans, this set of genes is known as the HLA complex (for human leukocyte antigens) and is situated on the short arm of the chromosome 6 (Figure 1).

The HLA complex codes for cell-surface glycoproteins of two types. The HLA class I molecule is a protein chain of approximately 350 amino acids and a weight of 45 kilodaltons (kDa). On the cell surface, the HLA class I chain is associated with β_2-microglobulin. The major class I genes are HLA-A, B, and C, and they are all polymorphic. There are a number of additional HLA class I genes (e.g., HLA-E, G, H, and J), but these seem to be nonpolymorphic and are expressed at a low rate on the cell surface.

The HLA class II molecule is made up of two polypeptides, one α and one β chain, of 30 to 34 and 26 to 29 kDa, respectively, which corresponds to 250 to 270 amino acids. These chains are encoded by closely linked genes (termed A and B genes) at three loci, HLA-DR, DQ, and DP. All of these genes are highly polymorphic except for the HLA-DRA gene. In addition, there are other genes in the class II region (HLA-DO, DN, and DM), which encode molecules expressed at low levels, whose function remains unknown.

HLA class I and class II molecules share several characteristics with regard to both structure and function, but there are also clear and important differences. Both are extremely polymorphic four-domain cell-surface molecules, with a similar groove on their outermost aspect. This groove is designed to bind a peptide, and the role of the HLA molecule is to present this peptide to cells of the immune system.

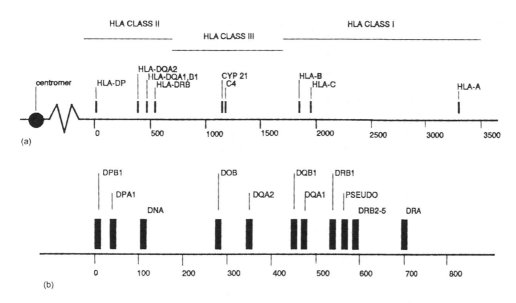

Figure 1   (a) An outline of the HLA gene complex on the short arm of chromosome 6. (b) A closeup of the HLA class II region. Distances are given in kilobase pairs.

However, there are also important differences. The HLA class I molecule is present on most nucleated cells and binds a peptide with a length of 8 to 9 amino acids in order to present it to CD8-positive cytotoxic T cells, the major effector cells of the cell-mediated immune response. On the other hand, the HLA class II molecule is found on only a limited number of specialized antigen-presenting cells and presents a slightly longer peptide of around 13 to 25 amino acids to CD4-positive T-helper cells. Another difference is that HLA class I molecules primarily present peptides that have been produced within the presenting cell—such as peptides produced during normal cellular processes or during neoplastic events or peptides derived from viral products (28); whereas class II molecules present peptides derived from proteins taken up and degraded by the antigen-presenting cell (29). In this way, class I and class II molecules take part in the surveillance of distinct immune compartments: the intracellular (class I) and the extracellular (class II) compartments.

For many years, immunologists were looking for an "immune response gene," a gene that determined whether an individual would be able to react immunologically against a certain peptide antigen. It now seems that the role ascribed to the products of immune response genes is in fact performed by the MHC class II molecule, through one or both of its principal functions (30). First, the molecule presents peptides to the T-helper cell in the first stage of the immune response. Since different HLA class II alleles have different affinities for a given peptide, the efficiency of this presentation will be determined by the HLA class II phenotype of the individual (31). In addition, the class II phenotype is also thought to further influence the "response phenotype" by educating T cells during their thymic selection (32). Therefore, the final repertoire of T-cell specificities is decisively influenced by the MHC class II phenotype.

As mentioned above, the MHC genes are extremely polymorphic. The number of recognized HLA alleles continues to increase steadily as new populations are investigated. At present, 328 HLA-B alleles, 289 DRB alleles, and 44 DQB alleles are known to exist (IMGT/HLA Database, http://www3.ebi.ac.uk/Services/imgt/hla/cgi-bin/statistics.cgi; February 18, 2000). Another characteristic feature of the MHC genes is strong linkage disequilibrium, which in humans is most evident between HLA-DR and -DQ. As a result, a certain HLA-DRB allele will occur together with only a limited set of DQA and DQB alleles. Such combinations are referred to as haplotypes. The extension of the HLA-DR-DQ haplotypes varies greatly. The haplotype DR3,DQ2, for instance, is very well conserved across the HLA class III region to the HLA class I region, resulting in the frequent occurrence of the "extended" haplotype HLA-A1,B8,DR3,DQ2. Another frequently seen haplotype is A3,B7,DR2,DQ6, at least some parts of which are associated with MS.

The HLA class III region is the chromosomal region located between the HLA class I and class II regions. It contains a number of genes; some code for components of the immune system—such as complement factors and tumor necrosis factors α and β—and others for proteins with no relation to immune functions, such as cytochrome P21. However, in this region, no genes coding for peptide-presenting HLA molecules are found.

C. HLA and Disease Associations

Beginning in the late 1960s, it was repeatedly observed that certain HLA-A and -B alleles were more common than expected in groups of patients with various diseases. When HLA class II alleles were discovered, it was revealed that several of the established associations were stronger with regard to these genes and that the class I associations were secondary and due to linkage disequilibrium between class I and II alleles. This turned out to be the case for MS (33) as well as for rheumatoid arthritis (34) and insulin-dependent diabetes mellitus (IDDM) (35). For other diseases, such as ankylosing spondylitis, the class I association was revealed to be stronger and thus primary (36), while for still others there is as yet no general agreement as to where the strongest association lies. An example of this is myasthenia gravis, which is associated with the highly conserved HLA-B8,DR3,DQ2 haplotype (37).

Why are such a large number of diseases associated with alleles of HLA genes? Although the phenomenon has been known for over 30 years, no satisfying answer to this question has been given. If one looks at a list of HLA-associated diseases, it is clear that the majority of these conditions show inflammatory characteristics, which suggests an involvement of immune mechanisms in their pathophysiology. Many of them are also considered autoimmune diseases. Typical examples are ankylosing spondylitis, MS, rheumatoid arthritis, systemic lupus erythematosus (SLE), and myasthenia gravis. For IDDM, the discovery of an HLA association was one of the first indications that this disease also possessed autoimmune features, something that has become increasingly clear since. Yet, other HLA-associated conditions seem to lack inflammatory characteristics completely, such as narcolepsy, which nonetheless occurs almost exclusively in patients positive for DR2 (38).

In autoimmune conditions, it might be considered reasonable to assume that "immune response genes" influence the ability of an individual to raise such a response. The mechanism by which this would happen is less obvious. A well-known hypothesis is that of "molecular mimicry," according to which structural homology between a peptide of the invading microorganism and a self antigen of the invaded host results in a misdirected immune response against host tissues expressing the "mimicked" self antigen. A more general explanation for HLA associations is that, somehow, the presentation of a specific peptide is of importance. This presentation could take place in the thymus during the maturation of T cells, thus affecting the composition of the T-cell repertoire, or peripherally in the mature immune system. An additional possibility is that the actual association is with another, non-HLA gene, located in the vicinity of, and thus in linkage disequilibrium with, specific HLA alleles. It is tempting to speculate that this mechanism could explain the strong DR2 association in narcolepsy. However, when discussing purportedly "autoimmune" diseases, it seems less relevant to speculate about other, yet unknown genes.

D. Typing Techniques and Nomenclature

HLA class II typing was initially performed by coculturing leukocytes from different individuals. In this way the HLA-Dw specificities were discovered and classified. This technique has the disadvantage of being slow and expensive and of having less than satisfying reproducibility. Therefore, it was a great improvement when antisera with specificities corresponding to the Dw types were identified. In the mid-1980s, the HLA class II genes were cloned (39), and since then class II polymorphism has been studied by genomic methods. Typing is now usually performed using various PCR-based techniques.

Even though cellular, serological, and genomic techniques aim to describe the same biological structures and related functions, the typing results of one technique are difficult to express in the terminology of another. Thus, they each require a specific nomenclature, a fact that makes reading HLA studies from different periods strikingly confusing to the nonexpert. Nucleotide sequence–based terminology, by which the Dw2 haplotype is defined as DRB1*1501,DRB5*0101,DQA1*0102,DQB1*0602, is clearly the most explicit.

E. Characterization of the HLA-Dw2 Haplotype in MS

Early Results

In 1972, Jersild and coworkers reported that MS was associated with the class I alleles A3 and B7 (40). In 1973, the same authors reported an increase of the cellular specificity Dw2 among Danish MS patients (33), the frequency being 70% among patients and 25% among controls, and it became clear that the class I associations were secondary to the linkage disequilibrium with this marker. In the following years, the Dw2 association was confirmed in a number of studies. It was thus recognized that Dw2 confers an increased risk for MS among individuals of western European origin.

As mentioned above, serological studies soon came to dominate the field, and a large number of groups of MS patients were investigated. As expected, the pattern was similar in most studies, with DR2 being more common among MS patients than controls. Typical DR2 frequencies in Europe are 60% among MS patients and 30% among healthy controls, corresponding to a relative risk of 3.5. However, differences in Dw2 frequencies between patients and controls are in general wider, especially in populations from northwestern Europe.

HLA-Dw2: Findings by Genomic Typing

Genomic HLA class II typing techniques have permitted specifications regarding the MS-associated haplotype. First, DR2 can serologically be split into DR15 and DR16. At the sequence level, there are at least seven DRB1 sequences, each associated with a specific set of DQA1 and DQB1 alleles. In addition, DR2 haplotypes also carry an expressed DRB5 gene, for which four possible allelic variants exist (DRB5*0101, *0102, *0201, and *0202), each linked to a specific haplotype.

The basic achievement of genomic techniques in MS has been to specify the HLA association as being to the DRB1*1501,DQA1*0102,DQB1*0602 haplotype. By using the PCR-SSP typing technique (PCR with sequence-specific primers), we have recently found that it is possible to add DRB5*0101 to this haplotype (41). In other words, DRB1*1501,DRB5*0101,DQA1*0102,DQB1*0602 is the full genomic designation of the MS-associated Dw2 haplotype.

Table 1 lists a number of studies in which genomic HLA class II typing techniques have been carried out on groups of MS patients and controls. The table clearly shows a universal pattern of increase of the Dw2 haplotype among MS patients in all ethnic groups. The only exceptions from the pattern are the reports from Sardinia, where the Dw2 haplotype is extremely uncommon (47,48). Interestingly, in North America as well as Europe, the frequency of MS varies with the distribution of the Dw2 haplotype, which is regarded by some to be marker for a pool of genes of Scandinavian origin (49).

HLA-DR or DQ in MS?

In several other HLA-associated diseases, most clearly in IDDM (50) and celiac disease (51), there is evidence that either the DR or DQ part of the associated haplotypes is of primary importance for the association. In MS, it has been suggested that the DQ genes (22,52,53), or even specific segments of the DQ molecule (54,55), are responsible. However, though tested, these hypotheses have never been independently confirmed (56–59).

Table 1   Phenotypic Frequencies of Dw2 Haplotype Among MS
Patients and Controls of Various Ethnic Backgrounds, as Determined by
Genomic or Cellular Typing

	% Positive	
Population (ref.) (no. of patients)	MS Patients	Controls
USA (42) ($n = 330$)	52	18
USA, blacks (23) ($n = 31$)	35	0
Norway (55) ($n = 69$)	72	33
Sweden (43) ($n = 245$)	60	30
England (57) ($n = 71$)	63	32
Northern Ireland (85) ($n = 54$)	63	30
Northern France (52) ($n = 44$)	70	—
Southern France (44) ($n = 170$)	29	10
Sardinia (47) ($n = 103$)	5	7
Hungarian Gypsies (22) ($n = 10$)	30	0
Israel (45) ($n = 45$)	13.5	6.4
Japan (46) ($n = 60$)	22	7
Hong Kong (61)[a] ($n = 11$)	54	17

[a]Of DR2-positives only.

In most populations, all parts of the Dw2 haplotype are unique to this specific haplotype; thus it is not possible to determine which part of the haplotype is responsible for the association or whether it is due to the haplotype in its entirety. Recently, however, Caballero and coworkers (60), comparing a group of Brazilian MS patients of African origin to ethnically matched controls, observed in patients a distinctly increased frequency of DQ6 (DQA1*0201,DQB1*0602) in the absence of DR15. This indicates that it may in fact be the DQ molecule rather than the DR molecule that is functionally responsible for the disease-predisposing association in MS. Similar observations have also been made in a small study from the Far East (61).

Mode of Inheritance

Analysis of 179 Swedish MS patients has shown that the distribution of patients homozygous and heterozygous for Dw2 is similar to what one would expect if this haplotype were acting dominantly, and that it is incompatible with a recessive model (59). However, other studies, in ethnically similar populations, have indicated that a recessive model may in fact be correct (62).

F.   Other HLA Haplotypes in MS

In the numerous studies of HLA alleles in MS that have been performed in the past 25 years, many alleles or haplotypes have been reported to have this or that effect. In particular, DR3, DR4, and DR6 have been suggested to be susceptibility factors in addition to Dw2.

HLA-DR3

Occasionally in MS studies, the DR3 association is with the DR17,DQ2 haplotype, designated in genomic nomenclature as HLA-DRB1*0301,DRB3*0101,DQA1*0501,DQB1*

Table 2 Phenotypic Frequencies of the HLA-DR3,DQ2 Haplotype
in a Number of Studies Using Genomic Typing Techniques

Population (ref.) (no. of patients)	% Positive	
	MS Patients	Controls
USA (56) ($n = 21$)	43	22
Sweden (59) ($n = 179$)	22	17
Norway (55) ($n = 69$)	33	27
Northern Ireland (85) ($n = 54$)	32	25
England (57) ($n = 71$)	24	20
Hungarian Gypsies (22) ($n = 10$)	30	24

0201 (63). Table 2 lists a number of studies in which frequencies for DR3 are given for MS patients and controls, most of them having been determined using serology but some using genomic techniques. Since, in Caucasians, DR3 is practically synonymous with the DR17,DQ2 haplotype, differences between serological and genomic findings are less pronounced than for DR2.

In some of these studies, an increase of DR3 was noted among patients, but the differences are small and may not seem very convincing and have therefore frequently evaded attention. However, in studying a possible second association when a stronger association already is present, one must take into consideration the fact that the most strongly associated haplotype will affect the frequency of the other haplotypes.

If DR3 were to have no influence on the occurrence of MS, its frequency should be somewhat lower among MS patients than controls, since twice as many patient chromosomes already carry DR2; but Table 2 shows clearly that this is not the case. Payami et al. (64) have described a way to compensate for this—namely, by calculating the genotypic difference after subtraction of the primarily associated haplotypes. If this were to be done, several of the differences in Table 2 might become significant. Furthermore, a metanalysis of all the studies in Table 2 reveals a significant increase for DR3 in patients compared to controls ($p = 0.001$), even without compensation for the increase in DR2 (in this approximative calculation, all studies are weighted equally). In fact, using the method of Payami et al., we recently observed a significant increase in DR3 in a large group of Swedish MS patients ($n = 816$) (65). Thus, it is possible that this haplotype is also of importance for MS.

HLA-DR4

In a study by Kurdi et al. (66), Jordanian Arabs with MS were found to have an increased frequency of DR4 compared to controls, and similar results were reported for MS patients from Sardinia (48). However, these findings have not yet been confirmed in either of these ethnic groups. On the other hand, more recent data from the Middle East, as well as data from the majority of studies conducted in Mediterranean Europe (67), do not show any such increase. Yet some very recent observations again raise the possibility of a DR4 association (68,69). However, as the specificity DR4 includes at least 15 different haplotypes, an association will probably turn out to be restricted to one or a few of these, as in rheumatoid arthritis. Analysis with haplotype-level resolution remains to be performed in these populations.

G. HLA and MS Heterogeneity

HLA and Prognosis

Jersild et al. (33), in describing the Dw2 association, suggested that Dw2 might serve as a marker for a worse prognosis, and several similar attempts to correlate prognosis to HLA phenotypes have been made since. The findings, however, have varied. Some studies have shown association of Dw2/DR2 with worse prognosis (70,71), others with a more benign course (72). However, a study in which a cohort of MS patients was followed for 30 years—an optimal design for this type of analysis—failed to find any evidence to suggest that the Dw2 haplotype influences prognosis (73). Likewise, HLA-DR3 has been reported to be associated both with malignant (72,73) and benign (70,71) course. We have recently readdressed this question in a large dataset of 816 Swedish MS patients. Our data fail to support a role in disease progression for any of the HLA-DRB alleles (65).

Clinical Subtypes of MS

Several attempts have been made to uncover possible HLA associations with different clinical forms of MS. In recent years, a number of reports have addressed the question whether primary chronic progressive MS (characterized by steady progression from onset, without relapse-like deterioration) differs from relapsing/remitting MS with regard to association to HLA alleles. In particular, a difference originally observed in Swedish and Norwegian patients, indicating a very low frequency of DR3 in patients with primary chronic progressive MS (74,75), has not been confirmed in subsequent studies in these or any other populations (65).

In recent years, however, Japanese researchers have reported a distinction between opticospinal MS and what they refer to as western-type MS. Interestingly, the HLA-Dw2 association is only present in western-type MS (76–78). In addition, the opticospinal form may be associated with the DPB1*0501 allele (79). The opticospinal form also differs from the western type in showing a lower frequency of oligoclonal immunoglobulin bands in cerebrospinal fluid and fewer intracerebral lesions as visualized by magnetic resonance imaging. Thus, in this instance, HLA associations may in fact, at the group level, distinguish two distinct disease entities, illustrating the potential usefulness of genetic analysis in complex disorders.

H. HLA–DP Alleles in MS

Typing for HLA-DP remained methodologically complicated until the development of PCR-based typing techniques. Thus, it is hardly surprising that two early reports of possible associations in MS (80,81) were later followed by clearly negative reports (55,82–85). Accordingly, there is currently a consensus that HLA-DP alleles do not confer susceptibility to MS. As previously stated, an exception may be the DPB1*0501 association in opticospinal MS patients of Japanese origin (79).

I. Other Genes in the HLA Gene Complex in MS

HLA Class I Genes in MS

Although the original report of an HLA association in MS concerned HLA-A, the importance of HLA class I genes and molecules has not been studied much since. However, in a recent study, we have found striking associations in MS with two HLA-A alleles (86).

HLA-A3 (HLA-A*0301) was found to confer a relative risk of 2 in MS (41% in MS patients, 25% in controls), whereas HLA-A2 (HLA-A*0201) decreased the risk by 50% (45% in MS, 61% in controls). This influence was surprisingly independent of the HLA-Dw2 association. The existence of a modifier gene close to the susceptibility factor HLA-Dw2 may explain some of the inconsistencies in previous association and linkage studies.

TNF-α and TNF-β (Lymphotoxin α)

The genes coding for the important cytokines tumor necrosis factor (TNF)-α and TNF-β (also known as lymphotoxin-α) reside between the HLA class I and II regions and are obvious candidates for the true source of the genetic-analytic signals emanating from the HLA region in MS. Numerous studies have been performed on these genes, and numerous claims made for their independent role in MS. However, most of these reports have failed to take into account the importance of the flanking class II genes. When this has been done, conclusions regarding the relevance of the TNF-α and β genes in MS have usually been negative (87,88). In addition, there are only a limited number of known polymorphisms within these genes, far fewer than in the neighboring HLA genes, and few additional ones have been identified in spite of ambitious screening (88). However, the identification of the influence of HLA-A alleles on MS susceptibility may make a renewed assessment of this issue necessary.

TAP, LMP, and DM Genes

Transporters associated with antigen processing and presentation (TAP1 and TAP2), large molecular proteins (LMP1 and LMP2), and the atypical HLA-DM molecule are all functionally involved in the processing and the presentation on class I or II molecules of antigenic peptides. Their genes are located in the HLA class II region between the DQ and DP loci and possess a few polymorphisms that have been studied for a role in MS (89–95). At present, the impression is that these genes are unlikely to be relevant for the risk for MS.

J.   How Important Are HLA class II Genes in MS?

Clearly, HLA class II genes, or at least the HLA-Dw2 haplotype, confer some degree of increased risk of developing MS, but the importance of this role is controversial. On the one hand, linkage studies, with their limitations, have frequently shown some degree of cosegregation of HLA genes and MS. Further, a simple algorithm, used to calculate the "etiological fraction" of a given risk factor in a given disease, indicates that 40% of MS cases would disappear if it were not for the influence of HLA-Dw2. However, linkage studies have sometimes given very low LOD scores for markers in the HLA region, casting doubt on the universality of its importance (7). However, in other studies, analysis of the HLA region has yielded formally significant LOD scores (6,96,97), and a metanalysis of the published genome screens (see below) shows very clearly that the HLA region contains what is by far the most important genetic factor in MS. On the other hand, the region does not seem as important for MS as it is for IDDM, in which the HLA complex contributes around half of the genetically determined susceptibility.

K.   HLA Genes in MS: How?

The mechanisms underlying the disease associations with HLA alleles are not known. One conclusion often drawn from the association with the HLA class II phenotype Dw2 is that CD4-positive T-helper cells are crucial for the etiopathogenesis of MS, as they are in the MS-like animal model experimental autoimmune encephalomyelitis (EAE). Based on the principal functions of class II molecules, the Dw2 phenotype could exert its influence either by preferential presentation of antigenic peptides in the periphery or by orchestrating the selection of a certain repertoire of T-cell receptors in the thymus.

It is clear that HLA genes are neither necessary nor sufficient for the development of MS. Dw2 simply increases the risk for MS by a factor of three or four. If the effect of Dw2 in MS is exerted by the preferential presentation of a peptide, the MS-specific property of the Dw2 phenotype may be related to the fact that a certain peptide, presented unusually effectively by Dw2 heterodimers (encoded by either DRB1-DRA, DRB5-DRA, or DQA-DQB) to Dw2-restricted T-cell clones, is crucial for induction of the disease. It may then be the case that other peptides are also capable of inducing the disease, but that the Dw2-presented peptide is the one most prone to elicit such a reaction. Other questions concerning the initial triggering event—whether it is directed against a self peptide or against a foreign peptide of similar conformation, and whether it occurs within the central nervous system (CNS) or outside of it—are left unanswered by this hypothesis. And the low incidence of MS—even in the large population of Dw2-positive individuals, all of whom are seemingly genetically predisposed to MS—would also need to be explained.

The affinity of the binding of the T-cell receptor (TCR) to the peptide-bearing HLA class II molecule is low compared to the affinities of ordinary specific receptor-ligand interactions. Factors other than the TCR-peptide-HLA complex—including ''second signals'' delivered through the interaction of molecules on the antigen-presenting cell, such as B7-1 and B7-2, with molecules on the T cell, such as CD28 or CTLA-4—are also crucial for eliciting a T-cell response. Thus, even if, in the presence of a putatively contributory environmental factor, the structural prerequisites of a specific TCR and the appropriate HLA molecule are fulfilled, a random event may also be required in order to trigger the disease. To get MS, you may also need some bad luck.

V. NON-HLA CANDIDATE GENES IN MS

The study of other, non-HLA candidate genes in MS has a long history, beginning with the study of blood groups and the analysis, at the protein level, of immunoglobulin ''Gm allotypes.'' Due to the ease provided by DNA technology and the identification of numerous polymorphisms, the opportunities to perform such studies have increased dramatically in recent years. The results of countless studies have been reported and many claims of association have been made.

However, from past experience, it is fair to state that the a priori odds that a reported association is due to a statistical type I error are overwhelming. Thus, each new claim should be viewed with great skepticism until independent studies have provided confirmation. A few candidate genes have been the focus of a great deal of research and will be mentioned in some detail below.

A. T-Cell–Receptor Genes

Shortly after the cloning of the TCR genes in the middle of the 1980s, a number of polymorphisms were identified in and around the genes, and soon after, associations with various inflammatory or autoimmune conditions began to be reported. In MS, associations were reported with both the TCR α-chain (98) and TCR β-chain (99,100) genes, and for the β-chain gene, linkage was also reported (101). However, studies reporting negative results soon followed, and in other diseases, a similar pattern of occasional, but unreplicable, positive findings was observed (reviewed in Ref. 102). In the wake of the predominantly negative findings for the chromosomal regions containing these genes in the genomic screens in MS, interest in the TCR genes has now waned.

B. Immunoglobulin Genes

In MS, intrathecal immunoglobulin production is detectable in a very high percentage of patients. In addition, autoantibodies to CNS antigens have been found in the cerebrospinal fluid of MS patients. Therefore, it may seem reasonable to investigate whether the inheritance of specific alleles of the immunoglobulin genes could influence susceptibility to MS. Several reports have described associations between MS and Gm allotypes (103–105). These studies have been performed using traditional Gm allosera. However, a closer look at these associations has shown that they are largely contradictory. Thus, it is not surprising that renewed analysis of Gm allotypes with DNA-based techniques has failed to confirm any of the original associations (106).

In 1991, Walter and coworkers (107) reported an association between MS and the VH2-5 gene segment of the variable region of the immunoglobulin heavy-chain gene on chromosome 14q. Later, however, the same group failed to find evidence for increased allele sharing in an affected sibling-pair study (108). Interestingly, a British sib-pair study reported increased sharing of marker alleles in the same region (109), a finding paralleled by evidence for linkage with microsatellite markers in the region in a genome screen including the same dataset (8). However, other genome screens have not confirmed the British findings, and an independent study in the Swedish population also failed to find evidence for linkage or association with an intragenic marker in this region (110). Thus, it is still an open question whether these genes add to the genetically determined risk for MS.

C. Myelin Basic Protein Gene

As the traditional autoantigen in experimental allergic encephalomyelitis (EAE) and one of the suspected autoantigens in MS, myelin basic protein (MBP) is a natural target for genetic studies in MS. After the first report of an association in 1990 (111), both association and linkage were described in a study from Finland in 1992 (112). However, several subsequent studies in other ethnic groups have failed to confirm these findings (113–116); nor did any of the large MS genome screens identify the MBP locus on chromosome 18 as important (6–8). Presently, there is widespread doubt about the involvement of the MBP gene in MS.

D. Mitochondrial DNA

Leber's hereditary optic neuropathy (LHON) is characterized by a subacute visual deterioration usually affecting young males and known to be caused by mutations of mitochondrial DNA (mtDNA). In 1992 Harding and coworkers (117) described families in which females carrying the same mutation as their affected male relatives suffered from a clinical syndrome indistinguishable from MS. This discovery prompted a search for mtDNA mutations in MS families and sporadic MS cases, a search that so far has turned up occasional aberrations absent in healthy controls (118,119). Thus, although relevant in only a small minority of MS patients, the phenomenon of LHON-associated mtDNA mutations seems to be the second genetic factor convincingly tied to MS. This finding is also of interest from theoretical and nosological points of view, since it suggests a definition of MS as a syndrome with several possible triggers, both genetic and environmental.

E. CTLA-4

The CTLA-4 molecule is a member of the immunoglobulin superfamily and is expressed on the surface of activated T cells; it shares extensive amino-acid sequence homology with CD28 and, like CD28, interacts with B7-1 and B7-2 on the surface of antigen-presenting cells. However, unlike the CD28-B7 interaction, which activates the T cell and results in the proliferation of an antigen-specific T-cell clone, the binding of B7 by CTLA-4 serves to downregulate T-cell clonal expansion and thus appears to be essential for both the termination of an ongoing immune response and the peripheral acquisition of tolerance to self antigens (120,121). Indeed, CTLA-4-deficient mice rapidly succumb to a multiorgan inflammatory disorder caused by the unchecked proliferation of lymphocyte clones (122), and administration of CTLA-4-blocking antibodies has been shown to exacerbate the severity of murine EAE (123).

The gene encoding CTLA-4 is located in proximity to the CD28 gene on chromosome 2q33, a region that scored positively for linkage in both the Canadian and Finnish MS genome screens (7,9) (see below), as well as in candidate-locus screens in IDDM (124,125), Graves' disease (126), and celiac disease (127). The CTLA-4 gene is known to contain three polymorphisms—biallelic single-base substitutions in the promoter and in exon 1, and a dinucleotide repeat in the 3′-untranslated region of exon 4.

The G allele of the A-G dimorphism in exon 1 has been shown to be associated with an impressively varied array of autoimmune diseases, including IDDM (125,128–131), thyroid diseases (126,128,129,132), rheumatoid arthritis (133), SLE (134), Addison's disease (135), and autoimmune hepatitis (136). At the same time, attempts to replicate these positive linkage and association findings in new datasets or different populations have sometimes failed (137–141); but, given the multifactorial nature of these disorders—the presumed presence of locus and allelic heterogeneity and the expectedly subtle effects of each disease-predisposing gene—such inconsistency is nonetheless reconcilable with a true susceptibility-conferring role for CTLA-4.

The initial positive findings for the CTLA-4 gene in MS have recently been corroborated in two independent Scandinavian studies. Flinstad Harbo et al. (142) found that the frequency of the exon 1 A/G genotype was increased in a group of Norwegian MS patients compared to controls; and our group (143) demonstrated association of homozygosity for the exon 1 G allele with sporadic MS in an analysis of Swedish cases and controls as well as excessive transmission of the same allele from parents to affected offspring in 31 Swedish MS families.

As will be discussed in the next section, it has been observed from linkage studies that human autoimmune disorders and their animal models share many candidate loci and thus seem to have a number of risk-bestowing genes in common. Vyse and Todd (144) have speculated that these shared genes may turn out to encode molecules regulating general immune functions—such as immune-cell differentiation or apoptosis—and that the generally disease-specific MHC associations in these disorders and models may simply determine the target organ for a dysregulated immune response. If that indeed is the case then the CTLA-4 gene is a compelling candidate—positionally as well as functionally— for the role of universal autoimmune susceptibility gene.

F.   Possible Influence on the Prognosis of MS: IL-1ra and APOE

In a series of studies published between 1993 and 1995, investigators in Sheffield (U.K.) demonstrated that an allele of the gene encoding the interleukin-1 receptor antagonist (IL-1ra) was associated with both susceptibility to and the increased severity of a number of chronic epithelial inflammatory disorders, including psoriasis (145), ulcerative colitis (146), systemic lupus erythematosus (SLE) (147), alopecia areata (148), and lichen sclerosus (149).

IL-1ra inhibits the effects of the key proinflammatory cytokine IL-1 by blocking its receptor. The IL-1ra gene (IL1RN) is located on 2q13-21, in a complex of genes that also includes those coding for the IL-1 α and β isoforms. IL1RN contains a variable number of tandem repeats (VNTR) of an 86-base-pair DNA sequence. The IL-1α and IL-1β genes are polymorphic as well, and the IL-1 complex haplotype has been shown to regulate plasma levels of IL-1ra (150).

In 1995 Crusius et al. (151) reported that the epithelial inflammation-associated IL-1ra allele—designated IL1RN*2—was more common in Dutch MS patients than in controls. Three subsequent attempts to confirm this finding—in the Swedish (152), Finnish (153), and French (154) populations—produced negative results, while a fourth, Spanish study (155) reported that IL1RN*2 in combination with HLA-DR15 increased the risk for the relapsing/remitting form of MS fourfold. Recent studies from Italy (156) and Holland (157) examining the influence of IL-1ra alleles on disease progression and prognosis in MS have produced conflicting results; the Italian group reported an association between the more common IL1RN*1 allele and MS severity, whereas in the Dutch study, IL1RN*2 was found to predispose to rapid disease progression, but only in the absence of a specific IL-1β allele.

Despite the confusing results in the case of MS, gene variants of the IL-1 cluster appear to serve as markers of disease severity across a broad range of inflammatory disorders; indeed, alleles from the cluster have recently been found to be associated with conditions as seemingly diverse as diabetes nephropathy (158,159), advanced periodontitis (160,161), vulvar vestibulitis (162), and single-vessel coronary heart disease (163).

Another gene that has been studied with respect to its effect on MS prognosis is the gene that encodes apolipoprotein E (ApoE) on chromosome 19q13, a region that scored positively in the British and American MS genome screens (6,8). In 1991 the same region was found to be linked to late-onset familial Alzheimer's disease (AD), and subsequent studies demonstrated an association of the ApoE ϵ4 allele with both early- and late-onset familial AD as well as with sporadic AD (reviewed in Ref. 164). The ApoE protein binds to cell-surface receptors and thereby allows the uptake of plasma lipoproteins, which are vital for membrane repair; it may also have neurotrophic, antioxidant and immunomodulatory effects (reviewed in Ref. 165).

Clinical and experimental evidence suggests that ApoE influences recovery from CNS injury in an allele-specific manner. Neuropathological studies have indicated that individuals carrying the ϵ4 allele are more likely to die after severe head trauma; other studies have demonstrated that ApoE genotype is correlated with the degree of recovery after both intracerebral hemorrhage and thromboembolic stroke, though the gene does not seem to alter the risk for either disease (reviewed in Ref. 166). In addition, when subjected to transient focal ischemia and reperfusion, mice transgenic for the human ε4 allele were found to have larger infarct volumes than mice transgenic for the more common ε3 allele (167).

Although none of the case-control studies performed thus far in MS has suggested that the ApoE gene is associated with a risk for developing the disease (168–173), there is less consensus concerning its impact on disease severity. Ferri et al. (171) found that neither the ε2-4 polymorphism nor an A-T biallelic polymorphism in position −491 of the gene promoter was associated with disability in MS, as assessed by the Expanded Disability Status Scale (EDSS). In a study by Evangelou and coworkers (172), however, the ε4 allele was found to predispose to more rapid disease progression (defined as duration in days divided by EDSS score); Oliveri et al. (174) reported that homozygosity for the A allele of the promoter dimorphism was associated with cognitive impairment in MS patients. In our own preliminary, unpublished data, comparing ApoE ε2-4 genotype and phenotype frequencies in a large dataset's ($n = 816$) most disparate duration-adjusted EDSS octiles, ε4 occurred at a higher rate in severe MS than in benign MS [$p = 0.18$; odds ratio (OR) = 1.5], and was significantly more common in patients than controls ($p = 0.025$; OR = 1.5).

VI.   GENOME SCREENS IN MS

A.   Three Large Screens

As described briefly above, the availability of large numbers of microsatellite markers spanning the genome has opened up the possibility to perform unbiased genetic screens of all parts of the genome in large numbers of families. In 1996, three such genomic screens in MS were published simultaneously: a British study of 128 affected sibling pairs as well as Canadian and American screens of 52 and 61 sib pairs, respectively (for loci giving indications of importance, additional families were included such that the final totals were 251, 222, and 126 sib pairs, respectively) (6–8).

The most striking finding was the absence of any strong individual locus with formally significant evidence for linkage. Each study indicated the possible importance of a number of loci, but at first there seemed to be little overlap between the three studies. However, after more families were added, each of the studies provided evidence for the importance of the HLA complex region. In addition, each study showed some positivity for markers on the short arm or close to the centromere of chromosome 5. This locus was also found to be positive in a Finnish analysis of 21 multiplex MS families published at the same time (175). Interestingly, the Finnish group had selected the 5p region as a candidate locus due to its homology with a mouse chromosomal region of importance for EAE (176). In summary, however, the general conclusion from these studies was that the genetic risk in MS is likely to be due to a large number of weakly acting genetic factors.

In 1997, a Finnish genomewide screen was published (9). Apart from HLA and 5p, which had already been reported on separately, a locus on 17q22-24 appeared promising, reaching a LOD score of 2.8. This region also scored positively in the British screen but lacked support in the Canadian and American screens.

Performing a metanalysis on these four genomic screens and limiting it to the families that were investigated for all markers, Wise (177) concluded that there was significant evidence for linkage not only for 6p (HLA) ($p = 0.0004$), but also for 19q13 ($p = 0.002$), 5p ($p = 0.025$), 17q ($p = 0.029$), and 2p ($p = 0.05$).

In a seminal paper, Becker and coworkers (10) reported similarity in location for candidate loci identified in genomic screen studies not only in MS but also in the putatively autoimmune disorders Crohn's disease, psoriasis, asthma, and IDDM. This clustering of susceptibility loci was quite similar to that observed in experimental animal models of autoimmune disease (EAE and the models for IDDM, SLE, and rheumatoid arthritis). Even more interestingly, the authors observed that the clustered animal model loci frequently were homologous to the clustered human autoimmune loci, again strengthening the impression that several weakly linked loci observed in the early MS screens were not merely replicated artifacts but rather true positives with relevance for the disease.

Since 1996, additional studies have directly addressed the significance of these shared loci. The overall impression is one of surprising consistency for a number of them. Table 3 shows a summary of the most promising of the loci. Some of them may be considered to be of special interest and are discussed in more detail below.

5p

Although this locus was originally thought to be very promising, with unusual congruity between the early screens, it was soon realized that the peaks in the various studies did not overlap. In particular, the peaks of the British and American studies were located well within the chromosome's centromeric regions or even proximally on the long arm, whereas the Canadian and Finnish peaks were located close together, more telomerically, in the 5p region. A subsequent study from the Nordic countries (62) reported a minor peak, with a maximum LOD score of 1.1, which overlapped with these telomeric peaks. An Italian study (139), on the other hand, revealed two peaks: one on 5p, specific to continental Italians; and another, which overlapped with the British peak on the first stretch of 5q, in the Sardinian ethnic group. Thus, it is possible that 5p represents not one but two separate loci.

17q

This locus was identified in the British screen and supported by findings in the Finnish families (8,9). Both studies had peaks at the same markers, and a subsequent Nordic study had a small peak very close to the first two (181). There are several attractive candidate genes for MS on 17q, and studies targeting a couple of these genes have already been performed. For example, in a large set of British MS patients, Chataway et al. (182) reported an association with alleles of the myeloperoxidase gene (MPO) on 17q23 but negative data for other markers and genes close by. However, Nelissen et al. (183) reported lack of association with MPO but found, instead, an association with PECAM-1 close by. Thus, although this is an interesting locus, data are at this point not quite consistent.

7p

Although at first glance this locus did not appear to be particularly strong, with maximum LOD scores of 1.7 in the British study (8) and less than 1 in the Canadian screen (7), subsequent studies have been rather positive. Thus, an Italian study (139) showed a formally significant nonparametric linkage (NPL) score of 1.66 ($p = 0.05$), whereas a Swedish study of 46 families showed a weaker NPL score of 0.73 but also a positive transmission distortion test (184). In addition, an update of the British screen still identifies this

Table 3 Summary of MS Candidate Loci*

Locus	Candidate gene	UK[a]	USA[b]	Canada[c]	Finland[d]	Italy[e]	Nordic[f]
Confirmed locus							
6p21	HLA	+	+	+	+	+	+
Likely loci (supported by at least 4 reports)							
2p11		+	+	+	−	+	−
5pter-cen		+	+	+	+	+	+
7pter-15		+	−	+	−	+	+
17q21-24	MPO	+	−	−	+	+	+
Suggestive loci (supported by 3 reports)							
3p13-cen		+	−	+	−	−	(+)
2q33	CTLA4	−	−	+	+	+	(+)
Possible loci (supported by 2 reports)							
7q35	TCRβ	−	+	−	−	(+)	+
11q21-23		−	−	+	+	−	+
12p13	CD4	+	−	−	(+)	−	+
12q24	SCA2	(+)	+	−	−	−	+
14q32	IgHeavy	+	−	−	+	−	−
17pter-cen		+	−	−	−	(+)	(+)
19q13.1	APOC/E	+	+	(+)	−	−	−
22q13.1		+	−	+	−	+	−
Xq21		+	−	+	−	−	−

* A summary of MS candidate loci identified in genome screen studies and receiving support in at least two of these, or in subsequent studies. Candidate genes within these loci are genes that have been reported, at least once, to be associated with MS. Thus, the CTLA-4 gene has been reported twice to be associated with MS in Nordic populations (142,143), although there was not evidence for linkage in these populations. This parallels the findings for SCA2, which was found to be associated with MS in a British study (178), but for which no evidence of linkage was found in the same population.

a Ref. 8.
b Ref. 6.
c Ref. 7.
d Refs. 9, 112, 175.
e Ref. 139.
f Refs. 62, 96, 179, 180, 184.

region as promising (185). Candidate genes in this region include those encoding interleukin-6 and the TCR γ chain.

In summary, it has been easier than originally thought to attain additional support for the weakly linked loci identified in the first screens. However, all these loci are poorly characterized with regard to both their physical delineation and the exact nature of their involvement in MS susceptibility.

VII. PROSPECTS

The strategy of attempting to identify genes in polygenic disease by linkage analysis based on affected relative pairs clearly has its limitations. First, the power of the analysis is poor, which is illustrated by the failure to identify genetic factors at a formally significant level in spite of large datasets. Second, the physical resolution is very crude. The typical size of an identified region is 10 to 20 centimorgans (cM), equaling roughly 10 to 20 million base pairs of genetic code. A region of this size is likely to contain several hundred genes, of which, until the completion of the Human Genome Project, only a minority will have been characterized. Identifying the factor responsible for a positive linkage signal can therefore be a tremendous task. Consequently, it is not surprising that a number of alternative approaches have been proposed.

The major alternative to linkage analysis in polygenic diseases is likely to be refined versions of association analysis, in this context often referred to as linkage disequilibrium analysis. This approach is based on the fact that even the general population may be viewed as a large pedigree. Since two seemingly unrelated individuals may have common ancestors a long way back in time—perhaps up to several hundred generations—the number of recombination events on a chromosome surrounding a disease-predisposing gene is likely to have been high. Therefore, the remaining chromosomal segment inherited together with the risk of disease and shared by affected individuals of the present generation will of necessity be small. However, if a genetic marker allele can be shown to be transmitted together with the risk of disease—i.e., to be in linkage disequilibrium with the disease—then the susceptibility allele itself is in all probability very close by.

Therefore, an association study may ultimately define a chromosomal region of such limited size that the responsible gene can be readily identified. Again, this high level of resolution has a price, in the form of the number of markers (i.e., polymorphisms) that needs to be investigated. Thus, a genomewide association study may require thousands of markers. Since microsatellite markers may occur at a rate as low as one every 0.5 cM, the resulting marker map may be insufficient if the average linkage disequilibrium in the genome is shorter than this, even if 7000 markers are used. Therefore, much interest is now being focused on the possible use of single nucleotide polymorphisms (SNPs)—biallelic, one-base substitutions that occur frequently in the genome, probably at a rate as high as one every 1000 base pairs—as genetic markers.

An SNP-based genomewide screen would have to be carried out using high-throughput technology, which would allow the rapid determination of millions of genotypes. So far, no such study has been performed in MS or in any other polygenic disease.

As mentioned above, association studies in which patients are compared with healthy controls run the risk of producing false-positive results due to the presence of ethnic admixture in the studied population. Therefore, the procedure of studying the transmission of marker alleles from parents to their affected offspring has rapidly become the new standard for association studies. In short, an allele that is found to be transmitted to an affected offspring more often then expected by chance is suspected of being in linkage disequilibrium with a disease-promoting sequence nearby. Thus, large groups of trios (two parents and one affected child) are now being recruited for a number of different polygenic diseases.

Whether these efforts will be successful depends essentially on a number of poorly known conditions—most importantly, on the degree of underlying genetic heterogeneity characterizing the disease in question, the actual contribution of each predisposing gene, and the extent of linkage disequilibrium around these genes. In fact, there is a risk that, in the end, these limitations will prevent us from identifying susceptibility genes in a purely genetic fashion (186,187). Thus, functional characterization of the products of genes in candidate loci may prove to be a necessary complement to genetic analysis.

An additional complementary approach may be the identification of autoimmune genes in animal models. The possibility of controlling genetic elements by selective breeding—in particular by producing so-called congenic strains (which differ from the background strain at only a single, specific locus)—may be an efficient way to delineate regions of interest, such that relevant genes may be definitively identified (188).

At any rate, when, as will soon be the case, the entire human genetic sequence is known, we will have the opportunity to test directly the importance of a great number of newly identified genes within the loci that we suspect contain MS genes. It is hoped that these developments will provide us with new information on disease mechanisms, which in turn will allow us to develop new therapeutic procedures for patients with MS.

REFERENCES

1   Mumford CJ, Wood NW, Kellar-Wood H, Thorpe JW, Miller DH, Compston DA. The British Isles survey of multiple sclerosis in twins. Neurology 1994; 44(1):11–15.

2. Sadovnick AD, Baird PA, Ward RH. Multiple sclerosis: Updated risks for relatives. Am J Med Genet 1988; 29(3):533–541.

3. Sadovnick AD, Armstrong H, Rice GP, Bulman D, Hashimoto L, Paty DW, Hashimoto SA, Warren S, Hader W, Murray TJ, Seland TP, Metz L, Bell R, Duquette P, Gray T, Nelson R, Weinshenker B, Brunet D, Ebers GC. A population-based study of multiple sclerosis in twins: Update. Ann Neurol 1993; 33(3):281–285.

4. Ebers GC, Sadovnick AD. The role of genetic factors in multiple sclerosis susceptibility. J Neuroimmunol 1994; 54(1–2):1–17.

5. Hillert J. Human leukocyte antigen studies in multiple sclerosis. Ann Neurol 1994; 36(suppl): 15–17.

6. Haines JL, Ter-Minassian M, Bazyk A, Gusella JF, Kim DJ, Terwedow H, Pericak-Vance MA, Rimmler JB, Haynes CS, Roses AD, Lee A, Shaner B, Menold M, Seboun E, Fitoussi RP, Gartioux C, Reyes C, Ribierre F, Gyapay G, Weissenbach J, Hauser JL, Goodkin DE, Lincoln R, Usuku K, Garcia-Merino A, Gatto N, Young S, Oksenberg JR. A complete genomic screen for multiple sclerosis underscores a role for the major histocompatability complex: The Multiple Sclerosis Genetics Group. Nature Genet 1996; 13(4):469–471.

7. Ebers GC, Kukay K, Bulman DE, Sadovnick AD, Rice G, Anderson C, Armstrong H, Cousin K, Bell RB, Hader W, Paty DW, Hashimoto S, Oger J, Duquette P, Warren S, Gray T, O'Connor P, Nath A, Auty A, Metz L, Francis G, Paulseth JE, Murray TJ, Pryse-Phillips W, Nelson R, Freedman M, Brunet D, Bouchard J-P, Hinds D, Risch N. A full genome search in multiple sclerosis. Nature Genet 1996; 13(4):472–476.

8. Sawcer S, Jones HB, Feakes R, Gray J, Smaldon N, Chataway J, Robertson N, Clayton D, Goodfellow PN, Compston A. A genome screen in multiple sclerosis reveals susceptibility loci on chromosome 6p21 and 17q22. Nature Genet 1996; 13(4):464–468.

9. Kuokkanen S, Gschwend M, Rioux JD, Daly MJ, Terwilliger JD, Tienari PJ, Wikstrom J, Palo J, Stein LD, Hudson TJ, Lander ES, Peltonen L. Genomewide scan of multiple sclerosis in Finnish multiplex families. Am J Hum Genet 1997; 61(6):1379–1387.

10. Becker KG, Simon RM, Bailey-Wilson JE, Freidlin B, Biddison WE, McFarland HF, Trent JM. Clustering of non-major histocompatibility complex susceptibility candidate loci in human autoimmune diseases. Proc Natl Acad Sci USA 1998; 95(17):9979–9984.

11. Sadovnick AD, Baird PA. The familial nature of multiple sclerosis: age-corrected empiric recurrence risks for children and siblings of patients. Neurology 1988; 38(6):990–991.

12. Heltberg A, Holm NV. Concordance in twins and recurrence in sibships in multiple sclerosis (letter). Lancet 1982; 1(8280):1068.

13. Sadovnick AD, Bulman D, Ebers GC. Parent-child concordance in multiple sclerosis. Ann Neurol 1991; 29(3):252–255.

14. Sadovnick AD, Ebers GC, Dyment DA, Risch NJ. Evidence for genetic basis of multiple sclerosis: The Canadian Collaborative Study Group. Lancet 1996; 347(9017):1728–1730.

15. Ebers GC, Sadovnick AD, Risch NJ. A genetic basis for familial aggregation in multiple sclerosis: Canadian Collaborative Study Group. Nature 1995; 377(6545):150–151.

16. Risch N. Linkage strategies for genetically complex traits. I. Multilocus models. Am J Hum Genet 1990; 46(2):222–228.

17. Phillips JT. Regression analysis of multiple sclerosis population data predicts multigenic interaction and minor combined effects of HLA and T-cell receptor genes (abstr). Neurology 1993; 43(suppl 2):205.

18. Skegg DC, Corwin PA, Craven RS, Malloch JA, Pollock M. Occurrence of multiple sclerosis in the north and south of New Zealand. J Neurol Neurosurg Psychiatry 1987; 50(2):134–139.

19. Gronning M, Mellgren SI. Multiple sclerosis in the two northernmost counties of Norway. Acta Neurol Scand 1985; 72(3):321–327.

20. Palffy G, Czopf J, Gyodi E. Multiple sclerosis in Baranya County in Hungarians and in Gypsies. In: W Firnhaber, K Lauer, eds. Multiple Sclerosis in Europe: An Epidemiological Update. Darmstadt: Leutchturm Verlag/LTV Press, 1993, pp. 274–278.

21. Kurtzke JK, Beebe GW, Norman JE Jr. Epidemiology of multiple sclerosis in U.S. veterans: 1. Race, sex, and geographic distribution. Neurology 1979; 29(9 pt 1):1228–1235.

22. Takacs K, Kalman B, Gyodi E, Tauszik T, Palffy G, Kuntar L, Guseo A, Nagy C, Petranyi G. Association between the lack of HLA-DQw6 and the low incidence of multiple sclerosis in Hungarian Gypsies. Immunogenetics 1990; 31(5–6):383–385.

23. Dupont B, Lisak RP, Jersild C, Hansen JA, Silberberg DH, Whitsett C, Zweiman B, Ciongoli K. HLA antigens in black American patients with multiple sclerosis. Transplant Proc 1977; 9(1 suppl 1):181–185.

24. Vogel F, Motulsky AG. Human Genetics: Problems and Approaches. Berlin: Springer-Verlag, 1979, pp. 173–186.

25. Phillips DI. Twin studies in medical research: can they tell us whether diseases are genetically determined? Lancet 1993; 341(8851):1008–1009.

26. Poser CM. The dissemination of multiple sclerosis: a Viking saga? A historical essay. Ann Neurol 1994; 36(suppl 2):231–243.

27. Reed PW, Davies JL, Copeman JB, Bennett ST, Palmer SM, Pritchard LE, Gough SC, Kawaguchi Y, Cordell HJ, Balfour KM, Jenkins SC, Powell EE, Vignal A, Todd JA. Chromosome-specific microsatellite sets for fluorescence-based, semi-automated genome mapping. Nature Genet 1994; 7(3):390–395.

28. Monaco JJ. A molecular model of MHC class-I-restricted antigen processing. Immunol Today 1992; 13(5):173–179.

29. Neefjes JJ, Ploegh HL. Intracellular transport of MHC class II molecules. Immunol Today 1992; 13(5):179–184.

30. Benacerraf B. Biological function of HLA molecules. In: BG Solheim, S Ferrone, E Möller,

eds. The HLA System in Clinical Transplantation. Berlin: Springer-Verlag, 1993, pp. 109–118.

31. Buus S, Sette A, Colon SM, Miles C, Grey HM. The relation between major histocompatibility complex (MHC) restriction and the capacity of Ia to bind immunogenic peptides. Science 1987; 235(4794):1353–1358.

32. Blackman M, Kappler J, Marrack P. The role of the T cell receptor in positive and negative selection of developing T cells. Science 1990; 248(4961):1335–1341.

33. Jersild C, Fog T, Hansen GS, Thomsen M, Svejgaard A, Dupont B. Histocompatibility determinants in multiple sclerosis, with special reference to clinical course. Lancet 1973; 2(7840): 1221–1225.

34. Stastny P. Mixed lymphocyte cultures in rheumatoid arthritis. J Clin Invest 1976; 57(5): 1148–1157.

35. Svejgaard A, Platz P, Ryder LP. Joint report: Insulin-dependent diabetes mellitus. In: PI Terasaki, ed. Histocompatibility Testing. Los Angeles: UCLA Tissue Typing Laboratory, 1980, p. 238.

36. Tiwari JL, Terasaki PI. Multiple sclerosis. In: HLA and Disease Associations. New York: Springer-Verlag, 1985, pp. 85–100.

37. Morita K, Moriuchi J, Inoko H, Tsuji K, Arimori S. HLA class II antigens and DNA restriction fragment length polymorphism in myasthenia gravis in Japan. Ann Neurol 1991; 29(2): 168–174.

38. Juji T, Satake M, Honda Y, Doi Y. HLA antigens in Japanese patients with narcolepsy: All the patients were DR2 positive. Tissue Antigens 1984; 24(5):316–319.

39. Larhammar D, Schenning L, Gustafsson K, Wiman K, Claesson L, Rask L, Peterson PA. Complete amino acid sequence of an HLA-DR antigen-like beta chain as predicted from the nucleotide sequence: Similarities with immunoglobulins and HLA-A, -B, and -C antigens. Proc Natl Acad Sci USA 1982; 79(12):3687–3691.

40. Jersild C, Svejgaard A, Fog T. HL-A antigens and multiple sclerosis. Lancet 1972; 1(7762): 1240–1241.

41. Fogdell A, Hillert J, Sachs C, Olerup O. The multiple sclerosis- and narcolepsy-associated HLA class II haplotype includes the DRB5*0101 allele. Tissue Antigens 1995; 46(4):333–336.

42. Gogolin KJ, Kolaga VJ, Baker L, Lisak RP, Zmijewski CM, Spielman RS. Subtypes of HLA-DQ and -DR defined by DQB1 and DRB1 RELPs: Allele frequencies in the general population and in insulin-dependent diabetes (IDDM) and multiple sclerosis patients. Ann Hum Genet 1989; 53(pt 4):327–338.

43. Hillert J, Kall T, Olerup O, Soderstrom M. Distribution of HLA-Dw2 in optic neuritis and multiple sclerosis indicates heterogeneity. Acta Neurol Scand 1996; 94(3):161–166.

44. Waubant E, Abbal M, Cambon-Thomsen A, Clanet M, Ohayon E, Roth MP. HLA class II genes and susceptibility to multiple sclerosis: a case-control study in the southwest of France (abstr). Sixth European Histocompatibility Conference, Strasbourg, 1992.

45. Brautbar C, Amar A, Cohen N, Oksenberg J, Cohen I, Kahana E, Bloch D, Alter M, Grosse-Wilde H. HLA-D typing in multiple sclerosis: Israelis tested with European homozygous typing cells. Tissue Antigens 1982; 19(3):189–197.

46. Hao Q, Saida T, Kawakami H, Mine H, Maruya E, Inoko H, Saji H. HLAs and genes in Japanese patients with multiple sclerosis: Evidence for increased frequencies of HLA-Cw3, HLA-DR2, and HLA-DQB1*0602. Hum Immunol 1992; 35(2):116–124.

47. Marrosu MG, Muntoni F, Murru MR, Costa G, Pischedda MP, Pirastu M, Sotgiu S, Rosati G, Cianchetti C. HLA-DQB1 genotype in Sardinian multiple sclerosis: Evidence for a key role of DQB1 *0201 and *0302 alleles. Neurology 1992; 42(4):883–886.

48. Marrosu MG, Muntoni F, Murru MR, Spinicci G, Pischedda MP, Goddi F, Cossu P, Pirastu M. Sardinian multiple sclerosis is associated with HLA-DR4: A serologic and molecular analysis. Neurology 1988; 38(11):1749–1753.

49. Ebers GC, Bulman D. The geography of MS reflects genetic susceptibility. Neurology 1986; 36(suppl 147):132–147.

50. Todd JA, Bell JI, McDevitt HO. HLA-DQ beta gene contributes to susceptibility and resistance to insulin-dependent diabetes mellitus. Nature 1987; 329(6140):599–604.

51. Sollid LM, Markussen G, Ek J, Gjerde H, Vartdal F, Thorsby E. Evidence for a primary association of celiac disease to a particular HLA-DQ alpha/beta heterodimer. J Exp Med 1989; 169(1):345–350.

52. Marcadet A, Massart C, Semana G, Fauchet R, Sabouraud O, Merienne M, Dausset J, Cohen D. Association of class II HLA-DQ beta chain DNA restriction fragments with multiple sclerosis. Immunogenetics 1985; 22(1):93–96.

53. Francis DA, Batchelor JR, McDonald WI, Hing SN, Dodi IA, Fielder AH, Hern JE, Downie AW. Multiple sclerosis in north-east Scotland: An association with HLA-DQw1. Brain 1987; 110(pt 1):181–196.

54. Vartdal F, Sollid LM, Vandvik B, Markussen G, Thorsby E. Patients with multiple sclerosis carry DQB1 genes which encode shared polymorphic amino acid sequences. Hum Immunol 1989; 25(2):103–110.

55. Spurkland A, Ronningen KS, Vandvik B, Thorsby E, Vartdal F. HLA-DQA1 and HLA-DQB1 genes may jointly determine susceptibility to develop multiple sclerosis. Hum Immunol 1991; 30(1):69–75.

56. Sinha AA, Bell RB, Steinman L, McDevitt HO. Oligonucleotide dot-blot analysis of HLA-DQ beta alleles associated with multiple sclerosis. J Neuroimmunol 1991; 32(1):61–65.

57. Francis DA, Thompson AJ, Brookes P, Davey N, Lechler RI, McDonald WI, Batchelor JR. Multiple sclerosis and HLA: Is the susceptibility gene really HLA-DR or -DQ? Hum Immunol 1991; 32(2):119–124.

58. Hillert J, Olerup O. Multiple sclerosis is associated with genes within or close to the HLA-DR-DQ subregion on a normal DR15,DQ6,Dw2 haplotype. Neurology 1993; 43(1):163–168.

59. Olerup O, Hillert J. HLA class II-associated genetic susceptibility in multiple sclerosis: A critical evaluation. Tissue Antigens 1991; 38(1):1–15.

60. Caballero A, Alves-Leon S, Papais-Alvarenga R, Fernandez O, Navarro G, Alonso A. DQB1*0602 confers genetic susceptibility to multiple sclerosis in Afro-Brazilians. Tissue Antigens 1999; 54(5):524–526.

61. Serjeantson SW, Gao X, Hawkins BR, Higgins DA, Yu YL. Novel HLA-DR2y-related haplotypes in Hong Kong Chinese implicate the DQB1*0602 allele in susceptibility to multiple sclerosis. Eur J Immunogenet 1992; 19(1–2):11–19.

62. Oturai A, Larsen F, Ryder LP, Madsen HO, Hillert J, Fredrikson S, Sandberg-Wollheim M, Laaksonen M, Koch-Henriksen N, Sawcer S, Fugger L, Sorensen PS, Svejgaard A. Linkage and association analysis of susceptibility regions on chromosomes 5 and 6 in 106 Scandinavian sibling pair families with multiple sclerosis. Ann Neurol 1999; 46(4):612–616.

63. Bodmer JG, Marsh SG, Albert ED, Bodmer WF, Dupont B, Erlich HA, Mach B, Mayr WR, Parham P, Sasazuki T, Schreuder GMT, Strominger JL, Svejgaard A, Terasaki PI. Nomenclature for factors of the HLA system, 1990. Tissue Antigens 1991; 37(3):97–104.

64. Payami H, Joe S, Farid NR, Stenszky V, Chan SH, Yeo PP, Cheah JS, Thomson G. Relative predispositional effects (RPEs) of marker alleles with disease: HLA-DR alleles and Graves' disease. Am J Hum Genet 1989; 45(4):541–546.

65. Masterman T, Ligers A, Olsson T, Andersson M, Olerup O, Hillert J. HLA-DR15 is associated with lower age of onset in multiple sclerosis (submitted).

66. Kurdi A, Ayesh I, Abdallat A, Maayta U. Different B lymphocyte alloantigens associated with multiple sclerosis in Arabs and North Europeans. Lancet 1977; 1(8022):1123–1125.

67. Ciusani E, Allen M, Sandberg-Wollheim M, Eoli M, Salmaggi A, Milanese C, Nespolo A, Gyllensten U. Analysis of HLA-class II DQA1, DQB1, DRB1 and DPB1 in Italian multiple sclerosis patients. Eur J Immunogenet 1995; 22(2):171–178.

68. Saruhan-Direskeneli G, Esin S, Baykan-Kurt B, Ornek I, Vaughan R, Eraksoy M. HLA-DR and -DQ associations with multiple sclerosis in Turkey. Hum Immunol 1997; 55(1):59–65.

69. Coraddu F, Reyes-Yanez MP, Parra A, Gray J, Smith SI, Taylor CJ, Compston DA. HLA associations with multiple sclerosis in the Canary Islands. J Neuroimmunol 1998; 87(1–2): 130–135.

70. Engell T, Raun NE, Thomsen M, Platz P. HLA and heterogeneity of multiple sclerosis. Neurology 1982; 32(9):1043–1046.

71. Duquette P, Decary F, Pleines J, Boivin D, Lamoureux G, Cosgrove JB, Lapierre Y. Clinical sub-groups of multiple sclerosis in relation to HLA: DR alleles as possible markers of disease progression. Can J Neurol Sci 1985; 12(2):106–110.

72. Madigand M, Oger JJ, Fauchet R, Sabouraud O, Genetet B. HLA profiles in multiple sclerosis suggest two forms of disease and the existence of protective haplotypes. J Neurol Sci 1982; 53(3):519–529.

73. Runmarker B, Martinsson T, Wahlstrom J, Andersen O. HLA and prognosis in multiple sclerosis. J Neurol 1994; 241(6):385–390.

74. Olerup O, Hillert J, Fredrikson S, Olsson T, Kam-Hansen S, Moller E, Carlsson B, Wallin J. Primarily chronic progressive and relapsing/remitting multiple sclerosis: Two immunogenetically distinct disease entities. Proc Natl Acad Sci USA 1989; 86(18):7113–7117.

75. Hillert J, Gronning M, Nyland H, Link H, Olerup O. An immunogenetic heterogeneity in multiple sclerosis. J Neurol Neurosurg Psychiatry 1992; 55(10):887–890.

76. Kira J, Kanai T, Nishimura Y, Yamasaki K, Matsushita S, Kawano Y, Hasuo K, Tobimatsu S, Kobayashi T. Western versus Asian types of multiple sclerosis: Immunogenetically and clinically distinct disorders. Ann Neurol 1996; 40(4):569–574.

77. Ma JJ, Nishimura M, Mine H, Saji H, Ohta M, Saida K, Uchiyama T. HLA-DRB1 and tumor necrosis factor gene polymorphisms in Japanese patients with multiple sclerosis. J Neuroimmunol 1998; 92(1–2):109–112.

78. Ono T, Zambenedetti MR, Yamasaki K, Kawano Y, Kamikawaji N, Ito H, Sakurai M, Nishimura Y, Kira J, Kanazawa I, Sasazuki T. Molecular analysis of HLA class I (HLA-A and -B) and HLA class II (HLA-DRB1) genes in Japanese patients with multiple sclerosis (Western type and Asian type). Tissue Antigens 1998; 52(6):539–542.

79. Ito H, Yamasaki K, Kawano Y, Horiuchi I, Yun C, Nishimura Y, Kira J. HLA-DP-associated susceptibility to the optico-spinal form of multiple sclerosis in the Japanese. Tissue Antigens 1998; 52(2):179–182.

80. Odum N, Hyldig-Nielsen JJ, Morling N, Sandberg-Wollheim M, Platz P, Svejgaard A. HLA-DP antigens are involved in the susceptibility to multiple sclerosis. Tissue Antigens 1988; 31(5):235–237.

81. Moen T, Stien R, Bratlie A, Bondevik E. Distribution of HLA-SB antigens in multiple sclerosis. Tissue Antigens 1984; 24(2):126–127.

82. Roth MP, Coppin H, Descoins P, Ruidavets JB, Cambon-Thomsen A, Clanet M. HLA-DPB1 gene polymorphism and multiple sclerosis: A large case-control study in the southwest of France. J Neuroimmunol 1991; 34(2–3):215–222.

83. Begovich AB, Helmuth RC, Oksenberg JR, Sakai K, Tabira T, Sasazuki T, Steinman L, Erlich HA. HLA-DP beta and susceptibility to multiple sclerosis: An analysis of Caucasoid and Japanese patient populations. Hum Immunol 1990; 28(4):365–372.

84. Morling N, Sandberg-Wollheim M, Fugger L, Georgsen J, Hylding-Nielsen JJ, Madsen HO, Rieneck K, Ryder L, Svejgaard A. Immunogenetics of multiple sclerosis and optic neuritis: DNA polymorphism of HLA class II genes. Immunogenetics 1992; 35(6):391–394.

85. Cullen CG, Middleton D, Savage DA, Hawkins S. HLA-DR and DQ DNA genotyping in multiple sclerosis patients in Northern Ireland. Hum Immunol 1991; 30(1):1–6.

86. Fogdell-Hahn A, Ligers A, Gronning M, Hillert J, Olerup O. Multiple sclerosis: A modifying influence of HLA class I genes in an HLA class II associated autoimmune disease. Tissue Antigens 2000; 55(2):140–148.

87. He B, Navikas V, Lundahl J, Soderstrom M, Hillert J. Tumor necrosis factor alpha-308 alleles in multiple sclerosis and optic neuritis. J Neuroimmunol 1995; 63(2):143–147.

88. Weinshenker BG, Wingerchuk DM, Liu Q, Bissonet AS, Schaid DJ, Sommer SS. Genetic variation in the tumor necrosis factor alpha gene and the outcome of multiple sclerosis. Neurology 1997; 49(2):378–385.

89. Kellar-Wood HF, Powis SH, Gray J, Compston DA. MHC-encoded TAP1 and TAP2 dimorphisms in multiple sclerosis. Tissue Antigens 1994; 43(2):129–132.

90. Bennetts BH, Teutsch SM, Buhler MM, Heard RN, Stewart GJ. HLA-DMB gene and HLA-DRA promoter region polymorphisms in Australian multiple sclerosis patients. Hum Immunol 1999; 60(9):886–893.

91. Bennetts BH, Teutsch SM, Heard RN, Dunckley H, Stewart GJ. TAP2 polymorphisms in Australian multiple sclerosis patients. J Neuroimmunol 1995; 59(1–2):113–121.

92. Bell RB, Ramachandran S. The relationship of TAP1 and TAP2 dimorphisms to multiple sclerosis susceptibility. J Neuroimmunol 1995; 59(1–2):201–204.

93. Liblau R, van Endert PM, Sandberg-Wollheim M, Patel SD, Lopez MT, Land S, Fugger L, McDevitt HO. Antigen processing gene polymorphisms in HLA-DR2 multiple sclerosis. Neurology 1993; 43(6):1192–1197.

94. Moins-Teisserenc H, Semana G, Alizadeh M, Loiseau P, Bobrynina V, Deschamps I, Edan G, Birebent B, Genetet B, Sabouraud O, Charron D. TAP2 gene polymorphism contributes to genetic susceptibility to multiple sclerosis. Hum Immunol 1995; 42(3):195–202.

95. Ristori G, Carcassi C, Lai S, Fiori P, Cacciani A, Floris L, Montesperelli C, Di Giovanni S, Buttinelli C, Contu L, Pozzilli C, Salvetti M. HLA-DM polymorphisms do not associate with multiple sclerosis: An association study with analysis of myelin basic protein T cell specificity. J Neuroimmunol 1997; 77(2):181–184.

96. Fogdell A, Olerup O, Fredrikson S, Vrethem M, Hillert J. Linkage analysis of HLA class II genes in Swedish multiplex families with multiple sclerosis. Neurology 1997; 48(3):758–762.

97. Tienari PJ, Wikstrom J, Koskimies S, Partanen J, Palo J, Peltonen L. Reappraisal of HLA in multiple sclerosis: close linkage in multiplex families. Eur J Hum Genet 1993; 1(4):257–268.

98. Oksenberg JR, Steinman L. The role of the MHC and T-cell receptor in susceptibility to multiple sclerosis. Curr Opin Immunol 1989; 2(4):619–621.

99. Beall SS, Concannon P, Charmley P, McFarland HF, Gatti RA, Hood LE, McFarlin DE, Biddison WE. The germline repertoire of T cell receptor beta-chain genes in patients with chronic progressive multiple sclerosis. J Neuroimmunol 1989; 21(1):59–66.

100. Martell M, Marcadet A, Strominger J, Dausset J, Cohen D. [Alpha genes of the T cell receptor: A possible implication in genetic susceptibility to multiple sclerosis]. C R Acad Sci III 1987; 304(5):105–110.

101. Seboun E, Robinson MA, Doolittle TH, Ciulla TA, Kindt TJ, Hauser SL. A susceptibility locus for multiple sclerosis is linked to the T cell receptor beta chain complex. Cell 1989; 57(7):1095–1100.

102. Hillert J, Olerup O. Germ-line polymorphism of TCR genes and disease susceptibility— Fact or hypothesis? Immunol Today 1992; 13(2):47–49.

103. Blanc M, Clanet M, Berr C, Dugoujon JM, Ruydavet B, Ducos SJ, Rascol A, Alperovitch A. Immunoglobulin allotypes and susceptibility to multiple sclerosis: An epidemiological and genetic study in the Hautes-Pyrenees county of France. J Neurol Sci 1986; 75(1):1–5.

104. Propert DN, Bernard CC, Simons MJ. Gm allotypes and multiple sclerosis. J Immunogenet 1982; 9(5):359–361.

105. Pandey JP, Goust JM, Salier JP, Fudenberg HH. Immunoglobulin G heavy chain (Gm) allotypes in multiple sclerosis. J Clin Invest 1981; 67(6):1797–1800.

106. Hillert J. Immunoglobulin gamma constant gene region polymorphisms in multiple sclerosis. J Neuroimmunol 1993; 43(1–2):9–14.

107. Walter MA, Gibson WT, Ebers GC, Cox DW. Susceptibility to multiple sclerosis is associated with the proximal immunoglobulin heavy chain variable region. J Clin Invest 1991; 87(4):1266–1273.

108. Hashimoto LL, Walter MA, Cox DW, Ebers GC. Immunoglobulin heavy chain variable region polymorphisms and multiple sclerosis susceptibility. J Neuroimmunol 1993; 44(1):77–83.

109. Wood NW, Sawcer SJ, Kellar-Wood HF, Holmans P, Clayton D, Robertson N, Compston DA. Susceptibility to multiple sclerosis and the immunoglobulin heavy chain variable region. J Neurol 1995; 242(10):677–682.

110. Ligers A, He B, Fogdell-Hahn A, Olerup O, Hillert J. No linkage or association of a VNTR marker in the junction region of the immunoglobulin heavy chain genes in multiple sclerosis. Eur J Immunogenet 1997; 24(4):259–264.

111. Boylan KB, Takahashi N, Paty DW, Sadovnick AD, Diamond M, Hood LE, Prusiner SB. DNA length polymorphism 5′ to the myelin basic protein gene is associated with multiple sclerosis. Ann Neurol 1990; 27(3):291–297.

112. Tienari PJ, Wikstrom J, Sajantila A, Palo J, Peltonen L. Genetic susceptibility to multiple sclerosis linked to myelin basic protein gene. Lancet 1992; 340(8826):987–991.

113. Wood NW, Holmans P, Clayton D, Robertson N, Compston DA. No linkage or association between multiple sclerosis and the myelin basic protein gene in affected sibling pairs. J Neurol Neurosurg Psychiatry 1994; 57(10):1191–1194.

114. Rose J, Gerken S, Lynch S, Pisani P, Varvil T, Otterud B, Leppert M. Genetic susceptibility in familial multiple sclerosis not linked to the myelin basic protein gene. Lancet 1993; 341(8854):1179–1181.

115. Graham CA, Kirk CW, Nevin NC, Droogan AG, Hawkins SA, McMillan SA, McNeill TA. Lack of association between myelin basic protein gene microsatellite and multiple sclerosis (letter, comment). Lancet 1993; 341(8860):1596.

116. He B, Yang B, Lundahl J, Fredrikson S, Hillert J. The myelin basic protein gene in multiple sclerosis: Identification of discrete alleles of a 1.3 kb tetranucleotide repeat sequence. Acta Neurol Scand 1998; 97(1):46–51.

117. Harding AE, Sweeney MG, Miller DH, Mumford CJ, Kellar-Wood H, Menard D, McDonald WI, Compston DA. Occurrence of a multiple sclerosis-like illness in women who have a Leber's hereditary optic neuropathy mitochondrial DNA mutation. Brain 1992; 115(pt 4): 979–989.

118. Olsen NK, Hansen AW, Norby S, Edal AL, Jorgensen JR, Rosenberg T. Leber's hereditary optic neuropathy associated with a disorder indistinguishable from multiple sclerosis in a male harbouring the mitochondrial DNA 11778 mutation. Acta Neurol Scand 1995; 91(5): 326–329.

119. Kellar-Wood H, Robertson N, Govan GG, Compston DA, Harding AE. Leber's hereditary optic neuropathy mitochondrial DNA mutations in multiple sclerosis. Ann Neurol 1994; 36(1):109–112.

120. Bluestone JA. Is CTLA-4 a master switch for peripheral T cell tolerance? J Immunol 1997; 158(5):1989–1993.

121. Karandikar NJ, Vanderlugt CL, Walunas TL, Miller SD, Bluestone JA. CTLA-4: A negative regulator of autoimmune disease. J Exp Med 1996; 184(2):783–788.

122. Tivol EA, Borriello F, Schweitzer AN, Lynch WP, Bluestone JA, Sharpe AH. Loss of CTLA-4 leads to massive lymphoproliferation and fatal multiorgan tissue destruction, revealing a critical negative regulatory role of CTLA-4. Immunity 1995; 3(5):541–547.

123. Perrin PJ, Maldonado JH, Davis TA, June CH, Racke MK. CTLA-4 blockade enhances clinical disease and cytokine production during experimental allergic encephalomyelitis. J Immunol 1996; 157(4):1333–1336.

124. Copeman JB, Cucca F, Hearne CM, Cornall RJ, Reed PW, Ronningen KS, Undlien DE, Nistico L, Buzzetti R, Tosi R, Pociot F, Nerup J, Cornelis F, Barnett AH, Bain SC, Todd

JA. Linkage disequilibrium mapping of a type 1 diabetes susceptibility gene (IDDM7) to chromosome 2q31-q33. Nat Genet 1995; 9(1):80–85.

125. Nistico L, Buzzetti R, Pritchard LE, Van der Auwera B, Giovannini C, Bosi E, Larrad MT, Rios MS, Chow CC, Cockram CS, Jacobs K, Mijovic C, Bain SC, Barnett AH, Vandewalle CL, Schuit F, Gorus FK, Tosi R, Pozzilli P, Todd JA. The CTLA-4 gene region of chromosome 2q33 is linked to, and associated with, type 1 diabetes: Belgian Diabetes Registry. Hum Mol Genet 1996; 5(7):1075–1080.

126. Vaidya B, Imrie H, Perros P, Young ET, Kelly WF, Carr D, Large DM, Toft AD, McCarthy MI, Kendall-Taylor P, Pearce SH. The cytotoxic T lymphocyte antigen-4 is a major Graves' disease locus. Hum Mol Genet 1999; 8(7):1195–1199.

127. Holopainen P, Arvas M, Sistonen P, Mustalahti K, Collin P, Maki M, Partanen J. CD28/ CTLA4 gene region on chromosome 2q33 confers genetic susceptibility to celiac disease: A linkage and family-based association study. Tissue Antigens 1999; 53(5):470–475.

128. Awata T, Kurihara S, Iitaka M, Takei S, Inoue I, Ishii C, Negishi K, Izumida T, Yoshida Y, Hagura R, Kuzuya K, Kanazawa Y, Katayama S. Association of CTLA-4 gene A-G polymorphism (IDDM12 locus) with acute-onset and insulin-depleted IDDM as well as autoimmune thyroid disease (Graves' disease and Hashimoto's thyroiditis) in the Japanese population. Diabetes 1998; 47(1):128–129.

129. Donner H, Rau H, Walfish PG, Braun J, Siegmund T, Finke R, Herwig J, Usadel KH, Badenhoop K. CTLA4 alanine-17 confers genetic susceptibility to Graves' disease and to type 1 diabetes mellitus. J Clin Endocrinol Metab 1997; 82(1):143–146.

130. Marron MP, Raffel LJ, Garchon HJ, Jacob CO, Serrano-Rios M, Martinez Larrad MT, Teng WP, Park Y, Zhang ZX, Goldstein DR, Tao YW, Beaurain G, Bach JF, Huang HS, Luo DF, Zeidler A, Rotter JI, Yang MC, Modilevsky T, Maclaren NK, She JX. Insulin-dependent diabetes mellitus (IDDM) is associated with CTLA4 polymorphisms in multiple ethnic groups. Hum Mol Genet 1997; 6(8):1275–1282.

131. Lee YJ, Huang FY, Lo FS, Wang WC, Hsu CH, Kao HA, Yang TY, Chang JG. Association of CTLA4 gene A-G polymorphism with type 1 diabetes in Chinese children. Clin Endocrinol (Oxf) 2000; 52(2):153–157.

132. Heward JM, Allahabadia A, Armitage M, Hattersley A, Dodson PM, Macleod K, Carr-Smith J, Daykin J, Daly A, Sheppard MC, Holder RL, Barnett AH, Franklyn JA, Gough SC. The development of Graves' disease and the CTLA-4 gene on chromosome 2q33. J Clin Endocrinol Metab 1999; 84(7):2398–2401.

133. Seidl C, Donner H, Fischer B, Usadel KH, Seifried E, Kaltwasser JP, Badenhoop K. CTLA4 codon 17 dimorphism in patients with rheumatoid arthritis. Tissue Antigens 1998; 51(1):62–66.

134. Pullmann R Jr, Lukac J, Skerenova M, Rovensky J, Hybenova J, Melus V, Celec S, Pullmann R, Hyrdel R. Cytotoxic T lymphocyte antigen 4 (CTLA-4) dimorphism in patients with systemic lupus erythematosus. Clin Exp Rheumatol 1999; 17(6):725–729.

135. Vaidya B, Imrie H, Geatch DR, Perros P, Ball SG, Baylis PH, Carr D, Hurel SJ, James RA, Kelly WF, Kemp EH, Young ET, Weetman AP, Kendall-Taylor P, Pearce SH. Association analysis of the cytotoxic T lymphocyte antigen-4 (CTLA-4) and autoimmune regulator-1 (AIRE-1) genes in sporadic autoimmune Addison's disease. J Clin Endocrinol Metab 2000; 85(2):688–691.

136. Agarwal K, Czaja AJ, Jones DE, Donaldson PT. Cytotoxic T lymphocyte antigen-4 (CTLA-4) gene polymorphisms and susceptibility to type 1 autoimmune hepatitis. Hepatology 2000; 31(1):49–53.

137. Hayashi H, Kusaka I, Nagasaka S, Kawakami A, Rokkaku K, Nakamura T, Saito T, Higashiyama M, Honda K, Ishikawa SE. Association of CTLA-4 polymorphism with positive anti-GAD antibody in Japanese subjects with type 1 diabetes mellitus. Clin Endocrinol (Oxf) 1999; 51(6):793–799.

138. Heward J, Gordon C, Allahabadia A, Barnett AH, Franklyn JA, Gough SC. The A-G polymorphism in exon 1 of the CTLA-4 gene is not associated with systemic lupus erythematosus. Ann Rheum Dis 1999; 58(3):193–195.

139. D'Alfonso S, Nistico L, Zavattari P, Marrosu MG, Murru R, Lai M, Massacesi L, Ballerini C, Gestri D, Salvetti M, Ristori G, Bomprezzi R, Trojano M, Liguori M, Gambi D, Quattrone A, Fruci D, Cucca F, Richiardi PM, Tosi R. Linkage analysis of multiple sclerosis with candidate region markers in Sardinian and Continental Italian families. Eur J Hum Genet 1999; 7(3):377–385.

140. Clot F, Fulchignoni-Lataud MC, Renoux C, Percopo S, Bouguerra F, Babron MC, Djilali-Saiah I, Caillat-Zucman S, Clerget-Darpoux F, Greco L, Serre JL. Linkage and association study of the CTLA-4 region in coeliac disease for Italian and Tunisian populations. Tissue Antigens 1999; 54(5):527–530.

141. Barton A, Myerscough A, John S, Gonzalez-Gay M, Ollier W, Worthington J. A single nucleotide polymorphism in exon 1 of cytotoxic T-lymphocyte-associated-4 (CTLA-4) is not associated with rheumatoid arthritis. Rheumatology (Oxford) 2000; 39(1):63–66.

142. Flinstad Harbo H, Celius EG, Vartdal F, Spurkland A. CTLA4 Promoter and exon 1 dimorphisms in multiple sclerosis. Tissue Antigens 1999; 53(1):106–110.

143. Ligers A, Xu C, Saarinen S, Hillert J, Olerup O. The CTLA-4 gene is associated with multiple sclerosis. J Neuroimmunol 1999; 97(1–2):182–190.

144. Vyse TJ, Todd JA. Genetic analysis of autoimmune disease. Cell 1996; 85(3):311–318.

145. Cork MJ, Tarlow JK, Blakemore AI, Mee JB, Crane AM, Stierle C, Bleehen SS, Duff GW. Psoriasis and interleukin-1: A translation. J R Coll Physicians Lond 1993; 27(4):366.

146. Mansfield JC, Holden H, Tarlow JK, Di Giovine FS, McDowell TL, Wilson AG, Holdsworth CD, GW Duff. Novel genetic association between ulcerative colitis and the anti-inflammatory cytokine interleukin-1 receptor antagonist. Gastroenterology 1994; 106(3):637–642.

147. Blakemore AI, Tarlow JK, Cork MJ, Gordon C, Emery P, Duff GW. Interleukin-1 receptor antagonist gene polymorphism as a disease severity factor in systemic lupus erythematosus. Arthritis Rheum 1994; 37(9):1380–1385.

148. Tarlow JK, Clay FE, Cork MJ, Blakemore AI, McDonagh AJ, Messenger AG, Duff GW. Severity of alopecia areata is associated with a polymorphism in the interleukin-1 receptor antagonist gene. J Invest Dermatol 1994; 103(3):387–390.

149. Clay FE, Cork MJ, Tarlow JK, Blakemore AI, Harrington CI, Lewis F, Duff GW. Interleukin 1 receptor antagonist gene polymorphism association with lichen sclerosus. Hum Genet 1994; 94(4):407–410.

150. Hurme M, Santtila S. IL-1 receptor antagonist (IL-1Ra) plasma levels are co-ordinately regulated by both IL-1Ra and IL-1beta genes. Eur J Immunol 1998; 28(8):2598–2602.

151. Crusius JB, Pena AS, Van Oosten BW, Bioque G, Garcia A, CD Dijkstra, CH Polman. Interleukin-1 receptor antagonist gene polymorphism and multiple sclerosis (letter). Lancet 1995; 346(8980):979.

152. Huang WX, He B, Hillert J. An interleukin 1-receptor-antagonist gene polymorphism is not associated with multiple sclerosis. J Neuroimmunol 1996; 67(2):143–144.

153. Wansen K, Pastinen T, Kuokkanen S, Wikstrom J, Palo J, Peltonen L, Tienari PJ. Immune system genes in multiple sclerosis: genetic association and linkage analyses on TCR beta, IGH, IFN-gamma and IL-1ra/IL-1 beta loci. J Neuroimmunol 1997; 79(1):29–36.

154. Semana G, Yaouanq J, Alizadeh M, Clanet M, Edan G. Interleukin-1 receptor antagonist gene in multiple sclerosis (letter, comment). Lancet 1997; 349(9050):476.

155. de la Concha EG, Arroyo R, Crusius JB, Campillo JA, Martin C, Varela de Seijas E, Pena AS, Claveria LE, Fernandez-Arquero M. Combined effect of HLA-DRBI*1501 and interleukin-1 receptor antagonist gene allele 2 in susceptibility to relapsing/remitting multiple sclerosis. J Neuroimmunol 1997; 80(1–2):172–178.

156. Sciacca FL, Ferri C, Vandenbroeck K, Veglia F, Gobbi C, Martinelli F, Franciotta D, Zaffaroni M, Marrosu M, Martino G, Martinelli V, Comi G, Canal N, Grimaldi LM. Relevance

of interleukin 1 receptor antagonist intron 2 polymorphism in Italian MS patients. Neurology 1999; 52(9):1896–1898.

157. Schrijver HM, Crusius JB, Uitdehaag BM, Garcia Gonzalez MA, Kostense PJ, Polman CH, Pena AS. Association of interleukin-1 beta and interleukin-1 receptor antagonist genes with disease severity in MS. Neurology 1999; 52(3):595–599.

158. Loughrey BV, Maxwell AP, Fogarty DG, Middleton D, Harron JC, Patterson CC, Darke C, Savage DA. An interluekin 1B allele, which correlates with a high secretor phenotype, is associated with diabetic nephropathy. Cytokine 1998; 10(12):984–988.

159. Blakemore AI, Cox A, Gonzalez AM, Maskil JK, Hughes ME, Wilson RM, Ward JD, Duff GW. Interleukin-1 receptor antagonist allele (IL 1RN*2) associated with nephropathy in diabetes mellitus. Hum Genet 1996; 97(3):369–374.

160. Galbraith GM, Hendley TM, Sanders JJ, Palesch Y, Pandey JP. Polymorphic cytokine genotypes as markers of disease severity in adult periodontitis. J Clin Periodontol 1999; 26(11): 705–709.

161. Gore EA, Sanders JJ, Pandey JP, Palesch Y, Galbraith GM. Interleukin-1beta+3953 allele 2: association with disease status in adult periodontitis. J Clin Periodontol 1998; 25(10):781–785.

162. Jeremias J, Ledger WJ, Witkin SS. Interleukin 1 receptor antagonist gene polymorphism in women with vulvar vestibulitis. Am J Obstet Gynecol 2000; 182(2):283–285.

163. Francis SE, Camp NJ, Dewberry RM, Gunn J, Syrris P, Carter ND, Jeffery S, Kaski JC, Cumberland DC, Duff GW, Crossman DC. Interleukin-1 receptor antagonist gene polymorphism and coronary artery disease. Circulation 1999; 99(7):861–866.

164. Sandbrink R, Hartmann T, Masters CL, Beyreuther K. Genes contributing to Alzheimer's disease. Mol Psychiatry 1996; 1(1):27–40.

165. Beffert U, Danik M, Krzywkowski P, Ramassamy C, Berrada F, Poirier J. The neurobiology of apolipoproteins and their receptors in the CNS and Alzheimer's disease. Brain Res Brain Res Rev 1998; 27(2):119–142.

166. Laskowitz DT, Horsburgh K, Roses AD. Apolipoprotein E and the CNS response to injury. J Cereb Blood Flow Metab 1998; 18(5):465–471.

167. Sheng H, Laskowitz DT, Bennett E, Schmechel DE, Bart RD, Saunders AM, Pearlstein RD, Roses AD, Warner DS. Apolipoprotein E isoform-specific differences in outcome from focal ischemia in transgenic mice. J Cereb Blood Flow Metab 1998; 18(4):361–366.

168. Barcellos LF, Thomson G, Carrington M, Schafer J, Begovich AB, Lin P, Xu XH, Min BQ, Marti D, Klitz W. Chromosome 19 single-locus and multilocus haplotype associations with multiple sclerosis: Evidence of a new susceptibility locus in Caucasian and Chinese patients. JAMA 1997; 278(15):1256–1261.

169. Gervais A, Gaillard O, Plassart E, Reboul J, Fontaine E, Schuller E. Apolipoprotein E polymorphism in multiple sclerosis. Ann Clin Biochem 1998; 35(pt 1):135–136.

170. Rubinsztein DC, Hanlon CS, Irving RM, Goodburn S, Evans DG, Kellar-Wood H, Xuereb JH, Bandmann O, Harding AE. Apo E genotypes in multiple sclerosis, Parkinson's disease, schwannomas and late-onset Alzheimer's disease. Mol Cell Probes 1994; 8(6):519–525.

171. Ferri C, Sciacca FL, Veglia F, Martinelli F, Comi G, Canal N, Grimaldi LM. APOE epsilon2-4 and -491 polymorphisms are not associated with MS. Neurology 1999; 53(4):888–889.

172. Evangelou N, Jackson M, Beeson D, Palace J. Association of the APOE epsilon4 allele with disease activity in multiple sclerosis. J Neurol Neurosurg Psychiatry 1999; 67(2):203–205.

173. Chapman J, Sylantiev C, Nisipeanu P, Korczyn AD. Preliminary observations on APOE epsilon4 allele and progression of disability in multiple sclerosis. Arch Neurol 1999; 56(12): 1484–1487.

174. Oliveri RL, Cittadella R, Sibilia G, Manna I, Valentino P, Gambardella A, Aguglia U, Zappia M, Romeo N, Andreoli V, Bono F, Caracciolo M, Quattrone A. APOE and risk of cognitive impairment in multiple sclerosis. Acta Neurol Scand 1999; 100(5):290–295.

175. Kuokkanen S, Sundvall M, Terwilliger JD, Tienari PJ, Wikstrom J, Holmdahl R, Petterson

U, Peltonen L. A putative vulnerability locus to multiple sclerosis maps to 5p14-p12 in a region syntenic to the murine locus Eae2. Nature Genet 1996; 13(4):477–480.

176. Sundvall M, Jirholt J, Yang HT, Jansson L, Engstrom A, Pettersson U, Holmdahl R. Identification of murine loci associated with susceptibility to chronic experimental autoimmune encephalomyelitis. Nature Genet 1995; 10(3):313–317.

177. Wise LH, Lanchbury JS, Lewis CM. Meta-analysis of genome searches. Ann Hum Genet 1999; 63:263–272.

178. Chataway J, Sawcer S, Coraddu F, Feakes R, Broadley S, Jones HB, Clayton D, Gray J, Goodfellow PN, Compston A. Evidence that allelic variants of the spinocerebellar ataxia type 2 gene influence susceptibility to multiple sclerosis. Neurogenetics 1999; 2(2):91–96.

179. Xu C, Dai Y, Hillert J. Linkage and association in multiple sclerosis with markers in 12p13 and 7q35: Synteny with experimental autoimmune disease loci (submitted).

180. Dai Y, Xu C, Holmberg M, Oturai A, Fredrikson S, Sandberg-Wollheim M, Ilonen J, Harbo H, Sörensen PS, Svejgaard A, Hillert J. Linkage analysis suggests a gene with importance in multiple sclerosis in 3p14-13 (submitted).

181. Larsen F, Oturai A, Ryder LP, Madsen H, Hillert J, Fredrikson S, Sandberg-Wollheim M, Laaksonen M, Harboe H, Sawcer S, Fugger L, Sörensen PS, Svejgaard A. Linkage analysis of a candidate region in Scandinavian sib pairs with multiple sclerosis reveals linkage to chromosome 17q (submitted).

182. Chataway J, Sawcer S, Feakes R, Coraddu F, Broadley S, Jones HB, Clayton D, Gray J, Goodfellow PN, Compston A. A screen of candidates from peaks of linkage: Evidence for the involvement of myeloperoxidase in multiple sclerosis. J Neuroimmunol 1999; 98(2):208–213.

183. Nelissen I, Fiten P, Vandenbroeck K, Hillert J, Olsson T, Marrosu MG, Opdenakker G. PECAM, MPO and PRKAR1A at chromosome 17q21-q24 and susceptibility for multiple sclerosis in Sweden and Sardinia. Neuroimmunol 2000; 108(1–2):153–159.

184. Xu C, Dai Y, Fredrikson S, Hillert J. Association and linkage analysis of candidate chromosomal regions in multiple sclerosis: indication of disease genes in 12q23 and 7ptr-15. Eur J Hum Genet 1999; 7(2):110–116.

185. Chataway J, Feakes R, Coraddu F, Gray J, Deans J, Fraser M, Robertson N, Broadley S, Jones H, Clayton D, Goodfellow P, Sawcer S, Compston DA. The genetics of multiple sclerosis: principles, background and updated results of the United Kingdom systematic genome screen. Brain 1998; 121(pt 10):1869–1887.

186. Kruglyak L. Prospects for whole-genome linkage disequilibrium mapping of common disease genes. Nature Genet 1999; 22(2):139–144.

187. Terwilliger JD, Weiss KM. Linkage disequilibrium mapping of complex disease: Fantasy or reality? Curr Opin Biotechnol 1998; 9(6):578–594.

188. Wakeland E, Morel L, Achey K, Yui M, Longmate J. Speed congenics: a classic technique in the fast lane (relatively speaking). Immunol Today 1997; 18(10):472–477.

4

Experimental Models of Virus-Induced Demyelination

MAURO C. DAL CANTO

Northwestern University Medical School, Chicago, Illinois

I. INTRODUCTION

During the past three decades, several laboratories have shown that viruses may induce demyelination of the central nervous system (CNS), with relative sparing of axons, in a pattern reminiscent of myelin destruction in human multiple sclerosis (MS). A number of experimental models have been published, utilizing both DNA and RNA viruses in a wide range of animal hosts (1,2).

Almost all published models show inflammation as part of the pathological picture; some have a rather acute monophasic course, while a few are characterized by chronic disease. Although each model can provide some useful insight into the complex viral-host interactions leading to myelin injury, viral infections producing chronic and even remitting-relapsing demyelination are obviously the most relevant to MS.

Because of space limitations, the acute viral models are mentioned only briefly in this review. Exception is made for Semliki Forest virus (SFV) infection, on which a rather extensive literature has accumulated in the last few years. The main focus of this review is on the chronic models of demyelination and their relevance to human disease.

II. CHRONIC VIRAL MODELS OF DEMYELINATION

A. Canine Distemper

Canine distemper virus (CDV) is a member of the genus *Morbillivirus* in the family Paramixoviridae. These viruses possess a single-stranded RNA genome of negative polarity, characterized by a leader sequence followed by six consecutive nonoverlapping genes, defined as N, P, L, M, F, and H. These genes encode six structural viral proteins, three complexed with the viral RNA (N, P, and L) and three involved in the formation of the envelope (M, H, and F) (3). After attachment of the virus to the target cell, virus infection is accomplished by fusion of the envelope to the cell plasma membrane, followed by viral entry. The viral genome is transcribed by a viral polymerase into complementary mRNA. Final maturation is accomplished by budding of assembled nucleocapsids through the cell membrane of the host cell. In vivo and in vitro studies have demonstrated the characteristic fusing properties of this virus by production of syncitia from infected cells (4,5). Fusion activity resides in the F peplomers, but it can be expressed only when F and H are complexed (3).

Canine distemper is a potentially important model of virus-induced demyelination, since the dog is the natural host for this virus. Infected animals show CNS disease, most commonly during the acute phase of infection, although in some cases several weeks of incubation may elapse (6). In the natural infection, which was the first to be investigated, CNS lesions are both demyelinating and destructive (7). Interestingly, initial demyelinating lesions are not necessarily associated with inflammatory infiltrates; they actually develop on a background of general immunosuppression, while demyelinating lesions in more advanced stages of the disease are associated with variable degrees of inflammation. Virus can be observed in both types of lesions (7). The initial absence of temporal relationship between inflammation and demyelination and the presence of virus in demyelinated areas suggested, at first, that the mechanism of demyelination was probably based on direct viral cytopathic effect rather than on immune-mediated mechanisms. In the past several years, however, a number of in vivo and in vitro studies have generated important data suggesting that the host immune response may play a primary role, not only in the establishment of the infection but also in the pathogenesis of demyelination.

In early in vitro studies of the cellular tropism of CDV, the main target for distemper virus was shown to be the astrocyte, while no viral antigen was demonstrated in oligodendrocytes (8). In later studies, however, Zurbriggen et al. unequivocally demonstrated the presence of CDV nucleocapsid sequences in oligodendrocytes of infected cultures by utilizing combined in situ hybridization and immunofluorescence techniques (9). However, only 1% of the oligodendrocytes that were positive for genomic material also contained viral antigen. Nevertheless, restricted oligodendroglial infection resulted in marked downregulation of myelin gene transcription (10) as well as reduction of oligodendrocyte-specific enzyme activity (11). On the basis of these in vitro studies, these authors suggested that restricted infection of oligodendrocytes may play a role in the persistence of virus in the CNS of infected animals. In addition, it was suggested that oligodendrocyte impairment following restricted viral infection could, at least in part, explain initial demyelinating lesions.

Despite the nonproductive nature of infection in oligodendrocytes and the rare occurrence of such infection, these cells were shown to undergo lytic changes in infected cultures, beginning around 20 days after viral inoculation and progressing to complete destruction in about 10 days (12). Interestingly, oligodendroglia degeneration in vitro could be equally obtained with either virulent demyelinating strains, such as A75/17 and CH84-CDV, virulent nondemyelinating strains, such as SH-CDV, or nonvirulent strains, such as OP-CDV (13). These results suggested that the capacity for in vitro indirect oligodendroglial injury is common to all strains of distemper virus despite the different outcome produced by different viral strains in vivo. Differences in outcome between the two systems, therefore, are most probably related to the more complex in vivo environment, particularly to interactions with the host immune response (14,15) and with other cell types such as astrocytes. In fact, both in vitro and in vivo studies have shown that, in contrast to the relative resistance of oligodendrocyte to CDV infection, astrocytes are highly susceptible. Since astrocytes have multiple important functions in the CNS (16), it was proposed that myelin alterations, at least in the acute lesions, could be secondary to severe compromise of astrocytic function following infection rather than to an attack on oligodendroglia (12,17,18). Recent studies support the hypothesis of indirect rather than direct oligodendroglial pathology in this model by clarifying the role of both apoptosis and necrosis in oligodendroglial injury. The authors conclude that demyelination in CDV infection does not directly result from either apoptosis or necrosis of oligodendrocytes but probably depends on some other mechanism, such as significant downregulation of myelin gene transcription in restrictively infected oligodendrocytes (22).

The in vitro data on the resistance of oligodendrocytes to infection correlate with numerous in vivo studies. Most authors, in fact, had been unable, initially, to consistently demonstrate direct oligodendroglial viral infection in either natural or experimental diseases, at least in the dog (18–21). Those studies have recently been extended with combined immunohoistochemical in situ hybridization studies in experimentally infected dogs (22). In such animals, the number of oligodendrocytes expressing viral mRNA was much larger than the number of antigen-positive oligodendrocytes, again suggesting that CDV infection in these cells is restricted. These in vivo studies also showed poor correlation between the presence of infected oligodendrocytes and demyelinating activity, since similar numbers of oligodendroglial cells expressing CDV mRNA were present in demyelinaed areas and in areas that were infected but not yet demyelinated. The lack of correlation between infected cells and demyelination supported the hypothesis of an indirect mechanism of myelin injury, since other cells having supporting function may be heavily infected.

The interactions between CDV and the host immune response have been extensively investigated. Rima et al. have addressed the role of the antibody response in experimental infection by using immunoprecipitation (15). They observed that dogs that developed white matter demyelination had a very restricted response to CDV proteins such as N, P, F, and H. On the other hand, dogs that did not develop disease or whose lesions resolved showed the presence of antibodies to the internal antigens N and P early in the disease and antibodies to surface glycoproteins H and F later on. The outcome of the infection, therefore, appears to be closely related to the ability of an animal to respond to viral antigens, particularly surface glycoproteins, since such responses are prerequisite for viral clearance (23).

Incomplete viral clearance may predispose animals to chronic white matter disease in which antibodies themselves may have a pathogenic role by participating in a process of antibody-dependent cell-mediated cytotoxicity (24). Macrophages appear to have a fundamental role in this process in various ways. For instance, studies in culture have shown that antigalactocerebroside antibody bound to oligodendrocytes may stimulate surrounding macrophages by interacting with their Fc receptors. Oligodendroglial damage may apparently result from this interaction as a consequence of the release of toxic factors, including tumor necrosis factor and reactive oxygen species, from the activated macrophages. In other studies, serum and cerebrospinal fluid containing anti-CDV antibodies were also able to induce the production of reactive oxygen species by macrophages in culture, causing oligodendroglial degeneration (25). These studies strongly suggest that myelin degeneration in CDV infection may be accomplished through a bystander type of mechanism in which macrophages play a central role, not only through cytokine production but through the generation of injurious oxygen radical species as well (25).

Other parameters of the inflammatory response have been recently studied. Alldinger et al., for instance, studied the distribution of MHC class II molecules in acute, subacute and chronic lesions in spontaneous CDV-induced encephalitis (26). They observed that in acute and subacute lesions, there was good correspondence between MHC class II expression and the presence of viral antigen, despite the paucity of inflammatory cells. In chronic lesions, on the other hand, there was widespread upregulation of MHC molecules even in areas where viral antigen had disappeared. Expression of MHC molecules was mostly on microglial cells. They concluded that while in acute lesions the virus may be the direct trigger for increased MHC expression, other antigens, possibly from myelin breakdown, could fuel MHC upregulation in the chronic phases of the disease. The same group of investigators later studied the distribution of CD4+, CD8+, and B cells in cerebellar lesions at varying stages of the disease (27). They observed a mild CD8+ infiltration in acute and subacute brains with noninflammatory encephalitis, probably suggesting their role in viral clearance and/or cytotoxicity. Also, CD8+, CD4+, and some B cells were present in subacute inflammatory and chronic lesions. On the other hand, when looking at perivascular inflammatory infiltrates, CD4+ lymphocytes clearly predominated, suggesting their role in delayed-type hypersensitivity (DTH) responses, and antibody-mediated cytotoxicity.

As previously noted, the initial demyelinating lesions in this model are not accompanied by overt inflammatory infiltrates, since they actually occur on a background of severe immunosuppression. A recent study has reexamined the presence of lymphocytes during this acute phase and has found that numerous T cells may actually be present in acute lesions and that there is diffuse upregulation of these cells throughout the CNS (28). The major fraction of these invading T cells was directed against the viral nucleocapsid protein, and the authors suggested that activated microglia probably recruited these T cells by secreting chomokines. They found, in fact, an increased IL-8 activity in the CSF of these dogs. The role of these invading T cells in demyelination has not been clarified. Interestingly, these cells remain in the CNS for long periods of time, and they may play a role in lesion formation later on in the disease process (28).

A very recent study has examined the expression of different cytokines in cells of the CSF from dogs with natural distemper and has correlated these cytokines with disease activity. IL-1β, IL-2, IL-6, IL-10, IL-12, TNF-α, TGF-β1, and INF-γ were investigated by reverse transcriptase–polymerase chain reaction (RT-PCR) in 12 dogs with lesions at different stages. The authors found simultaneous upregulation of multiple cytokines, of both pro- and anti-inflammatory type, suggesting a very complex interrelationship among them. Of all cytokines examined, however, IL-10 was the most frequently detected, suggesting a stage of inactivity in most of their animals (29).

Most authors exclude a mechanism of autosensitization—i.e., an autoimmune response against myelin components, in the pathogenesis of CDV-induced demyelination. For instance, immunoreactive myelin basic protein (MBP) was measured in the CSF of infected dogs at various time points after infection (30). Levels of MBP in the CSF showed variable degrees of correlation with the severity of pathological lesions. Similar results have been observed in humans (31), but no cause-and-effect relationship can be drawn from such findings, since MBP and even antibodies to MBP in the CSF may merely represent an epiphenomenon of myelin destruction.

Relevance to MS

Canine distemper has long interested investigators for several reasons. The virus has important similarities with measles virus, and the acute disease in the dog closely recalls the acute form of encephalitis which may complicate measles in humans. More importantly, the chronic form of CD shows remarkable similarities to human subacute sclerosing panencephalitis (SSPE) caused by persistent infection with measles virus (32). Canine distemper has also been proposed as a model of MS, due to its demyelinating pathology, and because of the early assumption that measles virus might be an etiological agent for this human disease. However, despite a burst of popularity, following reports of the possible association between MS and small dog ownership (33,34), CD is not as widely studied as other viral infections. The canine model is, in fact, rather cumbersome and, in adddition, not amenable to rigorous genetic and immunological investigations. Unfortunately, CDV infection in rodents has been generally disappointing in terms of its capacity to produce demyelinating lesions (35).

B. Coronavirus Infection

Coronaviruses are ubiquitous, being responsible for numerous infections in both animals and humans (36,37). About 25% of cases of the common cold may be due to coronavirus infection, and gastrointestinal infections have also been reported. The interest in coronaviruses has been stimulated by several papers in the arc of the last two to three decades, suggesting the presence of coronaviruses in the CNS of MS patients. For instance, Tanaka et al. described coronavirus-like particles in MS brains (38), coronaviruses were isolated from two MS brains after passage into mice (39), and coronavirus RNA and antigen were demonstrated in MS tissues by in situ hybridization and immunohistochemistry (40,41). Despite the obvious interest generated by such reports, there is still no general consensus that coronaviruses may in fact be involved in human MS. Coronaviruses utilized in MS models are derived from the natural mouse pathogen murine hepatitis virus (MHV).

The genome of these viruses is a single-stranded, nonsegmented, polyadenylated RNA having positive polarity (42). The virions are 60 to 200 nm in size and a phospholipid envelope containing glycoprotein peplomers surrounds the internal helical RNA-protein nucleocapsid. At least seven genes have been described along the 31-kb of the genome and a leader sequence at the 5′ end of the virus regulates transcription (43). Lavi et al. have addressed the genetic control of pathogenesis of murine coronaviruses by using recombinants between JHM virus, which, in 4-week-old C57BL/6 mice produces panencephalitis and mild hepatitis, and A59 virus, which, in contrast, produces focal encephalitis and severe hepatitis. They found that important biological properties of the virus—such as organ tropism, plaque morphology and replication in tissue culture, and distribution of CNS pathology—were all controlled by the 3′ portion of the viral genome, which codes for all the structural proteins, as well as some nonstructural proteins (44). The major structural proteins are the nucleocapsid protein N, associated with the genomic RNA, the membrane protein M, and the spike protein S. The S protein is crucial for viral entry into susceptible cells and for fusogenic activity. Most importantly, it appears to play a major role in the pathogenesis of viral persistence, as will be seen later.

The tropism of this virus for different CNS cells appears somewhat controversial and may depend on different viral isolates and on different developmental stages of the cells. For instance, Massa et al., studying JHM tropism for various rat neural cells in vitro, showed that the most susceptible cells were type I astrocytes and macrophages, while oligodendroglial cells appeared minimally susceptible (45). In the same study, astrocytes were shown to become persistently infected rather than succumbing to lysis. On the other hand, more recent studies by Pasick and Dales on primary brain cultures from neonatal rates suggest that type 1 astrocytes are resistant to infection, while O-2A cells—the oligo-dendrocyte type 2 astrocyte—would be the most susceptible (46). However, susceptibility is present only if O-2A cells' terminal differentiation is prevented, suggesting that permis-siveness of O-2A cells for the JHM virus is restricted to a relatively narrow window in their developmental stages (46). Ependymal cells may also be important in the development of the disease since, in a sequential study of virus spread after intracerebral inoculation of an antigenic variant of MHV-4, it was observed that these are the first cells to be infected. This study suggested that permissiveness of ependymal cells to viral infection was crucial to viral entry and to initiate the subsequent spread of the infection to other areas of the CNS (47).

In 1949 Cheever et al. first reported demyelinating lesions in the white matter of infected mice that had developed hind limb paralysis (48). The JHM strain of MHV was the first one shown to produce primary demyelination in mice after intracerebral infection (49,50). Those earlier studies concluded that the mechanism of demyelination was mainly dependent on a direct cytopathic effect on oligodendrocytes by the infecting virus. Immu-nosuppression of infected mice, in fact, was shown to exacerbate rather than prevent demy-elinating disease, a strong indirect indication that cell death was virus-induced rather than due to the host immune response (49). Subsequent studies, however, utilizing either tem-perature-sensitive mutants, small plaque mutants, or virus selected by neutralizing mono-clonal antibodies, clearly demonstrated that coronavirus-induced demyelination has also an important immune-mediated component. Such studies rendered this viral model quite relevant to human MS, in which an important immune pathogenetic component is now accepted by most investigators.

An important development of this model was the report of chronic active demyelin-ation in JHM-infected mice and the isolation of virus from the CNS several months after infection (51). The pathogenesis of viral persistence in this model is not fully understood and may depend on different factors. Stohlman and Weiner, for instance, studied the mech-anism of viral persistence of wild-type (WT) JHM in neuroblastoma cells (52). They suggested that the host immune response may be important in the establishment of viral persistence, since generation of plaque mutants, ts mutants, or production of interferon did not seem to play a role in their in vitro system. The addition of antiviral antibody, on the other hand, was able to produce a carrier culture with expression of viral antigen in the cells, but with no production of infectious virus.

Several in vivo studies, on the other hand, have suggested a role for ts mutants and plaque variants of coronaviruses in producing persistent infection and demyelination. Thus, small plaque variants of the virus were shown to be relatively avirulent, therefore allowing most of the animals to survive and to develop more frequent demyelination when compared to WT-JHM virus (53). The pathological features of disease produced by the small plaque variant were characterized by small subpial areas of demyelination with conspicuous gliosis, very few oligodendrocytes, and less remyelinating activity than in WT viral infection. There was no evidence of inflammation or viral particles (54). The authors suggested that this type of murine coronavirus infection has very close similarity to the chronic lesions of MS.

Another important in vivo mechanism of persistent CV infection is the generation of temperature sensitive mutants, such as ts8 virus (55). Again, ts mutations can modify the course of the infection, from highly cytolytic to chronic demyelinating. In contrast to the disease produced by the small plaque variant, ts8 infection is characterized by chronic active demyelination, with numerous macrophages in affected areas, and by viral persistence, since virus can be recovered in some mice as late as 12 months after infection (56).

Recent studies have shown that the spike (S) glycoprotein constitutes a major determinant of neurovirulence and viral persistence (57–59). This protein is important at several levels in virus-host interactions. It is the portion of the virus that binds to the cell surface receptor, allowing fusion of the virus to the cell membrane and viral entry. It also facilitates cell-cell fusion when expressed on the surface of infected cells. Finally, it has importance in the development of the immune response, since both neutralizing antibodies and cell-mediated responses are elicited by this protein. By utilizing the technique of targeted recombination, investigators have produced isogenic recombinant viruses containing either the S protein from the highly virulent MHV4 virus or the S protein of the less virulent MHV-A59 virus (60). Viruses with the MVH4 S gene showed striking increase in virulence when compared with those with the A59 S protein. Interestingly, the increase in virulence was accompanied by significant increase in antigen expression and inflammation, but there was no measurable increase in viral replication. The reasons for increased neurovirulence in MHV4 S gene recombinants are not clearly defined, but increased viral cytotoxicity, easier spread of virus from cell to cell, or a more destructive immune response to this recombinant virus have all been proposed. These studies correlate with investigations associating mutations in the S glycoprotein with alterations in neurovirulence. In this regard, Rowe et al. have studied the development of viral quasispecies characterized by various spike deletion variants in the S1 hypervariable region of the S protein during MIIV persistence (61,62). Frequent deletions in an isolated stem loop structure of the spike RNA were found. These studies suggest that high frequency recombinations at sites of RNA secondary structure of the spike protein may play an important role in the pathogenesis of persistent viral infection.

The role of mutations in the S1 hypervariable region has also ben studied in human coronaviruses. Talbot et al. have shown that several neural cell lines—including astrocytic, oligodendrocytic, microgllia, and neuroblastoma lines—may be infected in vitro by human coronaviruses, such as HuCV-OC43, normally a respiratory pathogen in humans. They also noted that after 130 days of culture, point mutations in the S1 gene were observed in all persistently infected cells, thus reproducing similar events to those in the murine system (63).

The role that mutations in the S protein may play in viral persistence has also been investigated by Perlman's group. They have shown that mutations in an immunodominant CD8+ T cell epitope (S-510-518), within the S surface glycoprotein, are found in all cases of persistent JHM virus infection (64). These mutations abrogated the recognition of the virus by virus-specific cytotoxic T cells in direct ex vivo cytotoxicity assays. Such mutations do not take place in SCID mice similarly infected, strongly suggesting that CTL escape mutants arise under the effect of immune pressure, and they contribute to the establishment of viral persistence and demyelinating disease. (64) This hypothesis is supported by a study by the same group of investigators that tested MHV-JHM variants showing epitope S-510-518 mutations, isolated from infected mice and inoculated into naïve mice. These showed delayed viral clearance resulting in higher mortality, morbidity, and neurological signs, in keeping with the hypothesis of escape from CD8+ mediated cyto-toxicity (65). Although the CD8+ T-cell immune response that pressures the origination of CTL escape mutants is polyclonal, this is largely monospecific and does not prevent the selection of CTL escape mutants. These authors used soluble MHC/peptide tetramers in direct ex vivo analysis of CNS derived lymphocytes to show that about 34% of CD8+ T cells in the CNS of mice with chronic demyelinating disease were specific for epitope S-510-518, although only virus expressing mutated epitope can be detected in these ani-mals. By sequence analysis of the beta-chain CD3 of several hundreds S-510-518–positive cDNA clones, they showed that a majority of clonotypes were identified in more than one mouse. In chronically infected mice, about 100 to 900 different CD8+ T cells clonotypes responsive to S-510-518 were identified in the CNS of each mouse. Therefore, epitope specific T cells may still be present at high levels even after the wild type sequence is no longer found (Pewe; in press).

The role of the immune response in the demyelinating pathology of this model has been intensely investigated during the past several years. It is generally held that the acute phase of myelin destruction, as originally demonstrated with the WT-JHM virus, is primar-ily dependent on direct oligodendroglial infection. Several studies, however, both in vivo and in vitro, would indicate that interactions between the virus and host immunity may be important in the chronic phase of the infection (68).

A number of studies have explored the pathogenetic role of virus-specific antibodies in the establishment of disease (69–73). Schwender et al. found that resistant Brown Nor-way (BN) rats were able to mount a very early viral neutralizing IgG antibody response in the CNS, while susceptible Lewis (LE) rats developed neutralizing antibody much later and with lower affinity than BN rats (74). The authors concluded that this differential antibody response in the two rat strains could help explain differences in development of demyelinating disease in the two strains. Thus, BN rats would be able to clear the virus before development of demyelinating lesions, while the initial absence of neutralizing antibodies in the LE rat would favor the spread of the infection in the CNS, with resultant severe demyelination (74).

Studies in the mouse, however, have shown a somewhat different picture. For in-stance, Lin et al. demonstrated that initial clearance proceeded normally in mice with a disrupted Ig mu gene, therefore being deprived of antibodies (75). Later on, however, increasing infectious virus was recovered from these mice. Absence of antibodies did not result in the emergence of mutant viruses and no alteration in cell-mediated immunity was observed. These results implicate antibodies in establishing and maintaining viral persistence, while it appears they have no significant role in controlling the virus in the acute phase of infection.

The role of cell-mediated immune responses has been defined in several studies. For instance, Wang et al. reported that general immunosuppression by irradiation in mice infected with JHM virus prevented the development of demyelination (68). In addition, adoptive transfer of MHC-restricted T cells from infected mice into irradiated, infected animals was able to restore their capacity to develop demyelinating lesions, therefore suggesting that T cells play a major role in the pathogenesis of the demyelinating process (68). Both CD4+ and CD8+ cells have been observed in infected animals (76). Both cell types appear to be important for effective clearance of virus. Recent studies have shown that CD8+ cells are particularly important for protective immunity in the rat, and the specificity of these cells has been demonstrated to be for the viral S protein (77). On the other hand, the same cells may participate in the pathogenesis of demyelination, particularly in view of the ability of CNS structures to express MHC molecules. Suzumura et al., for instance, reported interesting findings with A59 infection of glial cell cultures. They demonstrated that infection was able to stimulate expression of H2 class I antigens on astrocytes, and that this expression was not dependent on interferon-gamma (78). During persistent infection of glial cultures, however, when no detectable infectious virus is produced, class I antigens are not expressed by astrocytes unless IFN-gamma is added to the culture medium (79). Class I antigens may also be elicited on oligodendroglial cells, but a soluble factor, produced by infected cells, probably astrocytes, appears to be responsible for such induction, rather than direct viral activity. In vivo studies confirmed these results, by showing the expression of class I antigens on both astrocytes and oligodendrocytes following infection of mice with A59 virus (80). Almost simultaneously, Massa et al. demonstrated that infection of astrocytes with JHM virus elicited expression of class II molecules on these cells, apparently based on direct interaction between virus and targets (81). More recently, Gombold and Weiss demonstrated that infection of mixed glial cell cultures with mouse hepatitis virus A59 resulted in a significant increase in the level of class I mRNA in both infected and non-infected cells (82). In addition, increases in class I and class II mRNA also occurred in the CNS of infected mice in all portions of the brain, independently from the actual presence of infection or inflammation in any particular area (82). These results support the hypothesis that upregulation of MHC molecules in glial cells in this infection is mediated by soluble factors rather than by the obligatory presence of virus in the cells. These studies are important because the expression of class I and class II antigens on CNS cells may allow them to interact with T lymphocytes, and thus play a critical role in initiating and protracting an immune-mediated process of demyelination.

Recently, investigators have studied whether persistence of the virus influences the antigen specificity of CD8 lymphocytes. Initially, acute cytotoxic T-lymphocyte (CTL) clones had broad antigen specificity, thus being geared to better control the possible emergence of mutations; later on, however, clones with narrower, more selected specificity emerged, probably driven by selective pressure exerted by persisting antigen (83). Stohlman et al. investigated the role of CD4+ cells in cytotoxic activity and in altering the activity of CTLs (84). By using infected CD4+-depleted mice transferred with CTL, they found no changes in the ability of CD8+ cells to enter the CNS, and no differences in CTL activity between CD4+-depleted and control mice. However, they saw significant CTL apoptosis in CD4+-depleted mice, suggesting that, although not required for CTL induction, CD4+ lymphocytes may have an important role for maintaining CTL viability (84). Recent studies utilizing beta$_2$ microglobulin ''knockout'' mice have confirmed the importance of CD8+ lymphocytes for viral clearance (85). However, it appears that while these cells are very effective in clearing virus from endothelial cells, microglia, and inflammatory cells, they are not as effective on neurons and astrocytes. CD8+ cells are also important in preventing the spread of encephalitis (85). Lin et al. have also shown that CD4+ cells and IFN-γ but not TNF-α have a role in viral clearance (86).

It is of interest that IFN-γ is particularly important in controlling viral replication in oligodendroglia, while perforin-dependent CTL mechanisms are more important in controlling infection of astrocytes and microglia (85). Other interferon responses have been studied by Wang et al. in vitro. They saw that infection of primary astrocytes with either A59 or MHV-2 viruses resulted in upregulation of INF-β but not IFN-γ or IFN-α. This suggests that while astrocytes are capable of producing IFN-β, the other interferons are only produced by inflammatory cells, at least in this infection (87). Other cytokines have also been explored. IL-10, for instance, does not appear to have a role in viral clearance, while it may decrease the extent of inflammation in the CNS during the acute infection (88). However, it does not appear to have a role in the final resolution of the inflammatory process. Parra et al. have compared the cytokine response in mice infected with two different JHMV variants, one producing a nonlethal encephalitis, the other resulting in a fulminant lethal infection (89,90). In both cases, both Th1 and Th2 cytokines were represented in the CNS; however, they noted a prevalence of IL-2, IL-1β, and IL-6 in the nonlethal infection, while there was a prevalence of iNOS, and IL-1α in the lethal disease. According to these authors, however, the differences in these cytokines were not sufficient to distinguish lethal from nonlethal infections leading to persistence.

Studies of the development of lesions in the rat model of coronavirus infection have also shown the upregulation of a number of inflammatory molecules, especially in later stages of the disease. Increased expression of IFN-γ, TNF-α, and iNOS were seen in the areas of inflammatory demyelination, in addition to several regulatory calcium binding proteins and to a novel cytokine, the endothelial monocyte activating polypeptide II (EMAP II) (91).

A number of chemokines—such as MIP-1β, MIP-2, MCP-1, MCP-3, RANTES, and CRG-2—are also upregulated in the CNS of MHV-infected mice (92). CRG-2 (cytokine response gene 2) may be particularly important since it colocalizes with viral RNA and it is mainly expressed by astrocytes in association with demyelinating lesions. These chemokines are important in the initiation and maintenance of the inflammatory response, including the recruitment and activation of macrophages into the CNS, and underscore the importance of macrophages in the process of demyelination not only in this viral model but in others as well. These same authors have also studied the effects of NOS2 regulation on inflammation in MHV-infected mice (93). They have shown that inhibition of NOS2 results in lower levels of MCP-1 mRNA at day 7 postinfection. This difference disappears at day 12 postinfection. The reduction of this chemokine corresponded with a decrease in the severity of inflammation and demyelination, during the first three weeks of infection, suggesting NOS2 participates in the induction of inflammatory demyelination during the first phase of infection.

The role of inflammation in virus-induced demyelination was also investigated by Wu and Perlman in a study utilizing recombinase-activating gene function deficient mice (RAG1−/−), that are defective in both B- and T-cell maturation (94). When RAG1−/− infected mice were infected with an attenuated variant of JHMV, J2.2-v1, they became persistently infected but did not develop demyelination, despite the presence of some macrophages in areas of viral replication. In contrast, infected RAG1−/− mice, transferred with splenocytes from infected normal mice, developed extensive demyelination in concomitance with striking macrophage infiltration in the demyelinated areas. This study shows that in the presence of lymphocytes, presumably able to produce a number of chemokines, macrophages may be recruited and activated in the infected CNS and precipitate the process of demyelination. Interestingly, it appears that blood-borne macrophages may not be necessary in this model, since depletion of blood-borne macrophages does not have much effect on the demyelinating process. The authors suggest that perivascular macrophages or microglia may be sufficient to produce injury in the presence of considerable antigen load necessary for activation (95). Wu and Perlman also suggest that apoptosis, although occurring in animals infected with the JHM virus, mainly in noninfected cells, is not likely to have a significant role in the demyelinating process in this model (94).

The nature of the primary immunogenic antigen involved in the pathogenesis of demyelination in this model is still debated, and it may be different in different species. For instance, studies conducted in the rat would suggest a definite role for an autoimmune pathogenesis of demyelination in coronavirus infection. The rat has been utilized by several investigators because of its demonstrated ability to develop recurrent demyelination weeks or months after a first phase of subacute demyelinating encephalomyelitis and for the frequent presence of inflammatory cells in affected white matter (96–102). Watanabe et al. demonstrated that lymphocytes from weanling Lewis rats infected with JHM virus, become sensitized to myelin basic protein in addition to viral antigens (101). Such lymphocytes, after stimulation with MBP, appear to be capable to adoptively transfer disease resembling experimental allergic encephalomyelitis (EAE) in recipient animals (101). These authors have proposed that an autoimmune attack against myelin is probably responsible for the chronic phase of demyelination in JHM infection. Since astrocytes can express Ia molecules after JHM infection, it is possible that persistently infected astrocytes may serve as presenters of myelin antigens (i.e., MBP), to sensitized lymphocytes, thus playing a role in the immune process leading to demyelination. Interestingly, the capacity of Ia expression by astrocytes correlates with the susceptibility to demyelination of the rat strain from which such cells are derived (102).

These results suggest that a viral infection of the CNS can trigger an autoimmune reaction against myelin antigens, thus leading to a process of cell-mediated demyelination. This concept, however, is still controversial. It is puzzling that, thus far, a similar autoimmune reaction against myelin has not been demonstrated in the mouse system, considering that mice, like rats, also develop EAE when injected myelin antigens or myelin antigens-primed cells (103).

Relevance to MS

Coronaviruses are ubiquitous viruses that affect several animal species, including humans. In the latter species they mainly attack the respiratory and gastrointestinal systems, being probably responsible for as many as 15% of common colds (36). Previous data on possible involvement of coronavirus in MS and on the identification of coronavirus mRNA and antigen in MS brain tissues have stimulated interest in this animal model for its potential relevance to this human disease. Despite such reports, however, no cause-effect relationship has been demonstrated between the presence of coronavirus in human MS and the disease itself, and the possibility that this virus, even if found in more cases, may represent an irrelevant bystander has to be considered. In any case, because of the chronic course of coronavirus infection in experimental animals and because of an immune component in the pathogenesis of demyelination in mice and rats infected with this virus, the coronavirus model is considered as one of the best and most relevant to human MS.

C. Visna Virus Infection

Visna virus (VV) is a retrovirus of the lentivirus family and the prototype of conventional slow viruses (104). Slow virus infections, a term coined by Sigurdsson (105), are characterized by a long incubation period and a protracted course. Lentiviruses have recently received renewed attention, because human immunodeficiency virus (HIV), the etiological agent of AIDS, belongs to such family (106).

Like other viruses of this group, VV has an RNA genome which, upon infection of a cell, is transcribed to an intermediate DNA by a virion-associated reverse transcriptase. This proviral DNA is integrated into the host cell DNA. Progeny RNA is transcribed from provirus DNA and acts as a messenger RNA. The Tat protein is essential for efficient viral replication since it regulates transcription through an AP-1 site, proximal to the TATA box, within the viral long terminal repeat (LTR). Carruth et al. have recently reported that a Tat leucine-rich domain adjacent to the Tat activation domain is crucial for the targeting of the Tat protein to AP-1 sites in the LTR (107). This region of Tat, in addition, has shown a pattern similar to the leucine zippers in the bZIP family of DNA-binding proteins, thus suggesting an important role for Tat interactions with cellular proteins, such as Fos and Jun, that are known to contain bZIP domains. These authors hypothesize that the association between Tat protein, Jun, and Fos would be important in facilitating the positioning of Tat proximally to the TATA box, where the virus Tat activation domain could contact the transcription factor TBP, or TATA-binding protein, to activate viral transcription (108). Viral maturation takes place by budding through the host cell membrane, which expresses virus-coded glycoproteins (104). A clear-cut dicothomy exists between in vitro and in vivo infections with VV. This virus produces an acute lytic infection in cultivated cells (109); but in the sheep it produces persistent infection in the presence of a vigorous host immune reaction (110). Initially, it was believed that antigenic shift of viral surface glycoproteins during the infection was the principal mechanism for the establishment of viral persistence by allowing the virus to escape antibody neutralization (111). In the case of Visna, however, antigenic variants make only a small percentage of total virus and do not replace the infecting serotype (112). It is now believed that severe restriction of viral gene expression is the main explanation for virus persistence in this infection (106,113), a concept recently reiterated by Haase (114). This author hypothesizes that VV, similarly to other lentiviruses, is able to establish a covert infection is susceptible cells by restriction of gene expression, thus hiding from the immune system of the host. It is interesting that replication is severely restricted in the monocyte, perhaps the cell most susceptible to infection. Apparently, only when monocytes differentiate into macrophages does viral replication become more readily apparent, suggesting that cellular factors induced during cell maturation may act as important regulatory elements in the expression of the virus (115). Recently Eriksson et al. have studied the role of CD4+ lymphocytes in the infection of macrophages (116). By using CD4+-depleted sheep, they showed that CD4+ lymphocytes but not dendritic cells of the skin are important for the infection of macrophages by maedi-visna virus. Impaired infection of macrophages in CD4+-depleted animals resulted in greatly reduced viral loads in these sheep. This, together with the absence of T helper cells, contributed to greatly decreased virus-specific immune responses, such as delayed induction of cytotoxic T cell precursors, decrease in antiviral-specific proliferative responses and delayed antiviral antibodies. Chebloune et al. have also investigated the role of activated T cells in the penetration of virus into the central nervous system (117). They showed that when the virus was inoculated intrathecally rather than directly into the brain, it could not reach the CNS compartment on its own. When EAE was produced in these animals, on the other hand, virus could easily establish CNS infection. These studies strongly suggest that activated T cells are necessary in addition to infected macrophages for VV neuropathogenesis.

The prototypical infection occurs in the Icelandic sheep (110,118–121). Both short- and long-term experiments have been performed. In short-term experiments (118) lasting about 13 months, virus could be recovered from blood and CNS for the entire course of the experiments, but it could not be recovered from the CSF longer than 4 months postinfection. At such time, intrathecal synthesis of neutralizing antibody could be demonstrated

(122). Pathological lesions can be found in 50% of the cases, as early as 2 weeks postinfection and consist of inflammatory infiltrates in the CNS comprising lymphocytes, macrophages, and plasma cells. There may be a particularly severe inflammatory involvement in the choroid plexus. Lesions begin typically in a periventricular location, from which they extend into the spinal cord alongside the central canal. From the periventricular areas, more severe lesions may extend into the lobar white matter, where they may coalesce into large areas of necrosis encompassing both axons and myelin sheaths. This pattern of white matter destruction has been designated the "early" type lesion, but it may be found even years after infection. The second type of lesion has been found mainly in long-term experiments lasting up to 11 years (110). This lesion, designated "late" type, is characterized by very well demarcated areas of demyelination in the spinal cord, with axonal preservation (123). Plaques of primary demyelination may be quiescent, or they may show inflammatory activity with ongoing myelin breakdown at any time during the course of the chronic disease. These lesions bear a strong resemblance to those in human MS. As in other viral infections, evidence of remyelination by both oligodendrocytes and Schwann cells has been observed. "Early" and "late" lesions may be seen in the same sections (110).

Studies by Nathanson et al. and Petursson et al. strongly suggest that the "early" type lesions may be immune-mediated (124,125). These authors, in fact, were successful in preventing such lesions by immunosuppressing animals with antithymocyte serum and cyclophosphamide. In addition, they demonstrated an increase in the severity of the lesions by rechallenging animals several weeks after infection in order to amplify their immune response (126). These authors believe that the immune response in affected animals is mainly directed toward virus-specific antigens rather than toward myelin components. This conclusion has found recent support in studies investigating the possible phenomenon of molecular mimicry of MBP by VV (127). Although a sequence similarity was found between an MBP peptide and the viral polymerase, no T-proliferative responses and only weak antibody responses to the MBP peptide were demonstrated in sheep infected with the maedi-visna virus. The weak antibody responses were thought to represent epiphenomena, rather than having pathogenetic significance. On the other hand, the severity of lesions appears to be dependent on the dose of virus, and good correlation may be found between the degree of pathological changes and the presence of virus in tissues (110,114).

For a time it was not clear whether the "late" focal demyelinating lesions in spinal cord white matter are also immune-mediated. One of the major obstacles in studying these lesions was the length of time necessary for them to develop as well as the lack of regularity in their presentation (110). Recently, Lutley et al. have reported that the course of the disease may be dramatically accelerated by using more virulent strains of visna virus (128). Subsequently, Georgsson et al. injected sheep with such strains and were able to produce an accelerated disease, from 5 to 12 weeks postinfection characterized by severe lesions of both types (129). Demyelinating lesions were rich in lymphoid cells and macrophages, and differed from those in sheep infected with less virulent virus in having less demarcated margins. In order to investigate the relationship between viral localization and myelin breakdown, a detailed immunohistochemical analysis of viral antigen distribution was also performed. In brain parenchyma, viral antigen expression was maximal in areas with intense inflammation and most of the virus was localized in lymphocytes and macrophages. Initially no viral antigen was found in either neurons or glial cells while it was observed in endothelial cells—an interesting finding that may be relevant to lymphocyte homing into the CNS (129). However, immunohistochemical and in situ hybridization studies have uncovered a wide spectrum of susceptible cells including plasma cells, pericytes, fibroblasts, choroid plexus cells, as well as astrocytes and oligodendrocytes (130). It is important to realize, however, that despite the observed susceptibility of these cells to VV infection, both the number of infected cells and the extent of active viral replication in these cells are extremely low, even in the presence of very florid inflammatory lesions (131). The stricking dichotomy between severity of tissue changes on one hand and the limited ability of the virus to replicate and propagate from cell to cell on the other strongly supports the hypothesis that tissue injury in VV infection is probably not directly related to viral cytopathic effects but it is mediated through host immune responses.

Recent studies have addressed the possible immune mechanisms that may be involved in the pathogenesis of white matter lesions in VV infection and have compared the role of antibody-versus cell-mediated immune (CMI) responses (132). Results clearly indicate that only CMIs correlate with the severity of both clinical and pathological expressions of disease. Furthermore, by analyzing the distribution and numbers of CD4+ and CD8+ cells in both tissues and CSF of affected animals, Torsteinsdottir et al. have suggested that CD8+-positive lymphocytes may be the main effector cells in disease production (132). In fact, while CD4+ cells remain mainly localized around blood vessels, CD8+ cells migrate into the brain parenchyma as if pursuing their target (133). In the CSF, accordingly, there is a reversion of the CD4+/CD8+ ratio with preponderance of CD8+ cells, and their presence correlates quite closely with the severity of disease. It has been suggested, therefore, that cytotoxic CD8+ lymphocytes may represent the cell population most responsible for tissue injury (133). Subsequently, the role of MHC antigens expression in the development of lesions has also been explored (134). While only class I antigens were expressed in normal sheep, mainly on endothelial cells and also on ependyma, choroid plexus, and meanings, both class I and class II antigens were unregulated on microglia of infected sheep and correlated with the distribution of the lesions in the white matter. Interestingly, while class II antigens were unregulated in all diseased sheep, class I antigens were increased only on microglia in the most severe lesions. The correlation of increased MHC expression by microglia with the distribution of lesions in white matter suggests that microglia may also have a role in the pathogenesis of tissue destruction. In a study by Craig et al, TNF-α was expressed by perivascular macrophages in concomitance with class II upregulation in CNS lesions, suggesting a role of cytokines in microglia-mediated tissue injury (135).

A new and interesting hypothesis has been recently advanced regarding the contribution of viral products to lesion production. Vigne et al. (115) have suggested that the viral tat regulatory protein may have cytotoxic effects on CNS cells. An inflammatory reaction would follow this cytotoxic effect and cytokines liberated by both astrocytes and macrophages recruited to the lesions would precipitate the pathological expression of disease. Recently, Starling et al. have reported that application of dizolcipine (MK801) reduces the volume of lesions produced by injection of a synthetic peptide derived from the basic region of Maedi-Visno virus TAT (136). This suggests that production of tissue injury by this viral transactivating protein involves glutamate neurotoxicity via the N-methyl-D-aspartate (NMDA) receptors. Interestingly this type of neurotoxicity is quite rapid as it may occur just half an hour after stereotactic injection of the synthetic TAT peptide into the CNS of rats.

Relevance to MS

Visna is the prototype for slow viral infections and it is one of the best models to investigate mechanisms of viral persistence. The taxonomic relationship between VV and human immunodeficiency virus has recently increased the interest of the scientific community for this animal model (106).

The lesions in white matter, characterized by primary demyelination, have also attracted the attention of MS investigators. Lesions of ''late'' type are certainly reminiscent of those in this human disease. The most serious limitations of this model are in its host restriction, essentially limited to the Icelandic sheep, the lack of genetic purity in the sheep population, and therefore the limited scope of immunological manipulations which may be performed. The new type of infection with more virulent strains will simplify future experiments, but it is hard to deny that sheep are rather cumbersome as laboratory animals.

D. Herpes Simplex Virus Infection

Herpes simplex virus (HSV) belongs to the family Herpetoviridae (137). It has an icosahedral nucleocapsid containing a core, which appears as a ring of DNA surrounding a protein plug. The capsid is surrounded by a tegument, which is wrapped in an envelope characterized by projecting spikes. The maturation of the virus starts in the nucleus of the infected cell and continues inside the cytoplasm. Newly formed virions are released by budding. The viral genome is made of double-stranded, linear DNA molecules (137).

Two main serological types, HSV-1 and HSV-2, have been recognized (138). Type 1 infection generally occurs by oral contact before puberty. Both experimental and human studies have shown that virus may persist, producing a latent, subclinical infection in trigeminal, superior cervical, and autonomic ganglia (139–142). Reactivation of infection may produce recurrent ulcerations, particularly in perioral location, or acute necrotizing encephalitis. Type 2 HSV is generally acquired after puberty by sexual contact and, after an acute-phase of infection, it may remain latent in the sacral ganglia (143). This too may undergo reactivation, thus producing recurrent genital ulcerations. With liberalization of sexual mores, genital HSV-1 and facial HSV-2 are increasingly observed. There is about 50% base-pair homology between the two serotypes, which explain some degree of cross-protection provided by the respective infections.

HSV has been utilized very extensively for investigating viral cell interactions, both in vitro and in vivo. During the last several years, it has attracted considerable attention for his capacity to produce demyelination of the nervous system in experimental animals and perhaps in humans. The original studies utilized HSV type 1 virus, but more recently interesting observations have also accumulated on HSV type 2 virus. Since the last edition of this book, some interesting data have been collected, particularly on mechanisms of persistence of these viruses and the possible role that infected astrocytes may have in the demyelinating process.

HSV-1 Model

Infection of mice and rabbits, via the trigeminal nerve, produces an acute inflammatory demyelinating process involving the central portion of the trigeminal root while sparing the peripheral portion (144–147). Replicating virus has been identified in neurons, astrocytes, and oligodendrocytes, while defective maturation has been observed in Schwann cells of the peripheral portion of the root. The presence of oligodendroglial infection suggested, at first, that demyelination was due to a direct viral cytopathic effect on the myelinating cell. A number of studies, however, utilizing both nude mice and various regimens of immunosuppression, have provided evidence that the host immune response may also play a role in the production of demyelination in this model (147–154). Of particular interest are recent studies involving the use of different strains of mice treated with different immunosuppressive drugs and of nude mice with different backgrounds (155). These authors conclude that virus is necessary but not sufficient to produce demyelination, including during the first phase of infection, while the immune system appears to play a major role not only in limiting the spread of virus into the CNS but also in precipitating the development of demyelinating lesions. The nature of such immune mechanisms is not yet clear. While there could be development of an EAE-like pathogenesis of myelin injury, it is also possible that a protracted immune attack against persistent virus could involve myelin in the destructive process. In fact, while viral antigen could not be visualized beyond 12 days postinfection by simple immunohistochemistry, viral genome could be demonstrated by in situ hybridization in active demyelinating lesions of A/J mice up to 8 weeks after infection (156). This would suggest that in some murine strains, a limited viral production may take place in the chronic phase of the infection and the presence of virus may continue to stimulate the host immune response, with resultant myelin damage.

Kastrukoff et al. have looked at the role of genetic resistance to HSV-1 infection in the expression of demyelination. These authors have shown that, while a resistant animal develops only mild inflammation at the trigeminal root entry zone, a moderately resistant strain develops focal demyelination in the same area, and a susceptible strain develops multiple demyelinating lesions, not only at the root entry zone but also in the cerebellum and cerebral hemispheres (157). In addition, the pathological characteristics of the disease and the capacity of developing active demyelination during late disease are different in the various strains. For instance, A/J and PL/J mice show active demyelination for at least 8 and 28 weeks after viral inoculation, respectively, while SJL/J mice show new lesions only up to 24 days postinfection (156). Differences in susceptibility and in the pattern of pathological lesions among different murine strains may depend on multiple factors, some related to target tissue susceptibility to infection, some related to the host immune response. For instance, susceptibility of oligodendrocytes to infection must play a role, since a direct relationship was observed between the capacity of the virus to infect cultured oligodendroglial cells from different animal strains and its capacity to produce demyelinating lesions in the respective strains in vivo (157). In vitro studies of this different susceptibility to infection by oligodendrocytes from different murine strains have shown that major replicative blocks may be present either at the level of the cytoplasmic membrane, as in C57BL/6 cells, or at the level of the nuclear membrane as in BALB/cByJ cells (158). More recently, these same authors have analyzed differences in resistance to HSV-1 among oligodendrocytes from the murine strains C57BL/6J, BALB/cByJ, and A/J. The results of this study suggest that the innate cellular resistance of oligodendrocytes to HSV-1 infection is determined before the expression of immediate early (IE) viral antigens. Viral adsorption and viral penetration studies showed that while viral adsorption was not different in the three strains, viral penetration was more efficient in A/J mice than in the other two strains. This suggests that differences in virus-cell interactions in different murine strains may contribute to different outcomes of infection in different animals, including the development of CNS demyelination (159).

The genetics of CNS demyelination in multiple strains of mice was also examined by Kastrukoff et al. (156). Their study suggests that the MHC has no major role in determining whether a certain strain will develop multifocal demyelination; however, it appears to have a role in determining the pathological appearance of demyelinating lesions in the CNS. This H-2 influence on pathology appears to be multigenic in nature (156). The involvement of MHC in the pathological expression of disease supports the contention that host immune mechanisms play an important role in pathogenesis. Further studies to better define the possible immune-mediated mechanisms of demyelination in HSV-1 infection are needed.

HSV-2 Model

This virus has been used by both intracerebral (160) and genital routes (161,162). The latter infection has stimulated considerable interest for several reasons: the vaginal is the natural route of infection; one of the HSV-2 strains being used, the MS strain, had been originally isolated from an MS patient (163); and interesting findings regarding the effects of the infection on the lymphoid tissues of the host have been reported.

Vaginal inoculation in mice of HSV-2 may cause a spectrum of CNS diseases, ranging from an acute necrotizing encephalitis to nonfatal infection characterized by extensive foci of demyelination (161,164). The dose of the virus, the animal's age, and the immune state of infected animals all contribute to determine different outcomes of this infection. The most severe disease, with rapid death, is characterized by lesions in both gray and white matter of the spinal cord as well as severe alterations in lymphoid tissues, which can be shown to be directly infected by the virus (162).

Animals that develop mild clinical disease and survive the acute phase of the infection develop multiple demyelinating lesions in the spinal cord (161,164). Studies have demonstrated a decreasing gradient of virus distribution, from the caudal to rostral levels of the neuraxis, and a direct temporal and anatomical relationship between the presence of lesions in the spinal cord and previous infection of sensory roots at lumbosacral levels. These results strongly support the hypothesis that HSV is mainly transported and distributed to tissues by the axonal route rather than by the bloodstream (165,166).

The pathogenesis of the demyelinating lesions is still under scrutiny. Studies thus far have shown a direct correlation between the presence and amount of virus in glial cells and the presence and degree of the demyelinating lesions. Thus, with a decrease of the number of virus-infected cells at higher levels of the neuraxis, a corresponding decrease of demyelinating lesions from the lower spinal cord toward the brain was observed (165,166). In demyelinated areas, lesions tend to extend in long longitudinal columns, suggesting a cell-to-cell mode of virus spread starting from the initial neuronal infection. Martin et al. have proposed several mechanisms to explain the selective amplification of lesions in the white matter of surviving animals: (a) multiplicity of oligodendrocytes providing myelin internodes to each axon; (b) secondary spread of infection between oligodendrocytes in glial columns; and (c) loss of several internodes of myelin for every oligodendrocyte lost to the infection (164–166).

The constant association between myelin injury and infection of oligodendroglial and Schwann cells supports the hypothesis that HSV-induced demyelination is mainly due to direct viral attack on the myelinating cells, at least in the first phases of infection. Recent studies, however, have shown that alterations in immunological functions may also play a role in this model. HSV-induced lesions of lymphoid tissues, in fact, have been observed also in animals that survive the acute infection and go on to develop demyelination (162). It has been proposed, therefore, that immune alterations in this model may be important not only in modifying the course of the acute infection but later events as well, such as the severity of lesions that may accompany reactivation of latent infection (164). In this regard, recent studies of the use of immunosuppressive drugs to produce a reactivating model of genital HSV-2 infection are of particular interest (167,168). The propensity of demyelinating lesions to undergo remyelination quite promptly, with both

Schwann cells and oligodendrocytes (169), will help the study of possible differences in the pathogenesis of early versus late lesions in this relapsing model.

Mechanisms of HSV-2 persistence in the CNS, were mainly investigated after HSV-2 inoculation intracerebrally rather than intravaginally. By using immunosuppression in mice surviving intracerebral HSV-2 inoculation, Martin and Suzuki were able to induce recurrent infection of the CNS and concluded that neural connections were important determinants of sites of reactivated infection (170). The same authors later reported on the identification of HSV-2 transcripts in trigeminal ganglia during acute and latent infection of mice after intracerebral viral inoculation (171). In situ hybridization was used in tandem with immunohistochemistry for viral antigen in these studies. While during the acute infection there was clear correspondence between the presence of antigen and hybridization signals given by probes for immediate-early, delayed-early, or late viral genes, no antigen was present during latent infection, and the only positive genomic signal was given by one of the probes for immediate-early genes (171). The authors concluded that HSV-2 transcription is restricted during latency with transcripts localized in the nuclei of ganglionic neurons in a pattern similar to that described in HSV-1 infection. In the latest published work by Gressens and Martin, however, additional interesting findings were reported regarding HSV-2 latency in the CNS that were not expected (172). By using an in situ PCR technique, these authors demonstrated that astrocytes in the CNS can also present HSV-2 DNA in their nuclei in the absence of any viral antigen. Astrocytes, therefore, can also harbor latent HSV-2 infection, but apparently with a different pattern from neuronal cells. While neurons, in fact, show HSV latency-associated transcript (LAT) RNA during latent infection, astrocytes do not, suggesting that persistent HSV infection in astrocytes may depend on different molecular mechanisms than in neurons (172).

Relevance to MS

HSV is one of the viruses most intensively studied, in large part because of its demonstrated capacity to become latent in somatic and autonomic ganglia and to persist in such state for the life of the host (139–143,173). In addition, HSV-1 DNA sequences have been isolated from the brains of several individuals, both normal, and with neurological diseases, including cases with MS (174). However, as for coronaviruses, no causal relationship between the presence of virus and the disease itself has been proven.

Koenig et al. reported the development of an acute demyelinating disease similar to disseminated encephalomyelitis in a patient with recurrent HSV encephalitis, following a dramatic response to ara-A during a previous bout of cerebral infection (175). From this case, the authors suggested that HSV may produce, in humans, a demyelinating CNS disease very similar to EAE. In this respect, both animal models of HSV may appear quite relevant to human disease. Whether relevance is more to the acute process, known as postinfectious encephalomyelitis, or to MS is debatable. It is of interest that Martin et al. cite similar epidemiological distribution of HSV-2 infection and multiple sclerosis in the human population as an additional point in favor of the genital HSV model (176).

E. Theiler's Murine Encephalomyelitis Virus Infection

Theiler's murine encephalomyelitis virus (TMEV) is a picornavirus of the genus cardioviridae (177–179). It has four structural proteins, designated VP1 to VP4, surrounding a single-stranded RNA genome. These viruses are highly cytocidal in cell culture, yet some strains may produce persistent infections in animals. The mechanisms leading to viral persistence in these viruses are not yet clear. It does not appear that mechanisms known to occur in other viral infections—such as mutations or generation of defective interfering particles—are significant events in picornavirus infections (180). It has been suggested that either interferon and/or antibody may play some role in TMEV persistence by allowing only a small number of cells to be infected at any one time (181).

Picornaviruses are natural pathogens for mice, in which they produce enteric and neurological symptoms (182). There are two different subgroups of TMEV (183). One, designated "Theiler's original," or TO subgroup, includes strains which have low virulence, grow to relatively low titers, produce small plaques, and may cause persistent infection of white matter with extensive demyelination (184). The other subgroup includes GD VII and FA viruses. These grow to high titers, are highly virulent, produce large plaques, and induce acute fatal encephalitides in mice rather than chronic demyelination (184). In cell culture, GD VII virus appears in large crystalline arrays, while the TO subgroup appears to line up along infected cell membranes (185). Unfortunately, in the adult animal, the TO subgroup does not produce any characteristic inclusions. Because of its small size and low tissue titers, virus in infected cells of these animals can be identified only by immunohistochemical techniques or by in situ hybridization (186–188).

Pevear et al. sequenced the entire RNA genomes of a TO virus, designated BeAn8386, and of the highly virulent GDVII virus (189). They found that these viruses are 90.4% identical at the nucleotide level, and 95.7% identical at the aminoacid level. Almost half of the differences in aminoacids were found to be at the level of the three surface-coat proteins VP1, VP2, and VP3. Since differences were found to cluster in distinct regions on a three-dimensional model of the virus (190), these authors suggest that such mutation clusters may represent the neutralizing immunogenic epitomes of TMEVs. The availability of the complete sequence for both the highly virulent and less virulent subgroups of TMEV will facilitate further studies of the mechanisms underlying differences in their pathogenicity by allowing construction of recombinant BeAn-GDVII viruses (189).

Clinical and pathological studies on TMEV-induced demyelinating disease have utilized TO strains such as the Daniel's (DA), or the BeAn8386. Another tissue-culture-adapted, attenuated strain, designated WW, has also been utilized to produce a relapsing model of TMEV infection (191). When the DA strain is injected intracerebrally into SJL/J mice, it produces a biphasic illness characterized by an initial stage of gray matter involvement, similar to polio virus infection, followed by a chronic phase of inflammatory demyelination of spinal cord white matter (192). The polio-like phase lasts 2 to 4 weeks and is clinically characterized by flaccid paralysis. The second phase of infection, characterized by severe involvement of white matter, particularly of the spinal cord, is manifest clinically by spastic paralysis (192,193). In these animals, demyelinating lesions are well demarcated and are characterized by the presence, since inception, of lymphocytes, plasma cells, and macrophages. Axons are spared and oligodendrocytes appeared normal, at least in the initial phase of the demyelinating process (193). Involvement of the white matter is chronic, since fresh inflammatory demyelinating lesions may be found months after infection (192–194). Although virus can be isolated from clarified homogenates of the CNS, essentially for the life of the animal, viral titers are very low in the chronic phases of the disease (192,194). Pathological features in TMEV-infected animals closely resemble those of EAE, the prototype of immune-mediated models of demyelination. This suggested early on that an immune process was probably involved in the pathogenesis of myelin injury in this model (193). Immunosuppression experiments, using Cy and rabbit antithymocyte serum, strongly supported such hypothesis, since they were able to prevent inflammation and demyelination during the early phase of white matter involvement (195).

Most studies done at this institution in the last several years have utilized the BeAn8386 strain of TMEV because it produces the chronic, inflammatory-demyelinating phase of the disease, with minimal early involvement of gray matter (196). With this virus, demyelinating lesions have been shown to have a different appearance in different susceptible strains of mice. In SJL mice, BeAn produces a very severe inflammatory disease of white matter in which macrophages constitute the most important cellular elements both in terms of quantity and persistence in affected tissues. In these mice there is considerable destruction of both axons and glia-limiting membrane (GLM). Remyelination in these mice, therefore, is minimal and mainly accomplished by Schwann cells migrating through the damaged GLM (197,198). In other strains, such as SWR/J, NZW, and DBA 2, demyelination is accompanied by moderate inflammation with lower numbers of macrophages. Axons are well preserved and the GLM is minimally affected. Consequently, in these mice there is considerable remyelination, which is mainly carried out by oligodendrocytes with a minor Schwann cell component (197). A similar situation has recently been demonstrated in hybrids between resistant C57L/J and SJL/J animals (198). The resistant genotype in this strain combination appears capable of converting the severe form of disease, characteristic of SJL/J mice, into a more moderate disease characterized by moderate macrophage infiltration, almost no axonal compromise, and minimal damage of the GLM. These mice, therefore, show abundant successful oligodendroglia-mediated remyelination (198). These studies demonstrate how genetic regulation of susceptibility/resistance to the disease has direct bearing on the phenotypic expression of the disease process, not only in terms of demyelination but of remyelination as well. The role that the immune response may play in the remyelinating phase of the disease has also been explored. Miller et al. had shown that antibody to some yet unknown CNS epitope is able to stimulate remyelination by oligodendrocytes in DA-infected SJL/J mice (199). Such studies have been extended and the effects of a number of antibodies in promoting remyelination were recently explored. In general, these are IgM-kappa antibodies that recognize different oligodendrocyte antigens, and they all appear to promote remyelination. A similar antibody, but for a small region involved in oligodendroglial binding, is not able to bind to oligodendrocytes and does not stimulate remyelination. Since the targets of these different antibodies are different cell antigens, it does not appear that the promotion of remyelination is mediated through a single receptor; rather, it is most likely related to some immunological mechanism (200). These studies may have relevance to human disease as well, since stimulation of remyelination in MS patients could have an important therapeutic value.

Susceptibility and/or resistance to TMEV-induced demyelinating disease is genetically regulated and appears to be dependent on multiple genes. Both MHC and non-MHC genes have been found to have a role in determining susceptibility or resistance to the disease (201–204). While resistance may be dominant in certain hybrids between susceptible and resistant strains, in other hybrids, susceptibility can be the dominant trait. The most susceptible strains were found to be the SJL/J, DBA/1, and DBA/2, SWR, PL/J, and NZW. The most resistant strains are BALB/c, C57BL/6, C57BL/10, C57/L, and 129/J. Some strains with intermediate susceptibility are C3H, CBA, AKR, and C57BR (205,206). Several genetic loci associated with susceptibility to TMEV-induced demyelination have been mapped. The most critical loci for resistance/susceptibility map to the H-2D region of the major histocompatibility complex (MHC) (202,203). The H-2D-linked gene that controls resistance to the demyelinating disease, codes for a class I antigen and strongly suggests a role for CD8+ cells in clearing the virus. In general, strains that are resistant to demyelinating disease are able to clear the virus rather rapidly, in contrast to strains that are susceptible. Other loci with a role in susceptibility/resistance to TMEV-induced demyelination are the *Tmevd-1* locus on chromosome 6 (207,208), which has been mapped very near loci encoding the beta-chain of the T cell receptor, and the *Tmevd-2* locus on chromosome 3, found to be very close to the *Car-2* locus (209), and whose function is still unknown. It is of importance that two loci, that are related to susceptibility, i.e., *H-2D* and *Tmevd-1*, are also involved in T-cell regulation. This further supports the immune-mediated hypothesis of demyelination in this model. Another locus, *Tmevd-5*, located on chromosome 11, has recently been found to influence clinical disease (210). In fact, C57BL/6 mice with high viral loads, have higher probability to show symptoms when they are homozygous at *Tmvd-5*. Finally, two loci in a small area of chromosome 14 may be involved in controlling demyelination (211), and two loci. *Tmevp2* and *Tmevp3*, on the telomeric region of chromosome 10, appear to have a role in viral persistence (212). Finally, sex appears to have influence on susceptibility as well, since males have significantly higher incidence of disease than females (213)

Interestingly, resistance to the disease in some strains is not absolute and can be overcome with certain immunological manipulations. For instance, low-dose irradiation (214,215) or low-dose cyclophosphamide treatment (216) has been shown to turn a resistant strain to a susceptible one. However, resistance can be restored to cyclophosphamide-treated or irradiated animals by the adoptive transfer of syngeneic spleen cells from infected resistant, nontreated animals (217). It is possible that low-dose cyclophosphamide or irradiation may damage a suppressor cell population that normally keeps susceptibility in check, thus preventing the development of disease. This cell population appears to consist of CD8+-radiosensitive lymphocytes that act early during TMEV infection to establish resistance to demyelinating disease. This conclusion is supported by transfer studies of CD8+ lymphocytes from TMEV-resistant infected donors into resistant mice made susceptible by exposure to low-dose radiation. The recipient animals become again resistant to the disease (218).

The importance of CD8+ lymphocytes in resistance/susceptibility to disease is also supported by studies in β2M-deficient C57BL/6 mice, which lack class I expression and CD8+ lymphocytes. These normally resistant animals, without functional CD8+ cells, become susceptible and develop inflammatory-demyelinating lesions. Interestingly, they do not show clinical signs (219–221). These animals are less capable of clearing virus that the resistant control littermate; however, viral titers are not as high as seen in the susceptible SJL/J mice. Therefore, an increase in viral titers is not by itself responsible for the histological signs of disease. On the other hand, these mice show increased DTH responses as well as CD4+ cell proliferation to the virus, but apparently not to a sufficient degree to translate into clinical signs. If these animals are immunized with virus before infection, however, they develop both clinical and histological signs in parallel with further enhancement of TMEV-specific CD4+ T-cell responses without any effects on the viral load. The authors have suggested that viral immunization of β2M-deficient mice results in a magnification of the CD4+ T-cell response to a level sufficient for the expression of both clinical and pathological paramers of disease (221). The mechanism of induction of clinical signs in β2M-deficient mice is probably quite complex. For instance, recent studies comparing the clinical and pathological diseases in perforin-deficient mice, Fas mutation (lpr) mice, gld mice (carrying a Fas ligand mutation), and class II-deficient mice have suggested that perforin release by CD8+ lymphocytes may be implicated in the expression of clinical signs (222).

Persistence of the virus is necessary for chronic demyelination to take place. In addition to host factors, persistence may also be regulated at the viral level. Roos and his collaborators have shown that viral strains that produce chronic disease (the TO strains) have an additional initiation code to that observed in the acute GDVII virus. This initiation code, at nucleotide 1079, appears to direct the synthesis of a 17-kDa protein, designated L*, that seems to be important for the establishment of chronic TMEV infection (223). The same group of investigators has recently reported that L* protein has antiapoptotic activity in macrophages, thus promoting virus persistence in these cells (224). Another determinant of viral persistence has been localized to the leader P1 (capsid) sequences. Studies using recombinant viruses, in which BeAn sequences are progressively substituted for GDVII sequences, suggest that viral persistence may depend on a conformational determinant requiring homologous sequences in the regions of both the VP2 puff and the VP1 loop (225).

The genetic influence on host susceptibility to TMEV-induced demyelinating disease supports the hypothesis of immune-mediated myelin injury in this model. In addition, numerous studies in the last several years have strongly suggested that cell-mediated host immune responses play a major role in the development of disease. Such studies may be summarized as follows:

1.   No direct relationship between anti-TMEV antibody and development of disease has been found. In parallel with viral titers, anti-TMEV antibodies were analyzed in resistant, versus susceptible strains. Both showed a rise in the antiviral antibody response in a similar manner, indicating that serum immunity has a minor role in the establishment of white matter disease (196,204,206,226).

2.   Studies of the distribution of viral antigen in acute and chronic lesions of susceptible animals suggest that most cell types in the CNS are susceptible to infection. It appears that initially, the process of demyelination is not accompanied by the presence of viral antigen in oligodendroglial cells (186), while at later times viral antigen is found in these cells (227,228). The role of viral infection of oligodendrocytes is not clear and is being investigated in several laboratories. There are indirect data, however, suggesting that infection of myelin-producing cells does not have a primary role in the production of myelin degeneration in this model. Such data come from studies of recurrent demyelination in CD-1 mice infected with WW virus, and in C3H mice infected with DA virus. In these animals, prominent remyelination by Schwann cells was observed in spinal cord white matter, and recurrent demyelination was seen in several of these remyelinated areas. Again, immunohistochemical studies failed to show the presence of viral antigen in Schwann cells in areas undergoing recurrent demyelination (229). Also, a study of differential disappearance of MBP and myelin-associated glycoprotein (MAG) in early demyelinating lesions of TMEV infection showed that MAG was relatively preserved while MBP in central-type myelin and PO in peripheral-type myelin, could no longer be visualized (230). Since MAG is localized in the periaxonal oligodendroglial component of the myelin sheath, these findings support the contention that the oligodendroglial cell is still intact in the initial phases of myelin destruction. Iit appears that infection of oligodendrocytes, demonstrated both in vitro and in vivo (227,231,232), may be only a secondary factor in the process leading to myelin destruction. On the other hand, macrophages carry large amounts of viral antigen during both acute and chronic demyelinating phases of the

disease (186,233). This is important, since they are professional antigen-presenting cells and may therefore perpetuate a T cell–mediated immune response. In fact, macrophages have recently been recognized as the principal cells to express class II antigens in the CNS of mice with TMEV-induced demyelination. Macrophages also showed upregulation of both costimulatory molecules B7-1 and B7-2, in contrast to CD4+ T cells that only expressed B7-2. Most importantly, macrophages freshly isolated from the CNS of these mice were capable of activating a TMEV epitope-specific T-cell line without the need of added antigen. This is strong indication that a continuous endogenous processing and presentation of viral antigens is taking place in the CNS of TMEV persistently infected mice (234).

The importance of macrophages in the pathogenesis of the disease has also been underscored by experiments aimed at depleting macrophages with either silica or dichloromethylene diphosphonate. Animals treated with those substances show either greatly decreased or no demyelination (235,236). Recent studies have also shown that infected macrophages and microglia from susceptible animals but not from resistant animals secrete a serine protease with proteolytic degrading activity on myelin basic protein, suggesting a direct mechanism of injury by macrophage products on myelin sheaths (237). Cash et al. have shown that most infected cells of the CNS contain a low amount of viral RNA and do not synthetize detectable levels of capsid proteins (187). They suggest that such restriction of viral RNA and capsid protein synthesis may help explain TMEV persistence in infected tissues. The role of macrophages in viral persistence is being investigated in our and other laboratories. So far, data are mainly derived form in vitro studies with macrophage-like cells rather than primary cultures of microglia or macrophages. Studies with these macrophage-like cells suggest that mature differentiated cells, such as BSC-1 and M1 myeloid cells, develop a restricted viral infection as well as changes indicative of apoptosis (238,239). So far, studies in our laboratory with primary cultures of microglial cells and macrophages from SJL/J mice have failed to show significant viral replication in these cells; however, they undergo a limited amount of apoptosis. In contrast, active replication of virus has been observed in astrocytes, while no apoptosis has been observed in these cells. It appears, therefore, that apoptosis is mainly found in restrictive cells rather than in permissive cells.

3. A clear relationship between cell-mediated immune parameters and TMEV-induced demyelination has been proven. Among the various immunological parameters that have been investigated, the one most consistently correlating with susceptibility to TMEV-induced demyelinating disease is the capacity to develop a delayed-type hypersensitivity (DTH) response to viral antigens (204,206,226). Only susceptible strains, in fact, show consistent and significant levels of anti-TMEV DTH responses. During the first phase of the disease, only antiviral DTH responses are found, while no responses can be elicited to various myelin antigens such as MBP or proteolipid protein (PLP), both well recognized encephalitogens for the induction of EAE (240,241). There findings supports previous studies in which cells from infected susceptible animals repeatedly stimulated with CNS myelin but failed to demyelinate organotypic spinal cord syngeneic cultures (242); this speaks further against a role for an EAE-like mechanism of demyelination during the acute phase of TMEV infection.

The above studies suggest an important role for Th1 lymphocytes, a subpopulation of CD4+, class II–restricted T cells known to be involved in DTH responses in the pathogenesis of myelin injury. They correlate with recent investigations on the effects of intravenous tolerization to either myelin or viral antigens on the subsequent development of disease in EAE and TMEV infection respectively (243–248). While tolerization to myelin basic protein (MBP) was able to abolish the DTH response to this antigen and to prevent the development of EAE, tolerization to the same protein in TMEV-infected animals had no effect on the development of virus-induced demyelination. Conversely, tolerization of TMEV-infected animals with viral antigens prevented development of anti-virus DTH and dramatically decreased the frequency and severity of virus-induced demyelination, while the same treatment had no effect on EAE animals (248). These experiments suggest that myelin injury is mediated by DTH responses in both models. However, while the DTH response in EAE is driven by myelin antigens, it is mainly elicited by viral antigens in the first phase of TMEV infection.

In contrast to the limitation of the DTH response to viral epitopes during the first phase of the disease, there is significant spreading of epitope responses to myelin antigens during the chronic phase of the infection (249). This phenomenon must be the most exciting discovery in regard to this model since the last edition of this book. Starting 3 to 4 weeks after the onset of disease, there is an ordered progression of emerging CD4+ T-cell responses to several myelin epitopes as judged by T-cell stimulation assays and DTH responses to such epitopes. The first responses are noted at around day 50 postinfection against myelin proteolipid protein (PLP) 139–151, which is the major encephalitogenic epitope of PLP. By day 164, epitope spreading is noted against the less dominant PLP 56–70, PLP 178–191, and MOG 92–106 epitopes. This orderly emergence of different epitope responses recapitulates a similar spreading in the model of EAE, and, like in that model, it follows a hierarchical order of decreasing encephalitogenicity. Most recently, we investigated whether the emergence of a T-cell response to the major encephalitogenic epitope of PLP has functional significance. We tested lymphocytes from chronically infected TMEV animals for their capacity to demyelinate organotypic cultures after stimulation with the major encephalitogenic epitope of PLP and, as a comparison, MBP and ovalbumin. While cells stimulated with MBP or with ovalbumin produced no demyelination of the myelinated cultures, cells stimulated with PLP produced severe demyelination, supporting a functional role for epitope spreading from viral to myelin antigens during the chronic phase of TMEV infection (250).

A primary role for Th1 lymphocytes in this demyelinating model has also been supported by in vitro studies on lymphokine production by lymphocytes from TMEV-immunized mice. These studies have shown that lymphocytes from lymph nodes of mice immunized with TMEV produce IL-2, lymphotoxin, and IFN-γ but not IL-4, IL-6 or IL-10, suggesting they belong to the Th1 subset of CD4+ cells, the subset which is primarily responsible for DTH responses (247,251). Similarly, the antibody response in susceptible mice is mainly represented by antibodies of the IgG-2a subclass, which is characteristically dependent on Th1 stimulation (247,252). The situation is somewhat different in the CNS itself, as shown by more recent studies examining the differential expression of cytokines in the CNS of SJL/J mice infected with TMEV (253). There was expression of IFN-γ, TNF-α, IL-10, and IL-4 mRNA during the preclinical phase of TMEV infection. Afterwards, the levels of these cytokines continued to increase during the chronic phase of the disease, and this correlates with the continuous presence of both lymphocytes and macrophages in the CNS of affected animals. This contrasts with the situation in relapsing EAE, where both IFN-γ and TNF-α peak at the height of the acute disease while they decrease during remission. IL-10, on the other hand, was continuously expressed in both TMEV and EAE, suggesting that it does not have a significant regulatory role in either disease (253). In vivo studies comparing cytokine production in susceptible versus resistant mice were also done in the model produced by the DA strain of TMEV. During the chronic demyelinating phase of the disease, susceptible but not resistant animals showed the presence of both viral genome and Th1-type cytokines mRNA. The expression of Th2-type cytokine mRNA, on the other hand, was variable, and it did not correlate with susceptibility or resistance to the demyelinating disease (254). Karpus et al. have also looked at the expression of a number of chemokines during TMEV infection. They found that several chemokines increase as the infection proceeds, but two in particular appear to correlate quite well with the development of clinical signs: MCP-1 and MIP-1α (255). However, when antibodies to these chemokines were used, only antibody to MCP-1 decreased the clinical expression of the disease, suggesting that this chemokine may have functional significance (Karpus, personal communication).

The functional role of various inflammatory mediators on oligodendrocytes and astrocytes from susceptible mice was recently studied in vitro (256). These studies showed that oligodendrocytes from susceptible animals are susceptible to infection; however, they do not show effects of cytopathic activity. In contrast, immortalized oligodendrocytes, which are arrested at an early developmental stage, proved to susceptible to cytolysis. In addition, TNF-α, IL-1α, and INF-γ were tested for their capacity to kill immortalized or adult oligodendrocytes. TNF-α was the only one capable of inducing cytotoxicity in immortalized oligodendrocytes but not in primary adult oligodendrocytes. However, it caused significant decrease in expression of mRNA for MBP and MOG in the latter cells, indicating that it may cause dysfunction of adult oligodendrocytes. These results support the hypothesis of DTH-mediated virus-induced demyelination (256).

It is of interest that astrocytes have also been found to be potentially capable of antigen presentation during TMEV infection. Astrocytes treated with INF-γ, were capable of processing and presenting various TMEV epitopes to virus specific T-cell hybridomas as well as bulk T cells. In addition, astrocyte-mediated T-cell activation was followed by T cell–mediated apoptosis of the astrocytes (257). These studies suggest an immunoregulatory role by these cells in the process of TMEV-induced demyelination.

Several viral epitopes could be involved in eliciting DTH responses in infected mice, and it is possible that both major and minor epitopes may play a role in disease pathogenesis. One major epitope in susceptible SJL/J mice has been identified in the VP2 nucleocapsid protein, between amino acids 74 and 86 (258). In fact, 80 to 90% of the DTH response by SJL/J mice to TMEV is directed against this portion of the virus (252,258,259). The importance of this major epitope in disease pathogenesis was highlighted by recent studies demonstrating that a specific Th1 lymphocytic line raised against it was able to increase the incidence and severity of disease in mice injected with suboptimal doses of TMEV (251). Several studies have also suggested that epitopes on VP1 may be important in the process of demyelination (260–264). A recent study has investigated DTH viral epitopes on VP1, VP2, and VP3. While each of these capsid proteins has DTH epitopes, it is of interest that only T cells reactive to VP1 and VP2 accelerate the development of demyelination. Cytokine profiles of T cells specific for the three-capsid protein correlate with such findings, since T cells reactive to VP1 and VP2 secrete cytokines of the Th1 subtype while T cells reactive to VP3 show the profile of Th2 cells (265). Taken together, the above studies lend support to the important role of CD4+ T-cell responses in disease pathogenesis through DTH mediated mechanisms.

4.   Injection of immune-modulating monoclonal antibodies into infected animals strongly supports a role for helper T lymphocytes in the development of disease. Several attempts have been made to modify the clinical and pathological expression of the demye-

linating process, by using antibodies to T helper, T suppressor/cytotoxic cells, and to Ia antigens (class II antigens). Treatment with antibody to Ia antigen, at the time of virus inoculation, or after development of inflammation, partially suppressed demyelination, independently from alterations in viral or serum antibody titers (266,267). Ia molecules are predominantly expressed by B lymphocytes, certain activated T cells, macrophages, and possibly other antigen-presenting cells in the CNS. They are crucial for the process of antigen presentation, for the proliferation of class II–restricted T lymphocytes, and for some T cell–B cell as well as T cell–T cell interactions, that are part of the immune response. Decrease in demyelination after blocking of these surface antigens demonstrates that immune mechanisms are, in fact, crucial for the production of myelin injury.

Experiments with antibodies to more specific cell populations have given somewhat mixed results. Thus, Welsh et al. reported that treatment of TMEV infection with anti-L3T4 antibody—specific for T helper cells—before the demyelinating phase of the disease significantly reduced the incidence of demyelination in CBA mice (268). Treatment prior to infection, on the other hand, produced high mortality, possibly because of failure of the animals to clear the virus. Similar results were reported in BeAn-infected SJL/J mice after depletion of CD4+ cells. A significant decrease in the number of mice developing disease and milder disease in the animals that became sick were observed in these experiments (251). These studies further support a role for CD4+ cells in the pathogenesis of the disease and correlate with studies indicating that essentially all lymphocytes expressing IL-2 receptors in the CNS of TMEV-infected mice are CD4+, while CD8+ lymphocytes found in the same infiltrates do not express IL-2 receptors (251). Since expression of IL-2 receptors is an important indicator of lymphocyte activation, these results strongly support an important effector role for T helper cells in TMEV-induced demyelination and suggest that CD8+ cells may represent a bystander cell population with no significant involvement in the process of demyelination. Contrasting results were obtained, however, by Rodriguez and Sriram, who reported the prevention of disease after inoculation of antibody to CD8+ cells, rather than CD4+ lymphocytes (269). Such discrepancy is probably due to the use of different strains of mice and different viral isolates and antibody preparations.

A number of possibilities may be considered among immune mechanisms of myelin injury (202). The best-known mechanism is autoimmune sensitization against myelin antigens, such as MBP and/or PLP, as classically postulated in EAE (103,271). Such a mechanism, as discussed earlier, does not appear to play a role during the acute phase of TMEV-induced demyelinating disease, but it may have an important role during the chronic phase, when DTH responses begin to emerge against PLP and MOG epitopes (249).

Another mechanism could be injury to oligodendrocytes following a cytotoxic T-cell attack on viral antigens expressed on the surface of these cells. We believe this mechanism is not the primary cause of myelin injury in this model (2,193,226). TMEV is a nonenveloped virus, which does not mature by budding through the cell surface of infected cells. However, it is known that cytotoxic T cells may be able to kill virus-infected cells, which are not known to express glycosylated viral proteins on their surface (272). Moreover, in vitro T-cytotoxic activity has recently been demonstrated against cells infected with another picornavirus, Coxsackievirus group B (273). Since cytotoxic T cells are restricted by determinants of the H-2 class I region, such as H-2D, which are involved in disease susceptibility in this model, a role for direct cytotoxic T-cell attack on oligodendrocytes cannot be excluded and needs further study.

It has recently been suggested that myelin could be destroyed by an antiviral response because of the possibility of antigenic similarities between myelin proteins and viral proteins (274). Although such similarities have been noted both with viruses that may produce postinfectious encephalomyelitis and with viruses that do not, such a hypothesis of "molecular mimicry" has received considerable attention and deserves further study. Although not confirmed, cross-reactivity has recently been observed between TMEV and galactocerebroside (275).

We initially suggested that an important mechanism of myelin injury in Theiler's, and possibly other viral models may be that of nonspecific myelin injury, in the presence of an immune attack against viral antigens in the vicinity of myelinated axons (2,193,226). Recently, the discovery that DTH response to the virus is the parameter that best correlates with disease susceptibility has further strengthened this hypothesis and refined its possible mechanism of action (226). It is postulated that T cells involved in DTH interact with virus-infected macrophages, which, as previously noted, are cells carrying a large proportion of viral antigen for many months after viral inoculation (186,233). This cellular interaction would stimulate lymphokine release, with additional recruitment of macrophages in the infected areas and nonspecific macrophage-mediated demyelination. Although a bystander mechanism of demyelination could not been demonstrated in the peripheral nervous system (276), it was shown to be effective in the CNS by Wisniewski and Bloom (277) and by Holoshitz et al. (278). A mechanism of nonspecific myelin injury through a DTH response to viral antigens could explain the occurrence of similar myelin pathology in different, unrelated experimental viral infections and possibly in humans as well.

Relevance to MS

TMEV infection is considered among the best models of human MS for several reasons. Theiler's virus is a natural pathogen for mice and normally produces a chronic persistent infection in its natural host. There is great similarity in the pathological features of the two diseases in both the acute and chronic/relapsing phases. Although TMEV can be isolated from infected mice long after inoculation, there is no direct correlation between the amount of virus present in the tissue and the severity of the demyelinating disease. Such uncoupling, between presence of virus and demyelinating pathology parallels the situation in MS, in which viruses, although believed to play a role (279,280), cannot be isolated with regularity.

III. ACUTE VIRAL MODELS OF DEMYELINATION

Several models have been described, in which demyelinating pathology is short-lived, either because the infection is fatal in the span of a few weeks or because the demyelinating process itself may only lasts for a short period of time (2).

Viruses that have been reported to be associated with an acute, or subacute demyelinating course include ts mutants of vesicular stomatitis virus (VSV) (281,282), a ts mutant of Chandipura virus (283), Venezuelan equine encephalomyelitis virus (VEEV) (284), and Semliki Forest virus (SFV) (285). These models show varying degrees of primary demyelination associated with inflammatory infiltrates. An immune pathogenesis has been postulated in some of them based on both morphological and immunological data (2).

A. Semliki Forest Virus Infection

SFV is an alphavirus of the family Togaviridae (286). It is an enveloped virus, first isolated
from mosquitos in Uganda in 1942 (287). While the virulent WT-virus causes an acute
fatal encephalitis in young mammals, several avirulent strains have been isolated and
utilized by different investigators to produce a slower yet short-lived form of demyelinating disease of the CNS in adult mice (288–295). There are some important differences
between the demyelinating encephalitis produced by SFV and that produced by chronic
models, such as those of CV and Theiler's virus. The lesions produced by SFV are generally smaller, the inflammatory infiltrates are less prominent, and demyelinated axons are
generally mixed with additional alterations, such as vacuolar or outright necrotic changes
(288). A distinct advantage of this model over the others, however, is the possibility of
infecting animals by a peripheral route rather than by intracerebral injection.

The pathogenesis of demyelination in SFV infection is controversial and, in fact,
may be different for different strains of viruses or in mice of different ages. Thus, Sheahan
et al., utilizing the avirulent M136 and M9 viruses, concluded that the demyelinating
pathology is due to direct attack by the virus on oligodendroglial cells (288,289). In contrast, a group of investigators at the Rayne Institute in London, have proposed that demyelination produced by the avirulent A7(74) virus is immune-mediated (290–293). Berger
also favors an immune pathogenesis in this model (294). Data from experiments spanning
the last 15 years support such a hypothesis. For instance, the London group (295,296)
could not demonstrate the same degree of SFV tropism for oligodendrocytes, which Sheahan et al. had shown with M136 an M9 strains (288,289); morphological studies have
shown both anatomical and temporal relationships between lymphocytes and pathological
changes of myelin (296); virus is not detected after 10 days postinoculation, while demyelination is maximal after virus clearance at 14 to 21 days postinoculation (297); immunosuppression of infected mice by prior irradiation prevents inflammation and demyelination
(298,299); similarly, treatment with cycloleucine, a nonmetabolizable amino acid, which
produces thymic atrophy and abrogates thymus-dependent immune responses, prevents
demyelination (300); adoptive transfer experiments in nude mice suggest that T lymphocytes are necessary for demyelination (301). Recently, Webb et al. reported that brain-
derived SFV is recognized by antiglycolipid antibodies and suggested that glycolipids of
host-cell derivation on the viral surface may be able to trigger an autoimmune reaction
(302–304). Atkins and Sheahan concluded that a direct oligodendroglial attack is probably
important in the first phase of the infection, while later on demyelination may be produced
by an EAE-like, autoimmune attack against myelin components (305). In line with this
hypothesis, recent studies by Mokhtarian and Swoveland have shown that SFV infection
predisposes EAE-resistant mice to develop an EAE-like disease after immunization with
MBP (306). They suggest that the infection somehow primed the host for an autoimmune
reaction against CNS components. Similar results have been published by Wu et al., using
the avirulent A7 strain of SFV and BALB/c mice, which are ordinarily resistant to EAE
(307). Eralinna et al. and Soilu-Hanninen et al. have recently investigated this mechanism
of EAE facilitation by SFV infection. They demonstrated productive infection of endothelial cells, and concluded that SFV facilitates EAE development in resistant murine strains,
such as BALB/c, by increasing CNS vascular permeability to inflammatory cells, more
than by immunoregulatory changes (308,309).

One of the possible mechanisms for virus-induced demyelination is that of shared
epitopes between the virus and one of the myelin components (molecular mimicry). This

phenomenon has been investigated by Mokhtarina et al. in C57B16/J mice. Aminoacid homologies were identified between the E2 SFV peptide 115–129 and MOG peptide 18–32. Both these peptides were able to induce a later-onset EAE-like disease with pathology reminiscent of that observed in SFV infection. No cross-reactivity was observed with other myelin antigens, such as PLP or MBP. The authors conclude that the cross-reactivity between SFV E2 and MOG may be an important contributor to the process of demyelination in this model (310).

Jenkins et al. investigated the possible role of T cells or related factors in the axoplasmic transport of virus before production of myelin injury. They suggest that the immune response may be important in modulating both viral transport and the pathological process leading to demyelination (311). Subsequent studies by these investigators on optic nerves from mice infected with the A7(74) virus have shown that oligodendrocytes in demyelinating lesions are not necessarily killed by direct cytopathic effect. Changes in these cells would rather suggest dedifferentiation, with the possibility that the same cells could be involved in remyelination of the characteristic focal demyelinating lesions (312). The role of the immune response in demyelination produced by SFV has been investigated by several groups. Mokhtarian et al. analyzed the immune responses during SFV infection of SJL/J and C57BL/6 mice, which are susceptible and resistant to EAE respectively. Their studies supported an important role for the host immune response in this infection since, following viral clearance, immune responses to both SFV and myelin basic protein (MBP) were significantly higher and more prolonged in SJL/J mice than in the EAE resistant strain (313). More recently, it has been determined that CD8+ cells are the most important lymphocytes in the pathogenesis of demyelination in this model. Depletion of CD8+ lymphocytes, in fact, prevents SFV-induced demyelination (314). A temporal study of both cellular and cytokines response in the CNS of mice infected with A7(74) virus has yielded interesting results. CD8+ cells dominated the mononuclear infiltrates in the brain from 3 days and were maximal during clearance of the virus. During the subsequent phase of demyelination, macrophages/microglia and CD45/B220+ B lymphocytes were the most numerous in the involved CNS. MHC class I antigens, IL-1α and β, IL-10, and TGF-β1 were upregulated early on day 3, while IL-2 and TNF-α were first observed at day 7 at the time of the most intense cellular infiltrates. Just prior to the demyelinating phase of the disease, at about day 10 postinfection, INF-γ and IL-6 were observed. No distinct bias toward either Th1 or Th2 cytokines was observed in this model; however, the temporal distribution of a number of cytokines that are known to be upregulated during various inflammatory demyelinating processes, including MS, strongly suggests a role for these soluble immune mediators in the pathogenesis of SFV-induced demyelination (315). These conclusions are consistent with a study that utilized the M9 mutant of SFV and compared susceptible and resistant mice in regards to viral persistence and cytokine profiles. While viral RNA could be seen up to 90 days in both BALB/c and SJL/J mice, there were significant differences in the presence of mRNA for INF-γ and TNF-α between the two strains. Cytokines mRNA was only seen up to 28 days in BALB/c mice, in which demyelination is rapidly repaired and does not persist, but for as long as 90 days in SJL/J mice in which demyelination may be present for longer times. The presence of proinflammatory cytokines in the absence of viral genome suggests a role for immune mechanisms of demyelination (316).

In the last few years, studies have focused on the molecular characterization of functional epitopes on the E-2 envelope glycoprotein of SFV, and on their possible role in eliciting immune responses. Both T cell and antibody responses have been explored and found to be mediated by specific sequences in the E2 envelope glycoprotein (317–319). Mutations in the E-2 envelope component have been studied to better define mechanisms of viral entry, viral maturation and viral pathogenicity for infected mice (320,321). An interesting conclusion from these studies is that mutations may affect pathogenicity by modulating the level of direct virus-induced neuronal damage and death. Recent studies have also looked at sequences that would result in avirulent variants of SFV, such as the demyelinating A7 strain. Results of sequencing studies and from the construction of various chimeras containing virulent SFV4 and avirulent SFV A7 sequences have shown that the determination of the avirulent phenotype is polygenic and depends on the additive effect of sequences form both the structural and nonstructural regions of the viral genome (322).

Relevance to MS

These infections, particularly the SFV model, are of interest because of their possible immune-mediated pathogenesis and deserve to be pursued further. Their only limitation is their relatively short course

IV. CONCLUSIONS

Epidemiological, virological, and immunological data suggest a possible combined viral-immune pathogenesis in multiple sclerosis (279,280,323–326). Although evidence is circumstantial, such a hypothesis enjoys considerable support and justifies the enthusiasm by several groups of investigators for viral models of demyelination. Because of the chronic nature of MS, chronic models of demyelination are obviously the most relevant. Some of these models, however, are cumbersome and limited to species that are not genetically defined, and, therefore, not amenable to sophisticated immunological manipulations. Visna and canine distemper infections are the best representatives of this group.

HSV is important because it has the capacity to persist in humans for the life of the individual. The pathological features of the lesions in its experimental models, however, and the course of the demyelinating disease produced by HSV infection are quite different from those of MS. Since the last edition of this book, models of HSV-induced demyelination have shown the least amount of progress.

There is little doubt that the murine models of CV and TMEV infection are, at present, the most relevant to human MS. They are both chronic, and relapses have been described in both infections. The pathological lesions in these models resemble those of MS. This may be especially appreciated in the TMEV model in which inflammation and demyelination are closely related, both temporally and anatomically, as in the acute lesions of MS (327). In view of the prevailing view that an environmental factor, most likely one or more viruses, could trigger the process of inflammatory destruction of myelin upon acting on the appropriate genetic background (279,325,326,328–330), it is not surprising that viral models of demyelination have been enjoying considerable increase in popularity during the last two decades.

ACKNOWLEDGMENTS

Supported by NIH grant NS-13011 and RG 2893 from the NMSS.

REFERENCES

1. Martin JR, Nathanson N. Animal models of virus-induced demyelination. In: Zimmerman HM, ed. Progress in Neuropathology. New York: Raven Press, 1979, pp. 27–50.
2. Dal Canto MC, Rabinowitz SG. Experimental models of virus-induced demyelination of the central nervous system. Ann Neurol 1982; 11:109–127.
3. Norrby E, Oxman MN. Measles virus. In: Fields BN, Knipe DM, eds. Fields Virology. New York: Raven Press 1990, pp. 1013–1044.
4. Koestner A, Long JF. Ultrastructure of canine distemper virus in explant tissue cultures of canine cerebellum. Lab Invest 1970; 23:196–201.
5. Raine CS. On the development of CNS lesions in natural canine distemper encephalomyelitis. J Neurol Sci 1976; 30:13–28.
6. Appel MJG. Pathogenesis of canine distemper. Am J Vet Res 1969; 30:1167–1182.
7. Wisniewski H, Raine CS, Kay WJ. Observations on viral demyelinating encephalomyelitis: Canine distemper. Lab Invest 1972; 26:589–599.
8. Vandevelde M, Zurbriggen A, Dumas M, Palmer D. Canine distemper does not infect oligodendrocytes in vitro. J Neurol Sci 1985; 69:133–137.
9. Zurbriggen A, Yamawaki M, Vandevelde M. Restricted canine distemper virus infection of oligodendrocytes. Lab Invest 1993; 68:277–284.
10. Graber HU, Muller CF, Vandevelde M, Zurbriggen A. Restricted infection with canine distemper virus leads to downregulation of myelin gene transcription in cultured oligodendrocytes. Acta Neuropathol 1995; 90:312–318.
11. Glaus T, Griot C, Richard A, Althaus U, Herschkowitz N, Vandevelde M. Ultrastructural and biochemical findings in brain cell cultures infected with canine distemper virus. Acta Neuropathol 1990; 80:59–67.
12. Zurbriggen A, Vandevelde M, Dumas M. Secondary degeneration of oligodendrocytes in canine distemper virus infection in vitro. Lab Invest 1986; 54:424–431.
13. Zurbriggen A, Vandevelde M, Bollo E. Demyelinating, non-demyelinating and attenuated canine distemper virus strains induce oligodendroglial cytolysis in vitro. J Neurol Sci 1987; 79:33–41.
14. Zurbriggen A, Vandevelde M, Bollo E. Demyelinating, non demyelinating and attenuated canine distemper virus strains induce oligodendroglial cytolysis in vitro. J Neurol Sci 1987; 79:33–41.
15. Rima BK, Duffy N, Mitchell WJ, Summers BA, Appel MJG. Correlation between humoral immune responses and presence of virus in the CNS in dogs experimentally infected with canine distemper virus. Arch Virol 1991; 121:1–8.
16. Duffy PE. Functional implications of astrocyte metabolism. In: Astrocytes: Normal, Reactive and Neoplastic. New York: Raven Press, 1983, pp. 39–41.
17. Zurbriggen A, Vandevelde M, Dumas M, Griot C, Bollo E. Oligodendroglial pathology in canine distemper virus infection in vitro. Acta Neuropathol (Berl) 1987; 74:366–373.
18. Summers BA, Greisen HA, Appel MJG. Early events in canine distemper demyelinating encephalomyelitis. Acta Neuropathol (Berl) 1979; 46:1–10.
19. Higgins RJ, Krakowka SG, Metzler AE, Koestner A. Primary demyelination in experimental canine distemper virus-induced encephalomyelitis in gnotobiotic dogs: Sequential immunologic and morphologic findings. Acta Neuropathol (Berl) 1982; 58:1–8.
20. Vandevelde M, Zurbriggen A, Higgins RJ, Palmer D. Spread and distribution of viral antigen in nervous canine distemper. Acta Neuropathol (Berl) 1985; 67:211–218.
21. Summers BA, Appel MJG. Demyelination in canine distemper encephalomyelitis: An ultrastructural analysis. J Neurocytol 1987; 16:871–881.
22. Zurbriggen A, Schmid I, Graber HU, Vandevelde M. Oligodendroglial pathology in canin distemper. Acta Neuropathol 1998; 95:71–77.
23. Bollo E, Zurbriggen A, Vandevelde M, Fankhauser R. Canine distemper virus clearance in chronic inflammatory demyelination. Acta Neuropathol 1986; 72:69–73.

24. Griot-Wenk M, Griot C, Pfister H, Vandevelde M. Antibody-dependent cellular cytotoxicity in anrtimyelin antibody-induced oligodendrocyte damage in vitro. J Neuroimmunol 1991; 33:145–155.

25. Griot C, Burge T, Vandevelde M, Peterhans E. Antibody-induced generation of reactive oxygen radicals by brain macrophages in canince distemper encephalitis: A mechanism of bystander demyelination. Acta Neuropathol 1989; 78:396–403.

26. Alldinger S, Wunschmann A, Baumgartner W, Voss C, Kremmer E. Up-regulation of major histocompatibility complex class II antigen expression in the central nervous system of dogs with spontaneous canine distemper encephalitis. Acta Neuropathol 1996; 92:273–280.

27. Wunschmann A, Alldinger S, Kremmer E, Baumgartner W. Identification of CD4+ and CD8+ T cell subsets and B cells in the brain of dogs with spontaneous acute, subacute, and chronic demyelinating distemper encephalitis. Vet Immunol Immunopathol 1999; 67:101–116.

28. Tipold A, Moore P, Zurbriggen A, Burgener I, Barben G, Vandevelde M. Early T cell response in the central nervous system in canine distemper virus infection. Acta Neuropathol 1999; 97:4–56.

29. Frisk AL, Baumgartner W, Grone A. Dominating interleukin-10 mRNA expression induction in cerebrospinal fluid cells of dogs with natural canine distemper virus induced demyelinating and nondemyelinating CNS lesions. J Neuroimmunol 1999; 97:102–109.

30. Summers BA, Whitaker JN, Appel MJG. Demyelinating canine distemper encephalomyelitis: Measurement of myelin basic protein in cerebrospinal fluid. J Neuroimmunol 1987; 14:227–233.

31. Lisak RP, Zweiman B, Whitaker JN. Spinal fluid basic protein immunoreactive material and spinal fluid lymphocyte reactivity to basic protein. Neurology 1981; 31:180–182.

32. Johnson RT. Inflammatory and demyelinating diseases. In: Viral Infections of the Nervous System. New York: Raven Press, 1982, pp. 247–251.

33. Cook SD, Dowling PC. A possible association between house pets and multiple sclerosis. Lancet 1977; 1:980–982.

34. Cook SD, Natelson BH, Levin BE, Chavis PS, Dowling PC. Further evidence of a possible association between house dogs and multiple sclerosis. Ann Neurol 1978; 3:141–143.

35. Gilden DH, Wellish M, Rorke LB, Wroblewska Z. Canine distemper virus infection of weanling mice: Pathogenesis of CNS disease. J Neurol Sci 1981; 52:327–339.

36. McIntosh K. Coronaviruses: A comparative review. Curr Top Microbiol Immunol 1974; 63:85–129.

37. Siddell SG, Wege H, ter Meulen V. The biology of coronaviruses. J Gen Virol 1983; 64:761–776.

38. Tanaka R, Iwasaki Y, Koprowski H. Intracisternal virus-like particles in brain of a multiple sclerosis patient J Neurol Sci 1976; 128:121–126.

39. Burks JS, DeVald BL, Jankovsky LD, Gerdes JC. Two coronaviruses isolated from central nervous system tissue of two multiple sclerosis patients. Science 1980; 209:933–934.

40. Murray RS, MacMillan B, Burks JS. Detection of coronavirus genome in the CNS of MS patients and control patients. Neurology 1987; 37(suppl 1):109.

41. Murray RS, Brown BS, Brian D, Cabirac GF. Detection of coronavirus RNA and antigen in multiple sclerosis brain. Ann Neurol 1992; 31:525–533.

42. Lai MMC, Stohlman SA. RNA of mouse hepatitis virus. J Virol 1978; 26:236–242.

43. Lai MMC, Baric RS, Brayton PR, Stohlman SA. Characterization of leader RNA sequences on the virion and mRNAs on mouse hepatits virus, a cytoplasmic RNA virus. Proc Natl Acad Sci USA 1984; 81:3626–3630.

44. Lavi E, Murray EM, Makino S, Stohlman SA, Lai MM, Weiss SR. Determinants of coronavirus MHV pathogenesis are localized to 3' portion of the genome as determined by ribonucleic acid–ribonucleic acid recombination. Lab Invest 1990; 62:570–578.

45. Massa PT, Wege H, ter Meulen V. Analysis of murine hepatitis virus (JHM strain) tropism toward Lewis rat glial cells in vitro. Lab Invest 1986; 55:318–327.

46. Pasick JM, Dales S. Infection by coronavirus JHM of rat neurons and oligodendrocyte-type-2 astrocyte lineage cells during distinct developmental stages. J Virol 1991; 65:5013–5028.

47. Wang FI, Hinton DR, Gilmore W, Trousdale MD, Fleming JO. Sequential infection of glial cells by the murine hepatitis virus JHM strain (MHV-4) leads to a characteristic distribution of demyelination. Lab Invest 1992; 66:744–754.

48. Cheever FS, Daniels JB, Pappenheimer AM, Bailey OT. A murine virus (JHM) causing disseminated encephalomyelitis with extensive destruction of myelin: I. Isolation and biological properties of the virus. J Exp Med 1949; 90:181–194.

49. LP. Weiner. Pathogenesis of demyelination induced by a mouse hepatitis virus (JHM virus). Arch Neurol 1973; 28:298–303.

50. Lampert PW, Sims JK, Kniazeff AJ. Mechanism of demyelination in JHM virus encephalomyelitis. Electron microscopic studies. Acta Neuropathol (Berl) 1973; 24:76–85.

51. Herndon RM, Griffin DE, McCormick U, Weiner LP. Mouse hepatitis virus-induced recurrent demyelination: A preliminary report. Arch Neurol 1975; 32:32–35.

52. Stohlman SA, Weiner LP. Stability of neurotropic mouse hepatitis virus (JHM strain) during chronic infection of neuroblastoma cells. Arch Virol 1978; 57:53–61.

53. Stohlman SA, Brayton PR, Fleming JO, Weiner LP, Lai MMC. Murine coronaviruses: isolation and characterization of two plaque morphology variants of the JHM neurotropic strain. J Gen Virol 1982; 63:265–275.

54. Erlich SS, Fleming JO, Stohlman SA, Weiner LP. Experimental neuropathology of chronic demyelination induced by a JHM virus variant (DS). Arch Neurol 1987; 44:839–842.

55. Haspel MV, Lampert PW, Oldstone MBA. Temperature sensitive mutants of mouse hepatitis virus produce a high incidence of demyelination. Proc Natl Acad Sci USA 1978; 75:4033–4036.

56. Knobler RL, Tunison LA, Lampert PW, Oldstone MBA. Selected mutants of mouse hepatitis virus type 4 (JHM strain) induce different CNS diseases. Am J Pathol 1982; 109:157–168.

57. Gallagher TM. A role for naturally occurring variation of the murine coronavirus spike protein in stabilizing association with the cellular receptor. J Virol 1997; 71:3129–3137.

58. Gallagher TM, Escarmis C, Buchmeier MJ. Alteration of pH dependence of coronavirus-induced cell fusion: Effect of mutations in the spike glycoprotein. J Virol 1991; 65:1916–1928.

59. Gombold JL, Hingley ST, Weiss SR. Fusion defective mutants of mouse hepatitis virus A-59 contain a mutation in the spike protein cleavage signal. J Virol 1993; 67:4504–4512.

60. Phillips JJ, Chua MM, Lavi E, Weiss SR. Pathogenesis of chimeric MHV4/MHV-A-59 recombinant viruses: The murine coronavirus spike protein is a major determinant of neurovirulence. J Virol 1999; 73:7752–7760.

61. Rowe CL, Baker SC, Nathan MJ, Sgro JY, Palmenberg AC, Fleming JO. Quasispecies development by high frequency RNA recombination during MHV persistence. Adv Exp Med Biol 1998; 440:759–765.

62. Rowe CL, Fleming JO, Nathan MJ, Sgro JY, Palmenberg AC, Baker SC. Generation of coronavirus spike deletion variants by high frequency recombination at regions of predicted RNA secondary structure. J Virol 1997; 71:6183–6190.

63. Arbour N, Cote G, Lachance C, Tardieu M, Cashman NR, Talbot PJ. Acute and persistent infection of human neural cell lines by human coronavirus OC43. J Virol 1999; 73:3338–3350.

64. Pewe L, Xue S, Perlman S. Cytotoxic T-cell-resistant variants arise at early times after infection in C57B1/6 but not SCID mice infected with a neurotropic coronavirus. J Virol 1997; 71:7640–7647.

65. Pewe L, Xue S, Perlman S. Infection with cytotoxic T lymphocyte escape mutants results

in increased mortality and growth retardation in mice infected with a neurotropic coronavirus. J Virol 1998; 72:5912–5918.

66. Pewe L, Perlman S. Immune response to the immunodominant epitope of mouse hepatitis virus is polyclonal, but functionally monospecific in C57B1/6 mice. Virology 1999; 255: 106–116.

67. Pewe L, Heard SB, Bergmann C, Dailey M, Perlman S. Selection of CTL escape mutants in mice infected with a neurotropic coronavirus: Quantitative estimate of TCR diversity in the infected central nervous system. J Immunol. In press.

68. Wang FI, Stohlman SA, Fleming JO. Demyelination induced by murine hepatitis virus JHM sttrain (MHV-4) is immunologically mediated. J Neuroimmunol 1990; 30:31–41.

69. Buchmeier MJ, Lewicki HA, Talbot PJ, Knobler RL. Murine hepatitis virus-4 (strain JHM) induced neurologic disease is modulated in vivo by monoclonal antibody. Virology 1984; 132:261–270.

70. Fleming JO, Trousdale MD, El-Zaatari FAK, Stohlman SA, Weiner LP. Pathogenicity of antigenic variants of murine coronavirus JHM selected with monoclonal antibodies. J Virol 1986; 58:869–875.

71. Dalziel RG, Lampert PW, Talbot PJ, Buchmeier MJ. Site-specific alteration of murine hepatitis virus type 4 peplomer glycoprotein E2 results in reduced neurovirulence. J Virol 1986; 59:463–471.

72. Wege H, Winter J, Meyermann R. The peplomer protein E2 of coronavirus JHM as a determinant of neurovirulence: definition of critical epitopes by variant analysis. J Gen Virol 1988; 69:87–98.

73. Yokomori K, Stohlman SA, Lai MM. The detection and characterization of multiple hemagglutinin-esterase (HE)-defective viruses in the mouse brain during subacute demyelination induced by mouse hepatitis virus. Virology 1993; 192:170–178.

74. Schwender S, Imrich H, Dorries R. The pathogenetic role of virus-specific antibody-secreting cells in the central nervous system of rats with different susceptibility to coronavirus-induced demyelinating encephalitis. Immunology 1991; 74:533–538.

75. Lin MT, Hinton DR, Marten NW, Bergmann CC, Stohlman SA. Antibody prevents virus reactivation within the central nervous system. J Immunol 1999; 162:7358–7368.

76. Zimprich F, Winter J, Wege H, Lassmann H. Coronavirus-induced primary demyelination: Indication for the involvement of a humoral immune response. Neuropathol Appl Neurobiol 1991; 17:469–484.

77. Flory E, Pfleiderer M, Stuhler A, Wege H, Wege H. Induction of protective immunity against coronavirus-induced encephalomyelitis. Evidence for an importanr role of CD8+ T-cells in vivo. Eur J Immunol 1993; 23:1757–1761.

78. Suzumura A, Lavi E, Weiss SR, Silberberg DH. Coronavirus infection induces H-2 antigen expression on oligodendrocytes and astrocytes. Science 1986; 232:991–993.

79. Correale J, Li S, Weiner LP, Gilmore W. Effect of persistent mouse hepatitis virus infection on MHC class I expression in murine astrocytes. J Neurol Sci 1995; 40:10–21.

80. Lavi E, Suzumura A, Lampson LA, Siegel RM, Murasko DM, Silberberg DH, Weiss SR. Expression of MHC class I genes in mouse hepatitis virus infection and in multiple sclerosis. Adv Exp Med Biol 1987; 218:219–222.

81. Massa PT, Dörries R, ter Meulen V. Viral particles induce Ia antigen expression on astrocytes. Nature 1986; 320:543–546.

82. Gombold JL and Weiss SR. Mouse hepatits virus A59 increases steady state levels of MHC mRNAs in primary glial cell sultures and in the murine central nervous system. Microb Pathogen 1992; 13:493–505.

83. Marten NW, Stohlman SA, Smith-Begolka W, Miller SD, Dimacali E, Yao Q, Stohl S, Goverman J, Bergmann CC. Selection of CD8 T cells with highly focused specificity during viral persistence in the central nervous system. J Immunol 1999; 162:3905–3914.

84. Stohlman SA, Bergmann CC, Cua DJ, Lin MT, Ho S, Wei W, Hinton DR. Apoptosis of

JHMV-specific CTL in the CNS in the absence of CD4 T cells. Adv Exp Med Biol 1998; 440:425–430.

85. Lavi E, J Das Sarma, Weiss SR. Cellular reservoirs for coronavirus infection of brain in beta2-microglobulin knockout mice. Pathobiology 1999; 67:75–83.

86. Lin MT, Hinton DR, Stohlman SA. Mechanisms of viral clearance in perforin-deficient mice. Adv Exp Med Biol 1998; 440:431–436.

87. Wang Q, Haluskey JA, Lavi E. Coronavirus MHV-A-59 causes upregulation of interferon-beta RNA in primary glial cell cultures. Adv Exp Med Biol 1998; 440:451–454.

88. Lin MT, Hinton DR, Parra B, Stohlman SA, van der Veen RC. The role of IL-10 in mouse hepatitis virus-induced demyelinating encephalomyelitis. Virology 1998; 245:270–280.

89. Parra B, Hinton DR, Marten NW, Bergmann CC, Lin MT, CS Yang, Stohlman SA. IFN-gamma is required for viral clearance from central nervous system oligodendroglia. J Immunol 1999; 162:1641–1647.

90. Parra B, Hinton DR, Lin MT, Cua DJ, Stohlman SA. Kinetics of cytokine mRNA expression in the central nervous system following lethal and nonlethal coronavirus-induced acute encephalomyelitis. Virology 1997; 233:260–270.

91. Wege H, Schluesener H, Meyermann R, Barac-Latas V, Suchanek G, Lassmann H. Coronavirus infection and demyelination: Development of inflammatory lesions in Lewis rats. Adv Exp Med Biol 1998; 440:437–444.

92. Lane TE, Asensio VC, Yu N, Paoletti AD, Campbell IL, MJ Buchmeier. Dynamic regulation of alpha- and beta-chemokine expression in the central nervous system during mouse hepatitis virus–induced demyelinating disease. J Immunol 1998; 160:970–978.

93. Lane TE, Fox HS, Buchmeier MJ. Inhibition of nitric oxide synthase-2 reduces the severity of mouse hepatitis virus-induced demyelination: Implications for NOS2/NO regulation of chemokine expression and inflammation. J Neurovirol 1999; 5:48–54.

94. Wu GF, Perlman S. Macrophage infiltration, but not apoptosis, is correlated with immune-mediated demyelination following murine infection with a neurotropic coronavirus. J Virol 1999; 73:8771–8780.

95. Xue S, Sun N, Van N Rooijen, Perlman S. Depletion of blood-borne macrophages does not reduce demyelination in mice infected with a neurotropic coronavirus. J Virol 1999; 73: 6327–6334.

96. Nagashima K, Wege H, Meyermann R, ter Meulen V. Coronavirus induced subacute demyelinating encephalomyelitis in rats: A morphological analysis. Acta Neuropathol 1978; 44: 63–70.

97. Wege H, Watanabe R, ter Meulen V. Relapsing subacute demyelinating encephalomyelitis in rats during the course of coronavirus JHM infection. J Neuroimmunol 1984; 6:325–336.

98. Sorensen O, Percy D, Dales S. In vivo and in vitro models of demyelinating diseases: III. JHM virus infection of rats. Arch Neurol 1980; 37:478–484.

99. Wege H, Koga M, Watanabe R, Nagashima K, ter Meulen V. Neurovirulence of murine coronavirus JHM temperature sensitive mutants in rats. Infect Immun 1983; 39:1316–1324.

100. Koga M, Wege H, ter Meulen V. Sequence of murine coronavirus JHM induced neuropathological changes in rats. Neuropathol Appl Neurobiol 1984; 10:173–184.

101. Watanabe R, Wege H, ter Meulen V. Adoptive transfer of EAE-like lesions from rats with coronavirus induced demyelinating encephalomyelitis. Nature (London) 1983; 305:150–153.

102. Massa PT, Brinkmann R, ter Meulen V. Inducibility of Ia antigen on astrocytes by murine coronavirus JHM is rat strain dependent. J Exp Med 1987; 166:259–264.

103. Wekerle H, Kojima K, Lannes-Viera J, Lassmann H, Linington C. Animal models. Ann Neurol 1994; 36:S47–S53.

104. Harter DH. The detailed structure of visna-maedi virus. In: Kimberlin RH, ed. Slow Virus Diseases of Animals and Man. Amsterdam and New York: North Holland, 1976, pp 45–60.

105. Sigurdsson B. Observations on three slow infections of sheep. Br Vet J 1954; 110:255–270.

106. Haase AT. Pathogenesis of lentivirus infections. Nature 1986; 322:130–136.

107. Carruth LM, Morse BA, Clements JE. The leucine domain of the visna virus Tat protein mediates targeting to an AP-1 site in the viral long terminal repeat. J Virol 1996; 70:4338–4344.

108. Carruth LM, Clements JE. Targeting of the visna virus Tat protein to AP-1 sites: Interaction with the bZIP domains of fos and jun in vitro and in vivo. J Virol 1999; 137–145.

109. Sigurdsson B, Thormar H, Palsson PA. Cultivation of visna virus in tissue culture. Arch Gesamte Virusforsch 1960; 10:368–381.

110. Georgsson G, Palsson PA, Petursson G. Pathogenesis of visna. In: Serlupi Crescenzi G, ed. A multidisciplinary approach to myelin disease. New York: Plenum, 1987, pp. 303–318.

111. Narayan O, Griffin DE, Chase J. Antigenic drift of visna virus in persistently infected sheep. Science 1977; 197:376–378.

112. Lutley R, Petursson G, Palsson PA, Georgsson G, Klein J, Nathanson N. Antigenic drift in visna virus variation during long term infection of islandic sheep. J Gen Virol 1983; 64: 1433–1440.

113. Haase AT, Stowring L, Narayan O, Griffin D, Price D. Slow persistent infection caused by visna virus: Role of host restriction. Science 1977; 195:175–177.

114. Haase AT. The role of active and covert infections in lentivirus pathogenesis. In: Bjornsson J, Carp RI, Love A, Wisniewski HM, eds. Slow Infections of the Central Nervous System. New York Annals of the New York Academy of Sciences, 1994; 724:75–86.

115. Vigne R, Neuveut C, Sire J, Philippon V, Filippi P. Involvement of viral regulatory gene products in the pathogenesis of lentivirus infections. In: Bjornsson J, Carp RI, Love A, Wisniewski HM, eds. Slow Infections of the Central Nervous System. New York: Annals of the New York Academy of Sciences, 1994; 724:107–124.

116. Eriksson K, McInnes E, Ryan S, Tonks P, McConnell I, Blacklaws B. CD4+ T cells are required for the establishment of maedi-visna virus infection in macrophages but not dendritic cells in vivo. Virology 1999; 248:355–364.

117. Chebloune Y, Karr BM, Raghavan R, Singh DK, Leung K, Sheffer D, Pinson D, Foresman L, Narayan O. Neuroinvasion by ovine lentivirus in infected sheep mediated by inflammatory cells associated with experimental allergic encephalomyelitis. J Neurovirol 1998; 4:38–48.

118. Petursson G, Nathanson N, Georgsson G, Panitch H, Palsson PA. Pathogenesis of Visna I. Sequential virologic, serologic and pathologic studies. Lab Invest 1976; 35:402–412.

119. Palsson PA. Maedi and visna in sheep. In Kimberlin RH, ed. Slow Virus Diseases of Animals and Man. Amsterdam and New York: North Holland, 1976, pp. 7–43.

120. Georgsson G, Nathanson N, Palsson PA, Petursson G. The pathology of visna and maedi in sheep. In: Kimberlin RH, ed. Slow Virus Diseases of Animals and Man. Amsterdam and New York: North Holland, 1976, pp. 61–96.

121. Nathanson N, Georgsson G, Palsson PA, Najjar JA, Lutley R, Petursson G. Experimental visna in islandic sheep: The prototype lentiviral infection. Rev Infect Dis 1985; 7:75–82.

122. Nathanson N, Petursson G, Georgsson G, Palsson PA, Martin JR, Miller A. Pathogenesis of visna: IV. Spinal fluid studies. J Neuropathol Exp Neurol 1979; 38:197–208.

123. Georgsson G, Martin JR, Klein J, Palsson PA, Nathanson N, Petursson G. Primary demyelination in visna: An ultrastructural study of islandic sheep with clinical signs following experimental infection. Acta Neuropathol (Berl) 1982; 57:171–178.

124. Nathanson N, Panitch H, Palsson PA, Petursson G, G Georgsson. Pathogenesis of visna: II. Effect of immunosuppression upon early central nervous system lesions. Lab Invest 1976; 35:444–451.

125. Petursson G, Nathanson N, Palsson PA, Martin J, Georgsson G. Immunopathogenesis of visna. A slow virus disease of the central nervous system. Acta Neurol Scand 1978; 57(suppl 67):205–219.

126. Nathanson N, Martin JR, Georgsson G, Palsson PA, Lutley R, Petursson G. Effect of post-infection immunization on the severity of experimental visna. J Comp Pathol 1981; 91:185–191.

127. Davies JM, Watt NJ, Torsteinsdottir S, Carnegie PR. Mimicry of a 21.5 kDa myelin protein peptide by a Maedi Visna virus polymerase peptide does not contribute to the pathogenesis of encephalitis in sheep. Vet Immunol Immunopathol 1996; 55:127–139.

128. Lutley R, Petursson G, Georgsson G, Palsson PA, Nathanson N. Strains of visna virus with increased neurovirulence. In: Sharp JM, Hoff-Jörgensen R, eds. Slow Viruses in Sheep, Goats and Cattle. Luxembourg: Commission of the European Communities, 1985, pp. 45–49.

129. Georgsson G, Houwers DJ, Palsson PA, Petursson G. Expression of viral antigens in the central nervous system of visna infected sheep: An immunohistochemical study on experimental visna induced by virus strains of increased neurovirulence. Acta Neuropathol. In press.

130. Stowring L, Haase AT, Petursson G, Georgsson G, Palsson P, Lutley R, Roos R, Szuchet S. Detection of visna virus antigens and RNA in glial cells in foci of demyelination. Virology 1985; 141:311–318.

131. Georgsson G. Neuropathologic aspects of lentiviral infections. In: Bjornsson J, Carp RI, Love A, Wisniewski HM, eds. Slow infections of the central nervous system. New York: Annals of the New York Academy of Sciences, 1994; 724:50–67.

132. Torsteinsdottir S, Georgsson G, Gisladottir E, Rafnar B, Palsson PA, Peturson G. Pathogenesis of central nervous system lesions in visna: Cell-mediated immunity and lymphocyte subsets in blood, brain and cerebrospinal fluid. J Neuroimmunol 1992; 41:149–158.

133. Torsteinsdottir S, Georgsson G, Gisladottir E, Rafnar B, Palsson PA, Peturson G. Pathogenesis of central nervous system lesions in visna. Cell-mediated immunity and lymphocyte subsets in blood, brain, and cerebrospinal fluid. In: Bjornsson J, Carp RI, Love A, Wisniewski HM, eds. Slow infections of the central nervous system. New York: Annals of the New York Academy of Sciences, 1994; 724:159–161.

134. Bergsteinsdottir K, Arnadottir S, Torsteinsdottir S, Agnarsdottir G, Andresdottir V, Pettursson G, Georgsson G. Constitutive and visna virus induced expression of class I and II major histocompatibility complex antigens in the central nervous system of sheep and their role in the pathogenesis of visna lesions. Neuropathol Appl Neurobiol 1998; 24:224–232.

135. Craig LE, Sheffer D, Meyer AL, Hauer D, Lechner F, Peterhans E, Adams RJ, Clements JE, Narayan O, MC. Pathogenesis of ovine lentiviral encephalitis: Derivation of a neurovirulent strain by in vivo passage. J Neurovirol 1997; 3:417–427.

136. Starling I, Wright A, Arbuthnott G, Harkiss G. Acute in vivo neurotoxicity of peptides from Maedi Visna virus transactivating protein Tat. Br Res 1999; 830:285–291.

137. Andrewes CH, Pereira HG, Wildy P. Herpetoviridae. In: Andrewes CH, Pereira HG, Wildy P, eds. Viruses of Vertebrates. London: Baillière Tindall 1978, pp. 312–355.

138. Nahmias AJ, Dowdle WR. Antigenic and biologic differences in herpesvirus hominis. Prog Med Virol 1968; 10:110–159.

139. Stevens JG, Cook ML. Latent herpes simplex virus in spinal ganglia of mice. Science 1971; 173:843–845.

140. Stevens JG, Nesburn AB, Cook ML. Latent herpes simplex virus from trigeminal ganglia of rabbits with recurrent eye infection. Nature 1972; 235:216–217.

141. Bastian FO, Rabson AS, Yee CL, Tralka TS. Herpes virus hominis: Isolation from human trigeminal ganglion. Science 1972; 178:306–307.

142. Warren KG, Brown SM, Wroblewska Z, Gilden D, Koprowski H, Subak-Sharpe J. Isolation of latent herpes simplex virus from the superior cervical and vagus ganglions of human beings. N Engl J Med 1978; 298:1068–1069.

143. Baringer JR. Recovery of herpes simplex virus from human sacral ganglions. N Engl J Med 1974; 291:828–830.

144. Kristensson K, Vahlne A, Persson LA, Lycke E. Neural spread of herpes simplex virus types 1 and 2 in mice after corneal or subcutaneous (footpad) inoculation. J Neurol Sci 1978; 35:331–340.

145. Townsend JJ, Baringer JR. Central nervous system susceptibility to herpes simplex virus infection. J Neuropathol Exp Neurol 1978; 37:255–262.
146. Kristensson K, Svennerholm B, Persson L, Vahlne A, Lycke E. Latent herpes simplex virus trigeminal ganglionic infection in mice and demyelination in the central nervous system. J Neurol Sci 1979; 43:253–264.
147. Townsend JJ, Baringer JR. Morphology of central nervous system disease in immunosuppressed mice after peripheral herpes simplex virus inoculation: Trigeminal root entry zone. Lab Invest 1979; 40:178–182.
148. Townsend JJ. The demyelinating effect of corneal HSV infections in normal and nude (athymic) mice. J Neurol Sci 1981; 50:435–441.
149. Kristensson K, Thormar H, Wisniewski HM. Myelin lesions in the rabbit eye model as a bystander effect of herpes simplex and visna virus sensitization. Acta Neuropathol (Berl) 1979; 48:215–217.
150. Kristensson K, Svennerholm B, Vahlne A, Nilheden E, Persson L, Lycke E. Virus induced demyelination in herpes symplex virus infected mice. J Neurol Sci 1982; 53:205–216.
151. Townsend JJ. The relationship of astrocytes and macrophages to CNS demyelination after experimental herpes simplex infection. J Neuropathol Exp Neurol 1981; 40:369–379.
152. Townsend JJ. Macrophage response to herpes simplex encephalitis in immune-competent and T-cell deficient mice. J Neuroimmunol 1985; 7:195–206.
153. Gudmundsdottir S, Svennerholm B, Kristensson K, Lycke E. Herpes simplex virus-enhanced production of autoantibodies against myelin basic protein in mice. Arch Virol 1986; 88:37–47.
154. Kristensson K, Svennerholm B, Lycke E. Herpes simplex virus-induced demyelination: Effect of reinfection and challenge with neuroantigens. J Neurol Sci 1983; 60:247–252.
155. Kastrukoff LF, Lau AS, Leung GY, Thomas EE. Contrasting effects of immunosuppression on herpes simplex virus type I (HSV I) induced central nervous system (CNS) demyelination in mice. J Neurol Sci 1993; 117:148–158.
156. Kastrukoff LF, Lau AS, Leung GY, Walker DG, Thomas EE. Herpes simplex virus type I (HSV-I)–induced multifocal central nervous system (CNS) demyelination in mice. J Neuropathol Exp Neurol 1992; 51:432–439.
157. Kastrukoff LF, Lau AS, Kim SU. Multifocal CNS demyelination following peripheral inoculation with herpes simplex virus type 1. Ann Neurol 1987; 22:52–59.
158. Thomas EE, Lau AS, Kim SU, Osborne D, Kastrukoff LF. Variation in resistance to herpes simplex virus type 1 of oligodendrocytes derived from inbred strains of mice. J Gen Virol 1991; 72:2051–2057.
159. Thomas EE, Lau AS, Morrison B, Kim SU, Kastrukoff LF. Differences in resistance to herpes simplex virus type 1 (HSV-1) among oligodendroglia derived from different strains of mice are determined after viral absorption but prior to the expression of immediate early (IE) genes. J Neurovirol 1997; 3:197–205.
160. Martin JR, Stoner GL, Webster H de F. Lethal encephalitis and non-lethal multifocal central nervous system demyelination in herpes simplex virus type 2 infections in mice. Br J Exp Pathol 1982; 63:651–666.
161. Martin JR, Stoner GL. The nervous system in genital herpes simplex type 2 infections in mice. Lethal panmyelitis or non-lethal demyelinative myelitis or meningitis. Lab Invest 1984; 51:556–566.
162. Martin JR, Reed EV, Striegel LC. Acute thymic atrophy in severe herpes simplex virus type 2 infection. In: Gilmore N, M Wainberg, eds. Viral mechanisms of immunosuppression. New York: Liss, 1985:185–190.
163. Gudnadottir M, Helgadottir H, Bjarnason O, Jonsdottir K. Virus isolated from the brain of a patient with multiple sclerosis. Exp Neurol 1964; 9:85–89.
164. Martin JR, Suzuki S, Webster H de F. Central nervous system demyelination in herpes sim-

plex virus type 2 infection. In: Serlupi-Crescenzi G, ed. A Multidisciplinary Approach to Myelin Diseases. New York and London: Plenum, 1987, pp. 329–340.

165. Martin JR. Intra-axonal virus in demyelinative lesions of experimental herpes simplex type 2 infection. J Neurol Sci 1984; 63:63–74.

166. Georgsson G, Martin JR, Stoner GL, Webster H de F . Virus spread and initial pathological changes in the nervous system in genital herpes simplex type 2 infection in mice. Acta Neuropathol (Berl) 1987; 72:377–388.

167. Martin JR, Reed EV. Central nervous system and genital infection with reactivation of latent herpes simplex virus type 2 in mice. Microb Pathog 1986; 1:181–189.

168. Martin JR, Suzuki S. Inflammatory sensory polyradiculopathy and reactivated peripheral nervous system infection in a genital herpes model. J Neurol Sci 1987; 79:155–171.

169. Soffer D, Martin JR. Remyelination of central nervous system lesions in experimental genital herpes simplex virus infection. J Neurol Sci 1988; 86:83–95.

170. Martin JR, Suzuki S. Targets of infection in a herpes simplex reactivation model. Acta Neuropathol 1989; 77:402–411.

171. Suzuki S, Martin JR. Herpes simplex virus type 2 transcripts in trigeminal ganglia during acute and latent infection in mice. J Neurol Sci 1989; 93:239–251.

172. Gressens P, Martin JR. HSV-2 DNA persistence in astrocytes of the trigeminal root entry zone: Double labeling by in situ PCR and immunohistochemistry. J Neuropathol Exp Neurol 1994; 53:127–135.

173. Subak-Sharpe J, Koprowski H. Isolation of herpes simplex virus from human trigeminal ganglia, including ganglia from one patient with multiple sclerosis. Lancet 1977; 2:637–639.

174. Nicoll JAR, Kinrade E, Love S. PCR-mediated search for herpes simplex virus DNA in sections of brain from patients with multiple sclerosis and other neurological disorders. J Neurol Sci 1992; 113:144–151.

175. Koenig H, Rabinowitz SG, Day E, Miller V. Post-infectious encephalomyelitis after successful treatment of herpes simplex encephalitis with adenine arabinoside: Ultrastructural observations. N Engl J Med 1979; 300:1089–1093.

176. Martin JR. Herpes simplex virus types 1 and 2 and multiple sclerosis. Lancet 1981; 2:777–781.

177. Pevear DC, Calenoff M, Rozhon E, Lipton HL. Analysis of the complete nucleotide sequence of the picornavirus Theiler's murine encephalomyelitis virus indicates that it is closely related to cardioviruses. J Virol 1987; 61:1507–1516.

178. Ozden S, Tangy F, Chamorro M, Brahic M. Theiler's virus genome is closely related to that of encephalomyiocarditis virus, the prototype cardiovirus. J Virol 1986; 60:1163–1165.

179. Ohara Y, Stein S, Fu J, Stillman L, Klaman L, Roos RP. Molecular cloning and sequence determination of DA strain of Theiler's murine encephalomyelitis viruses. Virology 1988; 164:245–255.

180. Roos RP, Richard OC, Ehrenfeld E. Analysis of Theiler's virus isolates from persistently infected mouse nervous tissue. J Gen Virol 1983; 64:701–706.

181. Roos RP, Richards OC, Green J, Ehrenfeld E. Characterization of a cell culture persistently infected with the DA strain of Theiler's murine encephalomyelitis virus. J Virol 1982; 43: 1118–1122.

182. Theiler M. Spontaneous encephalomyelitis of mice, a new virus disease. J Exp Med 1937; 65:705–719.

183. Lorch Y, Friedmann A, Lipton HL, Kotler M. Theiler's murine encephalomyelitis virus group includes two distinct genetic subgroups that differ pathologically and biologically. J Virol 1981; 40:560–567.

184. Lipton HL. Persistent Theiler's murine encephalomyelitis virus infection in mice depends on plaque size. J Gen Virol 1980; 46:169–177.

185. Friedmann A, Lipton HL. Replication of Theiler's murine encephalomyelitis viruses in BHK21 cells: An electron microscopic study. Virology 1980; 101:389–398.

186. Dal.Canto MC, Lipton HL. Ultrastructural immunohistochemical localization of virus in acute and chronic demyelinating Theiler's virus infection. Am J Pathol 1982; 106:20–29.
187. Cash E, Chamorro M, Brahic M. Theiler's virus RNA and protein synthesis in the central nervous system of demyelinating mice. Virology 1985; 144:290–294.
188. Brahic M, Stroop WG, Baringer JR. Theiler's virus persists in glial cells during demyelinating disease. Cell 1981; 26:123–128.
189. Pevear DC, Borkowski J, Calenoff M, Oh CK, Ostrowski B, Lipton HL. Insights into Theiler's virus neurovirulence based on a genomic comparison of the neurovirulent GDVII and less virulent BeAn strains. Virology 1988; 165:1–12.
190. Pevear DC, Luo M, Lipton HL. Three-dimensional model of the capsid proteins of two biologically different Theiler's virus strains: Clustering of aminoacis differences identifies possible locations of immunogenic sites on the virion. Proc Natl Acad Sci USA 1988; 85:4496–4500.
191. Dal Canto MC, Lipton HL. Schwann cell remyelination and recurrent demyelination in the central nervous system of mice infected with attenuated Theiler's virus. Am J Pathol 1980; 98:101–122.
192. Lipton HL. Theiler's virus infection in mice: An unusual biphasic disease process leading to demyelination. Infect Immun 1975; 11:1147–1155.
193. Dal Canto MC, Lipton HL. Primary demyelination in Theiler's virus infection. Lab Invest 1976; 33:626–637.
194. Lipton HL, Dal Canto MC. Chronic neurologic disease in Theiler's virus infection of SJL/J mice. J Neurol Sci 1976; 30:201–207.
195. Lipton HL, Dal Canto MC. Theiler's virus induced demyelination: Prevention by immunosuppression. Science 1976; 192:62–64.
196. HL Dal Canto, Dal Canto MC. The TO strain of Theiler's viruses cause "slow virus like" infection in mice. Ann Neurol 1979; 6:25–28.
197. Dal Canto MC, Melvold RW, Kim BS, Miller SD. Two models of multiple sclerosis: Experimental allergic encephalomyelitis (EAE) and Theiler's murine encephalomyelitis virus (TMEV) infection—A pathological and immunological comparison. J Micr Res Tech. In press.
198. Dal Canto MC, Melvold RW, Kim BS. A hybrid between a resistant and a susceptible strain of mouse alters the pattern of Theiler's murine encephalomyelitis virus-induced white matter disease and favors oligodendrocyte-mediated remyelination. Mult Scler 1995; 1:95–103.
199. Miller DJ, Sanborn KS, Katzmann JA, Rodriguez M. Monoclonal autoantibodies promote central nervous system repair in an animal model of multiple sclerosis. J Neurosci 1994; 14:6230–6238.
200. Asakura K, Miller DJ, Pease LR, Rodriguez M. Targeting of IgM kappa antibodies to oligodendrocytes promotes CNS remyelination. J Neurosci 1998; 18:7700–7708.
201. Clatch RJ, Melvold RW, Miller SD, Lipton HL. Theiler's murine encephalomyelitis virus (TMEV)-induced demyelinating disease in mice is influenced by the H2-D region: Correlation with TMEV-specific delayed-type hypersensitivity. J Immunol 1985; 135:1408–1414.
202. Rodriguez M, Leibowitz J, David CS. Susceptibility to Theiler's virus-induced demyelination. Mapping of the gene within the H-2D region. J Exp Med 1986; 163:620–631.
203. Melvold RW, Jokinen DM, Miller SD, Dal Canto MC, Lipton HL. H-2 genes in TMEV-induced demyelination, a model for multiple sclerosis. In: David C, ed. Major Histocompatibility Genes and Their Role in Immune Function. New York: Plenum, (1987), pp. 735–745.
204. Clatch RJ, Melvold RW, Dal Canto MC, Miller SD, Lipton HL. The Theiler's murine encephalomyelitis virus (TMEV) model for multiple sclerosis shows a strong influence of the murine equivalents of HLA-A, B, and C. J Neuroimmunol 1987; 15:121–135.
205. Lipton HL, Dal Canto MC. Susceptibility of inbred mice to chronic central nervous system infection by Theiler's murine encephalomyelitis virus. Infect Immun 1979; 26:369–374.

206. Lipton HL, Melvold RW. Genetic analysis of susceptibility to Theiler's virus induced demyelinating disease in mice. J Immunol 1984; 132:1821–1825.

207. Melvold RW, Jokinen DM, Knobler R, Lipton HL. Variations in genetic control of susceptibility to Theiler's murine encephalomyelitis virus (TMEV)-induced demyelinating disease: I. Differences between susceptible SJL/J and resistant BALB/c strains map near the T cell β-chain constant genes on chromosome 6. J Immunol 1986; 138:1429–1433.

208. Kappel CA, Dal Canto MC, Melvold RW, Kim BS. Hierarchy of effects of the major histocompatibility complex and the T cell receptor β-chain genes in susceptibility to Theiler's murine encephalomyelitis virus-induced demyelinating disease. J Immunol 1991; 147:4322–4326.

209. Melvold RW, Jokinen DM, Miller SD, Dal Canto MC, Lipton HL. Identification of a locus on mouse chromosome 3 involved in differential susceptibility to Theiler's murine encephalomyelitis virus (TMEV)-induced demyelinating disease. J Virol 1990; 64:686–690.

210. Aubagnac S, Brahic M, Bureau J-F. Viral load and a locus on chromosome 11 affect the late clinical disease caused by Theiler's virus. J Virol 1999; 73:7965–7971.

211. Bureau JF, Drescher KM, Pease LR, Vikoren T, Delcroix M, Zoecklein L, Brahic M, Rodriguez M. Chromosome 14 contains determinants that regulate susceptibility to Theiler's virus-induced demyelination in the mouse. Genetics 1998; 148:1941–1949.

212. Bihl F, Brahic M, Bureau JF. Two loci, Tmevp2 and Tmevp3, located on the telomeric region of chromosome 10, control the persistence of Theiler's virus in the central nervous system of mice. Genetics 1999; 152:385–392.

213. Kappel CA, Melvold RW, Kim BS. Influence of sex on susceptibility in Theiler's murine encephalomyelitis virus model for multiple sclerosis. J Neuroimmunol 1990; 29:15–19.

214. Rodriguez M, Patick AK, Pease LR. Abrogation of resistance to Theiler's virus-induced demyelination in C57BL mice by total body irradiation. J Neuroimmunol 1990; 26:189–199.

215. Nicholson MN, Paterson JD, Miller SD, Wang K, Dal Canto MC, Melvold RW. BALB/c substrain differences in susceptibility to Theiler's murine encephalomyelitis virus-induced demyelinating disease. J Neuroimmunol 1994; 52:19–24.

215. Olsberg C, Pelka A, Miller S, Waltenbaugh C, Creighton TM, Dal Canto MC, Lipton H, Melvold RW. Induction of Theiler's murine encephalomyelitis virus (TMEV)-induced demyelinating disease in genetically resistant mice. Reg Immunol 1993; 5:1–10.

217. Pelka A, Olsberg C, Miller S, Waltenbaugh C, Creighton TM, Dal Canto MC, Melvold R. Effects of irradiation on development of Theiler's murine encephalomyelitis virus (TMEV)-induced demyelinating disease in genetically resistant mice. Cell Immunol 1993; 152:440–455.

218. Nicholson S, Dal Canto MC, Miller SD, Melvold RW. Adoptively transferred CD8+ T lymphocytes provide protection against TMEV-induced demyelinating disease in BALB/c mice. J Immunol 1996; 156:1276–1283.

219. Fiette L, Aubert C, Brahic M, Rossi CP. Theiler's virus infection of beta 2-microglobulin-deficient mice. J Virol 1993; 67:589–592.

220. Rodriguez M, Dunkel AJ, Thiemann RL, Leibowitz J, Zijlstra M, Jaenisch R. Abrogation of resistance to Theiler's virus-induced demyelination in H-2^b mice deficient in B2-microglobulin. J Immunol 1993; 151:266–276.

221. Pullen LC, Miller SD, Dal Canto MC, Kim BS. Class I deficient resistant mice intracerebrally inoculated with Theiler's virus show an increased T cell response to viral antigens and susceptibility to demyelination. Eur J Immunol 1993; 23:2287–2293.

222. Murray PD, McGavern DB, Lin X, Njenga MK, Leibowitz J, Pease LR, Rodriguez M. Perforin-dependent neurologic injury in a viral model of multiple sclerosis. J Neurosci 1998; 18:7306–7314.

223. Chen HH, Kong WP, Zhang I, Ward PL, Roos RP. A picornaviral protein synthesized out of frame with the polyprotein plays a key role in a virus-induced immune-mediated demyelinating disease. Nature Med 1995; 1:927–931.

224. Ghadge GD, Ma L, Sato S, Kim J, Roos RP. A protein critical for a Theiler's virus-induced immune system-mediated demyelinating disease has a cell type-specific antiapoptotic effect and a key role in virus persistence. J Virol 1998; 72:8605–8612.

225. Adami C, Pritchard AE, Knauf T, Luo M, Lipton HL. A determinant for central nervous system persistence localized in the capsid of Theiler's murine encephalomyelitis virus by using recombinant viruses. J Virol 1998; 72:1662–1665.

226. Clatch RJ, Lipton HL, Miller SD. Characterization of Theiler's murine encephalomyelitis virus (TMEV)-specific delayed type hypersensitivity responses in TMEV-induced demyelinating disease: Correlation with clinical signs. J Immunol 1986; 136:920–927.

227. Rodriguez M, Leibowitz JL, Lampert P. Persistent infection of oligodendrocytes in Theiler's virus-induced encephalomyelitis. Ann Neurol 1983; 13:426–433.

228. Rodriguez M, Pease LR, David CS. Immune mediated injury of virus-infected oligodendrocytes. Immunol Today 1986; 7:359–363.

229. Dal Canto MC. Uncoupled relationship between demyelination and primary infection of myelinating cells in Theiler's virus encephalomyelitis. Infect Immun 1982; 35:1133–1138.

230. Dal Canto MC, Barbano RL. Immunocytochemical localization of MAG, MBP and Po protein in acute and relapsing demyelinating lesions of Theiler's virus infection. J Neuroimmunol 1985; 10:129–140.

231. Penney JB, Wolinsky JS. Neuronal and oligodendroglial infection by the WW strain of Theiler's virus. Lab Invest 1979; 40:324–330.

232. Rosenthal A, Fujinami RS, Lampert PW. Mechanism of Theiler's virus-induced demyelination in nude mice. Lab Invest 1986; 54:515–522.

233. Clatch RJ, Miller SD, Metzner R, Dal Canto MC, Lipton HL. Monocyte/macrophages isolated from the mouse CNS contain infectious Theiler's murine encephalomyelitis virus (TMEV). Virology 1990; 176:244–254.

234. Pope JG, Vanderlugt CL, Rahbe SM, Lipton HL, Miller SD. Characterization of, and functional antigen presentation by central nervous system mononuclear cells from mice infected with Theiler's murine encephalomyelitis virus. J Virol 1998; 72:7762–7771.

235. Rodriguez M, Quddus J. Effect of cyclosporin A, silica quartz and protease inhibitors on virus-induced demyelination. J Neuroimmunol 1986; 13:159–174.

236. Rossi CP, Delcroix M, Huitinga I, McAllister A, van Rooijen N, Claassen E, Brahic M. Role of macrophages during Theiler's virus infection. J Virol 1997; 71:3336–3340.

237. Liuzzi MG, Riccio P, Dal Canto MC. Release of myelin basic protein-degrading proteolytic activity from microglia and macrophages after infection with Theiler's murine encephalomyelitis virus: Comparison between susceptible and resistant mice. J Neuroimmunol 1995; 62: 91–102.

238. Jelachich ML, Bramlage C, Lipton HL. Differentiation of M1 myeloid precursor cells into macrophages results in binding and infection by Theiler's murine encephalomyelitis virus and apoptosis. J Virol 1999; 73:3227–3235.

239. Jelachich ML, Lipton HL. Theiler's murine encephalomyelitis virus kills restrictive, but not permissive cells by apoptosis. J Virol 1996; 70:6856–6861.

240. Endoh M, Tabira T, Kunishita T, Sakai K, Yamamura T, Taketomi T. DM-20, a proteolipid apoprotein, is an encephalitogen of acute and relapsing autoimmune encephalomyelitis in mice. J Immunol 1986; 137:3832–3835.

241. Miller SD, Clatch RJ, Pevear DC, Trotter JL, Lipton HL. Class II-restricted T cell responses in Theiler's murine encephalomyelitis virus (TMEV)-induced demyelinating disease: I. Cross-specificity among TMEV substrains and related picornaviruses, but not myelin proteins. J Immunol 1987; 138:3776–3784.

242. Barbano RL, Dal Canto MC. Serum and cells from Theiler's virus-infected mice fail to injure myelinating cultures or to produce in vivo transfer of disease: The pathogenesis of Theiler's virus-induced demyelination appears to differ from that of EAE. J Neurol Sci 1984; 66: 283–293.

243. Miller SD, Gerety SJ, Kennedy MK, Peterson JD, Trotter JL, Touhy VK, Waltenbaugh C, Dal Canto MC, Lipton HL. Class II restricted T cell responses in Theiler's murine encephalomyelitis virus (TMEV)-induced demyelinating disease: III. Failure of neuroantigen-specific immune tolerance to affect the clinical course of demyelination. J Neuroimmunol 1990; 26: 9–23.

244. Tan L-J, Kennedy MK, Dal Canto MC, Miller SD. Successful treatment of paralytic relapses in adoptive experimental autoimmune encephalomyelitis via neuroantigen-specific tolerance. J Immunol 1991; 147:1797–1802.

245. Miller SD, Tan L-J, Pope L, McRae B, Karpus WJ. Antigen-specific tolerance as a therapy for experimental autoimmune encephalomyelitis. Intern Rev Immunol 1992; 9:203–222. 35.

246. Tan L-J, Kennedy MK, Miller SD. Regulation of the effector stages of experimental autoimmune encephalomyelitis via neuroantigen-specific tolerance induction. II. Fince specificity of effector T cell inhibition. J Immunol 1992; 148:2748–2755.

247. Peterson JD, Karpus WJ, Clatch RJ, Miller SD. Split tolerance of Th1 and Th2 cells in tolerance to Theiler's murine encephalomyelitis virus. Eur J Immunol 1993; 23:46–55.

248. Karpus WJ, Pope JG, Peterson JD, Dal Canto MC, Miller SD. Inhibition of Theiler's virus-induced demyelination by peripheral immune tolerance induction. J Immunol 1995; 155: 947–957.

249. Miller SD, Vanderlugt CL, Smith W Begolka, Pao W, Yauch RL, Neville KL, Katz-Levy Y, Carrizosa A, Kim BS. Persistent infection with Theiler's virus leads to CNS autoimmunity via epitope spreading. Nature Med 1997; 10:1133–1136.

250. Dal Canto MC, Calenoff MA, Miller SD, Vanderlugt CL. Lymphocytes from mice chronically infected with Theiler's murine encephalomyelitis virus (TMEV) produce demyelination of organotypic cultures after stimulation with the major encephalitogenic epitope of myelin proteolipid protein (PLP): Epitope spreading in TMEV infection has functional significance. J Neuroimmunol. In press.

251. Miller SD, Karpus WJ, Pope JG, Dal Canto MC, Melvold RW. Theiler's virus-induced demyelinating disease. In: Cohen IR, Miller A, eds. Autoimmune Disease Models. San Diego and New York: Academic Press, 1994, pp. 23–38.

252. Peterson JD, Waltenbaugh C, Miller SD. IgG subclass response to Theiler's murine encephalomyelitis virus infection and immunization suggest a dominant role for Th1 cells in susceptible mouse strains. Immunology 1992; 75:652–658.

253. Begolka WS, Vanderlugt CL, Rahbe SM, Miller SD. Differential expression of inflammatory cytokines parallels progression of central nervous system pathology in two clinically distinct models of multiple sclerosis. J Immunol 1998; 161:4437–4446.

254. Sato S, Reiner SL, Jensen MA, Roos RP. Central nervous system cytokine mRNA expression following Theiler's murine encephalomyelitis virus infection. J Neuroimmunol 1997; 76: 213–223.

255. Hoffman LM, Fife BT, Begolka WS, Miller SD, Karpus WJ. Central nervous system chemokine expression during Theiler's virus-induced demyelinating disease. J Neurovirol 1999; 5:635–642.

256. Qi Y, Dal Canto MC. Effect of Theiler's murine encephalomyelitis virus and cytokines on cultured oligodendrocytes and astrocytes. J Neurosci Res 1996;45:364–374.

257. Palma JP, Yauch RL, Lang S, Kim BS. Potential role of CD4+ T cell-mediated apoptosis of activated astrocytes in Theiler's virus-induced demyelination. J Immunol 1999; 162:6543–6551.

258. Gerety SJ, Karpus WJ, Cubbon AR, Goswami RG, Rundell MK, Miller SD. Class II restricted T cell responses in Theiler's murine encephalomyelitis virus-induced demyelinating disease: V. Mapping of a dominant immunopathologic VP2 T cell epitope in susceptible SJL/J mice. J Immunol 1994; 152:908–918.

259. Gerety SJ, Rundell MK, Dal Canto MC, Miller SD. Class II restricted T cell responses in

Theiler's murine encephalomyelitis virus (TMEV) induced demyelinating disease: VI. Characteristics and fine specificity of an immuno-pathologic CD4+ T cell clone specific for an immunodominant VP2 epitope. J Immunol 1994; 152:919–929.

260. Roos RP, Stein S, Routbort M, Senkowski A, Bodwell T, Wollmann R. Theiler's murine encephalomyelitis virus neutralization escape mutants have a change in disease phenotype. J Virol 1989; 63:4469–4473.

261. Zurbiggen A, Hogle J, Fujinami R. Alteration of aminoacid 101 within the capsid protein VP1 changes the pathogenicity of Theiler's murine encephalomyelitis virus. J Exp Med 1989; 170:2037–2049.

262. Tangy F, McAllister A, Aubert C, Brahic M. Determinants of persistence and demyelination of the DA strain of Theiler's virus are found only in the VP1 gene. J Virol 1991; 65:1616–1618.

263. Yauch RL, Kim BS. A predominant viral epitope recognized by T cells from the periphery and demyelinating lesions of SJL/J mice infected with Theiler's virus is located within VP1(233–244). J Immunol 1994; 153:4508–4519.

264. Kim BS, Yauch RL, Bahk YY, Kang J-A, Dal Canto MC, Kappel Hall K. A spontaneous low-pathogenicity variant of Theiler's virus contains an amino acid substitution within the predominant VP1 233–250 T-cell epitope. J Virol 1998; 72:1020–1027.

265. Yauch RL, Palma JP, Yahikozawa H, Koh CS, Kim BS. Role of individual T cell epitopes of Theiler's virus in the pathogenesis of demyelination correlates with the ability to induce a Th1 response. J Virol 198; 72:6169–6174.

266. Rodriguez M, Lafuse WP, Leibowitz J, David CS. Partial suppression of Theiler's virus-induced demyelination in vivo by administration of monoclonal antibodies to immune-response gene products (Ia antigens). Neurology 1986; 36:964–970.

267. Friedmann A, Frankel G, Lorch Y, Steinman L. Monoclonal anti-I-A antibody reverses chronic paralysis and demyelination in Theiler's virus-infected mice: critical importance of timing of treatment. J Virol 1987; 61:898–903.

268. Welsh CJ, Tonks P, Nash AA, Blakemore WF. The effect of L3T4 T cell depletion on the pathogenesis of Theiler's murine encephalomyelitis virus infection in CBA mice. J Gen Virol 1098; 68:1659–1667.

269. Rodriguez M, Sriram S. Successful therapy of Theiler's virus-induced demyelination (DA strain) with monoclonal anti-Lyt-2 antibody. J Immunol 1988; 140:2950–2955.

270. Wisniewski HM. Immunopathology of demyelination in autoimmune diseases and virus infection. Br Med Bull 1977; 33:54–59.

271. Brocke S, Gijbels K, Steinman L. Experimental autoimmune encephalomyelitis in the mouse. In: Cohen IR and Miller A, eds. Autoimmune Disease Models—A Guidebook. San Diego, CA: Academic Press, 1994, pp. 1–14.

272. Gooding LR, KA O'Connell. Recognition by cytotoxic T lymphocytes of cells expressing fragments of the SV40 tumor antigen. J Immunol 1983; 131:2580–2586.

273. Huber SA, Job LP, Woodruff JF. In vitro culture of coxsackievirus group B, type 3 immune spleen cells and biologic activity of the cultured cells in vivo. Infect Immun 1984; 43:567–570.

274. Fujinami RS, Oldstone MBA. Aminoacid homology and immune responses between the encephalitogenic site of myelin basic protein and virus: A mechanism for autoimmunity. Science 1985; 230:1043–1045.

275. Oldstone MBA, Notkins AL. Molecular mimicry. In: Notkins AL, Oldstone MBA, eds. Concepts in Viral Pathogenesis II. New York: Springer-Verlag, 1986, pp. 195–202.

276. Powell HC, Braheny SL, Hughes RAC, Lampert PW. Antigen-specific demyelination and significance of the bystander effect in peripheral nerves. Am J Pathol 1984; 114:443–453.

277. Wisniewski HM, Bloom BR. Primary demyelination as a nonspecific consequence of a cell-mediated immune reaction. J Exp Med 1975; 141:346–359.

278. Holoshitz J, Naparstek J, Ben-Nun A, Marquardt P, Cohen IR. T Lymphocyte lines induce autoimmune encephalomyelitis, delayed hypersensitivity and bystander encephalitis and arthritis. Eur J Immunol 1984; 14:729–734.

279. Waksman B. Mechanisms in multiple sclerosis. Nature 1985; 318:104–105.

280. Booss J, Kim JH. Evidence for a viral etiology of multiple sclerosis. In: Cook SD ed. Handbook of Multiple Sclerosis. New York and Basel: Marcel Dekker, 1990, pp. 41–61.

281. Dal Canto MC, Rabinowitz SG, Johnson TC. Subacute infection with temperature-sensitive vesicular stomatitis virus mutant G41 in the central nervous system of mice:II. Immunofluorescent, morphologic and immunologic studies. J Infect Dis 1975; 139:36–51.

282. Dal Canto MC, Rabinowitz SG. Murine central nervous system infection by a viral temperature-sensitive mutant. Am J Pathol 1981; 102:412–426.

283. Dal Canto MC, Rabinowitz SG, Johnson TC. Virus-induced demyelination: Production by a viral temperature-sensitive mutant. J Neurol Sci 1979; 42:155–168.

284. Dal Canto MC, Rabinowitz SG. Central nervous system demyelination in Venezuelan equine encephalomyelitis virus infection: An experimental model of virus-induced myelin injury. J Neurol Sci 1981; 49:397–418.

285. Chew-Lim M, Suckling AJ, Webb HE. Demyelination in mice after two or three infections with avirulent Semliki Forest virus. Vet Pathol 1977;14:67–72.

286. Andrewes CH, Pereira HG, Wildy P. Togaviridae. In: Andrewes CH, Pereira HG, Wildy P, eds. Viruses of Vertebrates. London: Baillière Tindall, 1978, pp. 67–118.

287. Smithburn KC, Haddow AJ. Semliki Forest virus: I. Isolation and pathogenic properties. J Immunol 1944;49:141–148.

288. Sheahan BJ, Barrett PN, Atkins GJ. Demyelination in mice resulting from infection with a mutant of Semliki Forest virus. Acta Neuropathol (Berl) 1981; 53:129–136.

289. Sheahan BJ, Gates MC, Caffrey JF, Atkins GJ. Oligodendrocyte infection and demyelination produced in mice by the M9 mutant of Semliki Forest virus. Acta Neuropathol (Berl) 1983; 60:257–265.

290. Jagelman S, Suckling AJ, Webb HE, Bowen ETW. The pathogenesis of avirulent Semliki Forest virus infections in athymic nude mice. J Gen Virol 1978; 41:599–607.

291. Fazakerley JK, Amor S, Webb HE. Reconstitution of Semliki Forest virus infected mice induces immune mediated pathological changes in the CNS. Clin Exp Immunol 1983; 52: 115–120.

292. Pathak S, Illavia SJ, Webb HE. The identification and role of cells involved in CNS demyelination in mice after Semliki Forest infection: An ultrastructural study. Immunology of the nervous system. Progr Br Res 1983; 59:237–254.

293. Illavia SJ, Webb HE. The pathological effect on the central nervous system of mice following single and repeated infections of the demyelinating A7(74) strain of Semliki Forest virus. Neuropathol Appl Neurobiol 1988; 14:207–220.

294. Berger ML. Humoral and cell mediated immune mechanisms in the production of pathology in avirulent Semliki Forest virus encephalitis. Infect Immun 1980; 30:244–253.

295. Chew-Lim M, Scott T, Webb HE. An ultrastructural study of cerebellar lasions induced in mice by three inoculations of avirulent Semliki Forest virus. Acta Neuropathol (Berl) 1978; 41:55–59.

296. Kelly WR, Blakemore WF, Jagelman S, Webb HE. Demyelination induced in mice by avirulent Semliki Forest virus: Part 2. An ultrastructural study of focal demyelination in the brain. Br J Exp Pathol 1982; 2:43–53.

297. Webb HE, Chew-Lim M, Jagelman S, Oaten SW, Pathak S, Suckling AJ, Mackenzie A. Semliki Forest virus infection in mice as a model for studying acute and chronic CNS virus infections in man. In: Clifford Rose F, ed. Clinical Neuroimmunology. Oxford, UK: Blackwell Scientific Publications, 1979, pp. 369–390.

298. Chew-Lim M, Webb HE, Jagelman S. The effect of irradiation on demyelination induced by avirulent Semliki Forest virus. Br J Exp Pathol 1977; 58:459–464.

299. Fazakerley JK, Webb HE. Semliki Forest virus induced, immune mediated demyelination: The effect of irradiation. Br J Exp Pathol 1987; 68:101–113.

300. Amor S, Webb HE. The effect of cycloleucine on SFV A7(74) infection in mice. Br J Exp Pathol 1987; 68:225–235.

301. Fazakerley JK, Webb HE. Semliki Forest virus-induced, immune-mediated demyelination: Adoptive transfer studies and viral persistence in nude mice. J Gen Virol 1987; 68:377–385.

302. Webb HE, Mehta S, Gregson NA, Leibowitz S. Immunological reaction of the demyelinating Semliki Forest virus with immune serum to glycolipids and its possible importance to central nervous system viral auto-immune disease. Neuropathol Appl Neurobiol 1984;10:77–84.

303. Khalili-Shirazi A, Gregson N, Webb HE. Immunological relationship between a demyelinating RNA enveloped budding virus (Semliki Forest) and brain glycolipids. J Neurol Sci 1986; 76:91–103.

304. Evans NRS, Webb HE. Immunoelectron-microscopical labelling of glycolipids in the envelope of a demyelinating brain-derived RNA virus (Semliki Forest) by anti-glycolipid sera. J Neurol Sci 1986; 74:279–287.

305. Atkins GJ, Sheahan BJ. Semliki Forest virus neurovirulence mutants have altered cytopathogenicity for central nervous system cells. Infect Immun 1982; 36:333–341.

306. Mokhtarian F, Swoveland P. Predisposition to EAE induction in resistant mice by prior infection with Semliki Forest virus. J Immunol 1987; 138:3264–3268.

307. Wu L-X, Mäkelä MJ, Roÿttä M, Salmi A. Effect of viral infection on experimental allergic encephalomyelitis in mice. J Neuroimmunol 1988; 18:139–153.

308. Eralinna JP, Soilu-Hanninen M, Roytta M, Ilonen J, Makela A, Salonen R. Facilitation of experimental allergic encephalomyelitis by irradiation and virus infection: role of inflammatory cells. J Neuroimmunol 1994; 55:81–90.

309. Soilu-Hanninen M, Eralinna JP, Hukkanen V, Roytta M, Salmi A, Salonen R. Semliki Forest virus infects mouse brain endothelial cells and causes blood-brain barrier damage. J Virol 1994; 68:6291–6298.

310. Mokhtarian F, Zhang Z, Shi Y, Gonzales E, Sobel RA. Molecular mimicry between a viral peptide and a myelin oligodendrocyte glycoprotein peptide induces autoimmune demyelinating disease in mice. J Neuroimmunol 1999; 95:43–54.

311. Jenkins HG, Tansey EM, Macefield F, Ikeda H. Evidence for a T-cell related factor as the cause of demyelination in mice following Semliki Forest virus infection. Br Res 1988; 459: 145–147.

312. Butt AM, Tutton MG, Kirvell SL, Amor S, Jenkins HG. Morphology of oligodendrocytes during demyelination in optic nerves of mice infected with Semliki Forest virus. Neuropathol Appl Neurobiol 1996; 22:540–547.

313. Mokhtarian F, Shi Y, Zhu PF, Grob D. immune responses and autoimmune oucome during virus infection of the central nervous system. Cell Immunol 1994; 157:195–210.

314. Subak-Sharpe I, Dyson H, Fazakerley JK. In vivo depletion of CD8+ T cells prevents lesions of demyelination in Semliki Forest virus infection. J Virol 1993; 67:7629–7633.

315. Morris MM, Dyson H, Baker D, Harbige LS, Fazakerley JK, Amor S. Characterization of the cellular and cytokine response in the central nervous system following Semliki Forest virus infection. J Neuroimmunol 1997; 74: 185–197.

316. Donnelly SM, Sheahan BJ, Atkins GJ. Long term effects of Semliki Forest virus infection in the mouse central nervous system. Neuropathol Appl Neurobiol 1997; 23:235–241.

317. Grosfeld H, Velan B, Leitner M, Lustig S, Lachi BE, Cohen S, Shafferman A. Delineation of protective epitopes on the E2-envelope glycoprotein of Semliki Forest virus. Vaccine 1991; 9: 451–456.

318. Grosfeld H, Lustig S, Gozes Y, Velan B, Cohen S, Leitner M, Lachmi B, Katz D, Olshevski U, Shafferman A. Divergent envelope E2 alphavirus sequences spanning amino acids 297 to 352 induce in mice virus-specific protective immunity and antibodies with complement-mediated cytolytic activity. J Virol 1992; 66:1084–1090.

319. Snijders A, Benaissa-Trouw BJ, Visser-Vernooy HJ, Fernandez I, Snippe H, Kraaijeveld CA. A delayed-type hypersensitivity-inducing T cell epitope of Semliki Forest virus mediates effective T-helper activity for antibody production. Immunology 1992; 77:322–329.

320. Glasgow GM, Sheahan BJ, Atkins GJ, Wahlberg JM, Salminen A, Liljestrom P. Two mutations in the envelope glycoprotein E2 of Semliki Forest virus affecting the maturation and entry patterns of the virus alter pathogenicity for mice. Virology 1991; 185:741–748.

321. Glasgow GM, Killen HM, Liljestrom P, Sheahan BJ, Atkins GJ. A single amino acid change in the E2 spike protein of a virulent strain of Semliki Forest virus attenuates pathogenicity. J Gen Virol 1994; 75: 663–668.

322. Tarbatt CJ, Glasgow GM, Mooney DA, Sheahan BJ, Atkins GJ. Sequence analysis of the avirulent, demyelinating A7 strain of Semliki Forest virus. J Gen Virol 1997; 78:1551–1557.

323. Kurtzke JF. Epidemiologic contributions to multiple sclerosis: Am overview. Neurology 1980; 30:61–79.

324. Forghani B, Cremer NE, Johnson KB, Ginsberg AH, Likosky WH. Viral antibodies in cerebrospinal fluid of multiple sclerosis and control patients: Comparison between radioimmunoassay and conventional standards. J Clin Microbiol 1978; 7:63–69.

325. McFarlin DE, McFarland HF. Multiple sclerosis. N Engl J Med 1982; 307:1183–1188 and 1246–1251.

326. Johnson RT. The possible viral etiology of multiple sclerosis. In: Friedlander WJ, ed. Advances in Neurology, New York: Raven, (1975), vol. 13, pp. 1–46.

327. Prineas JW. Pathology of multiple sclerosis. In: Cook SD, ed. Handbook of Multiple Sclerosis. New York and Basel: Marcel Dekker, 1990:87–218.

328. Batchelor JR, Compston A, McDonald WI. The significance of the association between HLA and multiple sclerosis. Br Med Bull 1978; 34: 279–284.

329. Poser CM. The pathogenesis of multiple sclerosis: Additional considerations. J Neurol Sci 1993; 115(suppl):S3–S15.

330. Sadovnick AD. Genetic epidemiology of multiple sclerosis. Ann Neurol 1994; 36(S2):S194–S203.

5

Evidence for a Viral Etiology of Multiple Sclerosis

STUART D. COOK

University of Medicine and Dentistry of New Jersey and New Jersey Medical School, Newark, New Jersey

I. INTRODUCTION

Multiple sclerosis (MS) is an acquired inflammatory disease of the central nervous system (CNS) of unknown etiology. Based on available evidence, it seems probable that MS is a complex disease in which exposure to one or more environmental agents predisposes genetically susceptible individuals to develop immunologically mediated CNS demyelination and axonal injury. While the nature of the environmental agent(s) has not yet been defined, there is considerable indirect support for the role of infection in initiating and perhaps perpetuating the inflammatory pathology that results in neurologic symptoms and disability (1,2). Recently several novel exogenous agents have been identified in MS brain or cerebrospinal fluid (3–5), raising the possibility that antiviral or antibacterial drugs could alter disease prognosis. While the specificity of these findings remains in doubt, interest in an infectious cause of MS remains strong.

This chapter comprises a critical review of evidence for and against an infectious etiology of MS.

II. HISTORICAL PERSPECTIVE

The concept that MS may be caused or aggravated by an infectious agent is not new. Although both Charcot and Leyden suggested a relationship between an antecedent illness and the onset of MS, Pierre Marie more formally raised this possibility shortly after the clinical and pathological characteristics of MS were initially defined (6,7). In a paper published in 1884, Marie states ''I was struck by the coincidental occurrence of multiple sclerosis with infectious illnesses and by the close relationship that, from a theoretical point of view, unites these two afflictions; thus, I made an effort to renew the idea that multiple sclerosis often starts as an infectious process. . . .''

Over the past 116 years numerous, often highly publicized claims of isolation or identification of viruses, bacteria, and spirochetes from or in MS tissue have been made (8–10) (Table 1).

Unfortunately, independent attempts at verifying these reports or determining their specificity have been generally unsuccessful, leading to a pervasive skepticism over subsequent claims of linkage between MS and infectious agents.

Nevertheless, the suspicion remains high that an infectious agent is responsible for initiating the as yet imprecisely defined sequence of immunological and inflammatory events that lead to CNS demyelination in this enigmatic disease.

In recent years, with the advent of sophisticated molecular technology and the general failure of traditional isolation and culture techniques to identify conventional organisms, attention has been directed more toward viral candidates. Viruses can cause demyelinating disease in animals and humans, can remain latent in neural tissue for extended periods, and can cause chronic persistent infections of the CNS—characteristics attractive for a putative MS pathogen. However, the recent demonstration that bacterial or bacterialike organisms are responsible for cat scratch disease (*Rochalimaea* species), peptic ulcer (*Helicobacter pylori*), chronic Lyme arthritis (*Borrelia burgdorferi*), Whipple's disease (*Tropheryma whippelii*) and other diseases previously considered ''idiopathic'' should leave the reader with an open mind for the possible microbial spectrum of MS precipitants. In Whipple's disease, the bacterium, *T. whippelli*, was first cultured almost 100 years after the disease was initially described. While several reasons could be put forth to explain the delay in identifying this elusive organism, it is undoubtedly relevant that the agent has to be grown intracellularly in the absence of antibiotics and takes an extremely long time to grow (11). In this regard, Blaser (12) has pointed out that many infectious diseases have not been linked to their causative agent in a timely fashion, even in the modern era, because of technical barriers, including fastidious culture requirements or low tissue concentrations of the pathogen, or because of conceptual barriers, including the failure to recognize that the disease could be an uncommon complication of a common microbe or

Table 1 Negative, Unconfirmed, or Controversial Studies for Infectious Antigen or Genome in MS

Adenovirus	MS-associated agent
Borrelia burgdorferi	Measles virus
Canine distemper virus	Mumps virus
Chlamydia pneumoniae	Papovavirus
Coronavirus	Parainfluenza virus
Cytomegalovirus	Rabies virus
Epstein-Barr virus	Retrovirus
HHV-6	Rubella
HTLV-1 and/or 2	Scrapie agent
Herpes simplex 1 virus and/or 2	Simian virus 5
Human immunodeficiency virus	SMON-like virus

Key: HHV, human herpes virus; HTLV, human T-cell leukemia/lymphome virus; SMON, subacute myelo-optico neuropathy.
Source: Modified from Ref. 1.

because of a long latent period between infection and disease expression. Clearly, these same considerations could be relevant to MS.

III. EVIDENCE FOR AN INFECTIOUS ETIOLOGY

It seems safe to say that no convincing data yet exists linking a specific exogenous agent to MS. However, a persuasive body of evidence, albeit indirect, leads one to conclude that environmental factors undoubtedly play a role in determining risk for acquiring this disease. This evidence is based on studies of MS epidemiology, concordance rates in twins, pathology, and serology as well as the existence of viral models of demyelinating disease.

A. Epidemiology

One of the major clues to MS etiology comes from analysis of the remarkable worldwide pattern of MS. This shows a crude but inconsistent north-south gradient in North America and Europe; a low prevalence in most of Asia, Africa, and South America (although many of these studies are less than definitive because of uncertainty about the completeness of case ascertainment); and a smaller south-north gradient in Australia and New Zealand (see Chap. 2) (2,13–14). This nonrandom pattern is different from that seen with most other acute or chronic "immune-mediated disorders," including diseases of the central and peripheral nervous systems (PNS), such as acute disseminated encephalomyelitis (ADEM), the Guillain-Barré syndrome (GBS), and chronic inflammatory demyelinating polyneuropathy (CIDP).

When unusual worldwide patterns of disease are seen, interest heightens in the potential for identifying causative mechanisms. Some diseases with characteristic geographic features are genetic in origin. This would include Tay-Sachs disease, affecting primarily Ashkenazi Jews; β-thalassemia, occurring in populations originating in southern Italy, other Mediterranean countries, Africa, and Asia; and sickle cell disease in individuals with African ancestry. Other diseases caused by specific infectious agents may have a unique distribution because of environmental factors, including cultural characteristics of the population and degree of exposure to the vectors involved in transmission. Rabies and several parasitic diseases can be considered in this category. Yet other diseases—such as tuberculosis, paralytic poliomyelitis, and rheumatic heart disease—may have a restricted global pattern owing to a combination of environmental factors, including poor hygiene or crowded conditions, and genetic predisposition. Which of these possibilities best fits MS is debatable, but the latter two seem more likely than the former on the basis of available evidence.

There is also a consistent but not invariable effect of migration in altering MS risk in migrants or their offspring, depending on age at migration and whether movement is from high- to low-risk regions or the converse (see Chap. 2) (2,13,14). The effect of migration on disease risk has not been associated as clearly with other chronic "immune-mediated" diseases. In addition, controversial changes in MS incidence, up or down, or even frank clustering in some locales have been described, suggesting that MS is not always a stable endemic disease as would be predicted for a purely genetic disorder. Last, from an epidemiological point of view, multiple studies indicate that MS patients have had measles, Epstein-Barr virus (EBV), and other childhood infections at a later age than controls (15–21). Whether this indicates that late exposure to multiple, a few, or a single pathogen is a critical factor in triggering remains to be determined.

B. Twin Studies

Although genetic factors also seem important in determining MS susceptibility (see Chap. 3), the Canadian MS twin study showed a concordance rate of only 31% in monozygotic pairs, as compared with less than 5% in dizygotes, even with magnetic resonance imaging (MRI) brain scans to detect subclinical disease, and long-term follow-up evaluations (22). This means that in over two-thirds of identical twins, both twins do not develop MS, even when one of the pair does. It seems safe to conclude from this evidence that in most instances genetic factors alone are insufficient to cause MS.

Identical twins share not only genetic sameness but many common environmental exposures including diet, exposure to sunlight, vaccination schedules, and communicable diseases during the first 15 to 18 years of life. Assuming that an infectious agent is important in causing MS, one can speculate that either the agent is not readily spread from twin to twin (i.e., low infectivity, sexual spread, animal vector) or that host factors other than exposure are important (i.e., dose of infectious agent, route of infection, status of the individual's immune system). The relatively low concordance rate in identical twins, relatively narrow age of onset of MS, restricted geography, and migration effects appear to the author to be more suggestive of one or a few agents causing MS rather than a large number, as many experts believe. In this regard, a remarkably similar concordance rate in monozygotic as compared to dizygotic twins is seen with paralytic poliomyelitis (23).

C. CNS and Cerebrospinal Fluid Studies

CNS findings—including inflammatory lesions; abnormal profiles of chemokines, cytokines, and other effector molecules; and alterations in T- and B-cell concentrations (see Chaps. 7 and 12), as well as cerebrospinal fluid (CSF) changes in IgG, free light chains, and electrophoretically restricted bands (OCBs) in MS (see Chap. 14)—are compatible with the effect of either an infectious agent or an autoimmune process. Similar pathological changes can be seen with viral and nonviral encephalitides as well as in the animal model experimental allergic encephalomyelitis (EAE). Likewise, the CSF IgG abnormalities seen in MS are mirrored in many infectious disorders including subacute sclerosing panencephalitis (SSPE), neurosyphilis, Lyme disease, and viral encephalitis as well as in immune-mediated disorders such as EAE (24–30). Whereas in most viral infections the OCBs react with or can be adsorbed by disease-specific viral antigens (25,28,29), attempts at removing MS oligoclonal bands after exposure to measles and other candidate viruses have generally been unsuccessful (25,28) or, if positive (31), remain unconfirmed. It is currently unclear whether or not the OCBs in MS CSF react to an as yet undefined specific infectious agent or to host antigens.

D. Infectious Agents Causing Demyelination

Clues to the etiology of MS might come from considering viruses and other infectious agents capable of causing spontaneous demyelination in humans or animals (Table 2). Several DNA and RNA viruses can produce inflammatory myelin loss in the CNS or PNS. In humans, infection with measles, EBV, varicella, and other pathogens can result in ADEM or postinfectious encephalomyelitis (1), whereas infections with *Campylobacter jejuni*, EBV, *Mycoplasma pneumoniae*, and cytomegalovirus (CMV) are often associated with GBS (32). However, acute infection with these agents rarely produces recurrent or chronic demyelination, suggesting that either host factors are critical in this regard or that as yet unidentified agents are responsible for causing MS and CIDP. Persistent infection

Table 2 Spontaneous Human and Animal Viral Models of
Inflammatory Central Nervous System Demyelinating Diseases

Human	Animal
Acute disseminated encephalomyelitis	Canine distemper virus
Progressive multifocal leukoencephalopathy	Murine coronaviruses
HIV encephalopathy	Theiler's virus
HTLV-1	Visna virus
Other	Other

Key: HIV, human immunodeficiency virus; HTLV, human T-cell leukemia/
lymphoma virus.
Source: Modified from Ref. 1.

with other viruses—including papovavirus (progressive multifocal leukoencephalopathy),
human T-cell leukaemia/lymphonia virus type 1 (HTLV-1; tropical spastic paraparesis)
and human immunodeficiency virus (HIV)—result in chronic demyelination, although
there are distinct pathological differences between these encephalopathies and MS. Similarly, canine distemper virus (CDV) infection in dogs, Theiler's murine encephalomyelitis
virus, coronavirus infections in mice, and other animal viruses can cause demyelination
in their hosts, with an acute, exacerbating, or progressive course (see Chap. 4).

E. Serological Studies

Serological studies of MS serum and CSF show increased antibody titers to measles as
well as to other infectious agents when compared with controls (Table 3). Using a variety
of techniques, serum antibodies from MS sera are elevated to multiple measles peptides.
The measles antibody titer increase is modest (about twofold) and does not relate to disease
severity or duration (27). Increases in viral antibody titers have been reported to numerous
other agents, including vaccinia, herpes zoster, EBV, rubella, mumps, herpes simplex,
canine distemper, adenovirus, parainfluenza 2, and influenza viruses. Although any agent
inducing a consistent increase in antibody levels in MS patients could be considered a
potential causal agent, other reasons for increased antibody need to be considered. For
example, reactivation of a latent virus secondary either to the MS inflammatory process
or to the use of immunosuppressive drugs could in some instances explain these serological
findings. Alternatively, elevated antibody levels to multiple infectious agents in the same
patient could be attributable to nonspecific generalized B-cell hyperactivity. Such a phenomenon could also explain the presence of OCBs in MS CSF.

Similar to serum studies, an increase in CSF viral antibody titer or CSF/serum antibody ratio (after equalization of IgG levels in these two fluids) has been reported for
measles virus. However, such changes have also been reported in some but not all studies
for rubella, EBV, human coronavirus 229E, herpes zoster, and other agents. As with serum,
increased CSF titers to multiple viruses may be seen in the same CSF sample furthermore,
titers can fluctuate over time, indicating the potential problems inherent in attempts to
link a virus to MS by serological methods alone.

In summary, the occurrence of spontaneous human and animal models of virus-
induced demyelination as well as evidence from epidemiological, serological, and pathological studies provides strong support for the existence of an infectious trigger but not
as yet for a persistent CNS infection.

Table 3 Serum or CSF Antibody Titer Higher in
MS Patients Than Controls

Serum	
Adenovirus	Measles virus
Canine distemper virus	Mumps virus
Epstein-Barr virus	Parainfluenza virus
Herpes simplex	Rubella virus
HHV-6	Vaccinia virus
Influenza	Varicella zoster virus
CSF	
Adenoviruses	Measles virus
Chlamydia pneumoniae	Mumps virus
Cytomegalovirus	*Mycoplasma pneumoniae*
Epstein-Barr virus	Parainfluenza 1, 2, and 3
Human herpes virus 6	Respiratory syncytial virus
Herpes simplex	Rubella virus
Human coronavirus	Vaccinia virus
Influenza A and B	Varicella zoster virus

Source: From Ref. 1.

IV. POSSIBLE MECHANISMS OF VIRUS-INDUCED DEMYELINATION

If one assumes that MS is triggered by an infectious agent, at least two mechanisms by which the infectious agent could cause tissue injury can be considered (1,14,33).

A. Persistent Infection

The direct infection hypothesis implies that the virus persists in brain or perhaps in other organs, periodically seeding the brain. There are many examples of persistent infections or viral latency in the nervous system. In the former category are measles virus (SSPE), HIV, HTLV-1, papovavirus, and rubella virus encephalopathies. Herpes simplex, herpes zoster, certain retroviruses, and human herpes virus 6 (HHV-6) are examples of common viruses that persist in neural tissue, usually in a latent form. In these models, chronic low-grade infection, periodic reactivation of latent virus, or seeding of the brain through a hematogenous route could cause direct injury to glial or other neural cells. Alternatively, an immune response to the agent could trigger an autoimmune reaction because of agent-induced release or alteration of previously sequestered self-antigens with epitope spread; or a similar antigenic or structural relationship between agent and brain proteins or lipids could lead to host-induced self-injury (molecular mimicry) (34). In addition, the infectious agent could affect macrophages and lymphocytes, so that subsequently nonencephalito-genic activated T cells could enter the CNS, causing demyelination (bystander effect) (35). Last, the agent could act as a superantigen, directly stimulating encephalitogenic T-cell clones (36). Through any of these mechanisms, demyelination and axonal injury could arise.

If the agent does persist in the host, it should ultimately be identifiable using appropriate techniques, including the exquisitely sensitive polymerase chain reaction (PCR) or newer molecular techniques for identifying exogenous genes or proteins.

Further, if an infectious agent persists in the patient, it might be possible to show a serological association between pathogen and disease. Antibody to the agent might be extremely elevated compared with controls, even though the controls had been infected transiently by the same virus. For example, SSPE is a persistent measles virus infection of the brain, leading to very high serum and CSF measles antibody titers to most but not all viral proteins. However, even with persistent infection, viral antibody titers are not always elevated. For example, in progressive canine distemper encephalitis, viral antibody titers are often lower in animals with fulminant disease, perhaps related to virus-induced lymphopenia and immunosuppression (1,14).

Although discouraging, the failure to reproducibly culture an organism from or identify viral genome or antigens in MS tissues cannot be considered as proof that an infectious agent is not present (1,9,14). Nevertheless, the negative results to date indicate the need to consider alternative mechanisms for CNS lesions in MS.

B. Transient Infection

The second mechanism that can be considered for infection-induced lesion genesis in MS is the transient infection or hit-and-run hypothesis (1,33). In this scenario, the pathogen is present only briefly in the host, but this is sufficient for a persistent organ-specific autoimmune process to be established. The virus acts as a triggering agent only and may be undetectable when clinical symptoms develop. Demyelination could then be induced in several possible ways. As discussed previously, the infectious agent might contain structural sequences identical with a brain protein or other antigen (molecular mimicry). An immune response to the agent cross-reacts with the corresponding brain antigen, resulting in a chronic, self-perpetuating inflammatory disease, MS. Streptococcus-induced rheumatic heart disease may be an example of this type of autoimmune organ-specific disorder, where an antigenic similarity between bacterial M protein and cardiac myosin leads to cardiac valvular damage (1,14,37). Consistent with this mechanism, several bacterial and viral decapeptides have been identified with amino acid profiles similar to myelin proteins (16). These include hepatitis B virus, EBV, *Escherichia coli*, adenovirus, influenza, measles, and CDV. Using a different approach, Wucherpfennig and Strominger screened a large number of peptides for degeneracy of amino acid side chains required for major histocompatibility complex (MHC) class II binding and activation of myelin basic protein (MBP)–responsive T cells (38). A panel of 129 peptides satisfying these criteria was identified, of which herpes simplex virus, EBV, adenovirus type 12, influenza type A, and *Pseudomonas aeruginosa* peptides gave the greatest activation of MBP-specific T-cell clones derived from MS patients. Collectively, these studies support the concept that multiple common infectious agents have the potential for triggering MS by a molecular mimicry mechanism. An alternative possibility for tissue injury might also involve molecular mimicry between infectious agent and host protein, but instead of a myelin protein, a regulatory protein in the immune system or a critical host enzyme might be the target, resulting in altered immune function, disruption of the blood-brain barrier, or interference with myelin metabolism. This could lead to a less direct but equally devastating immunopathology. Additionally, transient CNS inflammation in a genetically susceptible host could also prime the host's CNS, leading to periodic bystander demyelination when the systemic immune response is activated. Another indirect mechanism for myelin injury could be through the effect of exogenus superantigens. In this scenario, infectious agents can activate T cells, including autoreactive T cells, by interacting directly with the Vβ receptor, resulting in a self-perpetuating autoimmune disease even after the agent is eliminated. Last, the agent could infect lymphocytes or other immunocompetent cells, altering delicately balanced control mechanisms and thereby allowing the emergence of aggressive autoimmune T- or B-cell clones (1,14). Measles and CDV are examples of viruses that produce transient profound immunosuppression and neurological illness in which MBP-responsive T cells can be found in peripheral blood (1,9,14,39,40).

If a virus triggers MS but is no longer present in the host when neurological disease is manifest, it will be extremely difficult to prove causation (1,14). In such a situation, it will be necessary to have persuasive epidemiological and serological evidence linking the virus to MS. However, several problems exist in attempting to use serology to link a virus to MS. If MS is caused by multiple viruses, there may be considerable variability in viral titers geographically and temporally. For example, CMV-induced GBS may occur in epidemics, with few GBS patients demonstrating positive CMV serology in the interepidemic period (41). Second, because MS is a chronic disorder with a variable, often long latent period before onset of neurological symptoms, one would not expect to see a four-fold rise or fall in antibody titers to the agent or a predominantly IgM antibody response, as usually occurs with an acute infectious process (42). Furthermore, if MS is an uncommon complication of a common infection and the agent does not persist, both MS patients and controls may have similar antibody titers to the agent in CSF and serum with no increase in the CSF to serum antibody index (1,14). For example, it is difficult to conclude whether an individual had early adult infectious mononucleosis or an asymptomatic childhood EBV infection, or paralytic or nonparalytic poliomyelitis, by measuring IgG antibody titers later in adult life. In addition, one would need to show some specificity of the antibody response by demonstrating no similar increase in antibody titers to other viral or nonviral antigens in these MS patients. Similarly, antibody titers should not be related solely to an increase in serum or CSF IgG. In contrast, if MS is caused by an agent that does not usually infect humans, it might be easier to demonstrate higher antibody titers to the agent in patients than in normal individuals (1). An example of this type of serological response is found with human rabies. In this situation, there should be fewer MS patients with low and more with higher antibody titers as compared to controls. Last, the presence of low antibody titers cannot be taken as proof that an individual has not been previously infected by the agent in question, because, after many infections, antibody titers fall over time.

V. CANDIDATE AGENTS IN MULTIPLE SCLEROSIS

It is conceivable that multiple infectious agents trigger MS. Unfortunately, if MS is caused by multiple agents, it is unlikely that measures will be available in the short term to decrease MS risk (14). Another possibility is that classic MS is caused primarily by an as yet unidentified single infectious agent or a known agent that has not yet been firmly linked to MS. In favor of the unitary hypothesis is the distinct worldwide distribution of MS, the effect of migration on MS risk, the relatively low concordance rate in identical twins who share a remarkably close childhood environment. In addition there are the reports, albeit controversial, of clustering of MS or changes in incidence in different locales. If only one or a few viruses are responsible for triggering MS, disease incidence may be alterable by development and deployment of appropriate viral vaccines (14).

Several infectious agents currently remain as viable candidate agents because they may be compatible with the unique worldwide distribution of MS, because they induce demyelination in humans or animals, because agent-specific antibodies are elevated in the serum or CSF of MS patients, or because, in unconfirmed studies, infectious genome has been identified in MS brain or CSF or the organism has been isolated from MS tissues (1,14). Measles, human coronavirus 226E, EBV, retroviruses, HHV-6, and *Chlamydia pneumoniae* have attracted the most interest in recent years in terms of known agents that commonly infect humans. Animal viruses currently most attractive are JHM, a mouse coronavirus; Theiler's murine encephalomyelitis virus, a picornavirus of mice; and CDV, a morbilliform virus of dogs and carnivores.

A. Human Infectious Agents

Measles Virus

Measles virus is an RNA morbilliform virus commonly linked to ADEM or postinfectious encephalomyelitis, although this disorder is now uncommonly seen in the western world due to the ubiquitous use of measles vaccine. Following postmeasles encephalomyelitis, myelin basic protein–reactive T cells circulate in the peripheral blood, suggesting a possible autoimmune mechanism of tissue injury in this disorder (9,43). However, patients with postmeasles encephalomyelitis rarely go on to develop MS. From an epidemiological point of view, measles virus infections often occur at a later age in MS patients than in controls, suggesting that a late age of infection may predispose to a different disease phenotype (15,16). A similar phenomenon has been noted to occur with EBV and poliovirus infections (14,21).

Since the original study by Adams and Imagawa (44), most serological studies have shown an increase in measles antibody titer in the serum and CSF of MS patients (14,27). Although absolute titers are only modestly elevated compared with controls, the consistency of these findings lends credence to the possible biological significance of the observation. A difference between MS patients and normal individuals has also been shown in cellular responses to measles virus. Lymphocytes obtained from MS patients appear to have a specific cytotoxic defect when reacted with measles-infected cell lines (45). This could theoretically lead to a persistent measles infection in MS patients. Consistent with this possibility, measles virus genome has been identified in some MS brain specimens, but other investigators, using a variety of techniques to identify measles genetic material or proteins, have been unable to confirm these observations (46–52). In terms of immunopathogenesis, measles virus decapeptides have amino acid sequences in common with myelin basic protein (MBP) and proteolipid protein (PLP), both components of myelin, suggesting a potential mechanism for molecular mimicry–induced tissue injury (16, 51).

Evidence against measles virus as the cause of MS, in addition to the failure to consistently identify the agent in MS tissue, is mainly epidemiological. There is a lack of correlation between measles infections worldwide and the incidence, prevalence, or clustering of MS. For example, MS prevalence is higher in northern United States and Canada than in the American South, although there appears to be no obvious difference in age of measles infection or measles vaccine exposure in these geographically disparate areas. Controversial epidemics of MS or changes in incidence have occurred in the Faroe (52), Orkney (53), and Shetland Islands (54) as well as elsewhere; these appear to bear no relation to the occurrence of measles infections in these locales. More importantly, there appears to be no decrease in the worldwide incidence of MS (13,55,56), despite increasing use of measles vaccines over the past 30 years, and individuals have been identified who have had typical measles infections after onset of MS (57). In contrast, measles vaccination has largely eradicated SSPE in the western world. Thus, measles is unlikely to be an important major primary cause of MS (1).

Coronavirus

Coronaviruses are single-stranded RNA viruses with positive polarity. Two human coronavirus serotypes have been identified, 229E and OC43 (58,59). Although not clearly documented to cause encephalitis or myelitis, these RNA viruses cause approximately 15 to 35% of all upper respiratory infections in humans. However, the potential for human neurotropism does exist, since a receptor for 229E has been demonstrated in brain synaptic membranes, and cultured human neural cells can be infected with this virus (60). In addition, evidence for molecular mimicry between nonstructural proteins of coronavirus 229E and MBP has been demonstrated. The mouse coronavirus JHM can cause demyelination in mice, rats, and primates (50), and both demyelination and mild neurological disease can be adoptively transferred from infected to normal rats (61) using MBP-stimulated donor lymphocytes.

With respect to MS, Tanaka et al. (62), in an unconfirmed study, observed coronavirus-like particles in the perivascular cuff of an MS plaque. In another unconfirmed study, an increase in CSF but not serum antibody to coronavirus 229E and OC43 was detected in 26 and 41% respectively of MS patients but not in neurological controls (63). In addition, coronavirus 229E viral RNA was identified by Stewart et al. in 4 of 11 MS brain specimens but in none of 11 controls using reverse transcriptase PCR (59). No OC43 nucleic acid was found in any specimens. Subsequently, Talbot et al. extended these studies, finding both the 229E and OC43 (36 vs. 14%) strains of coronavirus in MS brain samples, the latter significantly more than in controls but the former not (60). Unfortunately, these provocative observations have not yet been confirmed (Dowling, Personal communication, 64).

Confirmation of the presence of viral genome in MS brain tissue, further evidence that coronavirus strains 229E or OC43 cause human neurological disease, and additional demonstrations of higher serum or CSF antibody to 229E and OC43 in MS patients are needed before considering either of these coronaviruses more seriously as a candidate agent in MS causation (1).

Epstein-Barr Virus

There is much in favor of EBV as a candidate agent in MS. EBV, a DNA herpes family virus, causes infectious mononucleosis and has been linked to certain lymphomas, nasopharyngeal carcinoma, and a variety of acute neurological disorders, including GBS and ADEM (41,65–67). In one report, five patients with an acute EBV infection associated with neurological complications subsequently developed a more chronic MS-like illness (68). Epidemiological studies are also consistent with a relationship between EBV infections and MS. Similar to MS, the peak age for acquiring infectious mononucleosis is adolescence or early adulthood, and like MS, infectious mononucleosis is less common in underdeveloped countries, where exposure to EBV usually occurs at an early age (69). In several studies, a positive correlation has also been made between prior infectious mononucleosis and the subsequent development of MS, and the age at which infectious mononucleosis occurred may be relevant in this regard (21,70–72). Whether this indicates that EBV can trigger MS, predisposes to MS, or causes a flare-up of disease in a patient with underlying MS remains to be determined.

Immunological studies in support of an EBV-MS relationship have also been published. Several serological surveys have shown that MS patients have higher serum and CSF antibodies to multiple EBV antigens, with up to 100% of patients in some series seropositive to this agent (73–76). EBV peptide sequences can activate MBP responsive

T cells obtained from MS patients (38), and EBV has decapeptides homologous with bovine PLP and human MBP (16,51). In addition, B cells infected with EBV express ∝B crystallin and activate T cells reactive to ∝B crystallin, which is also present in myelin (77). Further antibodies in MS sera reactive to human transaldolase, expressed selectively in oligodendrocytes, cross-react with EBV capsid derived peptides (78). Thus, several potential mechanisms for EBV molecular mimicry induced autoimmune demyelination can be considered.

On the other hand, it is difficult to interpret the relevance of the serological findings because this virus is so ubiquitous. Indeed, 85 to 90% of controls also have positive serology (1). In addition, it is quite possible that latent EBV, like other herpes family viruses, is reactivated secondary to the altered immune system present in MS patients or to the use of immunomodulating drugs in this disease, resulting in a secondary increase in EBV antibody titers (1). In this regard, elevated antibody titers to numerous agents can be seen in MS sera and CSF, reflecting a generalized increase in B cell activity.

Unfortunately, it is difficult to prove or disprove the EBV-MS hypothesis, since attempts to identify EBV genome in MS brain tissue have either been negative or nonspecifically positive (79). It is also difficult to explain MS latitudinal gradients or migration effects on the basis of EBV, since no apparent difference in age of exposure to EBV has been unequivocally demonstrated between north and south in North America, and migration from high- to low-risk areas after age 15 should increase rather than decrease MS risk if EBV is more prevalent in areas of lesser hygiene. Despite these concerns, EBV remains a viable candidate for causing MS.

Retroviruses

Retroviruses, RNA viruses encoding for reverse transcriptase, have received considerable attention as possible causal agents in MS, because members of this genus of viruses—including visna, HTLV-1, and HIV—can cause chronic neurological disorders with demyelinating features. In the mid-1980s Koprowski et al. (80) reported increased serum and CSF HTLV-1 p24 antibody titers in MS patients as well as in other neurological disease controls. In addition, HTLV-1–specific RNA was demonstrated by in situ hybridization in cultured CSF cells obtained from some MS patients. Unfortunately, numerous attempts at reproducing these provocative findings have been unsuccessful or nonspecific (81). Furthermore, the pattern of HTLV-1 infections worldwide does not correlate well with the unique distribution of MS. Nevertheless, there has been a high degree of residual interest in this group of viruses in terms of MS causation.

Subsequently, additional reports claiming identification of other retroviruses or retroviral genomic sequences in biological material obtained from MS patients appeared. Perron et al. isolated a retrovirus (MSRV) in a leptomeningeal cell line obtained from the CSF of an MS patient (3,82). MSRV replicated in infected monocytes and both reverse transcriptase activity and a retrovirus like agent could be demonstrated in culture supernatants. Transcribed MSRV-pol gene sequences were also detected in the CSF of 5 of 10 MS patients but in none of 10 controls. MSRV RNA was also found in 9 of 17 MS patients but only 3 of 44 controls (83). Similar results were obtained when B cells from MS peripheral blood or choroid plexus cells from MS brain were cultured (3,82,84). Sequencing of MSRV genome showed similarities but also differences with the human endogenous retrovirus ERV-9 (85). MSRV was also found in EBV-transformed B cells obtained from MS patients, raising the possibility that a combination of EBV and MSRV could be cofactors in causing MS (85,86). It has recently been suggested that MSRV may belong to a new family of endogenous retroviruses designated HERV-W (87).

Serological studies in a few MS patients demonstrated serum antibodies reactive by Western blots with MSRV proteins (3). Further, human endogenous retrovirus peptides induced more proliferation and type 1 cytokine production in peripheral blood mononuclear cells from patients with active MS than in patients with stable disease or healthy controls (88).

Although the concept that a unique, endogenous retrovirus could cause MS is attractive, questions have been raised about the specificity of these viruses for MS (89), and some investigators using a different ultrasensitive reverse transcription technique, a modified product of enhanced reverse transcriptase (IMxPERT), have been unable to find a similar retrovirus in CSF, serum, or peripheral blood mononuclear cells obtained from MS patients (90). Additionally, autoantibodies cross-reactive with HERV proteins have been found in patients with other autoimmune diseases, including systemic lupus erythematosus and Sjögren's syndrome (88), suggesting a lack of serological specificity for MS.

Thus, the biological significance of MSRV and other retroviruses in MS is unknown and may merely represent a secondary activation of a common endogenous retrovirus, since HERVs are estimated to constitute up to 1% of human DNA (89), and sequences of endogenous retroviruses closely related to MSRV are expressed in both MS and control tissues (89,91). Alternatively, this or other retroviruses may be important exogenous agents in MS causation or may not initiate MS but may contribute to lesion development. More epidemiological, serological, and sequencing studies are needed to clarify the role of these viruses in MS.

Human Herpes Virus Type 6

Human herpes virus (HHV-6), a recently discovered DNA virus, causes exanthem subitum (roseola) in children. Two variants of HHV-6 have been described, A and B. HHV-6 typically causes rash and fever in children—but, in addition, this virus commonly enters the CNS during acute primary infections, occasionally resulting in meningitis or other neurological complications (4,92–94). HHV-6 has also been reported to cause encephalitis in immunosuppressed adults and has been linked in a few instances to encephalopathic and myelopathic disorders as well as to human demyelinating disease (95–101).

Almost all children are infected early in life by this ubiquitous virus, with HHV-6 seropositivity being seen in 90% of all children by 2 years of age (92–94). Like other herpes family viruses, HHV-6 persists lifelong in brain and other tissues in most normal individuals, and—as with other herpes viruses—HHV-6 can be reactivated in certain situations.

Interest in HHV-6 as a candidate agent in MS intensified following the report by Challoner et al. in 1995 demonstrating HHV-6 variant B group 2 in the brains of greater than 70% of patients with this disease (4). Although HHV-6 was found in a similar percentage of control brains, two viral proteins were identified by immunocytochemistry in oligodendrocytes from 12 of 15 MS brain samples but in none of 45 control brains. These proteins were preferentially expressed in MS plaques rather than in histologically uninvolved white matter. In this study, neurons from MS patients and controls also contained HHV-6 proteins. Similar immunocytochemical findings were found by Knox et al., who reported that 17 of 19 tissue sections that were undergoing active demyelination, obtained from six MS patients, contained HHV-6 proteins, versus none of 15 brain samples from patients with other inflammatory demyelinating diseases (102). In addition, Knox et al. found HHV-6 antigens in 6 of 9 MS lymph nodes but not in lymphoid tissue from 7 controls.

In contrast, other investigators, although finding HHV-6 genome or antigen in MS brain, have noted the lack of specificity for either MS CNS, brain cell types, or to areas of demyelination (103–104). Because herpes viruses can be activated nonspecifically by trauma or by alteration in immune status, it is conceivable that the intense inflammatory response, along with the cell death and proliferation that occurs in MS lesions (105), reactivates latent HHV-6. Similarly, HHV-6 could be nonspecifically reactivated in patients previously immunosuppressed with steroids or other drugs. This might explain why brain material from patients with SSPE, progressive multifocal leukoencephalopathy, and HIV can show similar HHV-6 brain findings as in MS (103–104).

HHV-6 variant A and B have also been identified in blood and CSF from a few MS patients (91,102,106,107) but others have not confirmed these findings or find them nonspecific (91,92,108–110).

As to serological responses, reports of higher IgG or IgM antibody titers to HHV-6 or HHV-6B in serum or CSF of MS patients versus controls have been found in several (92,93,106,107,112), but not all studies (113–115). In addition, an increased lymphoproliferative response to HHV-6A has been found in MS patients as compared to controls (116).

As has been stated previously, an increase in viral antibody titers in MS has been shown in serum and CSF to many agents, perhaps reflecting increased B-cell activity. In order to determine the specificity of HHV-6 serological findings, it would be desirable to compare viral titers in MS and inflammatory disease controls to HHV-6 and other candidate agents.

Although it is difficult to reconcile the pattern of early HHV-6 infection with the worldwide pattern of MS, twin studies, and migration effects, the ultimate test of the HHV-6 hypothesis awaits additional studies and attempts at modifying disease course with antiviral drugs. Although preliminary studies showed no clear evidence of clinical benefit in MS patients treated with acyclovir, trials with other antiviral therapies are ongoing (100). To date it seems more likely that HHV-6 is a passenger rather than the driver in MS causation, but even though it may be noncausative, it could contribute to lesion pathogenesis.

Chlamydia pneumoniae

Chlamydia pneumoniae, an obligate intracellular bacterium closely related to other chlamydial species including *C. psittaci, C. trachomatis*, and *C. pecorum*, was first described in 1986 by Grayston et al. (117). Seroepidemiological studies indicate that about 80% of the population has been exposed to this organism, usually in childhood and young adult life (118,119).

Chlamydial infections are typically mild or asymptomatic but because they may go unrecognized can cause a chronic low-grade infection. *Chlamydia pneumoniae* is thought to be responsible for approximately 10% of community-acquired pneumonias; other acute symptoms such as headache, abdominal complaints, pharyngitis and bronchitis are common (118–120). *Chlamydia* species may also cause neurological disease. For example, *C. pecorum* has been implicated as a possible causative agent in sporadic bovine encephalomyelitis, and a variety of neurological disorders including meningoencephalitis and GBS have been described with other chlamydial species, including *C. pneumoniae*. Natural infection with *Chlamydia* does not necessarily confer lasting immunity, so that reinfections can and do occur. In addition, following immunization against *C. trachomatis*, reinfections can be clinically more severe than in a primary infection (118).

Several lines of evidence suggest that *C. pneumoniae* may cause or contribute to atherosclerosis (119,120). For example, seroepidemiological studies suggest that the presence of antibodies to *C. pneumoniae* doubles one's risk for heart disease. In addition, *C. pneumoniae* has been found to be present in atherosclerotic lesions by a variety of techniques including PCR, immunocytochemistry, in situ hybridization, enzyme-linked immunosorbent assay (ELISA), and electron microscopy. *Chlamydia pneumoniae* has also been cultured from atherosclerotic arteries. These provocative studies have led to ongoing multicenter trials to determine if treatment with appropriate antibiotics alters the natural history of atherosclerotic complications.

Recently, two chronic neurological disorders have been associated with *C. pneumoniae*. Balin et al., using PCR, identified *C. pneumoniae* DNA sequences in the brain lesions of 17 of 19 patients with late-onset Alzheimers disease (AD) but in only 1 of 19 controls (121). Electron microscopy, immunoelectromicroscopy, reverse transcriptase PCR assays, and immunohistochemical studies also identified *C. pneumoniae* antigens, transcripts, or *C. pneumoniae*-like organisms in AD brain specimens, the latter being successfully cultured from AD but not control brains. The demonstration of *C. pneumoniae* in AD brains by multiple techniques has lent credence to the observation. Unfortunately, at lest two other groups using immunocytochemistry and PCR techniques have failed to confirm the findings of Balin et al. (122,123). While technical differences could explain the difference in results, enthusiasm for an AD-*Chlamydia* link has waned.

In 1999, Sriram called attention to a possible link between *C. pneumoniae* and MS (124). In their initial patient with rapidly progressive MS, *C. pneumoniae* was isolated from the CSF, and treatment with antibiotics resulted in marked neurological improvement. In a follow-up study of 37 patients with MS (17 relapsing-remitting, 20 progressive) and 27 patients with other neurological diseases, *C. pneumoniae* was isolated from the CSF of 64% of MS patients versus 11% of controls (5). By PCR, *C. pneumoniae* MOMP gene was identified in the CSF of 97% of MS patients as compared to 18% of controls; by ELISA, 86% of MS patients had *C. pneumoniae* antibody levels three standard deviations greater than those of controls. The specificity of the antibody response was confirmed with Western blot assays following isoelectric focusing of MS CSF. These assays revealed the presence of cationic antibodies in MS CSF reactive against several *C. pneumoniae* elementary body antigens, particularly to a 75-kDa protein. Sriram also reported that OCBs in MS CSF were partially or completely adsorbed following exposure to *C. pneumoniae* antigens but not to viral or neural antigens, whereas OCBs in CSF from patients with SSPE were adsorbed by measles but not *C. pneumoniae* antigens (125).

If confirmed, these provocative findings would suggest several possible roles for *C. pneumoniae* in MS. *Chlamydia pneumoniae* could cause MS, contribute to lesion pathogenesis due to entry of infected macrophages and monocytes into the CNS, or be an infections bystander of no particular relevance to MS lesion genesis or clinical prognosis. Unfortunately, several PCR studies over the past year have failed to identify *C. pneumoniae* in CSF, serum, peripheral blood mononuclear cells, or brain samples obtained from a large number of MS patients (Darling, Personal Communication, 126,127). In one of these studies, no increase in the ratio of CSF to serum antibody titers was found to suggest local production of *C. pneumoniae* antibody within the CNS (127). The possibility that technical differences between studies might have led to false-negative conclusions cannot be excluded; nevertheless, these findings cast doubt on the *Chlamydia* MS hypothesis. As yet, no studies have been carried out to confirm or refute Sriram's observation that MS CSF OCBs but not control OCBs react specifically with *C. pneumoniae*.

Sharing of coded samples between investigators, further studies on specificity of oligoclonal band adsorption by *C. pneumoniae* antigens, additional testing for the presence of *C. pneumoniae* in MS brain tissue, and assessing the response of MS patients to appropriate antibiotics should clarify the role, if any, of *C. pneumoniae* in MS.

B. Animal Infections Agents

Several animal viruses cause demyelination in their natural hosts (see Chap. 4). These include visna, Theiler's virus, murine coronavirus, and CDV. Even if not causative for MS, these animal models may provide valuable insight into mechanisms of virally induced demyelination.

Visna, an RNA lentivirus of sheep, seems unlikely to cause MS, since the worldwide pattern of MS is not compatible with a disease of sheep, and no reports of visna virus genome in MS brain or serological evidence for visna infections of humans have been forthcoming (1). Similarly, antibody titers to the mouse RNA viruses, mouse coronavirus, and Theiler's virus have not been increased in the serum or CSF of MS patients (1), and Theiler's virus genome has not yet been identified in MS brain samples. Although a murine-related coronavirus genome was identified in 12 of 22 MS brain specimens by in situ hybridization and coronavirus antigen was identified in brain material using immunocytochemical techniques from two patients with rapidly progressive MS (50), others have not been able to confirm the presence of mouse coronavirus genome or to isolate murine coronaviruses from MS tissues (1, Darling, Personal Communication). Thus, there is little in the way of epidemiological, serological, or microbiological evidence to indicate that these animal viruses are likely to cause MS.

Canine Distemper Virus

Canine distemper virus (CDV), a single-stranded RNA paramyxovirus of antimessage (negative) polarity, is a member of the *Morbillivirus* genus, which also includes measles, rinderpest, and the recently discovered seal plague (phocine) virus (1,14). These viruses are of great interest because they are highly contagious in their respective natural hosts (128,129); can be very neurotropic, causing CNS inflammation or demyelination in many species, including humans (1,14,130,131); and can jump species (1,14,127,132,133). A recent outbreak of a fatal disease in horses was thought to be caused by a new member of the *Morbillivirus* group. This virus was also apparently transmitted from horse to humans, causing a severe respiratory illness in two humans and death in one (134).

CDV infects dogs and other carnivores, including Japanese macaques. Susceptibility extends to a wide range of nondomestic animals and, more recently, CDV has been shown to produce disease in large cats, including lions, tigers, and leopards.

CDV can cause a subclinical disease in dogs but typically results in a febrile illness, with upper respiratory and gastrointestinal manifestations (128). Neurological sequelae are common either in close proximity to infection or after a variable latent period. Animals may develop optic neuritis, myelopathy, or encephalopathy. The neurological illness is commonly acute and monophasic but can be relapsing or progressive (1,14). In the former instance, virus can be readily identified in brain tissue, whereas in the latter situation, viral identification can be problematic (135). Some strains of CDV can cause demyelination in up to 90% of dogs, which makes it far more neurotropic in its natural host than measles is in humans (1,14,131). Pathologically, CDV can cause a panencephalitis or primary demyelination, occasionally with plaque-like lesions in periventricular white matter that are difficult to distinguish from MS (1,14,135).

The CDV-MS hypothesis implies that MS should be more common in geographic areas where genetically susceptible individuals have the greatest exposure to dogs (i.e., in areas where dog-human contact is closest and where CDV is common in the canine population) (1,14). Conversely, risk for MS would be expected to be diminished in areas where dogs are uncommon, where dog-human contact is low because of cultural attitudes toward dogs or because dogs are kept outdoors, and in isolated regions where distemper is not endemic (1,14). In this regard, both MS and dog density (and the indoor dog location for pet dogs) are higher in North America and Europe than in India (136) and, probably, in China and Japan (1,14). Moreover, dogs are more likely to be kept indoors in colder climates, such as the northern United States, compared with the American South (137); dogs are more likely to have epidemics of overt CDV infection in cold, damp climates (DiGiacomo, Personal Communication, 128); and CDV may survive longer at colder temperatures (138), conditions conductive to greater human–CDV-infected dog contact in regions of greatest MS prevalence (1,14). Examples of a geographic gradient for a dog-linked human infectious disease exists, with human hydatidosis being ten times more common in colder regions of Kenya, where dogs are kept indoors, than in warmer regions of this country (1,14,139).

If MS is a zoonosis, spread by CDV from dog to human, one would expect MS patients to have more dog exposure before onset of disease than matched controls. However, this might not be true for individual patients, because CDV, like measles, is an extremely contagious disease, typically spread by a respiratory route, and even brief exposure to an infected dog could be sufficient to cause infection (1,14). The problem with epidemiological studies of dog exposure is the high background noise, as 60 to 80% of controls in some American and European studies own dogs, indicating the need for large numbers of MS patients and controls to properly study this relationship (1,14).

Although most studies of MS patients (involving relatively few individuals) have not shown more dog ownership or dog exposure before onset or expected onset of MS, at least nine studies have shown such a temporal (139–149) correlation. However, if CDV is the agent and the dog the vector, then the more important relation is the contact between humans and dogs with distemper and the subsequent development of MS. Three reports of increased exposure of MS patients to dogs with a CDV-like illness before onset of MS have been published (140,150,151), in one of which exposure to dogs with a neurological illness was greater in MS patients than controls in the 5 years before onset of MS (144). Other studies, although not statistically significant, have shown a trend in this direction (156–158). Unfortunately, CDV infection still appears to be relatively common, even in dogs immunized with distemper vaccine (1,14,155), and epidemics of CDV have occurred over the last 15 years even in countries with high-level veterinary care, such as Switzerland and Australia.

Until recently, it was difficult to determine by serological methods whether a human had been infected by CDV because of the similar peptide homologies and antigenic relation between measles virus and CDV (156,157). Several early studies searching for serum antibodies to CDV showed higher titers in MS patients than in controls using a tissue culture neutralization assay (1,14,158). In one such study, the highest antibody titers in MS patients were to virulent rather than vaccine strains of CDV, and no significant increase in antibody titer was found to six other dog viruses (159). Smaller studies or those utilizing different techniques found no difference in serum CDV titers between patients and controls (1). Unfortunately, these serological studies were unable to definitively distinguish between CDV antibody and cross-reacting MV antibodies.

In 1995, following the publication of the entire nucleotide structure of CDV and measles, Rohowsky-Kochan et al. were able to select peptide sequences present in the surface CDV hemagglutinin H protein, which had predicted antigenic determinants that differed structurally from corresponding measles peptides (1,14,160). They synthesized three such CDV H peptides, each 15 to 16 amino acids in length, which—in addition to being structurally different from measles—were also structurally different from each other (1,14,160). In studies of animals and humans vaccinated or infected with measles virus and with high measles antibodies titers, the discriminatory capacity of the assay was demonstrated. None of these measles antibody–positive sera reacted with CDV in enzyme-linked immunosorbent assays (ELISA), whereas animals immunized with CDV reacted with all three CDV peptides (1,14,160). Subsequently, in a survey of large numbers of MS patients and age-sex–matched normal individuals and patients with other neurological and inflammatory diseases, a significant increase in serum CDV antibody titer to all three peptides was found only in the MS patients (1,14,160), with titers being significantly elevated over a wide age span (161). Some 70% of all high-titered CDV sera belonged to MS patients, indicating a relatively high degree of specificity, although not sensitivity, for this assay. A striking relationship was also observed between elevated CDV-H antibody levels and the diagnosis of MS. ($p < 0.0001$, odds ratio = 5.0) (166). In contrast, no increase in viral antibody titer was found to varicella zoster virus. In these studies, there was no relationship between CDV titer and serum IgG levels (1,14,160,161). These results indicate that humans can be infected by CDV, and they are consistent with, but do not prove the hypothesis that MS may in some instances be triggered by this agent (1,14,160,161).

The criticisms of the CDV-MS hypothesis include the failure to date to find CDV protein or genome in MS brain (49,162,163), the high titers of CDV antibody that can occur in individuals without MS, the low titers of CDV antibody in many patients with MS, lack of studies to show whether CSF OCBs bind to CDV, and no proof as yet of an elevated CDV CSF–serum antibody index.

In summary, the possibility that MS is a zoonosis remains viable and canine distemper remains a leading candidate agent for triggering MS in some patients.

V. CONCLUSION

In summary, we have reviewed the evidence favoring an infectious cause of MS. Possible mechanisms for infection-induced demyelination have been described. Epidemiological, serological, and other data in support of several human and animal candidate viruses have been presented. No single agent has yet been unequivocally linked to MS. Recommendations for further research are provided, but—as has been pointed out previously by Bernard and Simini—*sublata causa tollitur effectus* (164,165): a causal link can be invoked only after removal of the hypothetical cause has been shown to eliminate the effect.

REFERENCES

1. Cook SD, Rohowsky-Kochan C, Bansil S, Dowling PC. Evidence for multiple sclerosis as an infectious disease. Acta Neurol Scand Suppl 1995; 161:34–42.

2. Kurtzke JF. Epidemiologic evidence for multiple sclerosis as an infection. Clin Microbiol Rev 1985; 6:382–427.
3. Perron H, Lalande B, Gratacap B, Laurent A, Genoulaz O, Geny C, Mallaret M, Schuller E, Stoebner P, Seigneurin JM. Isolation of retrovirus from patients with multiple sclerosis. Lancet 1991; (337):862–863.
4. Challoner PB, Smith KT, Parker JD, et al. Plaque associated expression of human herpesvirus 6 in multiple sclerosis. Proc natl Acad Sci USA 1995; 92:7440–7444.
5. Sriram S, Stratton CW, Yao S, et al. Chlamydia penumoniae infection of the central nervous system in multiple sclerosis. Ann Neurol 1999; 46:6–14.
6. Marie P. Sclerose en plaques et maladies infectieuses. Prog Med Paris 1884; 12:287–289, 305–307, 349–351, 365–366.
7. Cook SD. Multiple sclerosis Arch Neurol 1998; 55:421–423.
8. McFarland DE, MacFarland HF. Multiple sclerosis. N Engl J Med 1982; 11:1246–1250.
9. Johnson RT. The virology of demyelinating diseases. Ann Neurol 1994; 36:554–560.
10. Rice GPA. Virus-induced demyelination in man: Models for multiple sclerosis. Curr Opin Neurol Neurosurg 1992; 5:188–194.
11. Raoult D, Birg M, La Scola B, Fournier P. Cultivation of the bacillus of Whipple's disease. N Engl J Med 2000; 342:620–625.
12. Blaser MJ. Bacteria and diseases of unknown cause. Ann Intern Med 1994; 121:144–145.
13. Kurtzke JF. MS epidemiology worldwide: One view of current status. Acta Neurol Scand Suppl 1995; 161:23–33.
14. Cook SD. Epidemiology of multiple sclerosis: Clues to etiology of a mysterious disease. Neuroscientist 1996; 2:172–180.
15. Alter M, Zhen-win Z, Davanipour Z, et al. Multiple sclerosis and childhood infections. Neurology 1986; 36:1386–1389.
16. Alvord EC, Jahnke U, Fischer EH, et al. The multiple causes of multiple sclerosis: The importance of infections in childhood. J Child Neurol 1987; 2:313–321.
17. Haile R, Smith P, Read D, et al. A study of measles virus and canine distemper virus antibodies and of childhood infections in multiple sclerosis patients and controls. J Neurol Sci 1982; 56:1–10.
18. Sullivan CB, Visscher BR, Detels R. Multiple sclerosis and age of exposure to childhood diseases and animals: Cases and their friends. Neurology 1984; 34:1144–1148.
19. Poskanzer DC, Sheridan JL, Prenny LB, et al. Multiple sclerosis in the Orkney and Shetland Islands: II. The search for an exogenous aetiology. J Epidemiol Commun Health 1980; 34:240–252.
20. Gronning M, Riise T, Kvale G, et al. Infections in childhood and adolescence in multiple sclerosis. Neuroepidemiology 1993; 12:61–69.
21. Operalski EA, Visscher BR, Malmgren R, Detels R. A case-control study of multiple sclerosis. Neurology 1989; 39:825–829.
22. Sadovnick AD, Armstrong H, Rice GPA, et al. A population based study of multiple sclerosis in twins: Update. Ann Neurol 1993; 33:281–285.
23. Eldridge R, Herndon CN. Multiple sclerosis in twins. N Engl J Med 1987; 318:50.
24. Chu AB, Sever JL, Madden DL, et al. Olilgoclonal IgG bands in cerebrospinal fluid in various neurological diseases. Ann Neurol 1983; 13:434–439.
25. Vartdal F, Vandvik B. Multiple sclerosis: Electrofocused "bands" of oligoclonal CSF IgG do not carry antibody activity against measles, varicella-zoster or rotaviruses. J Neurol Sci 1992; 54:99–107.
26. Norrby E, Link H, Olsson JE, Panelius M, Salmi A, Vandvik B. Comparison of antibodies against different viruses in cerebrospinal fluid and serum samples from patients with multiple sclerosis. Infect Immunol 1974; 10:688–694.
27. Norrby E. Viral antibodies in multiple sclerosis. Prog Med Virol 1978; 24:1–39.

28. Vartdal F, Vandvik B, Norrby E. Viral and bacterial antibody responses in multiple sclerosis. Ann Neurol 1979; 8:248–255.

29. Vandvik B, Nilsen RE, Vartdal F, Norrby E. Mumps meningitis: Specific and nonspecific antibody responses in the central nervous system. Acta Neurol Scand 1982; 65:468–487.

30. Gilden DH, Devlin ME, Burgoon MP, Owens GP. The search for virus in multiple sclerosis brain. Mult Scler 1996; 2:179–183.

31. Yao S-Y, Sriram S. Reactivity of oligoclonal bands seen in CSF to C. pneumoniae antigens in patients with multiple sclerosis. Neurology 1999; 52 (suppl 2):A559.

32. Cook SD, Dowling PC, Blumberg BM. Infection and autoimmunity in the Guillain. Barré syndrome. In: JA Aarli, WMH Behan, PO Behan, eds. Clinical Neuroimmunology. London: Blackwell Scientific, 1987, pp. 225–247.

33. Kennedy PGE, Steiner L. On the possible viral aetiology of multiple sclerosis. QJ Med 1994; 87:523–528.

34. Albert LJ, Inman RD. Molecular mimicry and autoimmunity. N Engl J Med 1999; 341:2068–2074.

35. Evans CE, Horowitz MS, Hobbs MV, Oldstone MBA. Viral infection of transgenic mice expressing a viral protein in oligodendrocytes leads to chronic central nervous system autoimmune disease. J Exp Med 1996; 184:2371–2384.

36. Rudge P. Does a retrovirally encoded superantigen cause multiple sclerosis? J Neurol Neurosurg Psychiatry 1991; 54:853–855.

37. Dale JB, Beachey EH. Epitopes of streptococcal M proteins shared with cardiac myosin. J Exp Med 1985; 162:583–591.

38. Wucherpfennig KW, Strominger JL. Molecular mimicry in T cell mediated autoimmunity: Viral peptides activate human T cell clones specific for myelin basic protein. Cell 1995; 80:695–705.

39. Krakowka S, Cockerell G, Koestner A. Effects of canine distemper virus on lymphoid function in vitro and in vivo. Infect Immun 1975; 11:1069–1078.

40. Cerruti-Sola S, Kristensen F, Vandevelde M, Bichsel P, Kihm U. Lymphocyte responsiveness to lectin and myelin antigens in canine distemper infection in relation to the development of demyelinating lesions. J Neuroimmunol 1983; 4:77–90.

41. Dowling PC, Cook SD. Role of infection in Guillain-Barré syndrome: Laboratory confirmation of herpesviruses in 41 cases. Ann Neurol 1981; 9(suppl):44–55.

42. Cook SD, Blumberg BM, Dowling PC. Potential role of paramyxoviruses in multiple sclerosis. In: G Thornton, J Booss, eds. Neurology Clinics: Infectious Diseases of the Nervous System. Philadelphia: Saunders, 1986, pp. 303–319.

43. Boos J, Kim JH. Evidence for a viral etiology of multiple sclerosis. In: Cook SD, ed. Handbook of Multiple Sclerosis. New York: Marcel Dekker, 1990.

44. Adams JM, Imagawa DT. Measles antibodies in multiple sclerosis. Proc Soc Exp Biol Med 1962; 3:562–566.

45. Jacobson S, Flerlage ML, McFarland HF. Impaired measles virus-specific cytotoxic T cell responses in multiple sclerosis. J Exp Med 1985; 162:839–850.

46. Haase AT, Ventura P, Gibbs CJ Jr, et al. Measles virus neucleotide sequences: detection by hybridization in situ. Science 1981; 212:672–675.

47. Crosby SL, McQuaid S, Taylor JM, et al. Examination of eight cases of multiple sclerosis and 56 neurological and non-neurological controls for genomic sequences of measles virus, canine distemper virus, simian virus 5 and rubella virus. J Gen Virol 1989; 70:2027–2036.

48. Stevens JG, Bastone VB, Ellison GW, Myers LW. No measles virus genetic information detected in multiple sclerosis-derived brains. Ann Neurol 1979; 8:625–627.

49. Dowling PC, Blumberg BM, Kolakofsky D, et al. Measles virus nucleic acid sequences in human brain. Virus Res 1986; 5:97–107.

50. Murray R, Brown B, Brain D, Cabirac G. Detection of corona virus RNA and antigen in MS brain. Ann Neurol 1992; 31:525–533.

51. Fujinami RS, Oldstone MBA. Amino acid homology between the encephalitogenic site of myelin basic protein and virus: Mechanism for autoimmunity. Science 1985; 230:1043–1045.

52. Kurtzke JF. Multiple sclerosis—An overview. In: Rose FC, ed. Clinical Neuroepidemiology. London: Pitman Medical, 1980, pp. 170–195.

53. Cook SD, Cromarty JI, Tapp W, Poskanzer D, Walker JD, Dowling PC. Declining incidence of multiple sclerosis in the Orkney Islands. Neurology 1985; 35:545–551.

54. Cook SD, Mac Donald J, Tapp W, Poskanzer D, Dowling PC. Multiple sclerosis in the Shetland Islands: An update. Acta Neurol Scand 1988; 77:148–151.

55. Lauer K. Multiple sclerosis in the old world: The new old map. In: W Firnhaber, L Lauer, eds. Multiple Sclerosis in Europe: An Epidemiological Update. Darmstadt: LTV Press, 1994, pp. 14–27.

56. Bansil S, Troiano R, Dowling PC, Cook SD. Measles vaccination does not prevent multiple sclerosis. Neuroepidemiology 1990; 9:248–254.

57. Ryberg B. Acute measles infection in a case of multiple sclerosis. Acta Neurol Scand 1979; 59:221–224.

58. Fleming JO, Zaatari FAK, Gilmore W, et al. Antigenic assessment of coronaviruses isolated from patients with multiple sclerosis. Arch Neurol 1988; 45:629–633.

59. Stewart JN, Mounir S, Talbot PJ. Human coronavirus gene expression in the brains of multiple sclerosis patients. Virology 1992; 191:502–505.

60. Talbot PJ, Ékandé S, Cashman NR, Mounir S, Stewart J. Neurotropism of human coronavirus. In: Laude H, Vautherot JF, eds. Coronaviruses. New York: Plenum Press, 1994.

61. Watanabe R, Wege H, ter Meulen V. Adoptive transfer of EAE-like lesions from rats with coronavirus-induced demyelinating encephalomyelitis. Nature 1983; 305:150–153.

62. Tanaka R, Iwasaki Y, Koprowski H. Ultrastructural studies of perivascular cuffing cells in multiple sclerosis brain. J Neurol Sci 1976; 28:121–126.

63. Salmi A, Zoila B, Hovi T, Reunanen M. Antibodies to coronaviruses OC43 and 229E in multiple sclerosis patients. Neurology 1982; 32:292–295.

64. Sorenson O, Collins A, Flintoff W, et al. Probing for the human coronavirus OC43 in multiple sclerosis. Neurology 1986; 36:1604–1606.

65. Evans AS, Niederman JC. Epstein-Barr virus. In: S Alfred, AS Evans, eds. Viral Infection of Humans: Epidemiology and Control, 3rd ed. New York: Plenum Press, 1989.

66. Henle G, Henle W, Diehl V. Relation of Burkitt tumor associated herpes-type virus to infectious mononucleosis. Proc Natl Acad Sci USA 1968; 59:94–101.

67. Paskavitz JF, Anderson CA, Filley CM, Kleinschmidt-DeMasters BK, Tyler KL. Acute arcuate fiber demyelinating encephalopathy following Epstein-Barr virus infection. Ann Neurol 1995; 38:127–131.

68. Bray PF, Culp KW, McFarlin DE, Panitch HS, Torkelson RD, Schlight JP. Demyelinating disease after neurologically complicated primary Epstein-Barr virus infection. Neurology 1992; 42:278–282.

69. Warner HB, Carp RI. Multiple sclerosis and Epstein-Barr virus. Lancet 1981; 2:1290.

70. Haahr S, Kochenriksen N, Mollerlarsen A, Eriksen LS. Increased risk of multiple sclerosis after late Epstein-Barr virus infection—a historical prospective study. Acta Neurol Scand 1997; 95(suppl 169):70–75.

71. Lindberg C, Andersen O, Vahlne A, Dalton M, Remarker B. Epidemiological investigation of the association between infectious mononucleosis and multiple sclerosis. Neuroepidemiology 1991; 10:62–65.

72. Martyn CN, Cruddas M, Compston DAS. Symptomatic Epstein-Barr virus infection and multiple sclerosis. J Neurol Neurosurg Psychiatry 1993; 56:167–168.

73. Bray PF, Bloomer LC, Salmon VC, Bagley MH, Larsen PD. Epstein-Barr virus infection and antibody synthesis in patients with multiple sclerosis. Arch Neurol 1983; 40:406–408.

74. Sumaya CV, Myers LW, Ellison GW. Epstein-Barr virus antibodies in multiple sclerosis. Arch Neurol 1980; 37:94–96.

75. Larsen PD, Bloomer LC, Bray PF. Epstein-Barr nuclear antigen and virus capsid antigen titers in multiple sclerosis. Neurology 1985; 35:435–438.

76. Bray PF, Luka J, Culp KW, Schlight JP. Antibodies against Epstein-Barr nuclear antigen (EBNA) in multiple sclerosis CSF, and two pentapeptide sequence identities between EBNA and myelin basic protein. Neurology 1992; 42:798–804.

77. van Sechel AC, Bajramovic JJ, van Stipdonk MS, et al. EBV-induced expression and HLA-DR-restricted presentation by human B cells of alpha B-crystallin, a candidate autoantigen in multiple sclerosis. J Immunol 1999; 162:129–135.

78. Esposito M, Venkatesh V, Otvos L, Weng Z, Vajda S, Banki K, Perl A. Human transaldolase and cross-reactive viral epitopes identified by autoantibodies of multiple sclerosis patients. Journal of Immunology 1999; 163:4027–4032.

79. Hilton DA, Love S, Fletcher A, Pringle JH. Absence of Epstein-Barr virus RNA in multiple sclerosis as assessed by in situ hybridization. J Neurol Neurosurg Psychiatry 1994; 57:975–976.

80. Koprowski H, DeFreitas EC, Harper ME, et al. Multiple sclerosis and human T-cell lympho-trophic retroviruses. Nature 1985; 318:154–160.

81. Rasmussen HB, Perron H, Clausen J. Do endogenous retroviruses have etiologic implications in inflammatory and degenerative nervous system diseases? Acta Neurol Scand 1993; 88:190–198.

82. Perron H, Geny C, Laurent A, et al. Leptomeningeal cell line from multiple sclerosis with reverse transcriptase activity and viral particles. Res Virol 1989; 140:551–561.

83. Garson JA, Tuke PW, Giraud P, Paranhos Baccala G, Perron H. Detection of virion-associated MSRV-RNA in serum of patients with multiple sclerosis (letter). Lancet 1997; 351:33.

84. Haahr S, Sommerelund M, Møller-Larsen A, Nielsen R, Hansen HJ. Just another dubious virus in cells from a patient with multiple sclerosis? Lancet 1991; 337:863–864.

85. Perron H, Garson JA, Bedin F, Beseme F, Paranhos-Baccala G, Komurian-Pradel F, Mallet F, Tuke PW, Voisset C, Blond JL, Lalande L, Seigneurin JM, Mandrand B. Molecular identification of a novel retrovirus repeatedly isolated from patients with multiple sclerosis. Proc Natl Acad Sci USA 1997; 94:7583–7588.

86. Haahr S, Sommerlund M, Christensen T, Jensen AW, Hansen HA, Møller-Larsen A. A putative new retrovirus associated with multiple sclerosis and the possible involvement of Epstein-Barr virus in this disease. Ann N Y Acad Sci 1994; 724:148–152.

87. Fujinami RS, Libbey JE. Endogenous retroviruses: are they the cause of multiple sclerosis? Trends Microbiol 1999; 7(7):263–264.

88. Clerici M, Fusi ML, Caputo D, Guerini FR, Trabattoni D, Salvaggio A, Cazzullo CL, Arienti D, Villa ML, Urnovitz HB, Ferrante P. Immune response to antigens of human endogenous retroviruses in patients with acute or stable multiple sclerosis. J Neuroimmunol 1999; 99:173–182.

89. Meinl E. Concepts of viral pathogenesis of multiple sclerosis (review). Curr Opin Neurol 1999; 12(3):303–307.

90. Hackett J, Swanson P, Leahy D, Anderson EL, Sato S, Roos RP, Decker R, Devare SG. Search for retrovirus in patients with multiple sclerosis. Ann Neurol 1996; 40:805–809.

91. Brahic M, Bureau JF. Multiple sclerosis and retroviruses (letter). Ann Neurol 1997; 42:984–985.

92. Wilborn F, Schmidt CA, Brinkmann V, Jendroska K, Oettle H, Siegert W. A potential role for human herpes virus type 6 in nervous system disease. J Neuroimmunol 1994; 49:213–214.

93. Sola P, Merelli E, Marasca R, et al. Human herpesvirus 6 and multiple sclerosis: Survey of anti-HHV-6 antibodies by immunofluorescence analysis and of viral sequences by polymerase chain reaction. J Neurol Neurosurg Psychiatry 1993; 56:917–919.

94. Saito Y, Sharer LR, Dewhurst S, Blumberg BM, Hall CB, Epstein LG. Cellular localization

of human herpes virus-6 in the brains of children with AIDS encephalopathy. J Neurovirol 1995; 1:30–39.

95. Asano Y, Yoshikawa T, Kajita Y, Ogura R, Suga S, Yazaki T, Nakashima T, Yamada A, Kurata T. Fatal encephalitis/encephalopathy in primary human herpesvirus-6 infection. Arch Dis Child 1992; 67:1484–1485.

96. Novoa LJ, Nagra RM, Nakawatase T, Edwards-Lee T, Tourtellotte WW, Cornford ME. Fulminant demyelinating encephalomyelitis associated with productive HHV-6 infection in an immunocompetent adult. J Med Virol 1997; 52:301–308.

97. Merelli E, Sola P, Barozzi P, Torelli G. An encephalitic episode in a multiple sclerosis patient with human herpesvirus 6 latent infection. J Neurol Sci 1996; 137:42–46.

98. Carrigan DR, Harrington D, Knox KK. Subacute leukoencephalitis caused by CNS infection with human herpesvirus-6 manifesting as acute multiple sclerosis. Neurology 1996; 47:145–148.

99. Kamei A, Ichinohe S, Onuma R, Hiraga S, Fujiwara T. Acute disseminated demyelination due to primary human herpesvirus-6 infection. Eur J Pediatr 1997; 156:709–712.

100. Bergström T. Herpesviruses—A rationale for antiviral treatment in multiple sclerosis. Antivir Res 1999; 41:1–19.

101. Mackenzie IRA, Carrigan DR, Wiley CA. Chronic myelopathy associated with human herpesvirus-6. Neurology 1995; 45:2015–2017.

102. Knox KK, Harrington D, Carrigan DR. Active human herpesvirus type 6 infections are present in the central nervous system, lymphoid tissues and peripheral blood of patients with multiple sclerosis. Ann Neurol 1998; 44:485.

103. Sanders VJ, Waddell AE, Felisan SL, Li X, Conrad AJ, Tourtellotte WW. Herpes simplex virus in postmortem multiple sclerosis brain tissue. Arch Neurol 1996; 53:125.

104. Gordon L, Mcquaid S, Cosby SL. Detection of herpes simplex virus (types 1 and 2) and human herpesvirus 6 DNA in human brain tissue by polymerase chain reaction. Clin Diagn Virol 1996; 6(1):33–40.

105. Dowling P, Husar W, Menonna J, Donnenfeld H, Cook SD, Sidhu M. Cell death and birth in multiple sclerosis brain. J Neurol Sci 1997; 149:1–11.

106. Ablashi DV, Lapps W, Kaplan M, et al. Human herpesvirus-6 (HHV-6) infection in multiple sclerosis: A preliminary report. Mult Scler 1998; 4:490–496.

107. Soldan SS, Berti R, Salem N, et al. Association of human herpes virus 6 (HHV-6) with multiple sclerosis: Increased IgM response to HHV-6 early antigen and detection of serum HHV-6 DNA. Nature Med 1997; 3:1994–1997.

108. Kim JS, Park JH, Lee KH, Lee KS, Shin WS. Detection of human herpes virus 6 variant a sequence in multiple sclerosis. Neurology 1999; 52(suppl 2):A491.

109. Goldberg SH, Albright AV, Lisak RP, Gonzalez-Scarano F. Polymerase chain reaction analysis of human herpesvirus-6 sequences in the sera and cerebrospinal fluid of patients with multiple sclerosis. J Neuro virology 1999; 5:134–139.

110. Martin C, Enbom M, Soderstrom M, et al. Absence of seven human herpesviruses including HHV-6, by polymerase chain reaction in CSF and blood from patients with multiple sclerosis and optic neuritis. Acta Neurol Scand 1997; 95:280–283.

111. Tenser RB, Hay KA, Hershey, PA. Herpes viruses in leukocytes of multiple sclerosis patients. Neurology 1999; 52(suppl 2):A558.

112. Ongradi J, Rajda C, Maródi CL, Csiszár A, Vécsci L. A pilot study on the antibodies to HHV-6 variants and HHV-7 in CSF of MS patients. J Neurovirol 1999; 5:529–532.

113. Nielsen L, Larsen AM, Munk M, Vestergaard BF. Human herpesvirus-6 immunoglobulin G antibodies in patients with multiple sclerosis. Acta Neurol Scand 1997; 169(suppl):76–78.

114. Nielsen L, Mollerlarsen A, Munk M, Vestergaard BF. Human herpesvirus-6 immunoglobulin G antibodies in patients with multiple sclerosis. Acta Neurol Scand 1997; 95(suppl 169): 76–78.

115. Fillet AM, Lozeron P, Agut H, et al. HHV-6 and multiple sclerosis (letter). Nature Med 1998; 4:537.

116. Soldan SS, Leist TP, Juhng KN, McFarland HF, Jacobson S. Increased lymphoproliferative response to human herpesvirus type 6A variant in multiple sclerosis patients. Ann Neurol 2000; 47:306–313.

117. Grayston JT, Campbell LA, Kuo CC, et al. A new respiratory tract pathogen: Chlamydia pneumoniae strain TWAR. J Infect Dis 1990; 161:618–625.

118. Danville T. Chlamydia. Pediatr Rev 1998; 19:85–91.

119. Shor A, Phillips JI. Chlamydia penumoniae and athlerosclerosis. JAMA 1999; 282:2071–2073.

120. Maass M, Gieffers J. Prominent serological response to Chlamydia pneumoniae in cardiovascular disease. Immunol Infec Dis 1996; 6:65–70.

121. Balin BJ, Gerard HC, Arking EJ, et al. Identification and localization of Chlamydia pneumoniae in the Alzheimer's brain. Med Microbiol Immunol 1998; 187:23–42.

122. Nochlin D, Shaw CM, Campbell LA, Kuo CC. Failure to detect Chlamydia pneumoniae in brain tissues of Alzheimer's disease. Neurology 1999; 53:1888.

123. Gieffers J, Reusche E, Solbach W, Maass M. Failure to detect Chlamydia pneumoniae in brain sections of Alzheimer's disease patients (abstr). Clin Microbiol Infect 1999; 5(suppl 3):90.

124. Sriram S, Mitchell W, Stratton C. Multiple sclerosis associated with Chlamydia pneumoniae infection of the CNS. Neurology 1998; 50:571–572.

125. Yao SY, Sriram S, Nashville TN. Reactivity of oligoclonal bands seen in CSF to C. pneumoniae antigens in patients with multiple sclerosis. Neurology 1999; 52(suppl 2):A559.

126. Poland SD, Rice GPA. Chlamydia pneumoniae and multiple sclerosis. Neurology 2000; 54(suppl 3):A165.

127. Boman J, Roblin PM, Sundström P, Sandström M, Hammerschlag MR. Failure to detect Chlamydia pneumoniae in the central nervous system of patients with MS. Neurology 2000; 54:265.

128. Appel MJG, Gillespie JH. Canine Distemper Virus. Vienna: Springer-Verlag, 1972, pp. 1–153.

129. Collins SD, Wheeler RE, Shannon RD. Occurrence of Whooping Cough, Chickenpox, Mumps, Measles, and German Measles in 200,000 Survey Families in 28 Large Cities. Bethesda, MD: National Institutes of Health, 1943.

130. Maurer KC, Neilsen SW. Neurological disorders in the raccoon in northeastern United States. J Am Vet Med Assoc 1981; 179:1095–1098.

131. Vandevelde M, Higgins RJ, Kristensen B, Kristensen F, Steck A, Kihm U. Demyelination in experimental canine distemper virus infection; immunological, pathologic and immunohistological studies. Acta Neuropathol (Berl) 1982; 56:285–293.

132. Blythe LL, Schmidtz JA, Roelke M, et al. Chronic encephalomyelitis caused by canine distemper virus in a Bengal tiger. J Am Vet Med Assoc 1983; 183:1159–1162.

133. Yoshikawa Y, Ochikubo F, Matsubara Y, et al. Natural infection with canine distemper virus in a Japanese monkey. Vet Microbiol 1989; 20:193–205.

134. Murray K, Selleck P, Hooper P, et al. A morbillivirus that caused fatal disease in horses and humans. Science 1995; 268:94–97.

135. Higgins RJ, Child G, Vandevelde M. Chronic relapsing demyelinating encephalomyelitis associated with persistent canine distemper virus infection. Acta Neuropathol 1989; 77:441–444.

136. Bansil S, Singhal BS, Ahuja GK, et al. Multiple sclerosis in India: A case control study of environmental exposures. Acta Neurol Scand 1997; 95:208–210.

137. Norman J, Cook SD, Dowling PC. Pilot survey of household pets among veterans with multiple sclerosis and age-matched controls. Arch Neurol 1983; 40:213–214.

138. Man, dogs and hydatid disease (editorial). Lancet 1987; 1:21–22.

139. Cook SD, Dowling PC. A possible association between house pets and multiple sclerosis. Lancet 1977; 1:980–982.

140. Cook SD, Natelson BH, Levin BE, et al. Further evidence of a possible association between house dogs and multiple sclerosis. Ann Neurol 1978; 3:141–143.

141. Compston DAS, Vakarelis BN, Paul E, McDonald WI, Batchelor JR, Mims CA. Viral infections in patients with multiple sclerosis and HLA-DR matched controls. Brain 1986; 109: 325–344.

142. Leibowitz U, Alter M. Multiple Sclerosis: Clues to Its Cause. Amsterdam: North-Holland, 1973.

143. Antonovsky A, Leibowitz U, Smith H, et al. Epidemiologic study of multiple sclerosis in Israel, part I (an overall review of methods and findings). Arch Neurol 1965; 13:183–193.

144. Jotkowitz S. Multiple sclerosis and exposure to house pets. JAMA 1977; 238:854.

145. Flodin U, Soderfeldt B, Noorlind-Brage H, Fredriksson M, Axelson O. Multiple sclerosis, solvents and pets: A case-referent study. Arch Neurol 1988; 45:620–623.

146. Landtblom AM, Flodin U, Karlsson M. Multiple sclerosis and exposure to solvents; Ionizing radiation, and animals. Scand J Work Environ Health 1993; 19:399–404.

147. Antonovsky A, Leibowitz U, Medalie JM, et al. Reappraisal of possible aetological factors in multiple sclerosis. Am J Public Health 1968; 58:836–848.

148. Mititelu G, Cernescu C, Bourceanu R. Dog ownership among multiple sclerosis patients and their level of measles antibodies: A case control study. Rev Med Chir Soc Med Nat Iasi 1986; 90:673–677.

149. Granieri E, Casetta I, Tola MR. Epidemiology of multiple sclerosis in Italy and southern Europe. Acta Neurol Scand Suppl 1995; 161:60–70.

150. Anderson LJ, Kibler RF, Kaslow RA, et al. Multiple sclerosis unrelated to dog exposure. Neurology 1984; 34:1149–1154.

151. Warren SA, Warren KG, Greenhill S, Paterson M. How multiple sclerosis is related to animal illness, stress and diabetes. Can Med Assoc J 1982; 126:377–385.

152. Read D, Nassim D, Smith P, Paterson C, Warlow C. Multiple sclerosis and dog ownership: A case-control investigation. J Neurol Sci 1982; 55:359–367.

153. Bauer HJ, Wikstrom J. Multiple sclerosis and house pets. Lancet 1978; 2:1029.

154. Hughes RAC, Russell WC, Froude JRL, Jarrett RJ. Pet ownership, distemper antibodies and multiple sclerosis. J Neurol Sci 1980; 47:429–432.

155. Zurbriggen A, Müller C, Vandevelde M. In situ hybridization of virulent canine distemper virus in brain tissue, using digozigenin-labeled probes. Am J Vet Res 1993; 54:1457–1461.

156. Sidhu SS, Husar W, Cook SD, Dowling PC, Udem SA. Canine distemper terminal and intergenic non-protein coding nucleotide sequences: completion of the entire CDV genome. Virology 1993; 193:66–72.

157. Sidhu SS, Menonna JP, Cook SD, Dowling PC, Udem SA. Canine distemper virus L gene: Sequence and comparison with related viruses. Virology 1993; 193:50–65.

158. Cook SD, Dowling PC, Russell WC. Neutralizing antibodies to canine distemper and measles virus in multiple sclerosis. J Neurol Sci 1979; 41:61–70.

159. Appel MJ, Glickman LI, Raine CS, et al. Viruses and multiple sclerosis. Neurology 1981; 31:944–949.

160. Rohowsky-Kochan C, Dowling PC, Cook SD. Canine distemper virus-specific antibodies in multiple sclerosis. Neurology 1995; 45:1554–1560.

161. Rohowsky-Kochan. Unpublished data.

162. Cook SD, Dowling PC, Prineas JW, et al. A radioimmunoassay search for measles and distemper antigens in subacute sclerosing panencephalitis and multiple sclerosis brain tissues. J Neurol Sci 1981; 51:447–456.

163. Hall WW, Choppin PW. Failure to detect measles virus proteins in brain tissue of patients with multiple sclerosis. Lancet 1982; 1:957.

164. Simini B. Measurement of posterior fossa neurovascular anomalies in essential hypertension (letter). Lancet 1995; 345:131.

165. Bernard C. Introduction à l' étude de la médecine expérimentale. Paris: Baillière, 1865. [Republished Paris: Garnier-Flammarion, 1966.]

6

Experimental Models of Autoimmune Demyelination

FRED D. LUBLIN

Mount Sinai School of Medicine, New York, New York

I. INTRODUCTION

Experimental allergic encephalomyelitis (EAE) is a cell-mediated autoimmune disorder of the central nervous system (CNS) that has served as a useful model of CNS inflammation, an animal model for the human disease multiple sclerosis (MS), and an easily evaluable and manipulable model for organ specific autoimmune diseases in general (1). EAE is the most commonly employed animal model of MS, despite differences in the two conditions. The primary difference between these disorders is that EAE must be induced in animals while MS occurs spontaneously in humans. A reliable spontaneously occurring inflammatory demyelinating animal model would enhance our experimental capabilities.

EAE was first described in monkeys by Rivers in 1933 (2). However, the disease itself was first induced accidentally in humans years before following the introduction of Pasteur's rabies vaccine (3). That vaccine was produced in brain tissue, which contaminated the vaccine, and led to induction of acute disseminated encephalomyelitis—an acute, monophasic, inflammatory demyelinating disease, the human form of EAE.

II. RELEVANCE TO MS

EAE, like MS, is an inflammatory, demyelinating disorder of the central nervous system. Both the clinical expression and pathological picture of EAE are similar to that seen in MS. As EAE is an autoimmune disorder, these similarities have provided strong evidence for MS also being an autoimmune disease. Similarly, as EAE is induced by specific myelin antigens—e.g., myelin basic protein (MBP) or proteolipid protein (PLP)—attention in MS has focused on autoimmunity to these molecules. Both EAE and MS appear to be

Table 1 Comparison of features of EAE and MS

	EAE	MS
CNS signs	+++	+++
Relapsing disease	++	+++
CNS perivascular inflammation	+++	+++
CNS demyelination	+ $->$ +++	+++
Antibody-mediated demyelination	++	++
CNS remyelination	++	++
Immunogen	MBP, PLP, MOG, others	Unknown
Genetic predisposition	++	++
Linked to MHC	++	++
Limited TCR heterogeneity	+	+
Microbial precipitant	+	++
Cytokine effects	++	?+
Response to immunomodulation	+++	++

Key: + = mild relationship; ++ = moderate relationship; +++ = strong relationship; ? = contradictory responses.

mediated by CD4$^+$ T cells; they are dependent on the expression of the appropriate MHC class II (HLA, la) antigens, specific T-cell receptor–bearing lymphocytes, adhesion molecule expression, and cytokine secretion. Both diseases are organ-specific, affecting solely myelin from the central nervous system, and require trafficking of lymphocytes from the periphery across the blood-brain barrier (BBB) into the CNS. New data suggest that antibodies to CNS antigens may play a similar role in the pathogenesis of both EAE and MS (Table 1).

In addition, EAE has served as a screening tool for potential therapies for MS. Most currently employed cytotoxic agents have been tested in EAE models [e.g., azathioprine (4), cyclophosphamide (5), mitoxantrone (6), methotrexate (7)]. MHC class II–directed therapies and T cell–receptor therapies were first tested in EAE models (8,9). Glatiramer acetate (copolymer I) was first reported to affect the course of EAE (10). Immunomodulating agents such as Linomide (11), cytokine-directed therapies, and anti–adhesion molecule therapies were all successfully utilized to impede the course of EAE before entering clinical trials in MS. Of interest, there was limited use of interferon-β in EAE prior to human studies, and the effect of interferon-γ on EAE is very different from its effect in patients with MS (see below).

III. INDUCTION PROTOCOLS

EAE is inducible in most mammalian species. The most commonly employed species are rat and mouse. Guinea pigs were frequently utilized in the past and develop particularly good demyelination (12). Nonhuman primates can also be used (13,14). EAE can be induced by either active or passive means. The method of inoculation determines whether an acute, monophasic illness or a relapsing form ensues. Originally, EAE was induced with whole CNS homogenate emulsified with an adjuvant, most commonly complete Freund's adjuvant, injected subcutaneously. Some models require the use of pertussis vaccine to enhance immunogenicity. More recently, the antigenic requirements of EAE have been better defined, with MBP and PLP or their component peptides serving as the commonest antigens for EAE induction. Other CNS antigens (e.g., MOG, S100) have been reported to induce CNS inflammation similar to that of the major myelin antigens (15,16), but they have not been as well characterized as the major myelin antigens. Passive forms of EAE are induced in naive recipients by transfer of encephalitogenic T cells from animals sensitized with CNS antigen. In addition to simplifying EAE induction, passive techniques have been instrumental in defining the immunological cellular requirements for EAE—e.g., CD4$^+$ T cells (17).

The immunodominant peptide fragment of either MBP or PLP is under immunogenetic control and varies among different species and strains. For example, SJL mice respond to the carboxyl-terminal peptide of MBP, while PL/J mice respond to the amino-terminal peptide (17). The type of T-cell receptor predominantly utilized in the EAE autoimmune response also differs among strains (see below).

The acute form of EAE most closely resembles the human disease acute disseminated encephalomyelitis, which, like acute EAE, is a monophasic inflammatory demyelinating disorder. Alterations of the induction procedure have led to relapsing forms of EAE that more closely resemble MS in their clinical and pathological expression. In mice, one form of induction leads to an acute form of EAE and then subsequent relapses (18). A second form has a delayed onset, similar to the postulated latency period in MS, followed by relapses (19). In both these forms, the pathological analysis of the CNS reveals both acute inflammatory lesions as well as areas of subacute and chronic demyelination, comparable to the lesions seen in brains from patients with MS (1,19,20).

IV. FEATURES OF EAE

A. Clinical Signs and Course

The clinical signs of EAE consist of hindlimb and tail paresis and paralysis—both flaccid and spastic—quadriparesis, hemiparesis, ataxia, abnormal righting responses, and incontinence. Tail flaccidity and hindlimb paresis are the commonest and earliest findings (Fig. 1).

Acute EAE develops 11 to 15 days after active induction protocols and 5 to 10 days after passive immunization protocols. The usual time course of R-EAE in the guinea pig and some mouse models is for an acute attack about 2 to 3 weeks after immunization, followed by recovery and then periodic relapses (1). In other mouse models and the hamster (1,19), there is a delayed onset of clinical signs of up to several months after immunization, followed by recovery and subsequent relapses.

In addition to a relapsing-remitting course, chronic progressive disease has been described in some mice and guinea pigs immunized as outlined above (21).

B. Histopathology

The pathological lesion of acute EAE consists of perivascular mononuclear cell inflammation with extension into CNS parenchyma and meninges (Fig. 2). In some forms of EAE, especially the relapsing models, there is also acute, subacute, and chronic demyelination (Fig. 3) with some remyelination. In the mouse, these lesions are most commonly seen in the white matter of the cerebellum, brainstem, and spinal cord (1,19). In demyelinated areas there is loss of myelin with relative preservation of axons, astrocytic gliosis, and loss of oligodendrocytes. In the murine form of EAE that employs a two-injection regimen without addition of pertussis, hemorrhagic lesions with influxes of polymorphonuclear

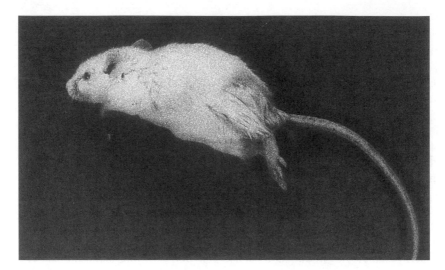

Figure 1   An SJL/J mouse with EAE. Notice the hindlimb spastic paresis and discoloration of the perineal skin secondary to incontinence.

leukocytes occur during acute episodes (20). Demyelination followed by remyelination also develops. In the guinea pig, the relapsing form of EAE follows a topographical distribution of lesions similar to MS (22). Periventricular lesions in the centrum semiovale are the commonest abnormality in the brain. Macroscopically visible plaques of demyelination can be seen in guinea pigs with relapsing EAE. The microscopic lesions are similar to

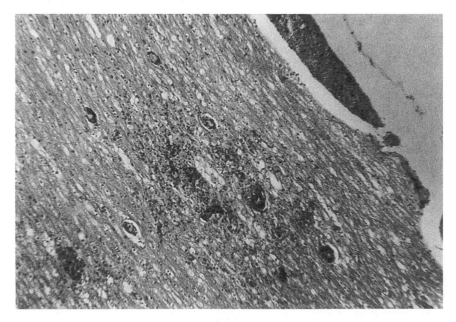

Figure 2   A photomicrograph of a section of mouse spinal cord demonstrating perivascular mononuclear cell infiltration with extension into the adjacent CNS parenchyma.

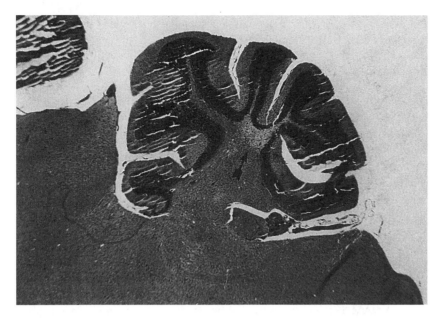

Figure 3 A photomicrograph of the cerebellum of a mouse with relapsing EAE demonstrating an area of chronic demyelination (arrow).

those of the mouse with perivenous inflammation, demyelination, oligodendrocyte loss, and gliosis. Older lesions tend to have fewer inflammatory cells. Areas of demyelination and remyelination occur in different areas of the same plaque. The degree of demyelination seen varies with the species utilized. Mice, guinea pigs, and monkeys all have considerable inflammation and demyelination. Rats show extensive inflammation but little demyelination, suggesting that demyelination is not the inevitable consequence of CNS inflammation alone. Demyelination can be induced in rats by the addition of antimyelin component antibodies along with the EAE induction protocol (23).

The development of pathological changes may ensue in the absence of clinical signs, but clinical signs rarely occur without corresponding pathological changes. Chronic demyelination is most prominent in animals that have more than one clinical attack. The pathological changes of EAE, especially the relapsing forms, closely resemble that of MS, with both acute perivascular inflammation and subacute-chronic areas of demyelination and remyelination. The nature of the induction protocol utilized and the species may affect the type of histopathological changes observed.

V. IMMUNOPATHOGENESIS

A. Cellular Components and Interactions

Following inoculation with a CNS antigen/adjuvant emulsion, the CNS antigen is processed by antigen presenting cells (APC) in draining lymph nodes. Once processed by an APC, the CNS antigen fragment in conjunction with the MHC class II molecule is presented to specific CD4$^+$ T cells, which become activated, proliferate, and home to the CNS. The exact mechanism by which these cells pass into the CNS is not fully understood.

Activated T cells are able to cross the BBB, without apparent restriction, in an antigen nonspecific manner (24,25). Those T cells not directed against an antigen expressed in the CNS presumably traffic out of the CNS without any further interaction. However, those T cells directed against CNS antigens will contact APCs in the CNS that present the appropriate antigen fragment and lead to stimulation, proliferation, and retention of these specific T cells in the CNS. The exact site of T-cell activation by APCs within the CNS is not entirely clear, but those T cells directed against myelin antigens appear to cluster in the perivascular spaces, leading to activation and recruitment of additional immune-reactive cells. There are several possible candidate APCs in the CNS. Cerebrovascular endothelial cells are able to express class II and present antigen to T cells (26). EAE susceptible strains of mice express more class II on their cerebrovascular endothelial cells than EAE-resistant strains. This is not a generalized phenomenon, as non-CNS vascular endothelial cells in these same strains do not show differential expression of class II. No strain differences occur in expression of class I or the adhesion molecule ICAM-1 (26). ICAM-1, which binds to leucocyte function–associated antigen 1 (LFA-1) on T cells, is expressed on CNS vessels during the inflammatory phase of EAE. ICAM-1 may nevertheless play a role in trafficking of encephalitogenic T cells, although the effects of anti-ICAM-1 or LFA-1 antibodies on EAE are contradictory (27,28). Another potentially important molecule is VCAM-1, which is expressed on endothelial cells and binds to the $\alpha 4$ integrin VLA-4 on T cells. Loss of VLA-4 on T cells leads to a reduced capacity to traffic into the CNS (29). Antibody to VLA-4 is able to prevent development of EAE (30). Of interest, PLP reactive T cells that do not express VLA-4 can mediate EAE if the hosts are treated with irradiation and pertussis vaccine (31). This may be due to alteration of the BBB, allowing easier access to the CNS. No specific CNS-homing molecule has been found, as yet. However, CNS directed lymphocytes may have distinct memory, integrin and selectin phenotypes (32). Antigen presentation/recognition may also occur in the perivascular region by astrocytes or perivascular microglia, both of which may express class II. Whichever site (vascular endothelial or perivascular) the initial T cell–APC interaction occurs, it leads to T-cell activation, cytokine release, upregulation of adhesion molecules, and attraction of non-specific lymphocytes—the cascade of events that characterize a delayed-type hypersensitivity (DTH), cell-mediated immune reaction, which in the case of EAE results in damage to myelin within the CNS.

The cellular requirements of the encephalitogenic response have been well characterized. T lymphocytes play a central role in mediating EAE. The primary effector cells of EAE are MHC class II restricted T-helper cells of the CD4$^+$ phenotype (17,33–35). EAE can be inhibited by specific antibodies to CD4 or by vaccination against CD4-bearing T cells (36–38). The other major T-cell subset, CD8$^+$ T cells, also plays a role in EAE, principally as a regulator of the encephalitogenic response. Mice lacking CD8$^+$ T cells develop more relapses of EAE and decreased resistance to subsequent reinduction of EAE (39,40). Therefore, the immunoregulatory activity of CD8$^+$ T cells appears to center around recovery from EAE. CD4$^+$ T cells also play a role in recovery from EAE and thus can serve as both effectors and suppressors of disease (41). The suppressor functions of CD4$^+$ T cells may involve secretion of IL-10 and/or transforming growth factor (42) (see below). Other suppressor populations have been described, including double-negative and double-positive (CD4$^+$CD8$^+$) T cells (43).

The role of specific T-cell receptors (TCR) in EAE, once controversial, appears to be better clarified in the MBP- or MBP peptide–specific immune response. In the PL/J mouse there is preferential usage of the V8 chain of the TCR by the encephalitic T cells

(44). However, if one deletes those TCR containing V8 from PL/J mice, EAE will still occur, in a smaller percentage of mice, utilizing TCR with other V chains (45). The lack of exclusivity of V8 is further demonstrated in other strains of mice that are capable of producing TCR with V8 chains, but do not utilize these TCRs exclusively or even predominantly in their MBP–specific immune response (46). Depending on the immuno-genetic background of a particular strain of mouse, V4, 6, 8, 13, and 17a may be utilized in the MBP response. The TCR response to PLP is even more heterogeneous (47). Similar diversity in the TCR V repertoire has been reported in the human MBP response, although there were initial reports of limited heterogeneity.

A more promising site for antigen-specific restriction of the TCR is at the CDR3 region, where there are reports of conserved motifs, both in animal models and in T cells obtained from the brains of patients with MS. However, this situation is also not universal, as some strains of mice show conservation while others do not (46).

$CD4^+$ T cells, as noted above, mediate the encephalitogenic course of EAE. The $CD4^+$ T-cell subset can be further subdivided into T helper (Th) 1 and 2 cells. Th1 cells mediate delayed-type hypersensitivity reactions, such as EAE. Th2 cells are involved with antibody-mediated events and tend to antagonize the effects of Th1 cells. This contraregu-lation is due, at least in part, to the differential cytokine secretion patterns of these T-cell subsets. Th1 cells secrete the proinflammatory cytokines IL-2, interferon (IFN)-γ and tu-mor necrosis factor (TNF)-α (lymphotoxin). Th2 cells secrete IL-4, IL-5, and IL-10. IL-4 and IL-10 have inhibitory effects on Th1 cells. Myelin antigen–reactive $CD4^+$ T cells of the Th1 subtype mediate EAE, while those of the Th2 subtype usually do not. Further, treatment of MBP-specific T cells with IL-4 transformed T-cell populations from Th1 to Th2 and ameliorated the effects of EAE (48). The EAE model has provided the best evidence for use of immune deviation techniques in treatment of autoimmune demyelin-ation. The logic of immune deviation involves a switch from a Th1–predominant immune response to a Th2 response, with the attendant switch in cytokine secretion from immune-enhancing to immunosuppressive. This approach is thought to underlie the use of oral antigen (49) and altered peptide ligand (50). One of the putative mechanisms of glatiramer acetate also invokes this mechanism (51). These therapeutic approaches have been demon-strated to produce an antigen-specific induction of Th2 cells, which then migrate to the CNS, where they "see" their cognate antigen and upregulate and secrete immunosuppres-sive cytokines, which turn off any immune response in the proximity to the Th2 cells, even responses directed against other CNS antigens. This is referred to as "bystander suppression."

Although much attention has been focused on the cellular aspects of EAE, there is a growing body of evidence suggesting an important role for antibody-mediated demyelin-ation in EAE and MS. In a MOG-induced EAE model in marmosets, demyelination was associated with MOG-specific autoantibodies (52). However, the finding of demyelination with EAE in B cell–deficient mice immunized with MOG suggests either species differ-ences in EAE pathology or diverse mechanisms for production of inflammatory demyelin-ation (53).

B. Cytokines and Chemokines in EAE

Cytokine secretion by activated T cells within the CNS appears to be involved in the pathogenesis of inflammatory demyelination and may be a key factor in EAE pathogenesis. During the acute phase of EAE, there is an increase in the levels of IL-1, IL-2, IL-4,

IL-6, and IFN-β. During the recovery phase there is an increase in the inhibitory interleukins, IL-10 and transforming growth factor beta (TGF-β) and downregulation of the proinflammatory cytokines (54,55). Listed below are details of the role of several of the major cytokines in EAE.

IFN-γ, a cytokine with multiple immunomodulatory activities, upregulates class II expression at a local level, which could initiate or augment a CNS directed immune response by activating CNS vascular endothelial cells, inducing class II expression on microglia and astrocytes, and inducing secretion of other immunostimulatory cytokines. IFN-γ also activates macrophages. During the early phases of EAE there is an increased number of IFN-γ–secreting cells (56). The role of IFN-γ is, however, more complicated when viewed from a systemic perspective rather than at the level of the CNS microenvironment. When administered systemically or intraventricularly to animals, IFN-γ does not enhance EAE but rather tends to ameliorate disease (57–59). Conversely, antibodies to IFN-γ enhance EAE (58,60,61). The mechanism for this action may relate to effects of IFN-γ on suppressor functions. This is in contradistinction to the one human study with IFN-γ in patients with MS, where disease was exacerbated by systemic administration of IFN-γ (62). The mechanism for this difference in response between patients with MS and animals with EAE likely is multifactorial, but may be related to the underlying suppressor cell defect in MS patients. Antibodies directed against an IFN-γ–inducing factor prevented development of EAE (63). Also to be considered in evaluating the role of cytokines in the pathogenesis of organ specific autoimmune disorders is the fact that these molecules act in the microenvironment of the cell-mediated immune response at the target organ and thus may behave quite differently and act on different cell populations when administered systemically.

Although many cytokines are involved in a cell-mediated reaction, as occurs in EAE, the one that is most implicated in the pathogenic process of EAE is the proinflammatory cytokine TNF. TNF-α, produced by activated macrophages, and TNF-β, produced by activated lymphocytes and activated microglia, have been implicated in CNS inflammation. TNF has been shown to be toxic for both oligodendrocytes and myelin, in tissue culture (64). The encephalitogenicity of T cells directed against MBP correlates with expression of TNF. In EAE, there is an increase in expression of TNFα and IFN-γ during the acute phase and during subsequent relapses (65). Antibodies against TNF or TNF receptor blockade inhibit development of EAE, both the acute and chronic relapsing variants (66–68). Therefore, demyelination may be the consequence of the proximity of the myelin sheath and/or oligodendrocytes to TNF secreted by lymphocytes, macrophages, microglia, and/or astrocytes as part of a cell-mediated immune response directed against a CNS antigen—e.g., MBP or PLP. In distinction to these results, in the MOG-induced model of EAE in mice, TNF appears to play an opposite role, ameliorating disease (69). Similar to the situation with IFN-γ, the translation of insights on pathogenesis of inflammatory demyelination obtained from TNF studies in EAE to MS has been problematic. TNF directed therapies have thus far been disappointing, suggesting that anti-TNF strategies might worsen the course of MS (70). This might be due to the way the anti-TNF therapy was applied, but it is also possible that this is another example of the difference between human MS and the animal model, EAE. As TNF-directed therapy has been successful in other autoimmune diseases (rheumatoid arthritis, Crohn's disease), this might also provide evidence that MS is not an autoimmune disorder. In general, cytokine-directed therapies will be limited by the method of delivery, as cytokine effects occur within the immunological micromillieu at the target organ, e.g., the CNS, which might be far removed from the site of systemic application of the anticytokine treatment.

IL-12 is a cytokine, produced by APCs, which promotes development of Th1 cells, cytotoxic T cells, and natural killer (NK) cells and induces secretion of both IFN-γ and TNF-α. Studies demonstrate that IL-12 enhances the severity of EAE while antibodies to IL-12 ameliorate EAE (71). This IL-12 action was not directly related to the action of IFN-γ or TNF-α (72). Of interest, male murine lymph nodes sensitized with MBP were less able to transfer EAE than female cells, an effect attributed to decreased production of IL-12, suggesting that this may be one cause for the sexual dimorphism of autoimmune demyelination in animals and humans (73).

IL-4 is primarily a Th2-type cytokine that had a beneficial effect when given to mice with adoptively transferred EAE (48). Preincubation of MBP-specific Th1 cells with IL-4 reduced their ability to mediate EAE.

The role of the inhibitory cytokines, TGF-β and IL-10, has also been demonstrated in EAE. TGF-β is a multifunctional peptide that has immunoregulatory properties, including inhibition of T cell activation, decreased cytokine production, inhibition of IFN-γ induced class II expression, and decrease in generation of cytotoxic lymphocytes. TGF-β inhibits the activation and proliferation of MBP specific T cells in vitro, reducing their ability to transfer EAE (74). Administration of TGF-β in vivo reduces the severity of clinical disease in EAE, even when administered after onset of clinical signs (75–78). TGF-β also reduces the occurrence of relapses of EAE. Animals treated with TGF-β show less inflammation and demyelination within the CNS following induction of EAE. There was also decreased expression of immune activation markers in the CNS, such as class II and LFA-1. Treatment with antibody to TGF-β causes a worsening of the clinical and pathologic expression of EAE (79). In addition to the actions of exogenously administered TGF-β, there is evidence for a role for this molecule in the natural course of EAE, as TGF-β has been found in the CNS inflammatory infiltrates of EAE during both the active disease and recovery phases. Taken together, these data implicate TGF-β in the immunoregulatory cascade of EAE. TGF-β has primarily anti-inflammatory actions, is present in the CNS during EAE, and inhibits the clinical and pathological signs of EAE, suggesting that it has a role in the recovery from EAE, perhaps by antagonizing the effects of proinflammatory cytokines such as TNF. CD4$^+$ suppressor cells that regulate the recovery of EAE in rats secrete TGF-β and inhibit the production of IFN-γ and TNF by EAE effector cells (74). TGF-β may also act by enhancing suppressor activity (80). In its ability to downregulate inflammatory cytokines and upregulate suppression, the activities of TGF-β have been likened to IFN-β, an agent that reduces the clinical expression of MS.

IL-10, a product of Th2 cells, B cells, and macrophages, inhibits lymphokine production by Th1 lymphocytes and macrophage/monocyte cells (81). During the recovery phase of EAE, there is a rise in messenger RNA for IL-10 in the CNS, suggesting a role for this cytokine in the resolution of EAE (54). IL-10 treatment of rats with EAE reduces clinical and pathological signs of disease (82). Encephalitogenic T cells treated in vitro with IL-10 show a marked decrease in TNF production without a loss of proliferative capacity. The suppression of EAE with IL-10 is associated with an increase in MBP specific antibody production (82). These data suggest a role for Th2-type cytokines in abrogating the inflammatory effects of Th1-mediated responses. IL-10 is not as effective an inhibitor of IFN-γ and TNF production by EAE effector cells as TGF-β (74). Not all studies support the regulatory role of Th2 cells in EAE (83).

IL-13 is produced by activated T cells, especially those of the Th2 subtype. IL-13 downregulates cytokine secretion (e.g., TNF, IL-1) by cells of macrophage/monocyte/microglial lineage and enhances B cell functions. In vivo treatment of rats with IL-13 suppresses development of EAE without significantly altering T-cell function, presumably by affecting the effector functions of macrophage/microglial cells (84).

Chemokines are a class of molecules that are secreted by a variety of cell types, predominantly immunologically active cells. There primary purpose appears to be chemo-attraction. Secretion of the chemokine MIP-1α was associated with the EAE inflammatory infiltrate and treatment of EAE with an antibody to MIP-1α ameliorated disease. The chemokine MCP-1 appears to have a regulatory rule in oral tolerance of EAE (85). A general review of the potential role of chemokines in EAE can be found in Ref. 86.

VI. SITE OF ATTACK IN EAE

In EAE, the animal is exposed initially to the sensitizing CNS antigen in the periphery, where the antigen is processed in draining lymph nodes and T cell activation occurs. These CNS antigen–activated T cells then home to the CNS where they "see" their target antigen and undergo further activation and recruitment of additional cellular immune effectors. In a DTH cell-mediated immune response, antigen recognition at the target organ by the activated T cells requires that the antigen be presented in association with an MHC class II molecule. This class II requirement raises some intriguing issues for CNS immune responses, as there is little constitutive or induced class II in the CNS. The putative target of EAE, CNS myelin and myelin-producing oligodendrocytes, do not express class II on their surfaces. In the CNS, class II can be expressed on microglia, astrocytes and cerebral vascular endothelium. For any of these to be the target, they also should express a processed CNS antigen, such as MBP. As CNS antigens undergo degradation and normal turnover, they can be phagocytized and processed within the CNS. All three of the above cell types are capable of presenting CNS antigens and therefore serving as a target for encephalitogenic T cells. However, if a nonmyelin structure is the target for encephalitogenic attack, how does demyelination occur?

The site of antigen recognition and presentation within the CNS during the course of the autoimmune inflammatory disease EAE has not been clearly identified. This disease can be produced by immunization with myelin proteins and their peptides (33,87,88). However, these antigens are not necessarily expressed in locations within the CNS that allow interface with immune effectors. For example, MBP, the most commonly utilized encephalitogenic myelin protein, is normally localized to an internal site on the cytoplasmic surface of the myelin membrane and not expressed on the surface of the myelin sheath (89). The actual mechanism of tissue damage in EAE has not been conclusively determined. Although there is convincing evidence that this disease is mediated by specific populations of T lymphocytes (33,90–92), it is not yet understood how these cells produce dysfunction within the CNS. Some have suggested that the production of disease was due to CNS-specific cytotoxic cells that may produce disease by direct attack on myelin (93), while others have implicated damage of CNS vasculature (94), recruitment of macrophages (95), or local edema formation (96) as important factors in disease production. In contrast, it has been proposed that the disease results from the proximity of neural tissue to lymphokines and other factors secreted during a delayed-type hypersensitivity response (a bystander response) (64,97). In support of this argument are studies with chimeric animals suggesting that the tissues of the CNS need not be syngeneic with the sensitized lymphocytes that mediate disease (98). These latter studies raise the possibility that the site of attack within the CNS in EAE may be directed against a component other than the myelin sheath.

Several studies demonstrate immunocompetent potential for certain CNS cell types. Over the past decade, there has been considerable interest in identifying which cell serves as the antigen-presenting cell of the CNS. The astrocyte, cerebrovascular endothelial cell, and microglia have all been proposed for this role. As outlined below, each of these may, under appropriate conditions, function in antigen presentation.

Astrocytes express MHC class II antigens in response to various cytokines and can serve as antigen-presenting cells (99–104). Astrocytes can secrete immunoreactive molecules (e.g., IL-1, IL-3, IL-6, TNF, TGF-β, interferon α/β and complement proteins) (105–116). Rat astrocytes cultured in vitro may serve as targets for encephalitogenic cytotoxic T lymphocytes (117). Lymphocytes from mice immunized with either whole CNS antigen or MBP show strong proliferative responses when cultured with astrocytes (118). Transplantation studies demonstrate that astrocytes can serve as targets for encephalitogenic T cells in vivo (119). In these experiments, aggregates of purified astrocytes transplanted into non-CNS sites developed perivascular inflammatory lesions following inoculation of the host animal with CNS antigen or MBP. These perivascular lesions develop at the same time as the onset of clinical and CNS pathological signs of EAE. Several studies report an increased immunological competence of astrocytes isolated from EAE susceptible strains of rats and mice as compared to EAE-resistant strains (120–122). There is a hyperinducibility of Ia antigen on astrocytes of EAE-susceptible but not EAE-resistant mice and rats (121). Similarly, astrocytes from EAE-susceptible mice (SJL) are better able to present MHC class II (Ia) to cell lines than astrocytes from EAE-resistant mice (B10.S) (120). Therefore, genetic control of the level of Ia expression on cells of the CNS may play an important role in the pathogenesis of CNS immune reactions. The actual immunological role of astrocytes in CNS inflammation is unclear at present, but they possess the potential properties to serve both as mediators of an immune response and as targets. In addition, there are data to suggest that astrocytes may serve a protective role in EAE by inhibiting both MBP reactive T and B cells (123). IFN-γ–stimulated astrocytes induced better suppression than unstimulated astrocytes, suggesting a possible mechanism for the disease ameliorating effects of IFN-γ, discussed above.

Several studies suggest an important and perhaps essential role for microglia in CNS autoimmunity (124–128). Microglia have antigen-presenting capacity and express Ia under a variety of conditions (129–131). Microglia are the major cells expressing MHC in the perivascular region (132). MHC class II expression in white matter from normal brain and from normal areas of brain from patients with MS occurs predominantly on microglia (133). Perivascular microglia may play a role in initial antigen recognition during the early phases of EAE (134). Microglia are the predominant CNS-based Ia-expressing cell in EAE and in the plaques of MS (135–137). Microglia can secrete IL-1 (138) and can produce lymphotoxin (139), which has been demonstrated in MS lesions (140). Microglia proliferate when exposed to IL-3 and can produce TNF (108). The role of strain differences in microglial Ia expression has received little attention. In one study, susceptible and resistant strains of rats were reported to express similar levels of Ia on microglia during EAE using either a chimeric immune system or a passive transfer protocol (141). In EAE, microglia and infiltrating macrophages produce TNF-α in response to cytokine secretion by infiltrating T cells (142).

The third major cell type within the CNS that has immunocompetent properties is the cerebrovascular endothelial cell. To reach targets within the CNS, lymphocytes must pass through or between the cerebrovascular endothelial cells of the BBB. Although there are data demonstrating that activated lymphocytes may freely pass through the BBB into the CNS (24,25), there is also evidence that lymphocytes activated against CNS antigens may interact with the cerebral vascular endothelial cells (143). Several laboratories report that CNS vascular endothelial cells can serve as in vitro targets when presenting CNS antigen to CD4$^+$ lymphocytes (144,145). Interaction between CD4$^+$ lymphocytes and vascular endothelial cells may play an important role in the early development of the lesion of EAE. Cerebral vascular endothelial cells are able to express Ia under certain circumstances and can serve as APCs to encephalitogenic T cells (146,147). Further, cerebrovascular Ia expression is upregulated during EAE (146).

Oligodendrocytes have not been thought to be immunocompetent cells. However, as the cell of origin of CNS myelin, oligodendrocytes might serve as targets for myelin based autoimmunity. Most reports fail to demonstrate class II expression on oligodendrocytes (148,149), although one study found Ia on cultured human oligodendrocytes (150). While in situ expression of class I or class II MHC molecules by oligodendrocytes has not been demonstrated, in vitro treatment with a combination of IFN-γ and the glucocorticoid dexamethasone can induce mRNA for the class II molecule and its protein product on the oligodendrocyte cell surface (151). The absence of class II expression on oligodendrocytes would make them less likely targets for a cell-mediated autoimmune disorder such as EAE. Nevertheless, oligodendrocytes have been reported to serve as targets for class II–restricted, encephalitogenic T cells (152–154). Oligodendrocytes are also reported to act as accessory cells in an Ia-independent T-cell mitogen response (155). Astrocytes and microglia can be induced to exhibit cytotoxic activity against oligodendrocytes. Oligodendrocytes or the myelin sheath may be damaged by the secreted immunoreactive products of a cell-mediated immune response—a bystander reaction (97). Experiments demonstrating that oligodendrocytes and myelin are damaged in culture when exposed to TNF (64) provide support for this mechanism. Of interest, oligodendrocytes that express an MHC class I transgene show dysmyelination (156). Therefore the cytokines secreted by activated immune cells could cause damage to oligodendrocytes either directly or through upregulation of MHC molecules.

VII. IMMUNOGENETICS OF EAE

Susceptibility to EAE is under immunogenetic control. Both outbred and inbred strains of the various species utilized in EAE models may vary in susceptibility to disease. EAE, like MS, is linked to specific class II major histocompatibility antigens (MHC). In the mouse these are the H2 antigens, which are analogous to the HLA antigens in humans. H2^s (e.g., SJL/J) and H2^u (e.g., PL/J) are the most susceptible H2 haplotypes (157). Other H2 groups can also develop EAE, and by boosting the inoculation procedure utilizing a combined active and passive immunization technique, one can induce EAE in most strains of mice, including those previously thought to be resistant (158). There are additional non-H2 gene loci that correlate with different clinical expression forms of EAE in mice, roughly corresponding to the clinical subtypes of MS (159). There are also genetic loci with gender-specific effects on EAE susceptibility (159). There are immunoregulatory genes that control susceptibility to multiple autoimmune disorders including EAE (160).

In the MOG-induced form of EAE in rat, there are graded MHC II effects on susceptibility that are modified by other MHC genes as well as non-MHC genes (161).

VIII. ENVIRONMENTAL INFLUENCES ON EAE

Although EAE is an autoimmune model for MS, there now is data to link environmental factors to autoimmunity. Superantigens, microbial byproducts such as staphylococcal en-terotoxin B (SEB), are molecules that stimulate and ultimately delete populations of T cells bearing specific TCR V chains. Superantigens have been shown to alter EAE, either by inducing disease or inhibiting it, depending on the timing of the exposure to the superan-tigen (45,162–168). As superantigens can have long-lasting effects on the immune system, exposure may explain the latency factor hypothesized for MS. Another example of poten-tial immune-environmental interaction comes from studies on transgenic mice constructed to express genes coding for a rearranged TCR specific for MBP (169). These mice sponta-neously develop EAE when housed in a non-germ-free environment or when inoculated with pertussis vaccine. These environmental-genetic interactions may afford important clues as to the precipitating factors in MS.

IX. TREATMENT STRATEGIES IN EAE

EAE has been most useful in developing treatment paradigms for autoimmune inflamma-tory disorders of the CNS. The availability of an easily inducible CNS inflammatory dis-ease provides the opportunity to screen a number of potential therapies for MS. EAE has the added advantage of assessing the effects of a given therapy on both the clinical expres-sion of disease and on the neuropathological consequences. More recently developed tech-niques for assessing brain MRI activity provide additional insights into pathogenesis and disease-monitoring potential. As noted above, the considerable knowledge of the underly-ing immunopathogenesis of EAE has allowed for therapies directed at specific aspects of the immune response—e.g., antigen presentation, T-cell activation, TCR interactions, and cytokine effects. In many instances, specific immunopathogenic mechanisms have been inferred by the response to therapies directed against their targets, e.g., anti-TNF-α therapy.

Therapies for EAE can be separated into those that prevent disease from occurring by inhibiting the initial attack, those that ameliorate ongoing episodes of EAE, i.e., treat-ment, and those that prevent relapses. Preventing disease is the easiest outcome to achieve but the least useful in predicting ability to treat MS, as at present we are unable to predict those at risk for MS or to treat them prior to onset of disease. Therefore, therapies that affect established EAE or prevent relapses are most readily applicable to treating MS. Most current treatment agents initially demonstrated an effect on limiting EAE prior to use in MS clinical trials.

Early EAE treatments centered on global immunosuppression—e.g., cytotoxic agents such as cyclophosphamide and methotrexate—which have not enjoyed universal acceptance as therapy for MS. New immunosuppressive therapies, based on initial EAE data are being utilized for specific forms of MS, as seen with mitoxantrone (6,170). In-creased understanding of the underlying immunopathogenesis of this disorder has led to newer therapies targeting various aspects of the trimolecular complex—e.g., anti-MHC class II, anti-CD4, anti-TCR, anti-adhesion molecule therapies, cytokine directed therapies, and therapies directed against putative CNS autoantigens. These defined approaches offer the hope of providing greater specificity against CNS autoimmune demyelination with fewer potential side effects.

As detailed above, there are apparent hazards in trying to translate the results of treating EAE into the human condition. Some of these problems relate to the still unanswered question as to whether MS is an autoimmune disorder. Others relate to the difficulty of directing a therapy to the target CNS without systemic toxicity. Nevertheless, there is no better model available to test new therapeutic hypotheses, keeping in mind the necessary precautions.

A new therapeutic approach to EAE centers on use of neural growth factors which have demonstrated both anti-inflammatory and potential remyelinating properties, a combination of benefits that is quite attractive. Insulinlike growth factor-1 (IGF-1), a growth factor for oligodendrocytes, reduces clinical disease in EAE and alters the underlying pathology, including changes at the BBB (171,172). Treatment of murine EAE with the neuregulin, glial growth factor 2 (GGF2), resulted in reduced clinical signs, increased remyelination, and increased expression of II-10 (173). Such a multidimensional response makes this an interesting therapeutic agent to consider in the treatment of MS.

X. SUMMARY

EAE is a readily inducible cell-mediated autoimmune model of CNS inflammatory demyelination. As such, EAE has allowed for dissection of the systemically induced, cell-mediated autoimmune response within the CNS, providing important details of autoantigen induction, processing, activation, and generation of CNS-targeted activated T cells, the nature of immune-BBB interactions, the activity of T cells within the CNS, T cell–macrophage/microglial interactions, and the role of cytokines/chemokines in the immune response and on CNS tissues. Experimental data obtained from manipulations of the EAE model have provided insights into both the immunogenetic and environmental aspects of CNS inflammatory demyelination. These careful observations of the various immunopathogenic components of EAE provide fertile analogies to human MS.

REFERENCES

1. Lublin FD. Relapsing experimental allergic encephalomyelitis: An autoimmune model of multiple sclerosis. Springer Seminars In Immunopathology 1985; 8:197–208.
2. Rivers TM, Sprunt DH, Berry GP. Observations on attempts to produce acute disseminated encephalomyelitis in monkeys. J Exp Med 1933; 58:39–53.
3. Remlinger J. Accidents paralytiques au cours du traitment anti-rabique. Ann Inst Pasteur 1919; 19:625–646.
4. Field EJ. Effect of imuran (azathioprine) on susceptibility of guinea pigs to allergic encephalomyelitis. Arch Int Pharmacodyn Ther 1967; 165:138–141.
5. Paterson PY, Drobish DG. Cyclophosphamide: Effect on experimental allergic encephalomyelitis in Lewis rats. Science 1969; 165:191–192.
6. Lublin FD, Lavasa M, Viti C, Knobler RL. Suppression of acute and relapsing experimental allergic encephalomyelitis with mitoxantrone. Clin Immunol Immunopathol 1987; 45:122–128.
7. Westarp ME, Wekerle H, Ben Nun A, Cohen IR, Vohl ML, Przuntek H. T lymphocyte line–mediated experimental allergic encephalomyelitis–A pharmacologic model for testing of im-

munosuppressive agents for the treatment of autoimmune central nervous system disease. J Pharmacol Exp Ther 1987; 242:614–620.

8. Sriram S, Steinman L. Anti I-A antibody suppresses active encephalomyelitis: Treatment model for diseases linked to IR genes. J Exp Med 1983; 158:1362–1367.

9. Offner H, Vainiene M, Gold DP, Morrison WJ, Wang RY, Hashim GA, Vandenbark AA. Protection against experimental encephalomyelitis: Idiotypic autoregulation induced by a nonencephalitogenic T cell clone expressing a cross-reactive T cell receptor V gene. J Immunol 1991; 146:4165–4172.

10. Teitelbaum D, Meshorer A, Hirshfeld T, Amon R, Sela M. Suppression of experimental allergic encephalomyelitis by a synthetic polypeptide. Eur J Immunol 1971; 1:242–248.

11. Karussis DM, Lehmann D, Slavin S, Vourka-Karussis U, Mizrachi-Koll R, Ovadia H, Ben-Nun A, Kalland T, Abramsky O. Inhibition of acute, experimental autoimmune encephalomyelitis by the synthetic immunomodulator linomide. Ann Neurol 1993; 34:654–660.

12. Lassmann H, Wisniewski HM. Chronic relapsing experimental allergic encephalomyelitis: Clinicopathological comparison with multiple sclerosis. Arch Neurol 1979; 36:490–497.

13. Rose LM, Richards T, Alvord EC Jr. Experimental allergic encephalomyelitis (EAE) in nonhuman primates: A model of multiple sclerosis (review). Lab Animal Sci 1994; 44:508–512.

14. Massacesi L, Genain CP, Lee-Parritz D, Letvin NL, Canfield D, Hauser SL. Active and passively induced experimental autoimmune encephalomyelitis in common marmosets: A new model for multiple sclerosis. Ann Neurol 1995; 37:519–530.

15. Kojima K, Berger T, Lassmann H, Hinze-Selch D, Zhang Y, Gehrmann J, Reske K, Wekerle H, Linington C. Experimental autoimmune panencephalitis and uveoretinitis transferred to the Lewis rat by T lymphocytes specific for the S100 beta molecule, a calcium binding protein of astroglia. J Exp Med 1994; 180:817–829.

16. Linington C, Berger T, Perry L, Weerth S, Hinze-Selch D, Zhang Y, Lu HC, Lassmann H, Wekerle H. T cells specific for the myelin oligodendrocyte glycoprotein mediate an unusual autoimmune inflammatory response in the central nervous system. Eur J Immunol 1993; 23:1364–1372.

17. Zamvil SS, Steinman L. The T lymphocyte in experimental allergic encephalomyelitis. Annu Rev Immunol 1990; 8:579–621.

18. Brown AM, McFarlin DE. Relapsing experimental allergic encephalomyelitis in the SJL/J mouse. Lab Invest 1981; 45:278–284.

19. Lublin FD, Maurer PH, Berry RG, Tippett D. Delayed, relapsing experimental allergic encephalomyelitis in mice. J Immunol 1981; 126:819–822.

20. Raine CS, Barnett LB, Brown A, Behar T, McFarlin DE. Neuropathology of experimental allergic encephalomyelitis in inbred strains of mice. Lab Invest 1980; 43:150–157.

21. Raine CS, Traugott U, Stone SH. Chronic relapsing experimental allergic encephalomyelitis: CNS plaque development in unsuppressed and suppressed animals. Acta Neuropathol 1978; 43:43–53.

22. Wisniewski HM, Keith AB. Chronic relapsing experimental allergic encephalomyelitis: An experimental model of multiple sclerosis. Ann Neurol 1977; 1:144–148.

23. Linington C, Bradl M, Lassmann H, Brunner C, Vass K. Augmentation of demyelination in rat acute allergic encephalomyelitis by circulating mouse monoclonal antibodies directed against a myelin/oligodendrocyte glycoprotein. Am J Pathol 1988; 130:443–454.

24. Wekerle H, Linington C, Lassmann H, Meyerman R. Cellular immune reactivity within the CNS. Trends Neurosci 1986; 9:271–277.

25. Hickey WF, Hsu BL, Kimura H. T-lymphocyte entry into the central nervous system. J Neurosci Res 1991; 28:254–260.

26. Jemison LM, Williams SK, Lublin FD, Knobler RL, Korngold R. Interferon-gamma–inducible endothelial cell class II major histocompatibility complex expression correlates

with strain- and site-specific susceptibility to experimental allergic encephalomyelitis. J Neuroimmunol 1993; 47:15–22.

27. Welsh CT, Rose JW, Hill KE, Townsend JJ. Augmentation of adoptively transferred experimental allergic encephalomyelitis by administration of a monoclonal antibody specific for LFA-1 alpha. J Neuroimmunol 1993; 43:161–167.

28. Cannella B, Cross AH, Raine CS. Anti-adhesion molecule therapy in experimental autoimmune encephalomyelitis. J Neuroimmunol 1993; 46:43–55.

29. Baron JL, Madri JA, Ruddle NH, Hashim G, Janeway CA Jr. Surface expression of alpha 4 integrin by CD4 T cells is required for their entry into brain parenchyma. J Exp Med 1993; 177:57–68.

30. Yednock TA, Cannon C, Fritz LC, Sanchez M, Steinman L, Karin N. Prevention of experimental autoimmune encephalomyelitis by antibodies against alpha 4 beta 1 integrin. Nature 1992; 356:63–66.

31. Kuchroo VK, Martin CA, Greer JM, Ju ST, Sobel RA, Dorf ME. Cytokines and adhesion molecules contribute to the ability of myelin proteolipid protein-specific T cell clones to mediate experimental allergic encephalomyelitis. J Immunol 1993; 151:4371–4382.

32. Engelhardt B, Martin-Simonet MT, Rott LS, Butcher EC, Michie SA. Adhesion molecule phenotype of T lymphocytes in inflamed CNS. J Neuroimmunol 1998; 84:92–104.

33. Pettinelli CB, McFarlin DE. Adoptive transfer of experimental allergic encephalomyelitis in SJL/J mice after in vitro activation of lymph node cells by myelin basic protein: Requirement for Lyt 1+ 2− T lymphocytes. J Immunol 1981; 127:1420–1423.

34. Ben Nun A, Lando Z. Detection of autoimmune cells proliferating to myelin basic protein and selection of T cell lines that mediate experimental autoimmune encephalomyelitis (EAE) in mice. J Immunol 1983; 130:1205–1209.

35. Ben Nun A, Cohen IR. Experimental autoimmune encephalomyelitis (EAE) mediated by T cell lines: Process of selection of lines and characterization of the cells. J Immunol 1982; 129:303–308.

36. Lider O, Reshef T, Beraud E, Ben Nun A, Cohen IR. Anti-idiotypic network induced by T cell vaccination against experimental autoimmune encephalomyelitis. Science 1988; 239: 181–183.

37. Ben Nun A, Wekerle H, Cohen IR. Vaccination against autoimmune encephalomyelitis with T-lymphocyte line cells reactive against myelin basic protein. Nature 1981; 292:60–61.

38. Waldor MK, Sriram S, Hardy R, Herzenberg LA, Lanier L, Lim M, Steinman L. Reversal of experimental allergic encephalomyelitis with monoclonal antibody to a T-cell subset marker. Science 1985; 227:415–417.

39. Koh DR, Fung-Leung WP, Ho A, Gray D, Acha-Orbea H, Mak TW. Less mortality but more relapses in experimental allergic encephalomyelitis in CD8−/− mice. Science 1992; 256: 1210–1213.

40. Jiang H, Zhang SI, Pernis B. Role of CD8+ T cells in murine experimental allergic encephalomyelitis. Science 1992; 256:1213–1215.

41. Karpus WJ, Swanborg RH. Protection against experimental autoimmune encephalomyelitis requires both CD4+ T suppressor cells and myelin basic protein-primed B cells. J Neuroimmunol 1991; 33:173–177.

42. Karpus WJ, Swanborg RH. CD4+ suppressor cells inhibit the function of effector cells of experimental autoimmune encephalomyelitis through a mechanism involving transforming growth factor-beta. J Immunol 1991; 146:1163–1168.

43. Sun D, Wekerle H, Raper K, Gold DP. CD4-CD8-splenic T cells from Lewis rats recovered from experimental autoimmune encephalomyelitis respond to encephalitogenic T cells that mediate this disorder. Cell Immunol 1991; 137:292–302.

44. Vainiene M, Offner H, Morrison WJ, Wilkinson M, Vandenbark AA. Clonal diversity of basic protein specific T cells in Lewis rats recovered from experimental autoimmune encephalomyelitis. J Neuroimmunol 1991; 33:207–216.

45. Kalman B, Lublin FD, Lattime E, Joseph J, Knobler RL. Effects of staphylococcal entero-toxin B on T cell receptor V beta utilization and clinical manifestations of experimental allergic encephalomyelitis. J Neuroimmunol 1993; 45:83–88.

46. Kalman B, Knobler RL, Lublin FD. Preferential but not exclusive T cell receptor V beta chain utilization of myelin basic protein and peptide-specific T cell clones in mice. Cell Immunol 1994; 153:206–213.

47. Sobel RA, Kuchroo VK. The immunopathology of acute experimental allergic encephalomy-elitis induced with myelin proteolipid protein: T cell receptors in inflammatory lesions. J Immunol 1992; 149:1444–1451.

48. Racke MK, Bonomo A, Scott DE, Cannella B, Levine A, Raine CS, Shevach EM, Rocken M. Cytokine-induced immune deviation as a therapy for inflammatory autoimmune disease. J Exp Med 1994; 180:1961–1966.

49. Al-Sabbagh A, Miller A, Santos LM, Weiner HL. Antigen-driven tissue-specific suppression following oral tolerance: Orally administered myelin basic protein suppresses proteolipid protein-induced experimental autoimmune encephalomyelitis in the SJL mouse. Eur J Immu-nol 1994; 24:2104–2109.

50. Ausubel LJ, Krieger JI, Hafler DA. Changes in cytokine secretion induced by altered peptide ligands of myelin basic protein peptide 85–99. J Immunol 1997; 159:2502–2512.

51. Aharoni R, Teitelbaum D, Arnon R, Sela M. Copolymer 1 acts against the immunodominant epitope 82–100 of myelin basic protein by T cell receptor antagonism in addition to major histocompatibility complex blocking. Proc Natl Acad Sci USA 1999; 96:634–639.

52. Genain CP, Cannella B, Hauser SL, Raine CS. Identification of autoantibodies associated with myelin damage in multiple sclerosis (see comments). Nature Med 1999; 5:170–175.

53. Hjelmstrom P, Juedes AE, Fjell J, Ruddle NH. B-cell-deficient mice develop experimental allergic encephalomyelitis with demyelination after myelin oligodendrocyte glycoprotein sensitization. J Immunol 1998; 161:4480–4483.

54. Kennedy MK, Torrance DS, Picha KS, Mohler KM. Analysis of cytokine mRNA expression in the central nervous system of mice with experimental autoimmune encephalomyelitis re-veals that IL-10 mRNA expression correlates with recovery. J Immunol 1992; 149:2496–2505.

55. Merrill JE, Kono DH, Clayton J, Ando DG, Hinton DR, Hofman FM. Inflammatory leuko-cytes and cytokines in the peptide-induced disease of experimental allergic encephalomyelitis in SJL and B10.PL mice. Proc Natl Acad Sci USA 1992; 89:574–578.

56. Mustafa MI, Diener P, Hojeberg B, Van der Meide P, Olsson T. T cell immunity and inter-feron-gamma secretion during experimental allergic encephalomyelitis in Lewis rats. J Neu-roimmunol 1991; 31:165–177.

57. Kalman B, Knobler RL, Perreault M, D'Imperio C, Marini J, Olender C, Joseph J, Korngold R, Lublin FD. Inhibition of EAE by intracerebral injection of interferon-gamma (IFN-gamma) (abstr). Neurology 1992; 42(suppl 3):346.

58. Lublin FD, Knobler RL, Kalman B, Goldhaber M, Marini J, Perrault M, D'Imperio C, Joseph J, Alkan SS, Korngold R. Monoclonal anti-gamma interferon antibodies enhance experimen-tal allergic encephalomyelitis. Autoimmunity 1993; 16:267–274.

59. Voorthuis JA, Uitdehaag BM, de Groot CJ, Goede PH, van der Meide PH, Dijkstra CD. Suppression of experimental allergic encephalomyelitis by intraventricular administration of interferon-gamma in Lewis rats. Clin Exp Immunol 1990; 81:183–188.

60. Duong TT, Finkelman FD, Singh B, Strejan GH. Effect of anti-interferon-gamma monoclonal antibody treatment on the development of experimental allergic encephalomyelitis in resistant mouse strains. J Neuroimmunol 1994; 53:101–107.

61. Billiau A, Heremans H, Vandekerckhove F, Dijkmans R, Sobis H, Meulepas E, Carton H. Enhancement of experimental allergic encephalomyelitis in mice by antibodies against IFN-gamma. J Immunol 1988; 140:1506–1510.

62. Panitch HS, Hirsch RL, Schindler J, Johnson KP. Treatment of multiple sclerosis with gamma

interferon: Exacerbations associated with activation of the immune system. Neurology 1987; 37:1097–1102.

63. Wildbaum G, Youssef S, Grabie N, Karin N. Neutralizing antibodies to IFN-gamma-inducing factor prevent experimental autoimmune encephalomyelitis. J Immunol 1998; 161:6368–6374.

64. Selmaj KW, Raine CS. Tumor necrosis factor mediates myelin and oligodendrocyte damage in vitro. Ann Neurol 1988; 23:339–346.

65. Begolka WS, Vanderlugt CL, Rahbe SM, Miller SD. Differential expression of inflammatory cytokines parallels progression of central nervous system pathology in two clinically distinct models of multiple sclerosis. J Immunol 1998; 161:4437–4446.

66. Ruddle NH, Bergman CM, McGrath KM, Lingenheld EG, Grunnet ML, Padula SJ, Clark RB. An antibody to lymphotoxin and tumor necrosis factor prevents transfer of experimental allergic encephalomyelitis. J Exp Med 1990; 172:1193–1200.

67. Selmaj K, Raine CS, Cross AH. Anti-tumor necrosis factor therapy abrogates autoimmune demyelination. Ann Neurol 1991; 30:694–700.

68. Baker D, Butler D, Scallon BJ, O'Neill JK, Turk JL, Feldmann M. Control of established experimental allergic encephalomyelitis by inhibition of tumor necrosis factor (TNF) activity within the central nervous system using monoclonal antibodies and TNF receptor-immunoglobulin fusion proteins. Eur J Immunol 1994; 24:2040–2048.

69. Liu J, Marino MW, Wong G, Grail D, Dunn A, Bettadapura J, Slavin AJ, Old L, Bernard CC. TNF is a potent anti-inflammatory cytokine in autoimmune-mediated demyelination. Nature Med 1998; 4:78–83.

70. The Lenercept Multiple Sclerosis Study Group and The University of British Columbia MS/MRI Analysis Group. TNF neutralization in MS: Results of a randomized, placebo-controlled multicenter study. Neurology 1999; 53:457–465.

71. Constantinescu CS, Wysocka M, Hilliard B, Ventura ES, Lavi E, Trinchieri G, Rostami A. Antibodies against IL-12 prevent superantigen-induced and spontaneous relapses of experimental autoimmune encephalomyelitis. J Immunol 1998; 161:5097–5104.

72. Leonard JP, Waldburger KE, Goldman SJ. Prevention of experimental autoimmune encephalomyelitis by antibodies against interleukin 12. J Exp Med 1995; 181:381–386.

73. Kim S, Voskuhl RR. Decreased IL-12 production underlies the decreased ability of male lymph node cells to induce experimental autoimmune encephalomyelitis. J Immunol 1999; 162:5561–5568.

74. Stevens DB, Gould KE, Swanborg RH. Transforming growth factor-beta 1 inhibits tumor necrosis factor-alpha/lymphotoxin production and adoptive transfer of disease by effector cells of autoimmune encephalomyelitis. J Neuroimmunol 1994; 51:77–83.

75. Montgomery IN, Rauch HC. Experimental allergic encephalomyelitis in mice: adoptive transfer of disease is modulated by the presence of natural suppressor cells. Neurochem Res 1984; 9:1399–1406.

76. Johns LD, Flanders KC, Ranges GE, Sriram S. Successful treatment of experimental allergic encephalomyelitis with transforming growth factor-beta 1. J Immunol 1991; 147:1792–1796.

77. Racke MK, Dhib J, Cannella B, Albert PS, Raine CS, McFarlin DE. Prevention and treatment of chronic relapsing experimental allergic encephalomyelitis by transforming growth factor-beta 1. J Immunol 1991; 146:3012–3017.

78. Kuruvilla AP, Shah R, Hochwald GM, Liggitt HD, Palladino MA, Thorbecke GJ. Protective effect of transforming growth factor beta 1 on experimental autoimmune diseases in mice. Proc Natl Acad Sci USA 1991; 88:2918–2921.

79. Johns LD, Sriram S. Experimental allergic encephalomyelitis: Neutralizing antibody to TGFβ1 enhances the clinical severity of the disease. J Neuroimmunol 1993; 47:1–8.

80. McGuire EJ, Savastano JA. Urodynamic findings and long-term outcome management of patients with multiple sclerosis-induced lower urinary tract dysfunction. J Urol 1984; 132: 713–715.

81. Fiorentino DF, Zlotnik A, Vieira P, Mosmann TR, Howard H, Moore KW, O'Garra A. IL-10 acts on the antigen presenting cell to inhibit cytokine production by Th1 cells. J Immunol 1991; 146:3444–3451.

82. Rott O, Fleischer B, Cash E. Interleukin-10 prevents experimental allergic encephalomyelitis in rats. Eur J Immunol 1994; 24:1434–1440.

83. Di Rosa F, Francesconi A, Di Virgilio A, Finocchi L, Santilio I, Barnaba V. Lack of Th2 cytokine increase during spontaneous remission of experimental allergic encephalomyelitis. Eur J Immunol 1998; 28:3893–3903.

84. Cash E, Minty A, Ferrara P, Caput D, Fradelizi D, Rott O. Macrophage-inactivating IL-13 suppresses experimental autoimmune encephalomyelitis in rats. J Immunol 1994; 153:4258–4267.

85. Karpus WJ, Kennedy KJ, Kunkel SL, Lukacs NW. Monocyte chemotactic protein 1 regulates oral tolerance induction by inhibition of T helper cell 1-related cytokines. J Exp Med 1998; 187:733–741.

86. Karpus WJ, Ransohoff RM. Chemokine regulation of experimental autoimmune encephalomyelitis: Temporal and spatial expression patterns govern disease pathogenesis. J Immunol 1998; 161:2667–2671.

87. Paterson PY. Molecular and cellular determinants of neuroimmunologic inflammatory disease. Fed Proc 1982; 41:2569–2576.

88. Sakai K, Zamvil SS, Mitchell DJ, Lim M, Rothbard JB, Steinman L. Characterization of a major encephalitogenic T cell epitope in SJL/J mice with synthetic oligopeptides of myelin basic protein. J Neuroimmunol 1988; 19:21–32.

89. Herndon RM, Rauch HC, Einstein ER. Immuno-electron microscopic localization of the encephalitogenic basic protein in myelin. Immunol Commun 1973; 2:163–172.

90. Ortiz O, Nakamura RM, Weigle WO. T cell requirement for experimental allergic encephalomyelitis induction in the rat. J Immunol 1976; 117:576–579.

91. Mokhtarian F, McFarlin DE, Raine CS. Adoptive transfer of myelin basic protein–sensitized T cells produces chronic relapsing demyelinating disease in mice. Nature 1984; 309:356–358.

92. Zamvil SS, Nelson PA, Mitchell DJ, Knobler RL, Fritz RB, Steinman L. Encephalitogenic T cell clones specific for myelin basic protein: An unusual bias in antigen recognition. J Exp Med 1985; 162:2107–2124.

93. Ben Nun A, Cohen IR. Genetic control of experimental autoimmune encephalomyelitis at the level of cytotoxic lymphocytes in guinea pigs. Eur J Immunol 1982; 12:709–713.

94. Sedgwick J, Brostoff S, Mason D. Experimental allergic encephalomyelitis in the absence of a classical delayed-type hypersensitivity reaction: Severe paralytic disease correlates with the presence of interleukin 2 receptor-positive cells infiltrating the central nervous system. J Exp Med 1987; 165:1058–1075.

95. Brosnan CF, Bornstein MB, Bloom BR. The effects of macrophage depletion on the clinical and pathologic expression of experimental allergic encephalomyelitis. J Immunol 1981; 126:614–620.

96. Goldmuntz EA, Brosnan CF, Norton WT. Prazosin treatment suppresses increased vascular permeability in both acute and passively transferred experimental autoimmune encephalomyelitis in the Lewis rat. J Immunol 1986; 137:3444–3450.

97. Wisniewski HM, Bloom BR. Primary demyelination as a nonspecific consequence of a cell-mediated immune reaction. J Exp Med 1975; 141:346–359.

98. Hinrichs DJ, Wegmann KW, Dietsch GN. Transfer of experimental allergic encephalomyelitis to bone marrow chimeras: Endothelial cells are not a restricting element. J Exp Med 1987; 166:1906–1911.

99. Selmaj KW, Farooq M, Norton WT, Raine CS, Brosnan CF. Proliferation of astrocytes in vitro in response to cytokines: A primary role for tumor necrosis factor. J Immunol 1990; 144:129–135.

100. Yong VW, Yong FP, Ruijs TC, Antel JP, Kim SU. Expression and modulation of HLA-DR on cultured human adult astrocytes. J Neuropathol Exp Neurol 1991; 50:16–28.

101. Cannella B, Raine CS. Cytokines up-regulate Ia expression in organotypic cultures of central nervous system tissue. J Neuroimmunol 1989; 24:239–248.

102. Benveniste EN, Sparacio SM, Bethea JR. Tumor necrosis factor-alpha enhances interferon-gamma-mediated class II antigen expression on astrocytes. J Neuroimmunol 1989; 25:209–219.

103. Fierz W, Endler B, Reske K, Wekerle H, Fontana A. Astrocytes as antigen-presenting cells: I. Induction of Ia antigen expression on astrocytes by T cells via immune interferon and its effect on antigen presentation. J Immunol 1985; 134:3785–3793.

104. Fontana A, Fierz W, Wekerle H. Astrocytes present myelin basic protein to encephalitogenic T-cell lines. Nature 1984; 307:273–276.

105. Lee JC, Simon PL, Young PR. Constitutive and PMA-induced interleukin-1 production by the human astrocytoma cell line T24. Cell Immunol 1989; 118:298–311.

106. Tobler I, Borbely AA, Schwyzer M, Fontana A. Interleukin-1 derived from astrocytes enhances slow wave activity in sleep EEG of the rat. Eur J Pharmacol 1984; 104:191–192.

107. Fontana A, Grob PJ. Astrocyte-derived interleukin-1-like factors. Lymphokine Res 1984; 3:11–16.

108. Frei K, Bodmer S, Schwerdel C, Fontana A. Astrocyte-derived interleukin 3 as a growth factor for microglia cells and peritoneal macrophages. J Immunol 1986; 137:3521–3527.

109. Frei K, Bodmer S, Schwerdel C, Fontana A. Astrocytes of the brain synthesize interleukin 3-like factors. J Immunol 1985; 135:4044–4047.

110. Benveniste EN, Sparacio SM, Norris JG, Grenett HE, Fuller GM. Induction and regulation of interleukin-6 gene expression in rat astrocytes. J Neuroimmunol 1990; 30:201–212.

111. Constam DB, Philipp J, Malipiero UV, ten Dijke P, Schachner M, Fontana A. Differential expression of transforming growth factor-beta 1, -beta 2, and -beta 3 by glioblastoma cells, astrocytes, and microglia. J Immunol 1992; 148:1404–1410.

112. Fontana A, Grob PJ. Lymphokines and the brain. Springer Semin Immunopathol 1984; 7:375–386.

113. Norris JG, Benveniste EN. Interleukin-6 production by astrocytes: Induction by the neurotransmitter norepinephrine. J Neuroimmunol 1993; 45:137–146.

114. Chung IY, Benveniste EN. Tumor necrosis factor-alpha production by astrocytes. Induction by lipopolysaccharide, IFN-gamma, and IL-1 beta. J Immunol 1990; 144:2999–3007.

115. Tedeschi B, Barrett JN, Keane RW. Astrocytes produce interferon that enhances the expression of H-2 antigens on a subpopulation of brain cells. J Cell Biol 1986; 102:2244–2253.

116. Levi S, Mallat M. Primary cultures of murine astrocytes produce C3 and factor B, two components of the alternative pathway of complement activation. J Immunol 1987; 139:2361–2366.

117. Sun D, Wekerle H. Ia-restricted encephalitogenic T lymphocytes mediating EAE lyse autoantigen-presenting astrocytes. Nature 1986; 320:70–72.

118. Jewtoukoff V, Bach MA. Lymphocyte proliferative response to glial cells in SJL/J mice immunized with rat whole spinal cord and rat myelin basic protein. J Neuroimmunol 1989; 21:81–86.

119. Lublin FD, Marini JC, Perreault M, Olender C, Dimperio C, Joseph J, Korngold R, Knobler RL. Autoimmune inflammation of astrocyte transplants. Ann Neurol 1992; 31:519–524.

120. Bimbaum G, Kotilinek L. Immunologic differences in murine glial cells and their association with susceptibility to experimental allergic encephalomyelitis. J Neuroimmunol 1990; 26:119–129.

121. Massa PT, ter Meulen V, Fontana A. Hyperinducibility of Ia antigen on astrocytes correlates with strain-specific susceptibility to experimental autoimmune encephalomyelitis. Proc Natl Acad Sci USA 1987; 84:4219–4223.

122. Chung IY, Norris JG, Benveniste EN. Differential tumor necrosis factor alpha expression

by astrocytes from experimental allergic encephalomyelitis-susceptible and -resistant rat strains. J Exp Med 1991; 173:801–811.

123. Xiao BG, Diab A, Zhu J, Van der Meide P, Link H. Astrocytes induce hyporesponses of myelin basic protein-reactive T and B cell function. J Neuroimmunol 1998; 89:113–121.

124. Matsumoto Y. Role of microglia in autoimmune encephalomyelitis. Neuropathol Appl Neurobiol 1994; 20:196–198.

125. Matsumoto Y, Ohmori K, Fujiwara M. Microglial and astroglial reactions to inflammatory lesions of experimental autoimmune encephalomyelitis in the rat central nervous system. J Neuroimmunol 1992; 37:23–33.

126. Matsumoto Y, Ohmori K, Fujiwara M. Immune regulation by brain cells in the central nervous system: Microglia but not astrocytes present myelin basic protein to encephalitogenic T cells under in vivo-mimicking conditions. Immunology 1992; 76:209–216.

127. Merrill JE, Ignarro LJ, Sherman MP, Melinek J, Lane TE. Microglial cell cytotoxicity of oligodendrocytes is mediated through nitric oxide. J Immunol 1993; 151:2132–2141.

128. Merrill JE, Zimmerman RP. Natural and induced cytotoxicity of oligodendrocytes by microglia is inhibitable by TGF beta. GLIA 1991; 4:327–331.

129. Poltorak M, Freed WJ. Immunological reactions induced by intracerebral transplantation: Evidence that host microglia but not astroglia are the antigen-presenting cells. Exp Neurol 1989; 103:222–233.

130. Steiniger B, van der Meide PH. Rat ependyma and microglia cells express class II MHC antigens after intravenous infusion of recombinant gamma interferon. J Neuroimmunol 1988; 19:111–118.

131. Giulian D. Ameboid microglia as effectors of inflammation in the central nervous system. J Neurosci Res 1987; 18:155–171.

132. Lassmann H, Zimprich F, Vass K, Hickey WF. Microglial cells are a component of the perivascular glia limitans. J Neurosci Res 1991; 28:236–243.

133. Hayes GM, Woodroofe MN, Cuzner ML. Microglia express MHC class II in normal and demyelinating human white matter. Ann NY Acad Sci 1988; 540.501–503.

134. Hickey WF, Kimura H. Perivascular microglial cells of the CNS are bone marrow-derived and present antigen in vivo. Science 1988; 239:290–292.

135. Matsumoto Y, Hara N, Tanaka R, Fujiwara M. Immunohistochemical analysis of the rat central nervous system during experimental allergic encephalomyelitis, with special reference to Ia-positive cells with dendritic morphology. J Immunol 1986; 136:3668–3676.

136. Konno H, Yamamoto T, Iwasaki Y, Saitoh T, Suzuki H, Terunuma H. Ia-expressing microglial cells in experimental allergic encephalomyelitis in rats. Acta Neuropathol 1989; 77: 472–479.

137. Boyle EA, McGeer PL. Cellular immune response in multiple sclerosis plaques. Am J Pathol 1990; 137:575–584.

138. Giulian D, Baker TJ, Shih LC, Lachman LB. Interleukin 1 of the central nervous system is produced by ameboid microglia. J Exp Med 1986; 164:594–604.

139. Frei K, Siepl C, Groscurth P, Bodmer S, Schwerdel C, Fontana A. Antigen presentation and tumor cytotoxicity by interferon-gamma–treated microglial cells. Eur J Immunol 1987; 17: 1271–1278.

140. Selmaj K, Raine CS, Cannella B, Brosnan CF. Identification of lymphotoxin and tumor necrosis factor in multiple sclerosis lesions. J Clin Invest 1991; 87:949–954.

141. Matsumoto Y, Kawai K, Fujiwara M. In situ Ia expression on brain cells in the rat: Autoimmune encephalomyelitis-resistant strain (BN) and susceptible strain (Lewis) compared. Immunology 1989; 66:621–627.

142. Renno T, Krakowski M, Piccirillo C, Lin JY, Owens T. TNF-alpha expression by resident microglia and infiltrating leukocytes in the central nervous system of mice with experimental allergic encephalomyelitis: Regulation by Th1 cytokines. Journal of Immunology 1995; 154: 944–953.

143. Sedgwick JD, Hughes CC, Male DK, MacPhee IA, ter Meulen V. Antigen-specific damage to brain vascular endothelial cells mediated by encephalitogenic and nonencephalitogenic CD4+ T cell lines in vitro. J Immunol 1990; 145:2474–2481.

144. McCarron RM, Racke M, Spatz M, McFarlin DE. Cerebral vascular endothelial cells are effective targets for in vitro lysis by encephalitogenic T lymphocytes. J Immunol 1991; 147: 503–508.

145. Lublin FD, Jemison L, Kalman B, D'Imperio C, Joseph J, Korngold R, Knobler RL. Susceptibility to EAE correlates with inducible Ia expression on cerebral endothelial cells but not astrocytes. Neurology 1992; 42:347.

146. McCarron RM, Spatz M, Kempski O, Hogan RN, Muehl L, McFarlin DE. Interaction between myelin basic protein-sensitized T lymphocytes and murine cerebral vascular endothelial cells. J Immunol 1986; 137:3428–3435.

147. Wilcox CE, Healey DG, Baker D, Willoughby DA, Turk JL. Presentation of myelin basic protein by normal guinea-pig brain endothelial cells and its relevance to experimental allergic encephalomyelitis. Immunology 1989; 67:435–440.

148. Lee SC, Raine CS. Multiple sclerosis: oligodendrocytes in active lesions do not express class II major histocompatibility complex molecules. J Neuroimmunol 1989; 25:261–266.

149. Grenier Y, Ruijs TC, Robitaille Y, Olivier A, Antel JP. Immunohistochemical studies of adult human glial cells. J Neuroimmunol 1989; 21:103–115.

150. Kim SU, Moretto G, Shin DH. Expression of Ia antigens on the surface of human oligodendrocytes and astrocytes in culture. J Neuroimmunol 1985; 10:141–149.

151. Bergsteindottir K, Brennan A, Jessen KR, Mirsky R. In the presence of dexamethasone, g interferon induces rat oligodendrocytes to express major histocompatibility complex class II molecules. Proc Natl Acad Sci USA 1992;89:9054–9058.

152. Kawai K, Heber K, Zweiman B. Cytotoxic effects of myelin basic protein-reactive T cell hybridoma cells on oligodendrocytes. J Neuroimmunol 1991; 32:75–81.

153. Kawai K, Zweiman B. Characteristics of in vitro cytotoxic effects of myelin basic protein-reactive T cell lines on syngeneic oligodendrocytes. J Neuroimmunol 1990; 26:57–67.

154. Kawai K, Zweiman B. Cytotoxic effect of myelin basic protein-reactive T cells on cultured oligodendrocytes. J Neuroimmunol 1988; 19:159–165.

155. Cashman NR, Noronha A. Accessory cell competence of ovine oligodendrocytes in mitogenic activation of human peripheral T cells. J Immunol 1986; 136:4460–4463.

156. Turnley AM, Morahan G, Okano H, Bernard O, Mikoshiba K, Allison J, Bartlett PF, Miller JF. Dysmyelination in transgenic mice resulting from expression of class I histocompatibility molecules in oligodendrocytes. Nature 1991; 353:566–569.

157. Zamvil SS, Steinman L. The T lymphocyte in experimental allergic encephalomyelitis. Annu Rev Immunol 1990; 8:579–621.

158. Shaw MK, Kim C, Ho KL, Lisak RP, Tse HY. A combination of adoptive transfer and antigenic challenge induces consistent murine experimental autoimmune encephalomyelitis in C57BL/6 mice and other reputed resistant strains. J Neuroimmunol 1992; 39:139–149.

159. Butterfield RJ, Sudweeks JD, Blankenhom EP, Korngold R, Marini JC, Todd JA, Roper RJ, Teuscher C. New genetic loci that control susceptibility and symptoms of experimental allergic encephalomyelitis in inbred mice. J Immunol 1998; 161:1860–1867.

160. Teuscher C, Hickey WF, Grafer CM, Tung KS. A common immunoregulatory locus controls susceptibility to actively induced experimental allergic encephalomyelitis and experimental allergic orchitis in BALB/c mice. J Immunol 1998; 160:2751–2756.

161. Weissert R, Wallstrom E, Storch MK, Stefferl A, Lorentzen J, Lassmann H, Linington C, Olsson T. MHC haplotype-dependent regulation of MOG-induced EAE in rats. J Clin Inves 1998; 102:1265–1273.

162. Soos JM, Hobeika AC, Butfiloski EJ, Schiffenbauer J, Johnson HM. Accelerated induction of experimental allergic encephalomyelitis in PL/J mice by a non-V beta 8-specific superantigen. Proc Natl Acad Sci USA 1995; 92:6082–6086.

163. Racke MK, Quigley L, Cannella B, Raine CS, McFarlin DE, Scott DE. Superantigen modulation of experimental allergic encephalomyelitis: Activation of anergy determines outcome. J Immunol 1994; 152:2051–2059.

164. Soos JM, Schiffenbauer J, Johnson HM. Treatment of PL/J mice with the superantigen, staphylococcal enterotoxin B, prevents development of experimental allergic encephalomyelitis. J Neuroimmunol 1993; 43:39–44.

165. Rott O, Wekerle H, Fleischer B. Protection from experimental allergic encephalomyelitis by application of a bacterial superantigen. Int Immunol 1992; 4:347–353.

166. Brocke S, Gaur A, Piercy C, Gautam A, Gijbels K, Fathman CG, Steinman L. Induction of relapsing paralysis in experimental autoimmune encephalomyelitis by bacterial superantigen. Nature 1993; 365:642–644.

167. Das MR, Cohen A, Zamvil SS, Offner H, Kuchroo VK. Prior exposure to superantigen can inhibit or exacerbate autoimmune encephalomyelitis: T-cell repertoire engaged by the autoantigen determines clinical outcome. J Neuroimmunol 1996; 71:3–10.

168. Crisi GM, Santambrogio L, Hochwald GM, Smith SR, Carlino JA, Thorbecke GJ. Staphylococcal enterotoxin B and tumor-necrosis factor-alpha-induced relapses of experimental allergic encephalomyelitis: Protection by transforming growth factor-beta and interleukin-10. Eur J Immunol 1995; 25:3035–3040.

169. Goverman J, Woods A, Larson L, Weiner LP, Hood L, Zaller DM. Transgenic mice that express a myelin basic protein-specific T cell receptor develop spontaneous autoimmunity. Cell 1993; 72:551–560.

170. Edan G, Miller D, Clanet M, Confavreux C, Lyon-Caen O, Lubetzki C, Brochet B, Berry I, Rolland Y, Froment JC, Cabanis E, Iba-Zizen MT, Gandon JM, Lai HM, Moseley I, Sabouraud O. Therapeutic effect of mitoxantrone combined with methylprednisolone in multiple sclerosis: A randomised multicentre study of active disease using MRI and clinical criteria (see comments). J Neurol Neurosurg Psychiatry 1997; 62:112–118.

171. Li W, Quigley L, Yao DL, Hudson LD, Brenner M, Zhang BJ, Brocke S, McFarland HF, Webster HD. Chronic relapsing experimental autoimmune encephalomyelitis: Effects of insulin-like growth factor-I treatment on clinical deficits, lesion severity, glial responses, and blood brain barrier defects. J Neuropathol Exp Neurol 1998; 57:426–438.

172. Yao DL, Liu X, Hudson LD, Webster HD. Insulin-like growth factor-I given subcutaneously reduces clinical deficits, decreases lesion severity and upregulates synthesis of myelin proteins in experimental autoimmune encephalomyelitis. Life Sci 1996; 58:1301–1306.

173. Cannella B, Hoban CJ, Gao YL, Garcia-Arenas R, Lawson D, Marchionni M, Gwynne D, Raine CS. The neuregulin, glial growth factor 2, diminishes autoimmune demyelination and enhances remyelination in a chronic relapsing model for multiple sclerosis. Proc Natl Acad Sci USA 1998; 95:10100–10105.

7

Evidence for Immunopathogenesis

UTE TRAUGOTT

New York Medical College, Valhalla, St. Agnes Hospital, White Plains, and Bronx Lebanon Hospital, Bronx, New York

I. INTRODUCTION

Although the clinical and pathological features of multiple sclerosis (MS) were described in detail by Charcot as early as 1868 (1), the etiology of this primary demyelinating disease of the central nervous system (CNS) remains largely unknown. In recent years, the application of highly sophisticated techniques has greatly facilitated the understanding of the complex mechanisms that lead to lesion formation in MS (2). In accord with the current concept on the pathogenesis of autoimmune diseases in general (3), in MS, it is proposed that in genetically predisposed individuals, viral or other infections can trigger a pathological white matter–specific cell-mediated immune response that, together with antibodies and complement, leads to selective destruction of myelin and oligodendrocytes and to some axonal damage. Immunological tolerance, which is normally maintained by various mechanisms such as suppressor cells and clonal deletion of T cells, can be overcome when activation of physiological low-affinity binding of autoreactive T cells by myelin antigen cross-reactive pathogens or by release of sequestered antigens leads to the generation of high-affinity binding of pathological autoreactive T cells, which can cause tissue damage. Polyclonal activation of T cells by proinflammatory cytokines produced during unrelated immune responses or by superantigens can also lead to high affinity-binding of autoreactive T cells (3). Proinflammatory cytokines can contribute to extravasation of leukocytes and to the development of inflammatory lesions in target organs by upregulating adhesion molecules, vascular addressins, chemokines, and matrix metalloproteases (MMP) and by inducing aberrant class II major histocompatibility complex (MHC) expression on endothelial cells and glial elements (4,5). Disease activation by cytokines in MS is strongly supported by the previously reported increased exacerbation rate following intercurrent viral infections (6) and after systemic administration of interferon (IFN)-γ (7). The specificity of the disease process for myelin and oligodendrocytes, the type IV delayed type hypersensitivity (DTH)-like features of inflammatory lesions, the presence of myelin-specific antibodies, the wide spectrum of immunological abnormalities in both blood and cerebrospinal fluid (CSF), and the similarities of these changes with those observed in other human autoimmune diseases and in the animal model experimental autoimmune encephalomyelitis (EAE) have provided strong support for the conclusion that MS is an immune-mediated disease. Classification of MS as an autoimmune disease may be possible according to criteria used in clinical settings, which require (a) presence of other autoimmune diseases in patients or their family members; (b) presence of lymphocytic infiltrates in the target organ;(c) statistical association with certain MHC haplotypes; and (d) a favorable response to immunosuppressive medications (8). Direct proof, as can be obtained for myasthenia gravis by passive transfer of the disease-mediating antibodies from a pregnant woman to her fetus, is difficult to obtain for T cell–mediated diseases due to the MHC restriction of T-cell functions (3,8). The following sections summarize immunological abnormalities in blood and CSF, report on the effect of cytokines on endothelial cells and glial elements in vitro, provide a detailed description of the lesion immunopathology, and discuss the findings as they relate to a possible autoimmune pathogenesis of MS.

II. IMMUNOLOGIC CHANGES IN BLOOD AND CEREBROSPINAL FLUID

A variety of quantitative and qualitative abnormalities of both the humoral and cellular immune system have been described in MS. Due to random enhancement of all inflammatory responses by cytokines, most of these changes are not specific for MS but can also be observed in other immune-mediated conditions (4,5).

A. Quantitative Immunologic Changes

Blood

Changes in peripheral blood leukocytes (PBL) reflect a generally low degree of immune activation.

T Cells. Percentages of CD3+ and CD4+ T cells are higher in MS than in normal controls (9–12). Numbers of CD8+ T cells may be decreased, but decreases do not reliably correlate to clinical disease activity (2). CD8+CD38+ cells are increased, CD8+CD28 (bind to B7 molecules)–positive cells are unchanged, and CD8+CD28− cells and CD8+CD11b (Mac)+ cells are decreased (10). Decreases in CD26 (dipeptidyl peptidase IV)–positive cells reportedly correlate to disability (2).

CD4+CD45RA+ (naive) and CD4+CD45RO+ (memory) T cells are either increased or decreased (2) and CD4+CD29 (β chain of β1 integrins)–positive cells are increased (2,11). Elevated numbers of CD4+SLAM (signaling lymphocyte activation molecule)–positive and CD4+CD7+ T cells, which produce Th1 cytokines, are consistent with a DTH response (13). Their preactivated state facilitates recirculation of CD4+CD45RO+ cells through organs and their potential for reactivation in the absence of costimulation by B7 molecules (3). Antigen-independent activation of CD4+ cells by IL-2, IL-6, IFN-γ, and TNF-α can precede clinical relapses and lesions determined to be active on magnetic resonance imaging (MRI) by about 1 month (11).

During early stages of the disease, the frequency of γ/δ T cell–receptor (TCR)-positive cells may be increased, while during chronic disease most T cells bear the α/β TCR (2). Oligoclonal expansion of V delta 2J delta 3+ gamma/delta TCR+ cells in blood as well as CNS lesions indicates an antigen-specific response (14,15). Polyclonal responses of γ/δ TCR+ cells can also be present (2). Gamma/delta TCR+ cells recognize hsp-70 in an MHC unrelated manner and can be stimulated by bacterial superantigens such as staphylococcal enterotoxin-B (SEB) and toxic shock toxin (TSST)-1 (16).

Numbers of *large granular lymphocytes* are normal, while those of *small mature natural killer (NK)* (CD3−, CD8−, CD56+, CD16+) cells and NK functional activity (NKFA) are lower in MS than in controls (2). NKFA shows fluctuations over time, and decreases may be followed by relapses with active MRI lesions (17). As sign of activation, mRNA levels for perforin, which mediates NK-dependent cell lysis, are increased (18).

ADHESION MOLECULES. CD2 leukocyte function–associated antigen (LFA)-1 (CD11a CD18), LFA-3 (CD58), and intercellular adhesion molecule (ICAM)-1 (CD54), which mediate cell-to-cell contacts, and the activation markers interleukin-2 receptor (IL-2R; CD25), class II MHC, and transferrin receptors (CD71) are increased on some lymphocytes (2). The $\beta1$-integrins VLA-4 (CDw49d), VLA-5 (CDw49e) and their common β chain CD29, which facilitate adhesion to extracellular matrix components, may be increased or decreased (2). Due to TNF-α activation–induced shedding of surface molecules, soluble (s) ICAM-1, sVCAM-1 and sCD8 levels are elevated in the presence of Gd+ MRI lesions (19,20). sE-selectin (CD62E), a marker for EC activation, may be unchanged or higher in primary progressive (PP) than relapsing-remitting (RR) and secondary progressive (SP) MS (21). During relapses, levels of s class I MHC are increased in both serum and CSF while s class II MHC levels are either increased or decreased in serum only (22). Soluble forms of adhesion molecules, vascular addressins, and MHC molecules may exert immunomodulatory effects by blocking their receptors without eliciting a biological effect.

In the presence of IL-2, strong antigen-directed activation of peripheral T cells leads to their clonal deletion by apoptosis. *Apoptosis* (programmed cell death, or PCD) is mediated by CD95 (Fas) /CD95L (FasL) interactions and characterized by DNA fragmentation (3). By contributing to peripheral tolerance, apoptosis can play an important role in limiting immune-mediated tissue damage. Numbers of CD95+ T cells and levels of sCD95 molecules may either be unchanged or increased, particularly during active disease. Increases in sCD95 can be associated with EDSS changes (23–27). In MS and controls, MBP and tetanus toxoid (TT)–specific T cells reportedly do not downregulate Bcl-2 and Bcl-X and thus are resistant to sCD95-mediated apoptosis (26). In addition to apoptosis, MBP-specific T cells can be eliminated by other perforin-producing cytotoxic MBP-specific T cells (24). These quantitative changes in CD95 expression and sCD95 concentrations may either indicate enhanced or impaired apoptosis, particularly, since binding of sCD95 to CD95L may fail to generate apoptotic signals (23,24).

Monocytes. Freshly isolated monocytes from active MS patients are activated. Accordingly, they contain increased levels of cAMP and display an increase in HLA-DP and HLA-DQ and a decrease in HLA-DR expression (2). Numbers of B7.2 (CD86)-positive monocytes are increased in MS over controls (28). While B7.2 is detectable in most samples, B7.1 (CD80)-positive monocytes appear to be associated with disease pathogenesis rather than with relapses (28). Binding of B7.1 to CD28 and CTL-4 on naive and activated T cells, respectively, leads to preferential activation of Th1 cells and to enhancement of the inflammatory response. Binding of B7.2 to CD28/CTL-4 preferentially triggers Th2 cells, which facilitate antibody production and downregulation of DTH responses (3). In MS, increases in both Th1- and Th2-derived cytokines reflect a mixed T and B cell response. Resistance of B7.1 and B7.2 to inhibitory regulation in chronic progressive (CP) MS reflects defective postthymic tolerance.

In active MS, monocytes spontaneously release larger amounts of IL-1β and IL-6 and produce even more TNF-α, IL-1α, IL-1β and IL-6 after lipopolysaccharide (LPS) activation than monocytes from stable MS, OND and normal controls (2). IFN-γ, TNF-α, IL-1β, immunomodulatory peptides and beta-endorphin trigger production of NO from arginin via inducable NO synthetase (iNOS). This process can be downregulated by IL-4 (29–31). In accord with monocyte activation, nitrate and nitrite levels are elevated in blood and CSF. Gd+ MRI lesions are associated with high NO, IFN-γ and TNF-α levels all of which concentrate to blood-brain-barrier (BBB) damage (31). While NO inhibits proliferation of Th1 cells in an autocrine manner, it leads to upregulation of HLA-DR on monocytes, increases their cytotoxic activity and contributes to the generation of new antigenic epitopes by nitrosination of proteins (30).

B Cells.   CD20+CD45RO+ B cells are increased in MS and Crohn's disease, two immune-mediated conditions that may coexist (32). CD19, a coreceptor for B cells is decreased in RR MS and increased on CD5+ cells in progressive MS. CD5+ cells produce low-affinity-binding IgM autoantibodies (2). During exacerbations, numbers of B7.1+ B cells and CD71+HLA-DR+ lymphocytes and monocytes are elevated. Increased IgG production correlates with high levels of IL-6 (2) and of the B cell growth factor sCD23 (33).

Cytokines.   Proinflammatory cytokines such as IL-1β, TNF-α, and IFN-γ activate immune cells and enhance expression of adhesion molecules, vascular addressins and chemokines on leukocytes and EC. Thus, they can render the BBB more permeable to soluble and cellular components of the immune system and facilitate the development of inflammatory lesions not only in MS but also in other immune-mediated conditions. Immunoregulatory cytokines such as IL-4, IL10 and TGF-β can downregulate the inflammatory response (3,4).

PROINFLAMMATORY CYTOKINES.   Serum levels of IL-2, sIL-2R, IFN-γ, TNF-α, TNF-β, and IL-2 may be increased just prior to or during exacerbations (2,34). IFN-γ and IL-12 are increased in CP MS during autumn and winter (35), and IL-2 is periodically elevated even during stable disease (2). Cells producing IFN-γ, TNF-α, IL-1α, IL-2, and sIL-2R are more numerous than those secreting IL-1β and IL-4 (2,36–38). IFN-γ-activated macrophages produce IL-12, IL-10, and matrix metalloproteases (MMP). Prevalence of mRNA expression for IFN-γ is noted in severe and of TGF-β in mild cases (2).

Circulating levels of TNF-α and neopterin produced by IFN-γ–stimulated monocytes are elevated (36). While short-term exposure to TNF-α is known to lead to immune cell activation, long-term exposure may result in immunosuppression (4). Increased TNF-α and decreased TGF-β levels precede exacerbations by about 4 weeks and correlate to severity of clinical signs and presence of Gd+ MRI lesions (37). Frequencies of TNF-α and LT-producing cells are comparable between MS and inflammatory neurologic diseases (IND) and are less common in blood than CSF (38). Levels of CD30, a member of the TNF superfamily derived from activated Th2 cells are unremarkable (39).

IL-12, produced by IFN-γ-activated macrophages and B cells activates NK cells and induces CD4+ cells to differentiate into Th1 cells (3). IL-12 levels and IL-12 mRNA expression are higher in CP and RR MS than in controls (40).

IMMUNOREGULATORY CYTOKINES.   IL-10 produced by activated macrophages and T cells exerts an anti-inflammatory effect by decreasing IFN-γ production and class II MHC expression on monocytes (3). In active and stable MS, serum IL-10 levels may be low (41,42). However, mRNA levels for IL-10 are higher in CSF than blood (41). Overall, the IL-10/IL12 baseline may be important for susceptibility to autoimmunity (43). Production of IFN-γ during bacterial infections can shift this balance in favor of IL-12 and thus can contribute to reactivation of the immune-mediated disease processes (44).

Levels of IL-4 and TGF-β can be decreased or increased (2). High levels are seen, particularly in short-term disease with minor disability, and are more common in RR than in SP MS. In progressive MS, mRNA levels for TGF-β (Th3) are increased (40). TGF-β is a potent anti-inflammatory cytokine which is produced by CD8+ and CD45RA+ cells. It suppresses expression of pro-inflammatory cytokines and counteracts IFN-γand TNF-α-mediated aberrant class II MHC expression.

Chemokines and Matrix-Metalloproteases (MMP).   Chemokines which attract leukocytes and MMP which degrade extracellular matrix (EM) components are produced by activated leukocytes and are essential for their extravasation into inflammatory sites. Levels for both groups of molecules may be increased in blood and CSF and may be associated with damage to the BBB and presence of Gd+ MRI lesions (45,46). mRNA levels for macrophage chemoattractant protein (MCP)-1 and RANTES (regulated upon activation, normal T cells expressed and secreted) are upregulated in blood and even higher in CSF cells. In both RR and progressive MS, CD3+ CXCR3+ cells are increased, while CD3+CCR5 + cells, which produce high levels of IFN-γ and IL-12, are elevated only in progressive MS (47). That a genetic deficiency in expression of CCR5, which serves as the major receptor for MIP-1α and MIP-1β, does not protect from developing MS reflects a redundancy in the function of chemokines (48).

Serum levels of gelatinase B (MMP-9) and tissue inhibitor of metalloprotease (TIMP)-1 and TIMP-2 fluctuate and are significantly higher in MS than in controls, particularly during relapses with Gd+ MRI lesions (46). During relapses, levels of TIMP-1 remain unchanged while TIMP-2 levels decrease. Abnormalities in the inhibition of MMPs by TIMPs may contribute to the chronicity of MS by promoting the development of inflammatory lesions (46).

Antibodies.   Serum concentrations for IgG are normal while those for IgA and IgM may be slightly increased. Oligoclonal bands and free light chains are virtually absent (2). Antibody titers to myelin antigens, other autoantigens (see Chap. 8), to viruses (2) (see Chap. 5) and to heat shock protein (hsp) 65 can be increased (2). Antibodies to MBP, PLP, MOG (49), 2′,3′-cyclic nucleotide 3′-phosphodiesterase (CNP), cerebroside (2), gangliosides (2), oligodendrocyte-associated transaldolase and cardiolipin (2) belong mainly to the IgG class although IgM antibodies to MBP, cerebroside and CNP can also be found (2). In both serum and CSF, antibodies to axolemnal fractions are increased (50). The wide spectrum of continuously increased antibody levels reflects a general dysregulation of the immune system rather than an antigen-specific response.

Complement activation and sera from MS and normal controls (2) mediate opsonization of myelin by macrophages equally well. Minor complement-induced alterations of myelin in vivo may result in a reversible conduction block while more extensive binding of complement leads to permanent damage. Clinically, these changes may correlate to transient and permanent neurologic deficits, respectively (2,51).

Cerebrospinal Fluid (CSF)

Although immunologic changes are similar in blood and CSF, they develop independently from each other and are frequently more pronounced in CSF. Since CSF communicates freely with extracellular fluid, it can reflect CNS immunopathology more accurately than blood (2).

Lymphocytes. CSF contains higher percentages of CD3+, CD4+, CD4+CD45RO+, CD8+CD45RO+, IL-2R+, CD26+ and CD5+ cells than blood (2,12). Numbers of CD3−, CD8+, class II MHC+ and CD16+ cells are decreased (2). CD95 expression may be increased on T cells, particularly during active demyelination (23).

Expression of *adhesion molecules* LFA-1, ICAM-1, CD2, LFA-3, VLA-3 (CD49wc), VLA-4, VLA-5 (CDw49e), VLA-6 (CDw49f), and CD29 (their common β chain) is upregulated (2). CD4+CD29+ cells are higher and CD8+CD11b (Mac)+ cells lower in CSF than blood (12). Levels of CD44, a homing receptor for hyaluronate-containing matrix components is commonly increased (2). Since during cell activation adhesion molecules and MHC antigens can be shed, concentrations of sICAM-1 and s class I MHC increase as their cell-bound forms decrease (19,47).

Gamma/delta TCR+ cells are more common in CSF than blood (2). Since oligoclonality of γ/δ TCR+ cells early during the disease indicates stimulation by specific antigen, this implies fundamental differences in the immunopathogenesis of acute versus chronic MS (2).

Monocytes. Percentages of class II MHC+ cells are unchanged during stable and decreased during active disease. CR1 (CD35), CR3, myeloperoxidase, KiM6, IOM3 and CD14 display lower levels in CSF than blood cells and decreases are even more pronounced in OND (2). Monocytes and B cells are B7.1+ and B7.2+ (52). B7.1 is prominent in less than 2 weeks disease duration but not during relapses (28).

Cytokines. Cytokine levels are also frequently higher in CSF than blood (2). During relapses, IL-2 and sIL-2R levels are increased (2). TNF-α, neopterin and nitrate production by IFN-γ-activated macrophages may be increased (53). Levels of TNF-α and LT are higher in CP than in stable MS and in normal controls (2,38). Freshly isolated CSF cells contain increased levels of mRNA for TNF-α, IFN-γ, IL-4, and TGF-β even without antigen stimulation in vitro (42). After stimulation with MBP and PLP, mRNA levels for IFN-γ, IL-4, and TGF-β increase more in CSF than in blood-derived cells (42). Involvement of biologically active TGF-β in disease resolution is suggested by its correlation to numbers and duration of acute relapses (54). Soluble CD30 is increased, particularly during remissions, possibly reflecting resolving lesions (39). mRNA expression for IL-12p70 and IL-12p40 in CSF and blood cells are higher and lower, respectively. In MS, cells expressing mRNA for IFN-γ and IL-10 and cells producing TNF-α and LT are more common in MS than in inflammatory neurologic diseases (IND) (47).

Chemokines. During relapses, MCP-1 is decreased and interferon-induced protein (IP)-10, RANTES, MIP-1a, and MMP-9 are increased (4). Increased levels of mRNA for MCP-1 and RANTES are present and indicate cell activation.

Antibodies. The most common findings in CSF are increased absolute and relative concentrations of IgG, oligoclonal bands and more free kappa than lambda light chains (2) (Chap. 8). IgG, IgA and IgM are continuously produced intrathecally and IgD is elevated particularly during active disease (2). CSF contains antibodies to MBP, MAG, MOG, and CNP (2). During relapses, free anti-MBP antibodies may transiently increase (2). In both CSF and white matter, peptide specificity patterns of myelin basic protein (MBP)-bound antibodies are identical and more restricted than those of free anti-MBP antibodies. Increased antibody titers to a variety of viruses may be due to immunodysregulation (2).

Oligoclonal Bands. In CSF, oligoclonal bands are present in more than 90% of MS patients. Although they are not specific for MS but are also seen in other chronic inflammatory CNS diseases, together with other CSF findings, they can support the clinical diagnosis of MS. That in encephalitis oligoclonal bands contain high-affinity binding antibodies to the causative virus raised the hope, that in MS they also may provide a clue to the underlying pathogen(s). However, only 1 % of oligoclonal bands are directed to specific antigens in MS (55). In addition to hsp, collagen proteins, 68-kDa neurofilamentous proteins, and proteins from herpes simplex virus, cytomegalovirus, and papillomavirus were found to interact with oligoclonal bands (56). The low affinity of these antigen-antibody interactions, however, indicates that the antibodies in question are nonsense antibodies, produced by polyclonal B cell activation rather than in response to specific antigens (2,57).

B. Qualitative Immunologic Changes

These include immunodysregulation and sensitization to myelin components and various pathogens.

Immunodysregulation

Dysregulation of the immune system is indicated by persistent immune activation, defective lymphocyte stimulation, ineffective apoptosis, and diminished NK cell function (2). Suppressor cell function may be reduced or normal (2). Together with continuous antigen and cytokine-induced stimulation, these abnormalities may contribute to T-cell activation and the apparently uninhibited production of antibodies to myelin components, other autoantigens, viruses, and hsp.

Reactivity to Myelin Antigens. Although proteins constitute only 30% of the dry weight of myelin, they are more potent immunogens than lipids. B and T cells in normal controls and in MS patients are sensitized to MBP, proteolipid protein (PLP), myelin-associated glycoprotein (MAG) and myelin oligodendrocyte associated glycoprotein (MOG, 2). Frequencies of myelin-reactive T cells are significantly higher in CSF than blood and may differ between diagnostic groups (2).

MYELIN BASIC PROTEIN (MBP). MBP 83-99 is an immunodominant epitope in HLA-DR2-positive individuals (2,58). There are apparently no differences in the selection of class II MHC restriction elements and MBP epitopes between MS patients, their unaffected identical twins, or other family members (2). Since in MS 84% of circulating MBP-reactive CD4+ T cells are memory cells, they may play a significant role in disease reactivation (59,60).

In addition to MBP in mature myelin, T-cell lines (TCL) from MS and controls are also sensitized to MBP variants of immature myelin present during remyelination, such as citrulline-containing MBP (MBP-C8; 2) and 2 exon-encoded MBP (X2 MBP; 2). Cross-reactivity between MBP and golli-MBP HOG7, which is present in peripheral lymphoid tissues, may contribute to immunologic tolerance (61). PBL activated by MBP express mRNA for IFN-γ, TNF-α, IL-4, TGF-β, IL-10, and GM-CSF (38). Although MBP-reactive CD4+ and CD8+ T cells are most prevalent during active disease, they persist even in stable MS at low levels for more than 12 months (2). While in individual patients, TCR Vα/Vβ usage is frequently mono- or oligoclonal, significant differences exist between patients, and MBP-reactive T-cell populations change during the course of MS (62). The observed increase in TCR heterogeneity in chronic disease may be shaped by degenerative antigen recognition of CD4+ cells, by the disease process itself, and by environmental factors and seems to be greatly unaffected by genetic factors (46,58,62). In MS and controls, 10 to 50% of MBP-reactive T cells can be expanded in a non-MHC restricted manner by the bacterial superantigens staphylococcal enterotoxin (SE) A, SEB, and toxic shock syndrome toxin (TSST) −1. Superantigens activate T cells by binding to certain Vβ chains of TCR outside the antigen combining site (3). In MS, proinflammatory cytokines produced by superantigen-activated T cells, together with defective apoptotis, may lead to disease activation.

PROTEOLIPIDPROTEIN (PLP). PLP is the most abundant protein in CNS myelin. MBP and PLP-reactive CD4+ cells, which display a marked heterogeneity in their TCR Vβ usage, have similar characteristics (2). The major epitope PLP (95–116) is presented in context with DR2w15 to TCR α/β+ cells. Cryptic epitopes generated extracellularly by proteolytic enzymes may contribute to epitope spreading as the disease progresses (63). During relapses, PLP-reactive CD4+ T cells produce high levels of IFN-γ and TNF-α, while during remissions, IL-10 and TGF-β levels may be increased. Class I MHC-restricted CD8+ cells producing IFN-γ, TNF-α, TNF-β and TGF-β can regulate PLP-reactive CD4+ cells either by recognizing their TCR Vβ chains or independent of their Vβ b chains involving anti-idiotypic and anti-ergotypic responses, respectively (64). Cerebrosides and gangliosides can elicit a cytotoxic CD8+T cell−mediated class I MHC−restricted response.

REACTIVITY TO HEAT SHOCK PROTEINS (HSP). Sensitization of peripheral blood leukocytes (PBL) to hsp is more common in MS than in normal controls and more prevalent for hsp70 than hsp65 (2,4). During early disease, frequencies of hsp-reactive T cells are higher in blood than CSF (14,15), while those of mycobacteria-reactive T cells predominate in the CSF (2). Molecular mimicry between bacterial and CNS-derived hsp may contribute to the activation of the intrathecal immune response and thus contribute to the chronicity of the disease process.

In recent years, tissue culture work has demonstrated that complex interactions can occur between cells of the immune system and endothelial cells and glial elements (2). The results of these studies are presented in the following paragraphs and discussed in regard to their significance for the immunopathogenesis of MS lesions.

III. TISSUE CULTURE STUDIES

Studies on the effect of cytokines on resident CNS tissue components—e.g., endothelial cells, astrocytes, oligodendrocytes, and microglia in vitro—have greatly facilitated the functional interpretation of immunopathological findings in MS lesions.

A. Endothelial Cells

Isolated microvessels from normal brain express class I MHC, factor VIII, low levels of transferrin receptors (CD71), urokinase plasminogen activator receptor (uPAR), and very little or no ICAM-1. They are negative for class II MHC, vascular cell adhesion molecule (VCAM)-1 (CD106), E-selectin, IL-10, and MCP-1 (2).

Class I MHC can be upregulated on EC by IFN-α/β (2). IFN-γ, soluble and cell-bound TNF-α (65), and IL-1 can enhance ICAM-1 and induce aberrant class II MHC, VCAM-1 and E-selectin expression in a dose-dependent manner. More than 50% of EC isolated from active MS lesions are positive for class II MHC, ICAM-1, and VCAM-1 (2). E-selectin, a marker for EC activation, is also present but less common and factor VIII is decreased. ICAM-1 and VCAM-1 are more frequently coexpressed with class II MHC than uPAR (2). According to the dual-signal theory, simultaneous expression of class II MHC and costimulatory molecules are needed for effective antigen presentation to naive T cells. However, preactivated memory T cells, which preferentially recirculate through organs, do not require B7 costimulation for reactivation. That IFN-γ-activated EC can indeed present MBP to specifically sensitized T cells, has been shown previously (2). Extravasation of leukocytes involves a series of steps which are mediated by cascade-like interactions between molecules on activated EC and activated circulating leukocytes. The first step in the adhesion cascade, a transient loose attachment of T cells that results in rolling of leukocytes along EC is mediated by L-selectin and its EC ligands CD34 and GlyCAM-1. In the second step, chemokine-induced conformational changes in LFA-1 lead to the arrest of LFA-1+ leukocytes and, in the third step, to their firm attachment to ICAM-1+ EC. In the fourth step, VLA-4+ leukocytes migrate through VCAM-1+ EC, basement membranes of EC, and astrocytes and enter the CNS parenchyma (64). In perivascular spaces, VLA-4+ leukocytes may attach to VCAM-1+ pericytes (2,66).

Accordingly, MS lymphocytes expressing VLA-4, CD29, and CD62L show stronger adherence to EC pretreated in vitro with IFN-γ, IL-β, and TNF-α than lymphocytes from patients with OND or from normal controls. At the onset of a relapse and in the presence of Gd+ MRI lesions, lymphocyte-EC adhesion is particularly strong and correlates to increased levels of TNF-α, sL-selectin, sICAM-1, and sVCAM-1 (67). CD4+ T cells and CD14+ monocytes adhere more strongly to MCP-1+ EC derived from MS brain than to EC from control brain (68).

B. Astrocytes

Astrocytes from normal brain are negative for MHC antigens and for ICAM-1, LFA-1, and LFA-3. They show faint labeling for hsp60 but are unreactive for hsp70 (2). Astroglia can express p80, a cell-specific hyaluronate binding protein of the CD44 family (2), and perforin which reflects cytotoxic properties of this cell type (69). Proinflammatory cytokines induce expression of surface molecules and some functional properties of macrophages in astrocytes. Expression of class I MHC can be triggered by IFN-α/β (2). IFN-γ, TNF-α, LT, and IL-1 induce class II MHC and ICAM-1 expression in a dose-dependent manner (2). Class II MHC expression can be downregulated by TGF-β1 and TGF-β2 (2). Together with IL-1β, IFN-γ can trigger TNF-α production. TNF-α and IL-1β can induce IL-6 and RANTES and their effect is potentiated by IFN-γ (2,70). Astrocyte-derived IL-3 stimulates microglia and induces IL-2 production by and IL-2R expression on T cells (2). Similar to EC, MHC-positive astrocytes can function as antigen-presenting cells (2). Different kinetics in MHC, IL-12, and ICAM-1 expression on astrocytes in vivo may contribute to immunoregulation of the local inflammatory response. While in short-term cultures, astrocytes are protected from apoptosis by high IL-8 levels, they are sensitive to CD95L-mediated apoptotic signals that involve the CPP32 cascade in long-term cultures (71).

C. Oligodendrocytes

Oligodendrocytes and myelin are susceptible to damage by various mechanisms. Both TNF-α and IFN-γ can trigger apoptotic signals in oligodendrocytes (2). TNF-α can also lead to vacuolar degeneration of myelin (2) and chronic exposure can interfere with oligodendrocyte differentiation, as indicated by lack of MBP expression (72). Oligodendrocytes and oligodendrocyte-astrocyte type-2 progenitor cells are highly sensitive to perforin and may be damaged by both MHC-unrestricted cytotoxic CD56+CD4+ T cells, by class I MHC-restricted CD8+ T cells (2), or by perforin-expressing astrocytes (69). Oligodendrocytes can be protected from TNF-α–mediated apoptosis but not from lysis by cytotoxic T cells by ciliary neurotrophic factor (CNTF) (73). IFN-α/β induce class I MHC, and IL-1 α, IFN-γ and TNF-α trigger hsp72 but not class II MHC expression (2). Hsp reactivity of oligodendrocytes may render them susceptible for lysis by γ/δ TCR+ cells (2).

Although oligodendrocytes in some species are highly sensitive to complement-mediated injury in the absence of specific antibodies, they can recover from sublethal damage by shedding membrane-bound C9 containing vesicles (2). Normal human oligodendrocytes may be protected from direct complement-mediated damage by expressing the complement regulatory protein CD59; they may become susceptible to damage due to low CD59 levels (74). Phagocytosis of myelin by microglia in the absence of specific antibodies is mediated by C3R and leads to increased production of TNF-α and NO. Remyelination occurs in the presence of ongoing demyelination and seems to be facilitated by various inflammatory mediators (2).

D. Microglia

Microglia can function as effector cells of CD4+ T cell-mediated DTH reactions. Freshly isolated microglia from adult brain express ICAM-1, LFA-1, LFA-3, CD11a, CD68 (macrosialine), and B7.2 but are negative for B7.1 and uPAR (75,76). UPAR and uPA interactions promote locomotion of microglia (76). Microglia can be activated by proinflammatory cytokines, cross-linking of its receptors and LPS (2). Activation leads to production of chemokines, proinflammatory cytokines, lysosomal enzymes, e.g. phosphatases and nonspecific esterases, a decrease in TGF-β levels and to increased phagocytic activity which is associated with activation of the oxidative burst and NO production (2,76). NO levels can also be increased by oligodendrocytes and can be down-regulated by TGF-β (2). Binding of VLA-4+ cells to VCAM-1+ microglia (77) or cross-linking of IFN-γ-induced CD40 by CD40L-positive T cells can trigger TNF-α production in microglia (78). Microglia are particularly actively involved in the phagocytosis of myelin during early stages of the disease (51). Myelin can be damaged by opsonization in the absence of specific antibodies, or by Fc receptor–mediated phagocytosis in the presence of specific antibodies.

These results document close interactions and complex modifications of EC and glial elements by activated immune cells and the pluripotential effects of their cytokines which may be essential for the development of inflammatory lesions but also are involved in downregulation of the inflammatory response and tissue repair.

IV. PATHOLOGY OF MS LESIONS

The pathology of MS lesions is outlined here briefly to facilitate correlations with immuno-pathologic findings in situ.

At the *macroscopic level*, chronic MS is characterized by multiple sharply demar-cated demyelinated plaques, which are frequently localized around ventricles and consist of astrocytic scar tissue (1,2). A pink, congested margin of chronic plaques indicates active disease. Silent chronic lesions represent the end stage of an inflammatory disease process during which myelin and oligodendrocytes are destroyed and axons are also damaged. Lesions in the rare form of rapidly progressive acute MS appear pink and congested and have a diffuse border.

By *light microscopy*, MS lesions can be classified as acute, active chronic, and silent chronic, depending on degree of inflammation, appearance of the lesion edge, and presence of myelin fragments or degradation products in macrophages (1,2,79).

Active chronic lesions are characterized by a zone of inflammation at the sharply demarcated lesion edge and the presence of hypertrophic, sometimes multinucleated astrocytes (Fig. 1). Inflammatory cells—e.g., macrophages, lymphocytes, and plasma cells—are numerous in Virchow-Robin spaces and in white matter parenchyma. Oligoden-drocytes and, particularly in highly active lesions, axons are reduced in numbers (80). Presence of myelin fragments in macrophages indicates ongoing demyelination, while foamy cells containing cholesterol esters, the end product of enzymatic myelin degrada-tion, reflect long-standing disease. Active lesions with their numerous inflammatory cells and reactive glial changes provide the most valuable information on immunopathological changes that lead to tissue damage.

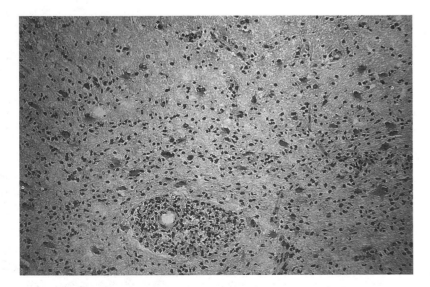

Figure 1 Brain, lesion edge, stained with hematoxylin and eosin (H&E). An area of inflammation containing many mononuclear cells in perivascular cuffs and in white matter parenchyma is shown. Note the hypertrophic sometimes multinucleated astrocytes. (×125) All photomicrographs were taken from 10-um-thick frozen sections of active chronic MS lesions. Sections were stained with hematoxylin and eosin (H&E) or with monoclonal antibodies (Mab) by the ABC technique.

Silent chronic lesions are sharply demarcated gliotic areas, which may contain some lipid-laden macrophages but lack lymphocytic infiltrates and significant reactive glial changes. Incomplete remyelination may be seen at the lesion edge.

Acute lesions have diffuse margins. Their parenchyma is filled with numerous randomly distributed mononuclear inflammatory cells between hypertrophic astrocytes. Perivascular cuffs appear small since they mainly contain lymphocytes and only a few macrophages.

V. IMMUNOPATHOLOGY OF MS LESIONS

A. Normal Central Nervous System

In normal brain, *endothelial cells* (*EC*) express class I MHC, ICAM-1, ICAM-2 (CD102), LFA-3, factor VIII, and TGF-receptor (R) type I and II (2,81). EC are weakly reactive for the chemokines RANTES and MIP-1β and for MMP-9 (gelatinase) (82). Brain EC are negative for class II MHC, VCAM-1 (CD106) and E-selection (2). *Microglia* are reactive for all three isoforms of TGF-β and for TGF-R type I and II (81) and are faintly stained for LFA-1, T-200 (CD45), MMP-7, MIP-1α, MIP-1β, and MCP-1 (82,83). MMPs and tissue inhibitors of MMP (TIMP) are frequently colocalized but latent in the absence of catalytic plasmin activity. Low levels of IL-4, IL-10, and TNF-α are occasionally seen (5). Constitutive expression of the active form of RelA(p65) and c-Rel (p50) NF-kappaB subunits in nuclei and cytoplasm, respectively, predisposes microglia for rapid activation (84). *Astrocytes* express CD44 (2). Apart from a few CD4+ and CD8 cells in perivascular location, hematogenous cells are virtually absent (2).

B. Active Chronic Lesions

Immunocytochemical studies reveal distinct distribution patterns of various types of inflammatory cells, deposits of immunoglobulin (Ig) and complement factors, and enhanced or abnormal expression of various immune markers on EC and glial elements which reflects their activation and participation in the local inflammatory response (2). Findings are consistent with complex immune-mediated inflammatory responses during which damage to myelin, oligodendrocytes and axons is caused not only by a CD4+ T cell–mediated delayed type hypersensitivity (DTH) reaction but also by antibody and complement-mediated and other cytotoxic mechanisms. This process leads not only to the formation of an astrocytic scar tissue but also induces remyelination, which, however, is commonly incomplete. CNS tissue from individual patients contains lesions with a wide spectrum of different stages of activity. Even in otherwise silent plaques, several restricted areas of active demyelination, which tend to extend along myelinated fibers, can be seen. This pattern may be reflected by the open ring image in Gd-enhanced MRI lesions (85).

Lesion Edge and Periplaque Area

Inflammatory Cells.   In active chronic plaques, macrophages are most numerous at the lesion edge while T cells predominate in the periplaque area (2). This composition and distribution pattern of inflammatory cells is characteristic of a DTH reaction in which CD4+ cells act as inducer and activated macrophages as effector cells, using immunoglobulins (Ig) as ligands to bind to their target (2). Vascular addressins, adhesion molecules, chemokines, and matrix metalloproteases (MMP) facilitate extravasation of leukocytes through EC, their migration within the parenchyma, and target cell interactions.

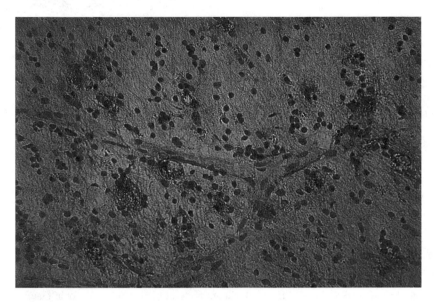

Figure 2 Brain, lesion edge, stained with MAb to class II MHC and counterstained for nuclear labeling with heamtoxylin. Between class II MHC-positive macrophages, a few class II MHC-positive hypertrophic astrocytes are seen. (×310.)

MACROPHAGES/MICROGLIA. Macrophages/microglia can serve as both scanvenger and professional antigen presenting cells. In accord with their activated state, macrophages show strong reactivity for class I and II MHC (Fig. 2), B7.2, LFA-1, LFA-3, CD11c (gp50/95; Fig. 3), VCAM-1, VLA-4 and for IL-1β, IL-12, TNF-α (Fig. 4), LT-α, IL-4 and for PGE-2 (2,86–88). ICAM-3+ cells can be seen closely apposed to LFA-1+ mi-

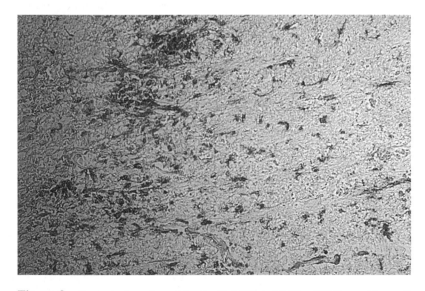

Figure 3 Brain, lesion edge, stained with MAb to CD11c. CD11c-positive cells are seen in perivascular cuffs and in the parenchyma (×160.)

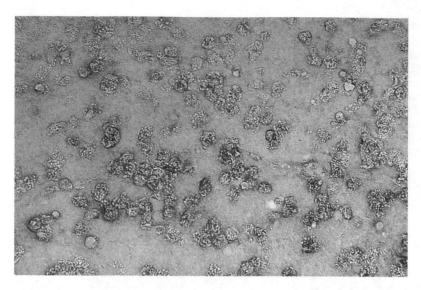

Figure 4   Brain, lesion edge, stained with polyclonal antibody to human IFN-α2. Some macrophages at the active lesion edge are IFN-α2–positive. (×200.)

croglia (89), which can express FasL and may trigger apoptotic signals in Fas+ cells. Although CNS tissue has a high inherent potential for generating apoptotic signals, a defect in this mechanism may contribute to the chronicity of inflammatory lesions in MS. Leukocyte chemoattractant factor (LCF), expressed on microglia at the lesion edge, can attract CD4+ cells (89,90). Labeling of some macrophages at the lesion edge for IFN-α and less commonly for IFN-β (2) may indicate local immunosuppression (2).

Elevated levels of Fc receptors type I (CD64), II (CDw32), and III (CD16) can facilitate myelin uptake via receptor-mediated endocytosis involving clathrin-coated pits and IgG as ligand (2,91). This process leads to intracellular myelin degradation by proteolytic enzymes such as proteases and lipases. In early active lesions, MRP154+ and 27E10+ macrophages contain MBP, PLP, and MOG-reactive myelin degradation products; while in late active lesions, debris in 27E10+ macrophages is stained for MBP and PLP only (79). Increased levels of reactive oxygen species (ROS) and NO enhance the cytotoxic effect of macrophages and contribute to the significant amount of local DNA damage (92). Peroxinitrite, derived from NO-superoxide interactions, can lead to peroxidation of myelin and oligodendrocyte membranes and to a reversible conduction block. Secondary degenerative changes induced by these mechanisms may contribute to irreversible tissue damage and clinical worsening even in the absence of inflammation. NO may also exert a protective effect by suppressing T cells and activated macrophages and by promoting outgrowth of neurites (53).

Chemokines, matrix metalloproteinases (MMP) and tissue inhibitors of MMP (TIMP) are widely distributed throughout lesions. Most chemokines are rapidly induced by PDGF, IL-1, TNF-α, IFN-γ, and IL-4 (93). Binding of CD40L+ T cells to CD40+ macrophages can trigger expression of MIP-1α, MIP-1β, RANTES and MCP-1 (47). Activation of *MMPs* by plasminogen triggers enhanced expression of integrins and leads to actin polymerisation and polarisation of lymphocytes involved in locomotion (5). Microvessels are reactive for MMP-9 (gelatinase) and macrophages express MMP-1, MMP-

2, MMP-3, MMP-7, and MMP-9 (94,95). That MMP-9 also facilitates outgrowth of oligo-dendrocyte processes and, together with IL-6, promotes remyelination of denuded axons, reflects a cell-specific effect of MMPs (94). Coexpression of MMPs and TIMPs is essential to balance their functions.

MIP-1α- and *MIP-1β*-positive microglia attract both CD8+ T cells as well as mac-rophages, and CD4+ cells, respectively (5,93,95). Reactivity of microglia for *MCP-1, MCP-2,* and *MCP-3* is variable and restricted to lesions. MCPs strongly attract T cells and monocytes, mediate cell-cell and cell-extracellular matrix (EM) contact, and stimulate production of cytokines and growth factors (93). Labeling for MCP-2 frequently predomi-nates over MCP-1 and MCP-3 reactivity (5,94). MCP-1 can also downregulate CD4+-T cell–mediated inflammatory responses by facilitating IL-4 production (93).

CHEMOKINE RECEPTORS.   Ligation of G-protein–coupled chemokine receptors re-sults in activation of T cells and microglial cells (93). Lymphocytes in perivascular cuffs express CXCR3, a receptor for IFN-γ inducible protein of 10 kDa (IP-10) and for monok-ine induced by IFN-γ (Mig) (96,97). Lymphocytes and microglia within lesions are labeled for CCR5, a receptor for RANTES which preferentially attracts memory T cells. MCP-1 and MCP-2–positive cells interact with CCR2 receptors on macrophages and on activated lymphocytes. Rapid downregulation of CCR2 by proinflammatory cytokines contributes to retention of inflammatory cells in the parenchyma (93).

T CELLS.   As the density of macrophage infiltrates decreases towards the periplaque area, T cells become more numerous. T cells are positive for CD3, CD2, LFA-1 (Fig. 5), ICAM-1, and ICAM-3 (2,90). B7.1 is preferentially expressed on CD2+ T cells and CD22+ B cells in pv cuffs but not in the parenchyma proper (86). Perivascular cuffs contain some CD1b+ cells, which act as class I MHC-like restriction factors for lipids (97). Numerous CD45+ (Fig. 6), CD4+, CD4+CD45RO+, VLA-4+, CD44+ and IL-2R+ cells penetrate from the active edge deeply into the periplaque area (2). CD8+ cells

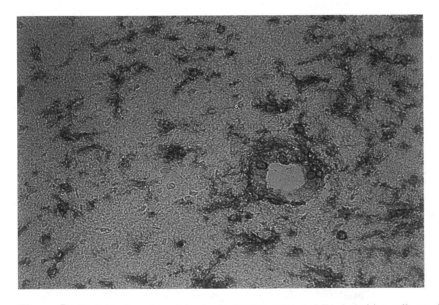

Figure 5   Brain, lesion edge, stained with MAb to LFA-1. LFA-1-positive cells are shown in the parenchyma and in perivascular distribution. (×200.)

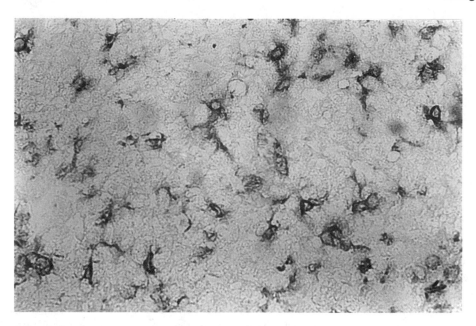

Figure 6   Brain, lesion edge, stained with MAb to CD45. Note intensive labeling of some infiltrating cells in clusters and fainter reactivity of glia. (×310.)

are also numerous in highly active plaques. CD4+CD45RA+ T cells and HNK 1 (CD57)+ cells are rare (2). In addition to their involvement in lesion pathogenesis, activated T and B cells may exert a neuroprotective effect by producing brain-derived neurotrophic factor (BDNF; 98).

T cells more frequently express γ/δ and α/β TCR (2,99). Preferential use of TCR V γ-2 and V δ-2 chains indicates their stimulation by a specific antigen (2). The close correlation between patterns of V δ-J δ re-arrangements of TCR genes in blood and MS lesions supports an important role of γ/δ TCR+ cells in the pathogenesis of MS (15). Accumulation of γ/δ TCR+ cells close to hsp-65- and hsp-70-positive oligodendrocytes (2,99) at the active edge indicates tissue damage by MHC unrestricted mechanisms (2). Lymphocytes are strongly reactive for LT-α, LT-β, and IFN-γ (4,5). Particularly in perivascular leukocytes, mRNA for IFN-γ, TNF-α, and IL-6 is more prevalent than for IL-1α, IL-2, IL-4, IL-10, TGF-β1, and TGF-β2 (2). IL-12p40 mRNA, which indicates secretion of bioactive IL-12, can be detected only in cases of short disease duration (86). In perivascular cuffs, cells are more commonly labeled for RANTES than for CCR5, CXCR3 (47,100), MIP-1α, MIP-1β (95), and amyloid precursor protein (APP) (100,101). Expression of RANTES on both EC and pv cells may provide a gradient along which memory T cells are preferentially attracted (100). Lymphocytes in the parenchyma proper express the RANTES receptor CCR5 and MIP-1α and MIP-1β (47,95). Leukocyte chemotactic factor (LCF) derived from CD4+ and CD8+ cells may regulate influx of CD4+ T cells and macrophages and immune functions of microglial (89).

IMMUNOGLOBULIN (IG)-POSITIVE CELLS, IG DEPOSITS, AND MAST CELLS.   Inflammatory infiltrates also contain immunoglobulin (Ig)-positive cells, CD19+, CD20+, and CD21+ mature circulating B cells are virtually absent due to terminal differentiation into plasma cells after extravasation (own observation). Expression of B7.1 and CD40 on pv

CD22+ B cells suggests their involvement in antigen-specific T cell activation. While most plasma cells are IgG-positive, some also stain for IgE (2). Presence of serum-derived or locally produced antimyelin antibodies and complement activation, as reflected in the intensive labeling of myelinated axons, particularly at the edge of lesions for IgG, C9 and C9 neo-antigen (2,91), supports their contribution to tissue damage (2). Mast cells, sometimes labeled for IL-4, are localized close to microvessels in demyelinated areas and less frequently seen in normal-appearing white matter. This reflects their potent effect on vascular permeability during cytokine activation (2).

Adhesion Molecules. Active chronic MS lesions are surrounded by a wide zone of diffuse ICAM-1 (Fig. 7) and LFA-3 (Fig. 8) reactivity. Staining is rather homogenous and encompasses the most peripheral parts of the astrocytic scar tissue, the lesion edge, and to a variable degree the adjacent normal-appearing white matter (2). Cellular labeling in this area is more common for LFA-3 than for ICAM-1. Enhanced expression of ICAM-1 and LFA-3 on endothelium and presence of a few LFA-1+, LFA-3+, and CD2+ cells may reflect early stages in lesion formation, followed by enhanced expression of adhesion molecules on glial cells (Fig. 9). As the local immune response progresses, both ICAM-1 and LFA-3, the ligands for LFA-1 and CD2, respectively, become widely distributed in the plaque and periplaque area. This may be due to binding of their soluble forms to extracellular matrix components.

Astrocytes. At the lesion edge, activated astrocytes show hypertrophy and express some immunological markers of macrophages. In highly active lesions, activation of astrocytes is accompanied by increased levels of mRNA for GFAP and by expression of class I class II MHC; ICAM-1, LFA-1, LFA-3; VCAM-1, VLA-4, and chemokines (2,62,102) (Figs. 10 and 11). Astrocytes also show strong reactivity for L-1, IL-2, IL-4, IL10, TNF-α, LT-β, LT-receptor, IFN-γ, all three isoforms of TGF-β, and both of their receptors (2,87).

Figure 7 Brain, gray-white matter border, stained with MAb to ICAM-1. A zone of ICAM-1 reactivity extends along the gray-white matter border. Labeling of endothelial cells is increased in white matter and decreased in gray matter (left bottom corner). (×125.)

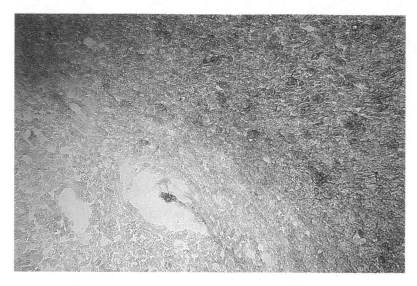

Figure 8 Brain, gray-white matter border, stained with MAb to LFA-3. Note selective labeling of white matter parenchyma for LFA-3 (on right) and unreactivity of gray matter (on left) (×125.)

Astrocyte labeling for IFN-β, however, is weak and less common. Astrocytes and oligodendrocytes are hsp-60–positive. Abnormal expression of these molecules on astrocytes in lesion areas suggests their induction by locally produced proinflammatory cytokines. While class I MHC is mainly expressed close to lymphocytic infiltrates early during lesion development, class II MHC is also detectable on astroglia in older lesions in the presence of numerous foamy macrophages (2). Expression of MHC antigens and of adhesion mole-

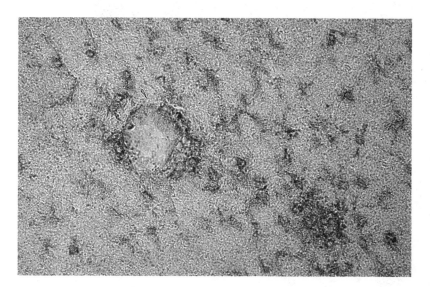

Figure 9 Brain, white matter remote from lesion, stained with MAb to LFA-3. In this rapidly progressive case, microfoci of LFA-3+ cells and faint labeling of glia can be seen remote from active lesions (×200.)

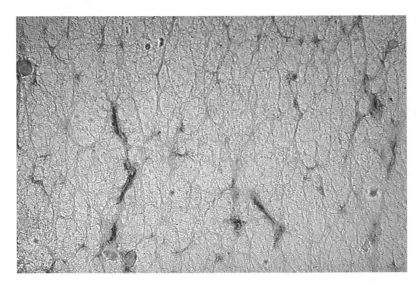

Figure 10   Spinal cord, normal white matter, stained with MAb to class I MHC. Segmental labeling of astrocytes is shown. (×310.)

cules on and presence of myelin fragments in astrocytes supports their ability to present specific antigen to T cells, as has been documented previously for MBP in vitro (2). Preferential migration of preactivated memory T cells into white matter parenchyma may facilitate astrocyte-mediated activation even in the absence of B7 costimulation. Strong labeling of hypertrophic astrocytes for CD1b, which is colocalized with colony stimulating factor (CSF), may reflect their ability to present lipids to T cells (Fig. 12). Differences in enzymatic degradation of myelin by astrocytes, macrophages, and extracellular proteolysis

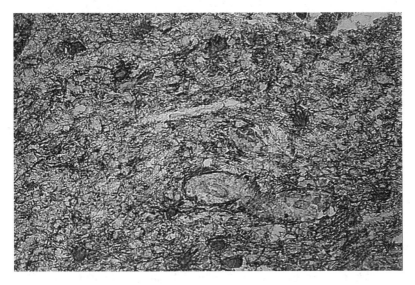

Figure 11   Brain, lesion edge, stained with MAb to GFAP. Note intensive labeling of astrocytic processes for GFAP (×125.)

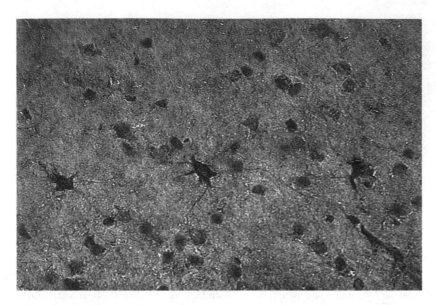

Figure 12 Brain, lesion edge, stained with polyclonal antibody to galactocerebroside and counterstained for nuclear labeling with heamtoxylin. In addition to diffuse labeling of white matter, some hypertrophic astrocytes are intensively stained for galactocerebroside. ($\times$200.)

by PA and MMPs (93) may contribute to epitope spreading and to the observed changes in TCR usage in chronic disease. By perpetuating or reactivating the local immune response, antigen-presenting astrocytes may contribute to lesion growth from the periphery.

Astrocytes express *MIP-1α* and low levels of *RANTES* (83). At the lesion edge and in the periplaque area, hypertrophic astrocytes are more intensively stained for MCP-1, MCP-2, and MCP-3 than inflammatory cells (83) and labeling is more pronounced for MCP-2 than for MCP-1 and MCP-3 (83). Reactive astrocytes also express CCR5, the CXCR3 ligand IP-10 (47), and the complement inhibitor CD59 (104). Presence of iNOS and nitrotyrosine in some reactive astrocytes indicates their ability to contribute to tissue damage (104).

Endothelial Cells.   For the development of inflammatory lesions, circulating leukocytes have to overcome the normally tight BBB and enter the CNS parenchyma. ICAM-1 expression is increased over normal controls and is present on 81 and 37% of microvessels in lesions and nonlesion areas, respectively, independently of lesion activity. ICAM-2 levels are comparable to controls (5). Strong labeling for VCAM-1 indicates EC activation by cytokines and mediates firm and prolonged attachment of intensively stained VLA-4+ cells. After shedding, sVCAM-1 may downregulate the inflammatory response by competitively inhibiting adhesion of circulating VLA-4+ leukocytes. Class I MHC is normal, enhanced, or downregulated in response to aberrant class II HC expression (2). Class II MHC + EC are randomly distributed throughout lesions and normal-appearing white matter. ICAM-1 and LFA-3 reactivity is particularly intensive in normal-appearing white matter. Double-labeling studies revealed coexpression of class II MHC and ICAM-1 or VCAM-1 on EC (2). While the majority of infiltrating cells are randomly recruited by adhesion molecules, presentation of antigen by EC may enrich for tissue-specific T cells (2). Stronger expression of these molecules at the lesion edge may reflect an additive effect of locally produced cytokines which reach the circulation by retrograde diffusion (2).

EC show increased expression of plasmin activator (PA), PA inhibitor (I)-1, uPA, vitronectin, fibronectin, MMP-9 (gelatinase), RANTES, and TGF-R type I and II (2,82,94,105). Some pv cells are MMP-7–positive and perivascular extracellular matrix (EM) may be stained for MMP-3. TIMP-1 expression on EC is induced by TGF-β and TIMP-2 counteracts TNF-α–mediated BBB damage. Reactivity of EC for RANTES is stronger in normal-appearing white matter than in lesions proper (94). Pericytes are reactive for MCP-1 and for C3R (47,106). Production of NO and of radical oxygen derivates by EC can activate microglia and enhance the inflammatory response (107).

Gliotic Lesion Center

The gliotic center contains only a few T cells and some foamy macrophages which commonly stain for IgG but are unreactive for MHC antigens, LFA-3, CD11c (gp150/95), ICAM-1, and IFN-α (2). EC express normal levels of ICAM-1, whereas LFA-3, class I MHC, and factor VIII may be decreased (2). The gliotic scar proper is unreactive for these markers. Close to the edge, oligodendrocytes and some remyelinated axons may be seen (79).

Normal White and Gray Matter

Normally, in both white and gray matter, a few CD2+, CD4+, CD8+, LFA-1+, LFA-3+, IgG+, and class I and class II MHC+ macrophages are consistently seen. Their presence indicates continuous low-grade inflammation, which may be due to enhanced expression of vascular addressins and MHC molecules on microvessels and may thus render them permissive for leukocyte diapedesis (2). Class I MHC, factor VIII, and LFA-3 may be decreased. Microglia stain for all three isoforms of TGF-β and TGF-R I and II (81) and show weak reactivity for Fc receptors (2). One of the earliest forms of myelin damage may be mediated by interaction of uPA with uPAR on microglia in the absence of blood-derived inflammatory leukocytes. Moreover, intensively labeled microglial cells (own observation) may surround microvessels strongly stained for adhesion molecule and vascular addressins, sometimes seen with leukocyte attached to their luminal surface. Particularly in rapidly progressive cases, this early event in lesion formation may be followed by small foci of LFA-1+, LFA-3+, CD45RO+, CD25+, and CD44+ cells close to ICAM-1 and LFA-3+ endothelial cells (2). Hematogeneous cells, attracted by chemokines, can be tightly packed in Virchow-Robin spaces, before they breach the glia limitans and enter the white matter parenchyma proper.

C. Silent Chronic Lesions

In accord with the gliotic nature of silent chronic lesions, immunopathological findings are rather limited. Most *macrophage/microglial* cells are negative for MHC antigens and IFNs but are weakly stained for MIP-1β (95). Labeling for the chronic stage inflammatory macrophage marker 24F9 increases with decreasing lesion activity (2,108). Some phagocytic cells continue to be Ig-positive and some are reactive for amyloid precursor protein (APP) (101).

A few *CD2+* as well as CD4+ and CD8+ cells are present in lesions and in normal CNS. Intensity of ICAM-1 and LFA-1 reactivity is higher and lower, respectively, and VCAM-1 and VLA-4 labeling of pv cells is comparable to active chronic plaques (109). IL-2R+, CD44+ and CD57 (HNK-1)+ NK cells are absent.

Levels of immunoregulatory *cytokines* are higher, and those of pro-inflammatory cytokines lower than in active plaques (109).

Class II MHC-positive *EC* are detectable throughout lesions and normal CNS, although at a lower frequency than in active chronic MS. Reactivity of EC for RANTES and MIP-1β is rather weak (94,96). After repeated immune attacks, perivascular fibrosis may facilitate edema formation by interfering with close contact between astrocytes and endothelial cells necessary for maintaining tight junctions (2).

Similar to active lesions, *Ig deposits* are prominent and may be due to locally produced specific antibodies or to increased permeability of the BBB (2).

Class II MHC and IFNs are virtually undetectable on *astroglia* in lesions and normal white and gray matter but some pv astrocytic foot processes are CD1b-positive (97). Although some hypertrophic astrocytes can express hsp-60, labeling for TGF-β and TGF-R (81), MCP-1, MCP-2, MCP-3, and CCR2 is negligible (47,102). Despite the virtual absence of inflammatory cells, most inactive chronic plaques are surrounded by a zone of diffuse ICAM-1 and LFA-3 reactivity. By providing appropriate ligands for LFA-1 and CD2, white matter–bound adhesion molecules may predispose previously affected CNS tissue for further immune attacks. Aberrant expression of class II MHC, vascular addressins, and adhesion molecules on EC facilitate preferential diapedesis of preactivated memory (CD45RO+) T cells. Secondary degenerative changes suggested by APP-reactivity in some hypertrophic astrocytes including their processes, in numerous axons, and in some 14E+ oligodendrocytes may contribute to worsening of neurologic signs in the absence of active inflammatory lesions (101).

D. Acute Lesions

In the rare variant of acute MS, the disease progresses rapidly and leads to death within 1 year. In contrast to their distinct distribution patterns in active chronic lesions, macrophages and lymphocytes are randomly distributed throughout acute plaques.

In accord with their state of activation, *microglia/macrophages* express class I and II MHC, CD11b, HAM65 (2) and are strongly-labeled for Ig and muramidase (2). Particularly in early lesions, expression of B7.1 and of IL-12p40 are increased. Labeling of pv and parenchymal cells in lesions and in normal white matter is consistently stronger for LFA-1 than for ICAM-1 (110. VLA-1 (CD49a)-positive cells outnumber VLA-4-positive cells (2,110). Within lesions, macrophages are MIP-1α and MIP-1β-positive. At the edge, MCP-1+ macrophages are more numerous and, together with some oligodendrocytes may express IL-4 (83,110). Except for TNF-α, levels of cytokines such as IL-βb, IFN-γ, IFN-α, IL-2, and IL-10 are higher than in active chronic plaques. TNF-α mRNA is detectable in a subgroup of macrophages reactive for the acute inflammatory macrophage marker MRP14 (110). IL-10 is particularly prominent on pv cells (109). Macrophages throughout lesions and scattered astrocytes contain iNOS, its cofactor neopterin, nitrotyrosin, and high levels of nitrate and nitrite (104) indicating their role in tissue damage.

In *normal white matter*, microglia are labeled for LFA-1, ICAM-1 and MIP-1β (83,109).

Lymphocytic infiltrates express CD2, CD4, CD8, IL-2R, CD44, and occasionally VLA-4, IFN-γ, and Ig (2,109). CD8+ cells consistently outnumber CD4+ cells in the plaque and only an occasional infiltrating cell is seen in white matter adjacent to lesions. Studies in VH germline segment use indicate that the *B cell response* in acute MS lesions is limited and antigen-specific (111).

Astrocytes, which reportedly become activated within 6 weeks after onset of signs, express class I and II MHC, IFN-γ, TNF-α, IFN-β (2) and show widespread staining for ICAM-1 and IL-10 (109). ICAM-1–positive astrocytes are present in lesions and normal-appearing white matter and occasionally also express TNF-α. Within lesions, at the edge, and in the periplaque area, astrocytes are MIP-1α+ and MCP-1+, respectively (83). Hypertrophic astrocytes, reactive macrophages and hyperplastic oligodendrocytes are strongly labeled for hsp60. In accord with the great potential of acute lesions for remyelination, oligodendrocyte hyperplasia is more prominent than in chronic plaques (2).

Endothelial cells show stronger labeling for ICAM-1 than for VLA-1 and occasionally express TNF-α (109). Scattered EC and perivascular extracellular matrix components may be labeled for TGF-β (109).

Immunoglobulin and Ig-Containing Cells

Similar to active MS lesions, there is extensive labeling of the parenchyma and of macrophages for Ig. Labeling for Ig, however, is uniform throughout the lesion and is not enhanced at the lesion edge.

VI. CONCLUSION

In MS there is evidence for sensitization of both B and T cells to myelin antigens and for a general dysregulation of the immune system. Because cytokines very effectively enhance immune responses in a random manner, many of the immunological abnormalities observed in MS can also be detected in other chronic immune-mediated and inflammatory diseases. Cytokine-induced upregulation of vascular addressins, adhesion molecules, chemokines, and MMP can facilitate random migration of activated immune cells into the CNS. Targeting of the inflammatory response to white matter may involve local antigen presentation by endothelial cells. Hyperexpression of immune markers on glial elements is essential for the development of inflammatory lesions and tissue damage. Upregulation of vascular addressins and class II MHC on CNS endothelial cells, and diffuse ICAM-1 and LFA-3 deposits at the lesion edge, may render the white matter parenchyma susceptible to further immune attacks. Together with tissue damage–associated sensitization of T cells to cryptic and immature MBP epitopes, activation of myelin-specific T cells by cross-reactive antigens, and superantigen-induced polyclonal T-cell stimulation, these changes contribute to the chronicity of the disease process. Inflammatory mediators not only promote the development of lesions but are also involved in downregulation of the inflammatory response and in remyelination. Interestingly, treatment with betaseron and methylprednisolone decreases leukocyte extravasation by downregulating Th1 and enhancing Th2 cytokine production. A similar effect was documented in fluoxetine (Prozac)-treated mice with chronic EAE (113,114). Sensitization of B and T cells to various myelin antigens, demyelination of organic CNS cultures by antibodies, lymphocytic infiltrates with restricted TCR heterogeneity in lesions, and a response to immunosuppressive therapy provide evidence that MS is an immune-mediated disease.

ACKNOWLEDGMENTS

The author thanks Drs. L.C. Scheinberg, M.B. Bornstein, J.P. Prineas, D. Horoupian, and D. Dickson for providing CNS tissue. This work was supported in part by a private donation from Leon Hirsch.

REFERENCES

1. Charcot J-M. Histologie de la sclerose en plaques, Gaz Hop (Paris) 1868; 41:554.
2. Traugott U. Evidence for immunopathogenesis. In: Cook, S, ed. Handbook of Multiple Sclerosis, 2nd ed. New York: Marcel Dekker, 1996, pp 157.
3. Janeway CA, Travers P. Autoimmunity: Responses to self antigens. In: Janeway CA, Travers P, eds. Immunobiology: The Immune System in Health and Disease, 2nd ed. New York: Garland, 1996, p 11:01.
4. Cope AP. Regulation of autoimmunity by proinflamamtory cytokines. Curr Opin Immunol 1998; 10:669.
5. Ransohoff RM. Mechanisms of inflammation in MS tissue: Adhesion molecules and chemokines. J Neuroimmunol. 1999; 98:57.
6. Sibley WA, Bamford CR, Clark K. Clinical viral infections and multiple sclerosis. Lancet 1985; 1313:13.
7. Panitch HS, Hirsch RL, Haley AS, Johnson KP. Exacerbations of multiple sclerosis in patients treated with gamma interferon. Lancet 1987; 8538:893.
8. Rose NR, Bona C. Defining criteria for autoimmune disease (Witebsky's postulates revisisted). Immunol. Today 1993; 14:426.
9. Traugott U, Scheinberg LC. Comparison between lymphocyte abnormalities in blood and cerebrospinal fluid and the immunopathology of lesions in multiple sclerosis and experimental autoimmune encephalomyelitis. In: Lowenthal A, Raus J, eds. Cellular and Humoral Immunological Components of Cerebrospinal Fluid in Multiple Sclerosis. New York: Plenum, 1987, p 17.
10. Bongioanni P, Fioretti C, Vanacore R, Bianchi F, Lombardo F, Ambrogi F, Meucci G. Lymphocyte subsets in multiple sclerosis: A study with two-colour fluorescence analysis. J Neurol Sci 1996; 139:71.
11. Calopa M, Bas J, Mestre M, Arbizu T, Peres J, Buendia E. T cell subsets in multiple sclerosis: A serial study. Acta Neurol Scand 1995; 92:361.
12. Oksaranta O, Tarvonen S, Ilonen J, Poikonen K, Reunanen M, Panelius M, Salonen R. T-cell subpopulations in the cerebrospinal fluid and peripheral blood of patients with multiple sclerosis: A follow-up study. Neurology 1996; 47:1542.
13. Ferrante P, Fusi ML, Saresella M, Caputo D, Biasin M, Trabattoni D, Salvaggio A, Clerici E, de-Vries JE, Aversa G, Cazzullo CL, Clerici M. Cytokine production and surface marker expression in acute and stable multiple sclerosis: Altered IL-12 production and augmented signaling lymphocytic activation molecule (SLAM)-expressing lymphocytes in acute multiple sclerosis. J Immunol 1998; 160:1514.
14. Liedtke W, Meyer G, Faustmann PM, Warnatz H, Raine CS. Clonal expansion and decreased occurrence of peripheral blood gamma delta T cells of the V delta 2J delta 3 lineage in multiple sclerosis patients. Int Immunol 1997; 9:1031.
15. Michalowska-Wender G, Nowak J, Wender M. Gamma/delta T cell receptor genes rearrangement in the blood and brain of multiple sclerosis patients. A preliminary study. Folia Neuropathol 1998; 36:1.
16. Richert JR, Robinson ED, Johnson AH, Cohn ML, McFarland HF, Hurley CK. Myelin basic protein–reactive human T-cell clones: Stimulation by diverse microbial antigens. Ann NY Acad Sci 1995; 756:319.
17. Kastrukoff LF, Morgan NG, Zecchini D, White R, Petkau AJ, Satoh J, Paty DW. A role for natural killer cells in the immunopathogenesis of multiple sclerosis. J Neuroimmunol 1998; 86:123.
18. Matusevicius D, Kivisakk P, Navikas V, Soderstrom M, Fredrikson S, Link H. Interleukin-12 and perforin mRNA expression is augmented in blood mononuclear cells in multiple sclerosis. Can J Immunol 1998; 47:582.
19. Kraus J, Oschmann P, Engelhardt B, Schiel C, Hornig C, Bauer R, Kern A, Traupe H, Dornd-

orf W. Soluble and cell surface ICAM-1 as markers for disease activity in multiple sclerosis. Acta Neurol Scand 1998; 98:102.

20. Mossner R, Fassbender K, Kuhnen J, Schwartz A, Hennerici M. Vascular cell adhesion molecule—A new approach to detect endothelial cell activation in MS and encephalitis in vivo. Acta Neurol Scand 1996; 93:118.

21. Giovannoni G, Thorpe JW, Kidd D, Kendall BE, Moseley IF, Thompson AJ, Keir G, Miller DH, Feldmann M, Thompson EJ. Soluble E-selectin in multiple sclerosis: raised concentrations in patients with primary progressive disease. J Neurol Neurosurg Psychiatry 1996; 60: 20.

22. Filaci G, Contini P, Brenci S, Gazzola P, Lanza L, Scudeletti M, Indiveri F, Mancardi GL, Puppo F. Soluble HLA class I and class II molecule levels in serum and cerebrospinal fluid of multiple sclerosis patients. Hum Immunol 1997; 54:54.

23. Zipp F, Faber E, Sommer N, Muller C, Dichgans J, Krammer PH, Martin R, Weller M. CD95 expression and CD95-mediated apoptosis of T cells in multiple sclerosis: No differences from normal individuals and no relation to HLA-DR2. J Neuroimmunol 1998; 81:168.

24. Ohsako S, Elkon KB. Apoptosis in the effector phase of autoimmune diabetes, multiple sclerosis and thyroiditis. Cell Death Differ 1999; 6:13.

25. Bansil S, Holtz CR, Cook SD, Rohowsky-Kochan C. Serum sAPO-1/Fas levels in multiple sclerosis. Acta Neurol Scand 1997; 95:208.

26. Zipp F, Martin R, Lichtenfels R, Roth W, Dichgans J, Krammer PH, Weller M. Human autoreactive and foreign antigen-specific T cells resist apoptosis induced by soluble recombinant CD95 ligand. J Immunol 1997; 159:2108.

27. Zipp F, Otzelberger K, Dichgans J, Martin R, Weller M. Serum CD95 of relapsing remitting multiple sclerosis patients protects from CD95-mediated apoptosis. J Neuroimmunol 1998; 86:151.

28. Windhagen A, Maniak S, Gebert A, Ferger I, Heidenreich D. Costimulatory molecules B7-1 and B7-2 on CSF cells in multiple sclerosis and optic neuritis. J Neuroimmunol 1999; 96: 112.

29. Santiago E, Perez-Mediavilla LA, Lopez-Moratalla N. The role of nitric oxide in the pathogenesis of multiple sclerosis. J Physiol Biochem 1998; 54:229.

30. Lopez-Moratalla N, Gonzalez A, Aymerich MS, Lopez-Zabalza MJ, Pio R, de-Castro P, Santiago E. Monocyte inducible nitric oxide synthase in multiple sclerosis: Regulatory role of nitric oxide. Nitric Oxide 1997; 1:95.

31. Giovannoni G. Cerebrospinal fluid and serum nitric oxide metabolites in patients with multiple sclerosis. Mult Scler 1998; 4:27.

32. Yacyshyn B, Meddings J, Sadowski D, Bowe-Yacyshyn MB. Multiple sclerosis patients have peripheral blood CD45RO + B cells and increased intestinal permeability. Dig Dis Sci 1996; 41:2493.

33. Zaffaroni M, Stampins LG, Ghezzi A, Baldini SM, Zibetti A. In vitro cytokine, sCD23 and IgG secretion in multiple sclerosis. J Neuroimmunol 1995; 61:1.

34. Calabresi PA, Fields NS, Farnon EC, Frank JA, Bash CN, Kawanashi T, Maloni H, Jacobson S, McFarland HF. ELI-spot of Th-1 cytokine secreting PBMCs in multiple sclerosis: Correlation with MRI lesions. J Neuroimmunol 1998; 85:212.

35. Balashov KE, Olek MJ, Smith DR, Khoury SJ, Weiner HL. Seasonal variation of interferon-gamma production in progressive multiple sclerosis. Ann Neurol 1998; 44:824.

36. Philippe J, Debruyne J, Leroux-Roels G, Willems A, Dereuck J. In vitro TNF-alpha, IL-2 and IFN-gamma production as markers of relapses in multiple sclerosis. Clin Neurol Neurosurg 1996; 98:286.

37. Chofflon M, Roth S, Juillard C, Paunier AM, Juillard P, Degroote D, Grau GE. Tumor necrosis factor production capacity as a potentially useful parameter to monitor disease activity in multiple sclerosis. Eur Cytokine Net 1997; 8:253.

38. Matusevicius D, Navikas V, Soderstrom M, Xiao BG, Haglund M, Fredrikson S, Link H.

Multiple sclerosis: the proinflammatory cytokines lymphotoxin-alpha and tumour necrosis factor-alpha are upregulated in cerebrospinal fluid mononuclear cells. J Neuroimmunol 1996; 66:115.

39. Navikas V, Martin C, Matusevicius D, Soderstrom M, Fredrikson S, Link H. Soluble CD30 levels in plasma and cerebrospinal fluid in multiple sclerosis, HIV infection and other nervous system diseases. Acta Neurol Scand 1997; 95:99.

40. Comabella M, Balashov K, Issazadeh S, Smith D, Weiner HL, Khoury SJ. Elevated interleukin-12 in progressive multiple sclerosis correlates with disease activity and is normalized by pulse cyclophosphamide therapy. J Clin Invest 1998; 102:671.

41. Navikas V, Link J, Palasik W, Soderstrom M, Fredrikson S, Olsson T, Link H. Increased mRNA expression of IL-10 in mononuclear cells in multiple sclerosis and optic neuritis. Scand J Immunol 1995; 41:171.

42. Monteyne P, Van-Laere V, Marichal R, Sindic CJ. Cytokine mRNA expression in CSF and peripheral blood mononuclear cells in multiple sclerosis: Detection by RT-PCR without in vitro stimulation. J Neuroimmunol 1997; 80:137.

43. Segal BM, Dwyer BK, Shevach EM. An interleukin (IL)-10/IL-12 immunoregulatory circuit controls susceptibility to autoimmune disease. J Exp Med 1998; 187:537.

44. Metz LM, McGuinness SD, Harris C. Urinary tract infections may trigger relapse in multiple sclerosis. Axone 1998; 19:67.

45. Kivisakk P, Teleshova N, Ozenci V, Huang Y, Matusevicius D, Fredrikson S, Soderstrom M, Link H. No evidence for elevated numbers of mononuclear cells expressing MCP-1 and RANTES mRNA in blood and CSF in multiple sclerosis. J Neuroimmunol 1998; 91:108.

46. Lee MA, Stabler JP, Ford J, Gearing A, Miller K. Serum gelatinase B, TIMP-1 and TIMP-2 levels in multiple sclerosis: A longitudinal clinical and MRI study. Brain 1999; 122:191.

47. Balashov KE, Rottman JB, Weiner HL, Hancock WW. CCR5(+) and CXCR3(+) T cells are increased in multiple sclerosis and their ligands MIP-1alpha and IP-10 are expressed in demyelinating brain lesions. Proc Natl Acad Sci USA 1999; 96:6873.

48. Bennetts BH, Teutsch SM, Buhler MM, Heard RN, Stewart GJ. The CCR5 deletion mutation fails to protect against multiple sclerosis. Hum Immunol 1997; 58:52.

49. Karni A, Bakimer-Kleiner R, Abramsky O, Ben-Nun A. Elevated levels of antibody to myelin oligodendrocyte glycoprotein is not specific for patients with multiple sclerosis. Arch Neurol 1999; 56:311.

50. Rawes JA, Calabrese VP, Khan OA, DeVries GH. Antibodies to the axolemma-enriched fraction in the cerebrospinal fluid and serum of patients with multiple sclerosis and other neurological diseases. Mult Scler 1997; 3:363.

51. Smith ME. Phagocytosis of myelin in demyelinative disease: A review. Neurochem Res 1999; 24:261.

52. Monteyne P, Guillaume B, Sindic CJ. B7-1 (CD80), B7-2 (CD86), interleukin-12 and transforming growth factor-beta mRNA expression in CSF and peripheral blood mononuclear cells from multiple sclerosis patients. J Neuroimmunol 1998; 91:198.

53. Cross AH, Manning PT, Keeling RM, Schmidt RE, Mishko TP. Peroxinitrite formation within the central nervous system in active multiple sclerosis. J Neuroimmunol 1998; 88:45.

54. Rollnik JD, Sindern E, Schweppe C, Malin JP. Biologically active TGF-beta 1 is increased in cerebrospinal fluid while it is reduced in serum in multiple sclerosis patients. Acta Neurol Scand 1997; 96:101.

55. Frederiksen JL, Sindic CJ. Intrathecal synthesis of virus-specific oligoclonal IgG, and of free kappa and free lambda oligoclonal bands in acute monosymptomatic optic neuritis: Comparison with brain MRI. Mult Scler 1998; 4:22.

56. Dybwad A, Flrre O, Sioud M. Probing for cerebrospinal fluid antibody specificities by a panel of random peptide libraries. Autoimmunity 1997; 25:85.

57. Luxton RW, Leman A, Holzel H, Harvey P, Wilson J, Kocen R, Morgan-Hughes J, Miller

DH, Compston A, Thompson EJ. Affinity of antigen-specific IgG distinguishes multiple sclerosis from encephalitis. J Neurol Sci 1995; 132:11.

58. Ristori G, Montesperelli C, Uccelli A, Giunti D, Buttinelli C, Bomprezzi R, Mancardi GL, Salvetti M. A major influence of the T cell receptor repertoire as compared to antigen processing-presentation in the selection of myelin basic protein epitopes in multiple sclerosis. J Neuroimmunol 1999; 96:241.

59. Burns J, Bartholomew B, Lobo S. Isolation of myelin basic protein-specific T cells predominantly from the memory T-cell compartment in multiple sclerosis. Ann Neurol 1999; 45:33.

60. Lovett-Racke AE, Trotter JL, Lauber J, Perrin PJ, June CH, Racke MK. Decreased dependence of myelin basic protein-reactive T cells on CD28-mediated costimulation in multiple sclerosis patients: A marker of activated/memory T cells [published erratum appears in J Clin Invest 1998 Apr 1;101(7):1542], J Clin Invest 1998; 101:725.

61. Tranquill LR, Skinner E, Campagnoni C, Vergelli M, Hemmer B, Muraro P, Martin R, McFarland HF, Campagnoni AT, Voskuhl RR. Human T lymphocytes specific for the immunodominant 83–99 epitope of myelin basic protein: Recognition of golli MBP HOG 7. J Neurosci Res 1996; 45:820.

62. Lovett-Racke AE, Martin R, McFarland HF, Racke MK, Utz U. Longitudinal study of myelin basic protein-specific T-cell receptors during the course of multiple sclerosis. J Neuroimmunol 1997; 78:162.

63. Markovic-Plese S, Fukaura H, Zhang J, al-Sabbagh A, Southwood S, Sette A, Kuchroo VK, Hafler DA. T cell recognition of immunodominant and cryptic proteolipid protein epitopes in humans. J Immunol 1995; 155:982.

64. Correale J, Rojany M, Weiner LP. Human CD8+ TCR-alpha beta(+) and TCR-gamma delta(+) cells modulate autologous autoreactive neuroantigen-specific CD4+ T-cells by different mechanisms. J Neuroimmunol 1997; 80:47.

65. Burger D, Lou J, Dayer JM, Grau GE. Both soluble and membrane-associated TNF activate brain microvascular endothelium: relevance to multiple sclerosis. Mol Psychiatry 1997; 2:113.

66. Verbeek MM, Westphal JR, Ruiter DJ, de-Waal RM. T lymphocyte adhesion to human brain pericytes is mediated via very late antigen-4/vascular cell adhesion molecule-1 interactions. J Immunol 1995; 154:5876.

67. Vora AJ, Kidd D, Miller DH, Perkin GD, Hughes RA, Ellis BA, Dumonde DC, Brown KA. Lymphocyte-endothelial cell interactions in multiple sclerosis: Disease specificity and relationship to circulating tumour necrosis factor-alpha and soluble adhesion molecules. Mult Scler 1997; 3:171.

68. Frigerio S, Gelati M, Ciusani E, Corsini E, Dufour A, Massa G, Salmaggi A. Immunocompetence of human microvascular brain endothelial cells: Cytokine regulation of IL-1beta, MCP-1, IL-10, sICAM-1 and sVCAM-1. J Neurol 1998; 245:727.

69. Gasque P, Jones J, Singhrao SK, Morgan B. Identification of an astrocyte cell population from human brain that expresses perforin, a cytotoxic protein implicated in immune defense. J Exp Med 1998; 187:451.

70. Barnes DA, Huston M, Holmes R, Benveniste EN, Yong VW, Scholz P, Perez HD. Induction of RANTES expression by astrocytes and astrocytoma cell lines. J Neuroimmunol 1996; 71:207.

71. Saas P, Boucraut J, Quiquerez AL, Schnuriger V, Perrin G, Desplat-Jego S, Bernard D, Walker PR, Dietrich PY. CD95 (Fas/Apo-1) as a receptor governing astrocyte apoptotic or inflammatory responses: A key role in brain inflammation? J Immunol 1999; 162:2326.

72. Cammer W, Zhang H. Maturation of oligodendrocytes is more sensitive to TNF alpha than is survival of precursors and immature oligodendrocytes. J Neuroimmunol 1999; 97:37.

73. D'Souza SD, Alinauskas KA, Antel JP. Ciliary neurotrophic factor selectively protects human oligodendrocytes from tumor necrosis factor-mediated injury. J Neurosci Res 1996; 43:289.

74. Scolding NJ, Morgan BP, Compston DA. The expression of complement regulatory proteins by adult human oligodendrocytes. J Neuroimmunol 1998; 84:69.

75. Dangond F, Windhagen A, Groves CJ, Hafler DA. Constitutive expression of costimulatory molecules by human microglia and its relevance to CNS autoimmunity. J Neuroimmunol 1997; 76:132.

76. Washington RA, Becher B, Balabanov R, Antel J, Dore-Duffy P. Expression of the activation marker urokinase plasminogen-activator receptor in cultured human central nervous system microglia. J Neurosci Res 1996; 45:392.

77. Chabot S, Williams G, Yong VW. Microglial production of TNF-alpha is induced by activated T lymphocytes. Involvement of VLA-4 and inhibition by interferon beta-1b. J Clin Invest 1997; 100:604.

78. Tan J, Town T, Paris D, Placzek A, Parker T, Crawford F, Yu H, Humphrey J, Mullan M. Activation of microglial cells by the CD40 pathway: relevance to multiple sclerosis. J Neuroimmunol 1999; 97:77.

79. Lassmann H. Neuropathology in multiple sclerosis: new concepts. Mult Scler 1998; 4:93.

80. Trapp B, Peterson J, Ransohoff R, Rudick R, Mork S, Bo L. Axonal transection in the lesions of multiple sclerosis. N Engl J Med 1998; 338:278.

81. De-Groot CJ, Montagne L, Barten AD, Sminia P, Van-Der-Valk P. Expression of transforming growth factor (TGF)-beta1, -beta2, and -beta3 isoforms and TGF-beta type I and type II receptors in multiple sclerosis lesions and human adult astrocyte cultures. J Neuropathol Exp Neurol 1999; 58:174.

82. Cossins JA, Clements JM, Ford J, Miller KM, Pigott R, Vos W, Van-der-Valk P, De-Groot CJ. Enhanced expression of MMP-7 and MMP-9 in demyelinating multiple sclerosis lesions. Acta Neuropathol Berl 1997; 94:590.

83. Simpson JE, Newcombe J, Cuzner ML, Woodroofe MN. Expression of monocyte chemoattractant protein-1 and other beta-chemokines by resident glia and inflammatory cells in multiple sclerosis lesions. J Neuroimmunol 1998; 84:238.

84. Gveric D, Kaltschmidt C, Cuzner ML, Newcombe J. Transcription factor NF-kappaB and inhibitor I kappaBalpha are localized in macrophages in active multiple sclerosis lesions. J Neuropathol Exp Neurol 1998; 57:168.

85. Masdeu JC, Moreira J, Tras S, Visinteiner P, Cavaliere R, Grundman M. The open ring. A new imaging sign in demyelinating disease. J Neuroimaging 1996; 6:104.

86. Windhagen A, Newcombe J, Dangond F, Strand C, Woodroofe MN, Cuzner ML, Hafler DA. Expression of costimulatory molecules B7-1 (CD80), B7-2 (CD86), and interleukin 12 cytokine in multiple sclerosis lesions. J Exp Med 1995; 182:1985.

87. Cannella B, Sizing ID, Benjamin CD, Browning JL, Raine CS. Antibodies to lymphotoxin alpha (LT alpha) and LT beta recognize different glial cell types in the central nervous system. J Neuroimmunol 1997; 78:172.

88. Raine CS, Bonetti B, Cannella B. Multiple sclerosis: Expression of molecules of the tumor necrosis factor ligand and receptor families in relationship to the demyelinated plaque. Rev Neurol Paris 1998; 154:577.

89. Schluesener HJ, Seid K, Kretzschmar J, Meyermann R. Leukocyte chemotactic factor, a natural ligand to CD4, is expressed by lymphocytes and microglial cells of the MS plaque. J Neurosci Res 1996; 44:606.

90. Bo L, Peterson JW, Mork S, Hoffman PA, Gallatin WM, Ransohoff RM, Trapp BD. Distribution of immunoglobulin superfamily members ICAM-1, -2, -3, and the beta 2 integrin LFA-1 in multiple sclerosis lesions. J Neuropathol Exp Neurol 1996; 55:1060.

91. Storch MK, Piddlesden S, Haltia M, Iivanainen M, Morgan P, Lassmann H. Multiple sclerosis: In situ evidence for antibody- and complement-mediated demyelination. Ann Neurol 1998; 43:465.

92. Vladimirova O, O'Connor J, Cahill A, Alder H, Butunoi C, Kalman B. Oxidative damage to DNA in plaques of MS brains. Mult Scler 1998; 4:413.

93. Cuzner ML, Opdenakker G. Plasminogen activators and matrix metalloproteases, mediators of extracellular proteolysis in inflammatory demyelination of the central nervous system. J Neuroimmunol 1999; 94:1.

94. Yong VW, Krekoski CA, Forsyth PA, Bell R, Edwards DR. Matrix metalloproteinases and diseases of the CNS. Trends Neurosci 1998; 21:75.

95. McManus C, Berman JW, Brett FM, Staunton H, Farrell M, Brosnan C. MCP-1, MCP-2 and MCP-3 expression in multiple sclerosis lesions: An immunohistochemical and in situ hybridization study. J Neuroimmunol 1998; 86:20.

96. Sorensen TL, Tani M, Jensen J, Pierce V, Lucchinetti C, Folcik VA, Qin S, Rottman J, Sellebjerg F, Strieter RM, Frederiksen JL, Ransohoff RM. Expression of specific chemokines and chemokine receptors in the central nervous system of multiple sclerosis patients. J Clin Invest 1999; 103:807.

97. Battistini L, Fischer FR, Raine CS, Brosnan CF. CD1b is expressed in multiple sclerosis lesions. J Neuroimmunol 1996; 67:145.

98. Kerschensteiner M, Gallmeier E, Behrens L, Leal VV, Misgeld T, Klinkert WE, Kolbeck R, Hoppe E, Oropeza-Wekerle RL, Bartke I, Stadelmann C, Lassmann H, Wekerle H, Hohlfeld R. Activated human T cells, B cells, and monocytes produce brain-derived neurotrophic factor in vitro and in inflammatory brain lesions: a neuroprotective role of inflammation? J Exp Med 1999; 189:865.

99. Battistini L, Salvetti M, Ristori G, Falcone M, Raine CS, Brosnan CF. Gamma delta T cell receptor analysis supports a role for HSP 70 selection of lymphocytes in multiple sclerosis lesions. Mol Med 1995; 1:554.

100. Hvas J, McLean C, Justesen J, Kannourakis G, Steinman L, Oksenberg JR, Bernard CC. Perivascular T cells express the pro-inflammatory chemokine RANTES mRNA in multiple sclerosis lesions. Scand J Immunol 1997; 46:195.

101. Gehrmann J, Banati RB, Cuzner ML, Kreutzberg GW, Newcombe J. Amyloid precursor protein (APP) expression in multiple sclerosis lesions. Glia 1995; 15:141.

102. Van Der Voom P, Tekstra J, Beelen RJ, Tensen CP, Van Der Valk P, De Grot CAJ. Expression of MCP-1 by reactive astrocytes in demyelinating multiple sclerosis lesions. Am J Pathol 1999; 154:45.

103. Zajicek J, Wing M, Skepper J, Compston A. Human oligodendrocytes are not sensitive to complement: Study of CD59 expression in the human central nervous system. Lab Invest 1995; 73:128.

104. Oleszak A, Zaczynska E, Bhattacharjee M, Butunoi C, Legido A, Katsetos CD. Inducible nitric oxide synthase and nitrotyrosine are found in monocytes/macrophages and/or astrocytes in acute but not in chronic multiple sclerosis. Clin Diagn Lab Immunol 1998; 5:438.

105. van-der-Maesen K, Hinojoza JR, Sobel RA. Endothelial cell class II major histocompatibility complex molecule expression in stereotactic brain biopsies of patients with acute inflammatory / demyelinating conditions. J Neuropathol Exp Neurol 1999; 58:346.

106. Gasque P, Singhrao SK, Neal JW, Wang P, Sayah S, Fontaine M, Morgan BP. The receptor for complement anaphylatoxin C3a is expressed by myeloid cells and nonmyeloid cells in inflamed human central nervous system: Analysis in multiple sclerosis and bacterial meningitis. J Immunol 1998; 160:3543.

107. Mayer AM. Therapeutic implications of microglia activation by lipopolysaccharide and reactive oxygen species generation in septic shock and central nervous system pathologies: A review. Medicina B Aires 1998; 58:377.

108. Bruck W, Sommermeier N, Bergmann M, Zettl U, Goebel HH, Kretzschmar HA, Lassmann H. Macrophages in multiple sclerosis. Immunobiology 1996; 195:588.

109. Cannella B, Raine CS. The adhesion molecule and cytokine profile of multiple sclerosis lesions (see comments). Ann Neurol 1995; 37:424.

110. Bitsch A, da-Costa C, Bunkowski S, Weber F, Rieckmann P, Bruck W. Identification of

macrophage populations expressing tumor necrosis factor-alpha mRNA in acute multiple sclerosis. Acta Neuropathol Berl 1998; 95:373.

111. Owens GP, Kraus H, Burgoon MP, Smith-Jensen T, Devlin ME, Gilden DH. Restricted use of VH4 germline segments in an acute multiple sclerosis brain. Ann Neurol 1998; 43:236.

112. Traugott U, Trejo, V. Fluoxetine greatly inhibits disease progression in chronic experimental allergic encephalomyelitis (EAE) in SJL/J mice. Neurology 1997; 48:A422.

113. Traugott U. Detailed analysis of the immuomodulatory properties of Fluoxetine (Prozac) in chronic experimental allergic encephalomyelitis (EAE) in SJL/L mice. Neurology 1998; 50: A105.

114. Lujan S, Masjuan J, Roldan E, Villar LM, Gonzalez-Porque P, Alvarez-Cermeno JC. The expression of integrins on activated T-cells in multiple sclerosis: Effect of intravenous methylprednisolone treatment. Mult Scler 1998; 4:239.

115. Corsini E, Gelati M, Dufour A, Massa G, Nespolo A, Ciusani E, Milanese C, La-Mantia L, Salmaggi A. Effects of beta-IFN-1b treatment in MS patients on adhesion between PBMNCs, HUVECs and MS-HBECs: an in vivo and in vitro study. J Neuroimmunol 1997; 79:76.

8

Autoantibodies in Demyelinating Disease

ANNE H. CROSS, JERI-ANNE LYONS, and JOHN L. TROTTER

Washington University School of Medicine, St. Louis, Missouri

I. INTRODUCTION

Since the 1940s it has been known that more than 90% of multiple sclerosis (MS) patients have increased intrathecal production of immunoglobulins (Ig) in an oligoclonal pattern (1). These Igs include IgG, IgA, IgD, and IgM antibodies. In support of a role for antibodies (Abs) in the pathogenesis of MS are studies suggesting that increased concentrations of Abs in CSF of MS patients correlates with episodes of MS worsening (2) and that MS patients lacking oligoclonal bands in CSF have a more benign course (3). For many years, research into the pathogenesis of MS focused on the humoral immune system. However, in recent years, emphasis has been placed on investigating the role of the T lymphocyte in the pathological process in MS, due to the findings of activated T lymphocytes in MS plaques, T cell–subset alterations in MS blood, and the fact that an animal model for MS, experimental allergic encephalomyelitis (EAE), is initiated by myelin-reactive T cells (4).

Since the previous edition of this book, new evidence has accumulated, which has once again focused investigations into the pathogenesis of MS upon the humoral immune system. The evidence comes from studies of the pathology of the MS lesion, cerebrospinal fluid (CSF) studies, and studies of the EAE model for MS. Studies reporting the successful treatment of MS with IVIG and plasma exchange have also implicated humoral mechanisms in the disease process (5–11). This chapter describes the new evidence implicating B cells and Abs in MS pathogenesis and reviews some of the older literature on this topic. We review data that suggests that autoantibodies (autoAbs) directed against central nervous system (CNS) myelin targets that are isolated behind the blood-CNS barrier may be specific to MS pathogenesis. However, we also point out that autoAbs may be secondary to the primary disease process due to the liberation of antigens with CNS damage or nonspecific due to nonspecific B-cell activation.

II. ANTIBODIES IN THE NEUROPATHOLOGY OF MS

B cells, plasma cells and myelin-specific Abs are present in chronic MS plaques and in areas of active myelin breakdown in MS patients (12,13), implicating their involvement in the pathogenesis of MS. Lucchinetti et al., in a detailed immunohistochemical study of active MS lesions from 83 biopsies and autopsies of MS patients, found that by far the most common pattern of pathology (>70% of active lesions) involved the prominent presence of Abs and complement, in addition to T cells and macrophages (14). Detailed counting of cells within MS-affected CNS has shown Ab-producing plasma cells to be extremely numerous in some chronic lesions and in the surrounding normal-appearing white matter (15). Since the accumulation of plasma cells at sites of chronic inflammation has been shown to depend upon antigen at the site as well as nonspecific activators, this suggests that the presence of plasma cells in MS lesions is antigen-driven (16,17).

A. Intrathecal Synthesis of Immune Globulins: Specific or Nonspecific Antibody Production?

Elevations in concentrations of cerebrospinal fluid IgG, IgM, IgD, and IgA are reported in MS (18–20) (for review, see Ref. 21). Cerebrospinal IgG and IgM in this disease are often found to demonstrate an oligoclonal pattern when the proteins are separated by a variety of electrophoretic methods (21). The oligoclonal pattern varies among different patients but may remain unchanged when the CSF of a given patient is followed over time (20). These quantitative (IgG concentration, IgG index, IgG synthesis rate) and qualitative (electrophoresis) abnormalities are used as diagnostic tools, described elsewhere in this volume.

   The major bands usually do not represent autoAbs against major recognizable myelin components or Abs against infectious agents when tested by immunoelectrophoretic techniques (21). When the separated Igs are examined by imprint fixation, Abs can be detected that are of limited heterogeneity and directed against a wide variety of infectious agents (22).

B. Antibodies Against Myelin Proteins

Bands that represent antimyelin basic protein have been identified by immunoblot in the CSF from some MS patients (23). AutoAbs that do not correspond to the major bands by electrophoresis have also been identified in the CSF using immunoassay techniques. Many of the published studies describing autoAbs to MBP in CSF come from the laboratories of Warren and Catz. These investigators separated presumed antigen-antibody complexes of MBP prior to searching for Abs to this antigen (24,25). When the IgG fraction of CSF from MS patients was isolated, neutralizing Abs to anti-MBP antibodies were also identified (26). Warren and Catz therefore hypothesized an MBP Ab cascade within the CSF compartment which may have a regulatory mechanism. Using immunoassay techniques, these investigators have also described Abs to myelin proteolipid protein in the CSF from MS patients with active disease who do not have Abs to MBP (27). On the other hand, other investigators using similar methods have not found Abs to MBP or PLP in the CSF from MS patients (28).

Myelin-oligodendrocyte glycoprotein (MOG) is another candidate autoantigen within CNS myelin, since it is highly immunogenic and can be used to induce EAE in animals. Xiao and colleagues used an enzyme-linked immunosorbent assay (ELISA) method to detect Abs to MOG in the CSF from 7 of 30 MS patients (29). The CSF from 2 of 30 other neurological disease controls and a single patient with tension headache also had Abs to MOG, but generally with a lower titer.

Another candidate autoantigen in MS is oligodendrocyte-specific protein (OSP), a recently identified CNS-specific myelin protein. Abs recognizing OSP have been found in CSF samples from relapsing-remitting MS (RRMS) patients in studies using Western blot analysis, peptide blots, and ELISA (30). Moreover, the peptide consisting of amino acids 114–120 of OSP has homologies with common viral proteins. Using OSP 114–120 as antigen, ELISAs were performed on CSF from 85 MS and 51 control patients. Eighty percent of the samples from RRMS patients had an ELISA reading above 0.55 optical density units, whereas all 20 control CSF samples had values less than 0.55 U. ELISAs performed on CSF using homologous viral peptides as antigen showed a close correlation with OSP 114–120 ELISA readings; in some, the readings were higher than those using OSP peptide. The overall conclusion was that there is an autoAb response in many RRMS patients that is directed against a specific region of OSP and that is cross-reactive with several common viral peptides.

C. Antibodies Against Other CNS Constituents

2′,3′-cyclic nucleotide 3′ phosphodiesterase (CNP) is a membrane-associated protein of the oligodendrocyte that is also expressed by lymphocytes and in the retina. Walsh and Murray reported that 74% of 70 MS patients tested had Abs to the CNP I isoform in serum and CSF samples (31). Only 3 of 33 controls subjects with other neurological diseases, and none of the 28 healthy controls tested had autoAbs to CNP. The autoAb was predominantly of the IgM isotype. In addition, these investigators reported that both isoforms of CNP (CNP I and II) bind C3 complement. Thus, CNP, which is located in oligodendrocyte processes and at paranodal myelin loops, but not in compact myelin, is a potential site of myelin opsonization.

Transaldolase is an enzyme which, in the CNS, is relatively specific to oligodendroglia. AutoAbs to this protein have been described in the serums and CSF of MS patients. The incidence of these Abs is higher in MS than in control subjects (32). T-cell responses have also been detected against transaldolase (33). There is evidence that there is cross-reactivity between some of the epitopes of transaldolase and some infectious agents, allowing for the possibility of molecular mimicry in the development of the autoAbs (34).

Elevated titers of serum IgM Abs directed against GM1 gangliosides have been found among patients with MS (35). These titers are not as great as those found in multifocal motor neuropathy but are similar to those found in other purported autoimmune diseases. Thus, these Abs are not specific for MS. Low-titer autoAbs against other myelin lipids—especially glycolipids such as galactocerebroside, GM4 gangliosides, as well as GM1 gangliosides—can be detected in the sera and cerebrospinal fluid (CSF) from a portion of MS patients (36–38). Patients in the progressive stage of disease are reported to have a higher incidence of antilipid Abs than patients with a relapsing-remitting course.

Often a higher incidence of autoAbs directed against glycolipids can be detected if immune complexes are disassociated (39,40). However, a comparison of the incidence of such autoAbs among MS patients when compared to normal or disease controls, especially stroke and trauma, has demonstrated no difference in some studies (41,42).

AutoAbs against arrestin protein found in the retina and CNS have been reported in sera from 8 of 14 MS patients and were highest in 2 patients undergoing clinical relapse (43). These autoAbs were not found in CSF specimens of MS patients and were absent in serum samples from normal or disease control subjects. In a second study, the same investigators noted serum autoAbs to arrestin in 2 of 7 patients with acute disseminated encephalomyelitis (ADEM), one of whom subsequently developed MS (44). These results must be considered preliminary, since so few MS patients have been examined. Other autoAbs described to be elevated in the sera or CSF from MS patients include "lymphocytotoxic" Abs, which react at reduced temperatures (45–47); Abs to pituitary peptides (48); and miscellaneous Abs that react with uncharacterized antigens in the CNS (49). A report of Abs to endothelial cells in MS (50) was intriguing in light of the breakdown of the blood-CNS-barrier that occurs in active MS lesions. Unfortunately many of these types of studies usually showed nonspecificity of Abs (due to autoimmunity in general or nonspecific tissue binding) when proper controls were performed. Furthermore, in none of these studies was tissue specificity–proven.

Due to the breakdown of the blood-CNS-barrier observed in active MS lesions and the ensuing contamination of CSF by serum proteins, interpretation of the meaning of the presence of autoAb within CSF may not always be straightforward. Determination of the CSF/serum albumin index (21) may help to prevent misleading interpretations of results.

D. Bound Oligoclonal Immunoglobulins in MS Plaques

One limiting factor in the search for autoAbs in serum and CSF samples is the possibility that autoAbs may be bound to CNS tissue. Igs eluted from CNS tissue could represent several sources including (a) nonspecific binding to tissue components; (b) Fc receptor binding to glial or mononuclear cells; or (c) specific binding to antigen with the formation of immune complexes (51). In addition to their studies of CSF, Warren and Catz isolated affinity-purified IgG recognizing MBP directly from MS plaques, and identified the epitopes of MBP recognized by many of the Abs (52). The dominant epitopes recognized were identified by using peptides of MBP to block Ab binding. The MBP (83–97) peptide appeared immunodominant since it inhibited autoAb binding to MBP almost 100% in all cases. Residues contributing to autoAb binding were located in a 10-amino acid segment (V86-T95) that also contained the MHC/T cell receptor contact residues of the main epitope recognized by MS T cells (53). Microbial peptides were identified that were also bound by purified autoAb from MS patients. Binding of microbial peptides required sequence identity at four or five contiguous residues in the epitope center. There was strong binding by autoAb from all 11 MS patients tested to peptides from papillomavirus as well as several other common viral and bacterial pathogens.

Using immunostaining techniques, Genain and colleagues identified Abs to MOG in lesions of MS and a marmoset EAE model, which were localized in areas of disrupted myelin (13). These investigators also localized Ab to MOG within macrophages that had engulfed myelin, suggesting that the Ab may have been involved in opsonization. In a subsequent report, Raine et al. demonstrated that human IgG, including IgG directed against peptides of myelin basic protein and myelin/oligodendrocyte glycoprotein (MOG), was colocalized with vesiculated CNS myelin within acute MS lesions (54). These studies build upon early work that had demonstrated the presence of Ab at sites of myelin uptake by macrophages in MS lesions (55–57).

Another method of identifying autoAbs in CSF of MS patients is to assay the specificity of B lymphocytes derived from CSF. Olsson and colleagues have assayed B lymphocytes from the CSF and blood of MS patients for cells secreting Abs to MBP (58,59), PLP (60), myelin-associated glycoprotein (MAG) (61), and MOG (62). Significant numbers of cells secreting Abs to MBP, PLP, and MAG were found in CSF of MS patients in comparison to such cells in peripheral blood. The incidence of cells secreting Abs to MOG was similar in CSF and blood from MS patients but higher in these two compartments in MS patients than in control subjects (62). The incidence of cells secreting Abs to PLP and MAG in the CSF from MS patients was significantly greater than in control subjects (60,61), as was the incidence of cells secreting Abs to an MBP peptide consisting of amino acids 70–89 (59). The frequencies of cells in CSF secreting Abs to the whole MBP molecule was similar in MS and control subjects.

As mentioned above, autoAbs may be bound to CNS tissues. In diseases such as subacute sclerosing panencephalitis, which is caused by a single virus (measles virus), elutions from different parts of the brain in each patient all have similar electrophoretic patterns (63). However, it has not been resolved whether each MS patient displays the same pattern in different plaques. Some investigators find this to be true (20,64,65), whereas others find different patterns in different plaques within the same MS brain (63,66). The resolution of this issue may be quite important, since it will have implications as to whether MS Ab production within the CNS is driven by a single antigen.

With regard to this issue, recent studies have utilized knowledge regarding how an Ab response to antigen develops to strongly suggest that production of Abs in MS CNS is antigen-driven, while not identifying the antigenic target (67–69). These studies relied on knowledge that an Ab response to Ag involves somatic mutation of the genes encoding the antigen contact areas (complementarity determining regions-CDRs). The results showed that somatic mutation was increased in genes encoding CDR regions in CSF and MS brain lesions as compared to germline, typical of an antigen-driven response.

E. Serum Demyelinating Antibodies

Much of the early impetus for research on humoral immunity in MS came from the reports that sera from some MS patients demyelinate CNS cultures (70). This subject has been reviewed (71). The mechanism of this phenomenon was thought to be complement-dependent, although fresh complement only partially reversed the effects of heat-inactivation of the serums. Interest in this subject was enhanced when it was reported that a similar finding occurred when myelinated cultures were exposed to sera from animals immunized with myelin. However, the "demyelinative factors" were not specific, since sera from some patients with amyotrophic lateral sclerosis, and some normal control subjects also demyelinated CNS cultures.

To determine whether serum-demyelinating activity in vitro correlated with the presence of Igs that bound myelin in serum samples, Johnson and Bornstein used an immunoperoxidase method to identify putative antimyelin Abs from sera of MS patients bound to organotypic cultures of fetal mouse spinal cord (72). Positive controls were sera from rabbits with EAE induced by whole CNS tissue or galactocerebroside, both of which stained myelin and had strong demyelination activity. Although the demyelinative effects of MS sera were confirmed, their effects were not asociated with immunostaining of my-elin. These findings are in contrast to reports of binding of Igs to frozen or fixed myelin, although binding was observed using serums from normal control subjects as well (73,74). Nonspecific binding has often proved to be due to binding by Fc fragments of IgG (75,76). The presence of Fc receptors for IgG, species-specific interactions, and staining by samples from control subjects have raised questions about many of the immunohistochemical stud-ies attempting to identify autoAbs directed against myelin or oligodendroglia (77,78).

F. Immune Complexes

The search for autoAbs often led to the detection of immune complexes. In the late 1980s, the search for immune complexes in the serums and CSF samples from MS subjects and controls was performed using a variety of methods. These methods included the C1q binding assay, the Raji cell assay, polyethelene glycol precipitation, radioimmunoassay, and protein A binding to capture the immune complexes. The immune complexes con-tained IgG, IgA, IgM, Abs to myelin basic protein, RNA and DNA from a variety of viruses, Abs to glycolipids, Abs to endothelial cells, and a variety of low molecular-weight materials (40,79–85). Immune complexes are found in a significant proportion of normal human populations (86). Complexes are rare in CSF except in situations associated with an intrathecal immune response (87). The incidence of immune complexes in serum and CSF samples from MS patients is elevated compared to those in normal subjects, but there is no correlation between the levels in the two compartments (reviewed in Ref. 82). Some investigators have reported a correlation between the presence of serum immune com-plexes and disease activity in MS (88). However, immune complexes were also found in the body fluids from control subjects with other neurological diseases and often did not correlate with the activity of disease. For these reasons, the relevance of the complexes for the pathogenesis of MS has been questioned (87,89).

III. COMPLEMENT IN MS

Immunostaining studies of MS tissues have emphasized the presence of complement in most acute MS lesions (14,90). In prior studies, complement deposition in the vessel walls within MS lesions was observed (91) and was subsequently shown to be associated with breakdown of the blood-CNS barrier (92). Evidence for a role of complement in MS also includes recent studies demonstrating increased CSF complement activation in MS pa-tients and a significant correlation of neurologic disability as measured by expanded dis-ability status scale (EDSS) and CSF concentration of terminal complement complex (93).

Interestingly, CNS myelin itself had been demonstrated to activate the classical com-plement pathway (94). A candidate myelin antigen for complement binding is MOG, which is expressed on the outermost lamellae of myelin and which contains a conserved motif similar to the C1q-binding site of IgG (95). Johns and Bernard showed that the extracellular portion of the CNS myelin-specific protein, MOG, binds C1q in a calcium- and dose-dependent manner (96). Another candidate complement binding protein is CNP, which binds C3, as mentioned above (31). Oligodendroglial cells may be especially sus-ceptible to complement damage (97). Although astrocytes appear to be protected against complement attack by their expression of complement-regulatory proteins (98,99), oligo-dendroglial cells lack expression of such complement-regulatory proteins (100).

IV. POTENTIAL PATHOGENIC MECHANISMS OF ANTIBODIES IN MS

Possible roles for Abs in the course of CNS inflammatory demyelination include (a) demyelination mediated via myelin opsonization for phagocytosis by Ab $+/-$ complement; (b) activation of the complement cascade, (c) remyelination, and (d) antigen uptake, processing, and presentation, which may involve both B cells acting as a critical antigen-presenting cells (APCs) and Abs acting in the uptake and processing of antigen.

A. Role of Antibodies in Myelin Opsonization

In addition to a potential role in directing specific antigen processing by B cells, Abs have been implicated in the opsonization of myelin and subsequent phagocytosis by macrophages in MS and EAE (101–103). Goldenberg et al. showed that anti-MBP, anti-galactocerebroside (GC), and anti-myelin antiserums all increased macrophage phagocytosis (101). Van der Laan et al. showed that binding and uptake by macrophages of CNS myelin was enhanced after opsonization with complement and that phagocytosis of myelin by macrophages activated the macrophages to produce TNF-α and nitric oxide (103). The latter substances have each been implicated in demyelination and/or toxicity toward oligodendroglia.

B. Binding of Antibody to FC Receptors

The main cell types involved in antigen presentation in the periphery and the CNS—macrophages, microglia, dendritic cells, and B cells—also express one or more Fc receptors (FcR) that bind the Fc portion of Igs, irrespective of the antigen specificity of the Ab (104). For the IgG isotype, three different classes of FcR (FcγR) exist. Engagement of most of the FcγRs encourages phagocytosis (reviewed in Ref. 105), and engagement of some of the FcγRs encourages cell activation, as measured by cytokine production and early activation events (e.g., protein tyrosine kinase activation and increased intracellular Ca^{2+}). However, as opposed to FcRs on other immune cell types, engagement of FcγRIIB1 expressed by B cells usually inhibits B-cell phagocytosis, endocytosis, and activation, with reported exceptions (105,106). Thus, ligation of FcRs on B cells delivers a negative signal, leading to B-cell inactivation and decreased Ab production. Parenthetically, this may be one mechanism by which IVIG may work in some neurological and autoimmune disorders, perhaps including MS.

C. Autoantibodies May Induce Remyelination

Rodriguez and colleagues demonstrated that the humoral immune response directed against certain CNS antigens enhances CNS remyelination in the Theiler's virus and EAE models of MS (107,108). Recently such Abs have been shown to be polyreactive toward a variety of intracellular antigens but also reactive to an unidentified surface antigen on oligodendrocytes. The authors point out that although Abs that recognize normal CNS components, especially oligodendrocytes or myelin, have traditionally been considered to be a disease marker or to be involved in the pathogenesis of MS, these autoAbs may be beneficial for myelin repair. Such autoAbs may be related to the reported benefit of IVIG in MS.

Cells as Antigen-Presenting Cells and the Role of Antibody in Antigen Processing

The uptake, processing, and presentation of antigen to T cells may involve both B cells acting as a critical APCs and Ab acting in the uptake and processing of antigen (109–111) (reviewed in Ref. 112). B cells express surface receptors that consist of the antigen-binding portion of the Ig they secrete. These B cell receptors (BCR) confer B cells with the ability to specifically bind and concentrate a given antigen with vastly greater efficiency than other cell types (111). The epitopes presented to T cells by B cells depend on the BCR expressed by the B cells. Following antigen binding to the BCR, the antigen-BCR complex moves to intracellular compartments containing MHC class II molecules (113). Previous studies demonstrated that the antigenic epitopes presented to T cells by a given B cell depend on the epitope to which the BCR is bound. Moreover, binding of additional Abs to the Ag at the time of endocytosis can further modify the epitopes presented to B cells (114). The stability of the BCR-antigen complex is another factor that regulates the epitope selection (115). Evidence indicates that Ab can either enhance or suppress the T-cell responses to certain epitopes based on their effect on Ag processing (116).

V. THE ROLE OF THE B CELL IN EXPERIMENTAL ALLERGIC ENCEPHALOMYELITIS

Some of the controversy surrounding the role of Abs in MS pathogenesis arises from contradictions in the data obtained from the animal model, experimental allergic encephalomyelitis (EAE). EAE, the prime autoimmune model for MS, is induced in susceptible animals following active immunization with various myelin proteins or passive transfer of T cells specific for these myelin proteins. B cells and Ab have been thought by many not to be important for EAE pathogenesis, as passive transfer of either was unable to induce EAE in susceptible animal strains (117). Furthermore, no direct correlation has been found between Ab titers and disease severity (117,118). Studies of EAE induction in mice genetically deficient in B cells found no requirement for B cells or Ab in disease induction or demyelination in models induced using peptides of MBP and MOG (119,120). On the other hand, early studies demonstrated that rats (121,122) or mice (123) depleted of B cells by repeated injection of anti-IgM Ab from birth were resistant to EAE induction by immunization with MBP or spinal cord homogenate. If, at the time of immunization, animals were also given an injection of serum from MBP-immunized mice, animals were again susceptible to EAE induction (124). While these studies suggested that Abs were important for EAE pathogenesis, subsequent studies showed that these animals were also deficient in other aspects of the immune response, including T-cell activity, making interpretation of the original data difficult (125).

Current studies in our laboratories have sought to address the discrepancies in the above data. Mice genetically deficient in B cells, and hence Ab, were immunized with either a recombinant form of the MOG protein (rMOG) or the encephalitogenic MOG(35–55) peptide, and the development of EAE was followed (126). As was observed in previous studies, peptide-immunized B cell–deficient mice were fully susceptible to EAE induction and demyelination that was similar in all ways to peptide-induced disease in wild-type

(WT) mice. However, whereas WT mice were susceptible to rMOG-induced EAE, B cell–deficient mice were resistant to disease induction by this protocol. Histological examination of the spinal cord demonstrated a lack of inflammation and demyelinating pathology in the B cell–deficient mice. These data suggest that B cells and Abs are important to the disease process when a more complex (protein) form of the antigen is used for EAE induction. These studies have important implications for the use of EAE as a model for MS, in which antigens involved are likely to be present in a more complex form.

Early studies demonstrated the presence of serum factors capable of causing demyelination and myelin swelling in serum of rabbits immunized with whole myelin white matter (127). Subsequently, Abs specific for a variety of myelin antigens and capable of potentiating disease or promoting demyelination have been identified (128–130). Most often implicated in disease pathogenesis are Abs to MOG. While the MOG protein is a minor component of myelin, it is prime candidate for direct interaction with auto Abs, as it is expressed on the outer surface of the myelin sheath (131). Abs to MOG have been demonstrated to be critical to EAE induction in a primate (marmoset) model (132) and potentiate MBP-induced EAE in Lewis rats (133–135), inducing demyelination in a model which is typically lacking in this aspect of CNS pathology. In a murine model of disease, both PLP- and MOG-induced EAE were accelerated and disease exacerbated in mice genetically engineered to produce high titers of anti-MOG antibodies (136).

Roles for Abs recognizing PLP and MBP, predominant encephalitogens in the EAE model, have also been investigated. Indirect evidence was found for a contribution of anti-PLP Abs to the extent of disease in PLP-induced EAE (137,138). Recently, an enhancing effect for anti-PLP Abs in PLP peptide-induced EAE has been suggested (128). These investigators first infected mice with a recombinant vaccinia virus encoding the PLP protein (VVplp) followed by challenge with one of three PLP peptides. With peptide challenge following VVplp infection, an increase in anti PLP titer and a shift in isotype from IgG1 to IgG2a and IgG2b was observed. These were associated with enhanced clinical and histological disease when compared with mice infected with a control construct lacking the PLP gene. Despite intensive investigation, some studies have not found a role for anti-MBP Abs in EAE (139,140). However, studies using B cell–depleted animals suggested a role for Abs directed against MBP in an adoptively transferred EAE model (123,124).

It is interesting to note that many times the epitope specificity of Abs recovered from animals with EAE is identical to that of the encephalitogenic epitope of the protein used for disease induction. PLP(139–151) is the predominant encephalitogenic epitope in SJL mice (141). In the PLP studies of Wang and Fujinami, anti-PLP(139–151) Abs appeared to comprise a larger portion of the anti-PLP titer than other specificities following VVplp immunization. Also, the anti-PLP(139–151) response was most elevated and enhancement of EAE was most pronounced following PLP(139–151)-challenge of VVplp-immunized mice (128). Liu et al. observed similar restriction of the anti-MOG response in a murine model of EAE, with the predominant Ab response directed against the encephalitogenic MOG(35–55) epitope (142). However, this is not always the case, as Abs recognizing conformational epitopes, carbohydrate epitopes, and responses to other MOG peptides have been identified (143,144).

In addition to anti-protein responses, Ab responses to myelin lipids have also been identified in EAE. The observation that EAE induced with intact whole myelin or total brain homogenate was more severe and induced more demyelination than EAE induced with MBP alone, coupled with the observation that antigalactocerebroside antiserum demyelinated organotypic cultures, led to the hypothesis and confirmation that anti-galactocerebroside antibodies would potentiate EAE (140). Studies comparing lipid-free MBP with lipid bound-MBP further indicated an enhancing effect of myelin lipids on the immune response and suggested that it might be related to Ab formation against lipids or against novel conformational epitopes of lipid-bound MBP (145,146).

Serum from animals with chronic EAE displays a higher incidence of demyelinating activity than serum from animal with acute or subacute EAE (117). These results are in agreement with the studies of Prineas and Wright suggesting that plasma cells are more prevalent in chronic MS lesions than acute lesions (147). Studies to characterize the production of auto Abs to MOG during MOG-induced EAE show that they are more prevalent during relapsing and chronic disease than during the acute phase (129). Abs in the CNS may be the result of in situ production by resident plasma cells (148) or serum Ab, which gains access to the CNS following damage to the blood-CNS barrier.

VI. MECHANISMS OF ANTIBODY IN EAE PATHOGENESIS

Both serum and CSF samples from animals with EAE augment the phagocytosis and metabolism of CNS myelin by macrophages in vitro (149,150). In both MS and EAE, receptor-mediated phagocytosis of myelin via clathrin-coated pits on macrophages has been demonstrated and implicated in the pathogenesis (147). Using the EAE model in guinea pigs and colloidal-gold labeled Abs, Moore and Raine identified IgG diffusely scattered over myelin, within macrophage lysosomes, and occasionally within coated pits (151). In the latter instances, it was suggested that the IgG might provide contact between the macrophage and myelin, leading to internalization and phagocytosis. More recently, Ab specific for MOG was shown to specifically bind to disintegrating myelin around axons in a marmoset model of EAE (13,54).

Another role for autoAbs in demyelinating disease has been suggested by work from the laboratories of Zhou and Whitaker (152,153). This group has developed monoclonal Abs that recognize the binding site of T-cell receptors on encephalitogenic lymphocytes. They provide evidence for an idiotypic network which may regulate autoimmune diseases such as EAE or possibly MS.

VII. THE ROLE OF COMPLEMENT IN EAE

The demyelinating potential of a given Ab in EAE has been correlated with its ability to fix complement (130,143,154). Linington and colleagues investigated the role of complement in both MBP-mediated EAE and in "Ab-mediated" demyelination (143,155). These models have been associated with the deposition of C9, indicative of membrane attack complex formation, although complement depletion studies in vivo suggest that these proteins are not essential to the pathogenesis of demyelination in the Ab-mediated disease. These findings have been extended recently in studies using transgenic mice with an astrocyte-targeted production of a soluble inhibitor of complement activation (156). These transgenic mice were protected from MOG peptide–induced EAE, indicating that complement activation has a critical role in the pathogenesis of this model. Activated complement factors have chemotactic effects as well as potentiating the production of proinflammatory cytokines and adhesion molecule expression. It was suggested that the major effector mechanism responsible for the beneficial effect of soluble complement inhibitor was its blockade of complement-mediated trafficking of inflammatory cells into the CNS.

VIII. CONCLUSION

In conclusion, new data from several laboratories, using a variety of methods, have once again focused research efforts in MS on the humoral immune system. The roles of B cells, plasma cells, and Ig in MS are likely to be complex and may include both pathogenic, regulatory, and reparative roles. The possibility remains that the intrathecal antibody response in MS patients is due to nonspecific immunodysregulation. Nonetheless, that autoAb production in MS patients might be driven or promoted by cross-reacting infectious antigens (e.g., molecular mimicry) is an especially appealing concept with accumulating support.

ACKNOWLEDGMENT

The authors were each supported by the National Multiple Sclerosis Society during preparation of this manuscript.

REFERENCES

1. Kabat EA, Glusman M, Knaub V. Quantitative estimation of albumin and gamma globulin in normal and pathologic cerebrospinal fluid by immunochemical methods. Am J Med 1948; 4:653–662.
2. Olsson JE, Link H. Immunoglobulin abnormalities in multiple sclerosis: Relation to clinical parameters: exacerbations and remission. Arch Neurol 1973; 28:392–399.
3. Zeman AZJ, Kidd D, McLean BN, Kelly MA, Francis DA, Miller DH, Kendall BE, Rudge P, Thompson EJ, McDonald WI. A study of oligoclonal band negative multiple sclerosis. J Neurol Neurosurg Psychiatry 1996; 60:27–30.
4. Pettinelli CB, McFarlin DE. Adoptive transfer of experimental allergic encephalomyelitis in SJL/J mice after in vitro activation of lymph node cells by myelin basic protein: Requirement for Lyt1+2+ T lymphocytes. J Immunol 1981; 127:1420–1423.
5. Achiron A, Gabbay U, Gilad R, Hassin-Baer S, Barak Y, Gornish M, Elizur A, Goldhammer Y, Sarova-Pinhas I. Intravenous immunoglobulin treatment in multiple sclerosis: Effect on relapses. Neurology 1998; 50:398–402.
6. Lisak RP. Intravenous immunoglobulins in multiple sclerosis (review). Neurology 1998; 51(6 suppl 5):S25–S29.
7. Sorensen PS, Wanscher B, Jensen CV, Schreiber K, Blinkenberg M, Ravnborg M, Kirsmeier H, Larsen VA, Lee ML. Intravenous immunoglobulin G reduces MRI activity in relapsing multiple sclerosis. Neurology 1998; 50:1273–1281.
8. Fazekas F, Deisenhammer F, Strasser-Fuchs S, Nahler G, Mamoli B. Randomised placebo-controlled trial of monthly intravenous immunoglobulin therapy in relapsing-remitting multiple sclerosis. Lancet 1997; 349:589–593.
9. Khatri BO, McQuillen MP, Hoffmann RG, Harrington GJ, Schmoll D. Plasma exchange in chronic progressive multiple sclerosis: A long-term study. Neurology 1991; 41(3):409–414.
10. Rodriguez M, Karnes WE, Bartleson JD, Pineda AA. Plasmapheresis in acute episodes of fulminant CNS inflammatory demyelination. Neurology 1993; 43(6):1100–1104.
11. Weinshenker BG, O'Brien PC, Petterson TM, Noseworthy JH, Lucchinetti CF, Dodick DW, Pineda AA, Stevens LN, Rodriguez M. A randomized trial of plasma exchange in acute central nervous system inflammatory demyelinating disease. Ann Neurol 1999; 46:878–886.
12. Esiri MM. Immunoglobulin-containing cells in multiple sclerosis plaques. Lancet 1977; 2:478–480.
13. Genain CP, Cannella B, Hauser SL, Raine CS. Identification of autoantibodies associated with myelin damage in multiple sclerosis. Nature Med 1999; 5:170–175.

14. Lucchinetti CF, Bruck W, Rodriguez M, Lassmannn H. Distinct patterns of multiple sclerosis pathology indicates heterogeneity in pathogenesis. Brain Pathol 1996; 6:259–274.
15. Prineas JW, Wright RG. Macrophages, lymphocytes and plasma cells in the perivascular compartment in chronic multiple sclerosis. Lab Invest 1978; 38:409–421.
16. Mallison SM, Smith JP, Schenkein HA, Tew JG. Accumulation of plasma cells in inflamed sites: Effects of antigen, nonspecific microbial activators, and chronic inflammation. Infect Immun 1991; 59:4019–4025.
17. Van Dinther-Janssen ACHM, Hofland L, Scheper RJ. Specific plasma cell accumulation in antigen-induced chronic inflammation in the guinea pig peritoneal cavity. Int Arch Allergy Appl Immunol 1986; 79:14–18.
18. Sharief MK, Thompson EJ. Intrathecal immunoglobulin M synthesis in multiple sclerosis. Brain 1991; 114:181–195.
19. Sharief MK, Hentges R. Importance of intrathecal synthesis of IgD in multiple sclerosis. Arch Neurol 1991; 48:1076–1079.
20. Walsh MJ, Tourtelotte WW, Roman J, Dreyer W. Immunoglobulin G, A, and M-clonal restriction in multiple sclerosis cerebrospinal fluid and serum-analysis by two-dimensional electrophoresis. Clin Immunol Immunopathol 1985; 35:313–327.
21. Trotter JL, Rust RS. Human cerebrospinal fluid immunology. In: Brumbach R, Herndon R, eds. Cerebrospinal Fluid. Amsterdam: Martinus Nijhoff 1989:179–226.
22. Sindic CJM, Monteyne PH, Laterre EC. The intrathecal synthesis of virus-specific oligoclonal IgG in multiple sclerosis. J Neuroimmunol 1994; 54:75–80.
23. Cruz M, Olsson T, Ernerudh J, Hojeberg B, Link H. Immunoblot detection of oligoclonal antimyelin basic protein IgG antibodies in cerebrospinal fluid in multiple sclerosis. Neurology 1987; 37:1515–1519.
24. Warren KG, Catz I. Diagnostic value of cerebrospinal fluid anti-myelin basic protein in patients with multiple sclerosis. Ann Neurol 1986; 20:20–25.
25. Warren KG, Catz I. A correlation between cerebrospinal fluid myelin basic protein and anti-myelin basic protein in multiple sclerosis patients. Ann Neurol 1987; 21:183–189.
26. Warren KG, Catz I. A myelin basic protein antibody cascade in purified IgG from cerebrospinal fluid of multiple sclerosis patients. J Neurol Sci 1990; 96:19–27.
27. Warren KG, Catz I. Relative frequency of autoantibodies to myelin basic protein and proteolipid protein in optic neuritis and multiple sclerosis cerebrospinal fluid. J Neurol Sci 1994; 121:66–73.
28. Brokstad KA, Page M, Nyland H, Haaheim LR. Autoantibodies to myelin basic protein are not present in the serum and CSF of MS patients. Acta Neurol Scand 1994; 89:407–411.
29. Xiao B-G, Linington C, Link H. Antibodies to myelin-oligodendrocyte glycoprotein in cerebrospinal fluid from patients with multiple sclerosis and controls. J Neuroimmunol 1991; 31:91–96.
30. Bronstein JM, Lallone RL, Seitz RS, Ellison GW, Myers LW. A humoral response to oligodendrocyte-specific protein in MS: a potential molecular mimic. Neurology 1999; 53:154–161.
31. Walsh MJ, Murray JM. Dual implication of 2′, 3′-cyclic nucleotide 3 phosphodiesterase as major autoantigen and C3 complement-binding protein in the pathogenesis of multiple sclerosis. J Clin Invest 1998; 101:1923–1931.
32. Banki K, Colombo E, Sia F, Halladay D, Mattson DH, Tatum AH, Massa PT, Phillips PE, Perl A. Oligodendrocyte-specific expression and autoantigenicity of transaldolase in multiple sclerosis. J Exp Med 1994; 180(5):1649–1663.
33. Colombo E, Banki K, Tatum AH, Daucher J, Ferrante P, Murray RS, Phillips PE, Perl A. Comparative analysis of antibody and cell-mediated autoimmunity to transaldolase and myelin basic protein in patients with multiple sclerosis. J Clin Invest 1997; 99(6):1238–1250.
34. Esposito M, Venkatesh V, Otvos L, Weng Z, Vajda S, Banki K, Perl A. Human transaldolase and cross-reactive viral epitopes identified by autoantibodies of multiple sclerosis patients. J Immunol 1999; 163(7):4027–4032.

35. Bansal AS, Abdul-Karim B, Malik RA, Goulding P, Pumphrey RS, Boulton AJ, Holt PL, Wilson PB. IgM ganglioside GM1 antibodies in patients with autoimmune disease or neuropathy, and controls. J Clin Pathol 1994; 47:300–302.

36. Acarin N, Rio J, Fernandez AL, Tintore M, Duran I, Galan I, Montalban X. Different antiganglioside antibody pattern between relapsing-remitting and progressive multiple sclerosis. Acta Neurol Scand 1996; 93(2–3):99–103.

37. Stevens A, Weller M, Wietholter H. CSF and serum ganglioside antibody patterns in MS. Acta Neurol Scand 1992; 6(5):485–489.

38. Arnon R, Crisp E, Kelley R, Ellison GW, Myers LW, Tourtellotte WW. Anti-ganglioside antibodies in multiple sclerosis. J Neurol Sci 1980; 46(2):179–186.

39. Kasai N, Pachner AR, Yu RK. Anti-glycolipid antibodies and their immune complexes in multiple sclerosis. J Neurol Sci 1986; 75(1):33–42.

40. Coyle PK, Procyk-Dougherty Z. Multiple sclerosis immune complexes: An analysis of component antigens and antibodies. Ann Neurol 1984; 16:660–667.

41. Rostami AM, Burns JB, Eccleston PA, Manning MC, Lisak RP, Silberberg DH. Search for antibodies to galactocerebroside in the serum and cerebrospinal fluid in human demyelinating disorders. Ann Neurol 1987; 22(3):381–383.

42. Endo T, Scott DD, Stewart SS, Kundu SK, Marcus DM. Antibodies to glycosphingolipids in patients with multiple sclerosis and SLE. J Immunol 1984; 132(4):1793–1797.

43. Ohguro H, Chiba S, Igarashi Y, Matsumoto H, Akino T, Palczewski K. Beta-arrestin and arrestin are recognized by autoantibodies in sera from multiple sclerosis patients. Proc Natl Acad Sci USA 1993; 90:3241–3245.

44. Ikeda Y, Sudoh A, Chiba S, Matsumoto H, Nakagawa T, Ohguro H. Detection of serum antibody against arrestin from patients with acute disseminated encephalomyelitis. Tohoku J Exp Med 1999; 187:65–70.

45. van den Noort S, Stjerholm RL. Lymphotoxic activity in multiple sclerosis serum. Neurology 1971; 21:783–793.

46. Rumbach L, Tongio MM, Warter JM, Mareocaux C, Mayer S, Rohmer F. Lymphocytotoxic and monocytotoxic antibodies in the serum and cerebrospinal fluid of multiple sclerosis patients. J Neuroimmunol 1982; 3:263–273.

47. Lisak RP, Mercado F, Zweiman B. Cold reactive anti-lymphocyte antibodies in neurological disease. J Neurol Neurosurg Psychiatry 1979; 42:1054–1057.

48. Moller A, Hansen BL, Hansen GN, Hagen C. Autoantibodies in sera from patients with multiple sclerosis directed against antigenic determinants in pituitary growth hormone-producing cells and in structures containing vasopressin/oxytocin. J Neuroimmunol 1985; 8:177–184.

49. Ryberg B. Antibrain antibodies in multiple sclerosis: relation to clinical variables. J Neurol Sci 1982; 54:239–261.

50. Tanaka Y, Tsukada N, Koh C-S, Yanagisawa N. Anti-endothelial cell antibodies and circulating immune complexes in the sera of patients with multiple sclerosis. J Neuroimmunol 1987; 17:49–59.

51. Arnason BGW, Antel JP, Reder AT. Immuno-regulation in multiple sclerosis. Ann NY Acad Sci 1984; 436:139–143.

52. Warren KG, Catz I. Autoantibodies to myelin basic protein within multiple sclerosis central nervous system tissue. J Neurol Sci 1993; 115:169–176.

53. Wucherpfenning KW, Catz I, Hausmann S, Strominger JL, Steinman L, Warren KG. Recognition of the immunodominant myelin basic protein peptide by autoantibodies and HLA-DR2-restricted T cell clones from multiple sclerosis patients. Identity of key contact residues in the B-cell and T-cell epitopes. J Clin Invest 1997; 100(5):1114–1122.

54. Raine CS, Cannella B, Hauser SL, Genain CP. Demyelination in primate autoimmune encephalomyelitis and acute multiple sclerosis lesions: A case for antigen-specific antibody mediation. Ann Neurol 1999; 46:144–160.

55. Esiri MM, Taylor CR, Mason DY. Application of an immunoperoxidase method to a study of the central nervous system: Preliminary findings in a study of human formalin-fixed material. Neuropathol Appl Neurobiol 1976; 2:233–246.

56. Prineas JW, Raine CS. Electron microscopy and immunoperoxidase studies of early multiple sclerosis lesions. Neurology 1976; 26:29–32.

57. Prineas JW, Graham JS. Multiple sclerosis: capping of surface immunoglobulin G on macrophages engaged in myelin breakdown. Ann Neurol 1981; 10:149–158.

58. Olsson T, Baig S, Hojeberg B, Link H. Antimyelin basic protein and antimyelin antibody-producing cells in multiple sclerosis. Ann Neurol 1990; 27:132–136.

59. Martino G, Olsson T, Fredrikson S, Hojeberg B, Kostulas V, Grimaldi LME, Link H. Cells producing antibodies specific for myelin basic protein region 70–89 are predominant in cerebrospinal fluid from patients with multiple sclerosis. Eur J Immunol 1991; 21:2971–2976.

60. Sun J-B, Olsson T, Wang W-Z, Xiao BG, Kostulas V, Fredrikson S, Ekre HP, Link H. Autoreactive T and B cells responding to myelin proteolipid protein in multiple sclerosis and controls. Eur J Immunol 1991; 21:1461–1468.

61. Baig S, Olsson T, Yu-Ping J, Hojeberg B, Cruz M, Link H. Multiple sclerosis: Cells secreting antibodies against myelin-associated glycoprotein are present in cerebrospinal fluid. Scand J Immunol 1991; 33:73–79.

62. Sun J, Link H, Olsson T, Xiao B-G, Andersson G, Ekre H-P, Linington C, Diener P. T and B cell responses to myelin-oligodendrocyte glycoprotein in multiple sclerosis. J Immunol 1991; 146:1490–1495.

63. Mattson DH, Roos RP, Arnason BG. Isoelectric focusing of IgG eluted from multiple sclerosis and subacute sclerosing panencephalitis brains. Nature 1980; 287:335–337.

64. Walsh MJ, Tourtellotte WW. Temporal invariance and clonal uniformity of brain and cerebrospinal IgG, IgA, and IgM in multiple sclerosis. J Exp Med 1986; 163:41–53.

65. Mehta PD, Miller JA, Tourtellotte WW. Oligoclonal IgG bands in plaques from multiple sclerosis brains. Neurology 1982; 32:372–376.

66. Mattson DH, Roos RB, Arnason BGW. Oligoclonal IgG in multiple sclerosis and subacute sclerosing panencephalitis brains. J Neuroimmunol 1982; 2:261–276.

67. Owens GP, Kraus H, Burgoon MP, Smith-Jensen T, Devlin ME, Gilden DH. Restricted use of VH4 germline segments in acute MS brain. Ann Neurol 1998; 43:236–243.

68. Qin Y, Duquette P, Zhang Y, Talbot P, Poole R, Antel J. Clonal expansion and somatic hypermutation of Vh genes of B cells from cerebrospinal fluid in multiple sclerosis. J Clin Invest 1998; 102:1045–1050.

69. Smith-Jensen T, Burgoon MP, Anthony J, Kraus H, Gilden DH, Owens GP. Comparison of IgG heavy chain sequences in MS and SSPE brains reveals an antigen-driven response. Neurology 2000; 54:1227–1232.

70. Bornstein MB. The immunopathology of demyelinative disorders examined in organotypic cultures of mammalian central nerve tissues. In: Zimmerman HM, ed. Progress in Neuropathology, vol 2. New York: Grune & Stratton, 1973: 69–90.

71. Seil FJ. Tissue culture studies of demyelinating disease: A critical review. Ann Neurol 1977; 2:345–355.

72. Johnson AB, Bornstein MB. Myelin-binding antibodies in vitro: Immunoperoxidase studies with experimental encephalomyelitis, anti-galacto-cerebroside and multiple sclerosis sera. Brain Res 1978; 159:173–182.

73. Allerand CD, Yahr MD. Gamma-Globulin affinity for normal human tissue of the central nervous system. Science 1964; 144:1141–1142.

74. Aarli JA, Aparicio SR, Lumsden CE, Tonder O. Binding of normal IgG to myelin sheaths, glia and neurons. Immunology 1975; 28:171–185.

75. Sindic CJM, Cambiaso CL, Masson PL, Laterre EC. The binding of myelin basic protein to the Fc region of aggregated IgG and to immune complexes. Clin Exp Immunol 1980; 41: 1–7.

76. Poston RN. Basic proteins bind immunoglobulin G: A mechanism for demyelinating disease? Lancet 1984; 1:1268–1271.

77. Traugott U, Snyder S, Raine CS. Oligodendrocytes staining by multiple sclerosis serum is nonspecific. Ann Neurol 1979; 6:13–20.

78. Pedersen JS, Walker M, Toh BH, DeAizpurua HJ, Lolact SJ, Bernard CCA. Flow microfluorometry detects IgM autoantibody to oligodendrocytes in multiple sclerosis. J Neuroimmunol 1983; 5:251–259.

79. Wiederkehr F, Wacker M, Vonderschmitt DJ. Analysis of immune complexes of cerebrospinal fluid by two-dimensional gel electrophoresis. Electrophoresis 1989; 10:473–479.

80. Procaccia S, Lanzanova D, Caputo D, Ferrante P, Papini E, Gasparini A, Colucci A, Bianchi M, Villa P, Blasio R. Circulating immune complexes in serum and in cerebrospinal fluid of patients with multiple sclerosis: Characterization and correlation with the clinical course. Acta Neurol Scand 1988; 77(5):373–381.

81. Tanaka Y, Tsukada N, Koh CS, Yanagisawa N. Anti-endothelial cell antibodies and circulating immune complexes in the sera of patients with multiple sclerosis. J Neuroimmunol 1987; 17(1):49–59.

82. Coyle PK. Detection and isolation of immune complexes in multiple sclerosis cerebrospinal fluid. J Neuroimmunol 1987; 15(1):97–107.

83. Kasai N, Pachner AR, Yu RK. Anti-glycolipid antibodies and their immune complexes in multiple sclerosis. J Neurol Sci 1986; 75:33–42.

84. Unger M, Wettergren A, Clausen J. Characterization of DNA and RNA in circulating immunocomplexes in multiple sclerosis, amyotrophic lateral sclerosis and normal controls. Acta Neurol Scand 1985; 72:392–396.

85. Araga S, Irie H, Takahashi K. Conglutinin microtiter plate ELISA system for detecting circulating immune complexes. J Neuroimmunol 1984; 6:161–168.

86. DiMario U, Guy K, Irvine WJ. The detection of circulating immune complexes in normal subjects using four different methods. J Clin Lab Immunol 1981; 5:95–99.

87. Rudick RA, Didlack JM, Knutson DW. Multiple sclerosis: Cerebrospinal fluid immune complexes that bind C1q. Arch Neurol 1985; 42(9):856–858.

88. Noronha ABC, Antel JP, Roos RP, Medof ME. Circulating immune complexes in neurologic disease. Neurology 1981; 31:1402–1407.

89. Arnadottir T, Kekomaki R, Lund GA, Reunanen M, Salmi AA. Circulating immune complexes in patients with multiple sclerosis: A longitudinal study of serum and CSF by C1q and platelet binding tests. J Neurol Sci 1982; 55(3):273–283.

90. Storch MK, Piddlesden S, Haltia M, Iivanainen M, Morgan P, Lassmann H. Multiple sclerosis: In situ evidence for antibody- and complement-mediated demyelination. Ann Neurol 1998; 43:465–471.

91. Compston DA, Morgan BP, Campell AK, Wilkins P, Cole G, Thomas ND, Jasani B. Immunocytochemical localization of the terminal complement complex in multiple sclerosis. Neuropathol Appl Neurobiol 1989; 15:307–316.

92. Gay D, Esiri M. Blood-brain barrier damage in acute multiple sclerosis plaques. Brain 1991; 114:557–572.

93. Sellebjerg F, Jaliashvili I, Christiansen M, Garred P. Intrathecal activation of the complement system and disability in multiple sclerosis. J Neurol Sci 1998; 157:168–174.

94. Vanguri P, Silverman B, Koski L, Shin ML. Complement activation by isolated myelin: Activation of the classical pathway in the absence of myelin-specific antibodies. Proc Natl Acad Sci USA 1982; 79:3290–3294.

95. Hilton AA, Slavin AJ, Hilton DJ, Bernard CC. Characterization of cDNA and genomic clones encoding human myelin oligodendrocyte glycoprotein. J Neurochem 1995; 65:309–318.

96. Johns TG, Bernard CC. Binding of complement component C1q to myelin oligodendrocyte glycoprotein: A novel mechanisms for regulating CNS inflammation. Mol Immunol 1997; 34:33–38.

97. Wren DR, Nobel M. Oligodendrocytes and oligodendrocyte/type-2 astrocyte progenitor cells of adult rats are specifically susceptible to the lytic effects of complement in the absence of antibody. Proc Natl Acad Sci USA 1989; 86:9025–9029.

98. Wu E, Brosnan CF, Raine CS. SP-40/40 immunoreactivity in inflammatory CNS lesions displaying astrocyte/oligodendrocyte interactions J Neuropathol Exp Neurol 1993; 52:129–134.

99. Sobel RA, Chen M, Maeda A, Hinojoza JR. Vitronectin and integrin vitronectin receptor localization in multiple sclerosis lesions. J Neuropathol Exp Neurol 1995; 54:202–213.

100. Scolding NJ, Morgan BP, Compston DA. The expression of complement regulatory proteins by adult human oligodendrocytes. J Neuroimmunol 1998; 84:69–75.

101. Goldenberg PZ, Kwon EE, Benjamins JA, Whitaker JN, Quarles RH, Prineas JW. Opsonization of normal myelin by anti-myelin antibodies an normal serum. J Neuroimmunol 1989; 23:157–166.

102. Trotter J, DeJong LJ, Smith ME. Opsonization with anti-myelin antibody increases the uptake and intracellular metabolism of myelin in inflammatory macrophages. J Neurochem 1986; 47:779–789.

103. Van der Laan, Ruuls SR, Weber KS, Lodder IJ, Dopp EA, Dijkstra CD. Macrophage phagocytosis of myelin in vitro determined by flow cytometry: phagocytosis is mediated by CR3 and induces production of tumor necrosis factor-α and nitric oxide. J Neuroimmunol 1996; 70:145–152.

104. Ulvestad E, Williams K, Matre R, Nyland H, Olivier A, Antel J. Fc receptors for IgG on cultured human microglia mediate cytotoxicity and phagocytosis of antibody-coated targets. J Neuropathol Exp Neurol 1994; 53:27–36.

105. Fridman WH. Regulation of B-cell activation and antigen presentation by Fc receptors. Curr Opin Immunol 1993; 5:355–360.

106. Liu C, Gosselin EJ, Guyre PM. FcγRII on human B cells can mediate enhanced antigen presentation. Cell Immunol 1996; 167:188–194.

107. Rodriguez M, Lennon VA. Immunoglobulins promote remyelination in the CNS. Ann Neurol 1990; 27:12–17.

108. Asakura K, Rodriguez M. A unique population of circulating autoantibodies promotes central nervous system remyelination (review). Mul Scler 1998; 4(3):217–221.

109. Constant SL. B lymphocytes as antigen-presenting cells for CD4+ T cell priming in vivo. J Immunol 1999; 162:5695–5703.

110. Fulcher DA, Lyons AB, Korn SL, Cook MC, Koleda C, Parish C, Fazekas de St Groth B, Basten A. The fate of self-reactive B cells depends primarily on the degree of antigen receptor engagement and availability of T cell help. J Exp Med 1996; 183:2313–2328.

111. Rock KL, Benacerraf B, Abbas AK. Antigen presentation by hapten-specific B lymphocytes: I. Role of surface immunoglobulin receptors. J Exp Med 1984; 160:1102–1113.

112. Schneider SC, Sercarz EE. Antigen processing differences among APC. Hum Immunol 1997; 54:148–158.

113. Cheng PC, Steele CR, Gu L, Song W, Pierce SK. MHC class II antigen processing in B cells: Accelerated intracellular targeting of antigens. J Immunol 1999; 1622:7171–7180.

114. Davidson HW, Watts C. Epitope-directed processing of specific antigen by B lymphocytes. J Cell Biol 1989; 109:85–92.

115. Aluvihare VR, Khamlichi AA, Williams GT, Adorini L, Neuberger MS. Acceleration of intracellular targeting of antigen by the B-cell receptor: importance depends on the nature of the antigen-antibody interactions. EMBO J 1997; 16:3553–3562.

116. Simitsek PD, Campbell DG, Lanzavecchia A, Fairweather N, Watts C. Modulation of antigen processing by bound antibodies can boost or suppress class II major histocompatibility complex presentation of different T cell determinants. J Exp Med 1995; 181:1957–1963.

117. Lassman H, Stemberger H, Kitz K, Wisniewski HM. In vivo demyelinating activity of sera

from animals with chronic experimental allergic encephalomyelitis: Antibody nature of the demyelinating factor and the role of complement. J Neurol Sci 1983; 59:123–137.

118. Paterson PY, Day ED, Whitacre CC. Neuroimmunologic diseases: Effector cell responses and immunoregulatory mechanisms. Immunol Rev 1981; 55:89–120.

119. Wolf SD, Dittel BN, Hardarottir F, Janeway CA. Experimental autoimmune encephalomyelitis induction in genetically B cell-deficient mice. J Exp Med 1996; 184:2271–2278.

120. Hjelmstrom P, Juedes AE, Fjell J, Ruddle NH. B cell-deficient mice develop experimental allergic encephalomyelitis with demyelination after myelin oligodendrocyte glycoprotein sensitization. J Immunol 1998; 161:4480–4483.

121. Willenborg DO, Prowse SJ. Immunoglobulin-deficient rats fail to develop experimental allergic encephalomyelitis. J Neuroimmunol 1983; 5:99–109.

122. Gausas J, Paterson PY, Day ED, Dal Canto MC. Intact B-cell activity is essential for complete expression of experimental allergic encephalomyelitis in Lewis rats. Cell Immunol 1982; 72: 360–366.

123. Myers KJ, Sprent J, Dougherty JP, Ron Y. Synergy between encephalitogenic T cells and myelin basic protein-specific antibodies in the induction of experimental autoimmune encephalomyelitis. J Neuroimmunol 1991; 41:1–8.

124. Willenborg DO, Sjollema P, Danta G. Immunoglobulin deficient rats as donors and recipients of effector cells of allergic encephalomyelitis. J Neuroimmunol 1986; 11:93–100.

125. Kim KY, Rollwagen F, Asofsky R, Lefkovits L. The abnormal funciton of T cells in chronically anti-µ treated mice with no mature B-lymphocytes. Eur J Immunol 1984; 14:476–482.

126. Lyons JA, San M, Happ MP, Cross AH. B-cells are critical to induction of experimental allergic encephalomyelitis by protein but not by a short encephalitogenic peptide. Eur J Immunol 1999; 29:3432–3439.

127. Grundke-Iqbal I, Raine CS, Johnson AB, Brosnan CF, Bornstein MB. Experimental allergic encephalomyelitis: Characterization of serum factors causing demyelination and swelling of myelin. J Neurol Sci 1981; 50:63–79.

128. Wang L-Y, Fujinami RS. Enhancement of EAE and induction of autoantibodies to T-cell epitopes in mice infected with a recombinant vaccinia virus encoding myelin proteolipid protein. J Neuroimmunol 1997; 75:75–83.

129. Morris MM, Piddlesden S, Groome N, Amor S. Anti-myelin antibodies modulate experimental allergic encephalomyelitis in Biozzi ABH mice. Biochem Soc Trans 1997; 25:168S.

130. Van der Goes A, Kortekaas M, Hoekstra K, Dijkstra CD, Amor S. The role of anti-myelin (auto)-antibodies in the phagocytosis of myelin by macrophages. J Neuroimmunol 1999; 101: 61–67.

131. Gardinier MV, Amiguet P, Lininton C, Matthieu J-M. Myelin/oligodendrocyte glycoprotein is a member of the immunoglobulin superfamily. J Neurosci Res 1992; 33:177–187.

132. Genain CP, Nguyen MH, Letvin NL, Pearl R, Davis RL, Adelman M, Lees MB, Linington C, Hauser SL. Antibody facilitation of multiple sclerosis-like lesions in a nonhuman primate. J Clin Invest 1996; 96:2966–2974.

133. Lassman H, Brunner C, Bradl M, Linington C. Experimental allergic encephalomyelitis: The balance between encephalitogenic T lymphocytes and demyelinating antibodies determines size and structure of demyelinated lesions. Acta Neuropathol 1988; 75:566–576.

134. Schluessner HJ, Sobel RA, Linington C, Weiner HL. A monoclonal antibody against a myelin oligodendrocyte glycoprotein induces relapses and demyelination in central nervous system autoimmune disease. J Immunol 1987; 139:4016–4021.

135. Linington C, Bradl M, Lassman H, Brunner C, Vass K. Augmentation of demyelination in rat acute allergic encephalomyelitis by circulating mouse monoclonal antibodies directed against a myelin/oligodendrocyte glycoprotein. Am J Pathol 1988; 130:443–454.

136. Litzenburger T, Fassler R, Bauer J, Lassmann H, Linington C, Wekerle H, Iglesias A. B lymphocytes producing demyelinating autoantibodies: Development and function in gene-targeted transgenic mice. J Exp Med 1998; 188:169–180.

137. Endoh M, Tabira T, Kunishita T. Antibodies to proteolipid apoprotein in chronic relapsing experimental allergic encephalomyelitis. J Neurol Sci 1986; 73:31–38.

138. van der Veen RC, Sobel RA, Lees MB. Chronic experimental allergic encephalomyelitis and antibody responses in rabbits immunized with bovine proteolipid apoprotein. J Neuroimmunol 1986; 11:321–338.

139. Schwerer B, Schuller-Lewis GB, Mehta PD, Madrid RD, Wisniewski HM. Cellular and humoral immune response to MBP during the course of chronic relapsing EAE. In: Alvord EC, Kies MW, Suckling AJ, eds. Experimental Allergic Encephalomyelitis: A Useful Model for Multiple Sclerosis. New York: Liss, 1984:187–192.

140. Tabira T, Endoh M. Humoral immune responses to myelin basic protein, cerebroside and ganglioside in chronic relapsing experimental allergic encephalomyelitis of the guinea pig. J Neurol Sci 1985; 67:201–212.

141. Whitham RH, Bourdette DN, Hashim GA, Herndon RM, Ilg RC, Vandenbark AA, Offner H. Lymphocytes from SJL/J mice immunized with spinal cord respond selectively to a peptide of proteolipid protein and transfer relapsing demyelinating experimental autoimmune encephalomyelitis. J Immunol 1991; 146:101–107.

142. Liu J, Marino MW, Wong G, Grail D, Dunn A, Bettadapura J, Slavin AJ, Old L, Bernard CCA. TNF is a potent anti-inflammatory cytokine in autoimmune-mediated demyelination. Nature Med 1998; 4:78–83.

143. Piddlesden SJ, Lassmann H, Zimprich F, Morgan BP, Linington C. The demyelinating potential of antibodies to myelin oligodendrocyte glycoprotein is related to their ability to fix complement. Am J Pathol 1993; 143:555–564.

144. Brehm U, Piddlesden SJ, Gardinier MV, Linington C. Epitope specificity of demyelinating monoclonal autoantibodies directed against the human myelin oligoendrocyte glycoprotein. J Neuroimmunol 1999; 97:9–15.

145. Lolli F, Liuzzi GM, Vergelli M, Massacesi L, Ballerini C, Amaducci L, Riccio P. Antibodies specific for the lipid-bound form of myelin basic protein during experimental autoimmune encephalomyelitis. J Neuroimmunol 1993; 44:69–76.

146. Massacesi L, Vergelli M, Zehetbauer B, Liuzzi GM, Olivotto J, Ballerini C, Uccelli A, Mancardi L, Ricco P, Amaducci L. Induction of experimental autoimmune encephalomyelitis in rats and immune response to myelin basic protein in lipid-bound form. J Neurol Sci 1993; 119:91–98.

147. Prineas JW, Connell F. The fine structure of chronically active multiple sclerosis. Neurology 1978; 28:68–75.

148. Knopf PM, Harling-Berg CJ, Cserr HF, Basu D, Sirulnick EJ, Nolan SC, Park JT, Keir G, Thompson EJ, Hickey WF. Antigen-dependent intrathecal antibody synthesis in the normal rat brain: Tissue entry and local retention of antigen-specific B cells. J Immunol 1998; 161:692–701.

149. Sadler RH, Sommer MA, Forno LS, Smith ME. Induction of anti-myelin antibodies in EAE and their possible role in demyelination. J Neurosci Res 1991; 30:616–624.

150. Sommer MA, Forno LS, Smith ME. EAE cerebrospinal fluid augments in vitro phagocytosis and metabolism of CNS myelin by macrophages. J Neurosci Res 1992; 32:384–394.

151. Moore GRW, Raine CS. Immunogold localization and analysis of IgG during immune-mediated demyelination. Lab Invest 1988; 59:641–648.

152. Whitaker JN, Sparks BE, Walker DP, Goodin R, Benveniste EN. Monoclonal idiotypic and anti-idiotypic antibodies produced by immunization with peptides specified by a region of human myelin basic protein mRNA and its complement. J Neuroimmunol 1989; 22:157–166.

153. Zhou S-R, Whitaker JN. Specific modulation of T cells and murine experimental allergic encephalomyelitis by monoclonal anti-idiotypic antibodies. J Immunol 1993; 150:1629–1642.

154. Ichikawa M, Koh C-S, Inaba Y, Seki C, Inoue A, Itoh M, Ishihara Y, Bernard CCA, Komi-

yama A. IgG subclass switching is associated with the severity of experimental autoimmune encephalomyelitis induced with myelin oligodendrocyte glycoprotein peptide in NOD mice. Cell Immunol 1999; 191:97–104.

155. Linington C, Morgan BP, Scolding NJS, Williams P, Piddlesden S. The role of complement in experimental autoimmune encephalomyelitis. Brain 1981; 112:895–911.

156. Davoust N, Nataf S, Reiman R, Holers MV, Campbell IL, Barnum SR. Central nervous system-targeted expression of the complement inhibitor sCrry prevents experimental allergic encephalomyelitis. J Immunol 199; 163:6551–6556.

9

Clinical Features

AARON E. MILLER

Maimonides Medical Center and State University of New York Health Science Center at Brooklyn, Brooklyn, New York

I. INTRODUCTION

Multiple sclerosis (MS) is a disease of central nervous system (CNS) white matter that causes clinical symptoms and signs by eliciting inflammation, local edema, and demyelination in the brain, spinal cord, and optic nerves. The disease afflicts persons almost worldwide, although with considerable epidemiological variation in incidence and prevalence rates. Women are more often affected than men, with ratios varying from 3:2 to 2:1 in various series (1,2). Young adults most frequently develop MS, but the disease may become evident at virtually any age.

The course of MS is highly variable. When disability results, it is most often a consequence of gait disturbance, impaired sphincteric function, and fatigue. The potential influence of a variety of factors on the natural history of the illness is discussed in this chapter.

II. DIAGNOSIS

The basis for the diagnosis of MS stems from the seminal clinicopathological observations of Charcot (3) and requires the demonstration of lesions disseminated over time and involving multiple, discrete anatomical loci in the white matter of the CNS. Schumacher et al. (4) proposed perhaps the first widely used scheme for the clinical diagnosis of MS in 1965. They categorized patients as "clinically definite, probable, or possible" MS, according to the number of the following criteria that were satisfied:

1. Age of onset between 10 and 50 years
2. Objective neurological signs present on examination

3. Neurological symptoms and signs indicative of CNS white matter disease
4. Dissemination in time: (a) two or more attacks (lasting at least 24 h) and separated by at least a month (an attack being defined as the appearance of new symptoms or signs or worsening of previous ones) or (b) progression of symptoms and signs for at least 6 months
5. Dissemination in space: two or more noncontiguous anatomical areas involved
6. No alternative clinical explanation

Patients were classified as "clinically definite MS" if they met five or six criteria, always including the last. Patients who satisfied fewer criteria were categorized as "probable" or "possible MS."

The Schumacher criteria depended solely on clinical history and examination for diagnosis. However, in the 1970s and 1980s technological advances permitted the demonstration of lesions that were clinically undetectable. Computer application allowed the development of evoked-response testing, a measure of electrophysiological dysfunction in the visual, brainstem auditory, or somatosensory pathways. In each of these domains, a repetitive stimulus is applied, and computed elimination of random background activity allows the appearance of an identifiable waveform time-locked to the stimulus. Analysis of these responses permits identification of lesions that are not apparent clinically.

Beginning with computed tomography (CT) in the early 1970s, revolutionary advances in neuroimaging have occurred. Magnetic resonance imaging (MRI) is a much more sensitive technique for the detection of MS lesions and is usually the imaging procedure of choice. These new imaging modalities have provided a means of demonstrating anatomical lesions that are not clinically evident (see Chap. 15). Indeed, cranial MRI demonstrates activity as much as five times more frequently than clinical relapse is apparent (5). Still newer MR techniques, such as MR spectroscopy (MRS) and magnetization transfer, promise further progress in our assessment and understanding of MS through neuroimaging.

In addition, increasingly sensitive methods for the study of cerebrospinal fluid (CSF) led to the recognition that most MS patients have evidence of abnormal immunoreactivity that can be demonstrated by CSF analysis. Abnormalities include elevated immunoglobulin IgG levels (6,7), increased IgG index (8), increased IgG synthesis rate (9), and oligoclonal bands (10–13) (see Chap. 13).

The opportunities created by these new techniques led to the formation of a committee, chaired by Charles Poser, to develop new criteria for the diagnosis of MS (14). The Poser criteria (Table 1) modify those of Schumacher by allowing the demonstration of *paraclinical* lesions (i.e., lesions detected by evoked-response testing or neuroimaging studies). In addition, the new criteria established a new category of laboratory-supported MS based on the inclusion of CSF abnormalities.

However, the Poser criteria were developed before the widespread use of MRI. This imaging modality has taught much about the biology of MS and may now require a reassessment of the criteria used to diagnose the disease. This has become critically important as new drug therapies have become available. Because it appears beneficial to initiate treatment early, before fixed neurological deficits develop, it is important to be able to diagnose the disease with *reasonable* certainty in the initial stages of the illness. Thus, it may prove wise to relax the stringent Poser criteria when MRI evidence provides very strong support for the diagnosis of MS. Although specific MRI criteria may be developed—a National MS Society task force is currently evaluating the issue—already many known MRI characteristics point to the high probability of MS. For example, Filippi et al. (15) have demonstrated that patients with monosymptomatic presentations consistent with a first attack of MS have an 86% chance of developing clinically definite MS within 5 years if the burden of disease on T2-weighted MRI images exceeds 1.23 cm^3. The presence of "black holes," low-signal lesions on T1-weighted images, implies chronic lesions suggesting disease activity in the past. Several criteria have been delineated that increase the specificity of MRI for MS. These include three or more lesions, at least one of which is periventricular in location; lesions greater than 5 mm in diameter; lesions in the posterior fossa; and lesions in the corpus callosum (16,17). With the advent of more effective and safe therapies, the physician and patient may be willing to sacrifice some specificity of diagnosis for increased sensitivity in order to achieve the greatest likelihood of benefit.

III. AGE OF ONSET

Although almost all MS patients develop their initial symptoms during young to middle adulthood, the disease can occur at virtually any age. Convincing cases in childhood have been reported as early as 15 months (18–20), with onset below age 10 occurring in about 0.3% of cases (21–23). The early-onset disease does not appear to differ clinically from that starting later, although there may be an even greater female preponderance in this age group (24).

Onset of the disease after the age of 50 has been considered rare, although a more recent report suggests that MS may be more common than suspected in older individuals (25). New techniques facilitating diagnosis are contributing to increased recognition of cases in this age population. When the disease begins after the age of 40, it tends more often to follow a progressive course particularly characterized by worsening spastic paraparesis (26–29).

IV. CLINICAL MANIFESTATIONS

A. Motor Symptoms

Corticospinal tract involvement occurs with the initial attack of MS in 32 to 41% of patients (30–33), but it is present to a significant degree in 62% (31–33) of patients with chronic disease. Symptoms may also include "heaviness," "stiffness," or even pain in an extremity. The legs are much more frequently involved than are the arms; when both are involved, symptoms in the legs usually appear earlier. Involvement often begins with one leg, but in most patients both are eventually affected, although the severity may be quite asymmetrical. Signs of corticospinal tract pathology may be as minimal as abnormal reflex activity, but the disease frequently progresses to severe spastic paraparesis. Hyperactivity of the deep tendon reflexes, often including crossed tibioadductor and puboadductor reflexes, is seen in most patients. Clonus, which may be sustained and severe, is often present. This is most common at the ankle, but it may be found at other sites as well. The Babinski reflex is frequently present, at times as the only manifestation of corticospinal tract dysfunction.

Spasticity is very commonly seen in the legs, but it may also occur in the arms. At times this abnormality actually helps a paretic patient walk (34,35), but in other patients it may produce discomfort or pain as well as flexor or extensor spasm (36,37) or interfere with personal hygiene (adductor spasticity). Patients complain of stiffness, cramps, spasm, or pain. The spastic paraparetic gait is also associated with an increased incidence of chronic low back pain (36,37).

In the upper extremity, weakness often predominates in the distal musculature. At times, this is accompanied by extensive atrophy, presumably reflecting demyelination in the root entry zones of the spinal cord (30).

Corticospinal tract involvement most often results from demyelination within the spinal cord, although other sites—including the medullary pyramids, basis pontis, cerebral peduncles, and deep hemispheric white matter—may also be involved (38). A hemiparetic pattern of motor weakness may be seen, but is uncommon. Indeed, on occasion MS may present with the acute onset of hemiparesis including the face (39). Although such cases initially appear to be vascular in etiology, MRI may lead to the diagnosis of MS, with lesions most often evident in the posterior limb of the internal capsule.

B. Somatosensory Symptoms

Sensory complaints are often the earliest symptoms of MS (21 to 55%) (30,31,33) and, during the entire course of MS, they occur in 52 to 70% of patients (29,31). The symptoms are often perplexing for the clinician, especially during the onset bout, because they are frequently unassociated with objective signs on the neurological examination. In addition, the anatomical distribution is often peculiar, not corresponding to recognized dermatomal, peripheral nerve, or homuncular patterns. Patients usually complain of numbness, but more often they are referring to a subjective positive sensation than to diminished or absent sensation. Common complaints including tingling, burning, tightness, a feeling like ''procaine (Novocaine) wearing off,'' or a sensation that a garment, such as a glove or a girdle, is being worn. Often the abnormal sensation occurs in a band-like fashion around a limb or the abdomen. Sometimes only a patch of abnormal sensation is reported.

These complaints are most often felt to reflect lesions of the myelinated posterior columns (fasciculi gracilis and cuneatus) rather than the spinothalamic tracts (30). Indeed, objective sensory signs usually indicate involvement of the former pathways. Impairment of vibratory sense is extremely common and almost always precedes detectable abnormality of joint position sense. The author has observed subtle reduction in the ability to perceive a vibrating tuning fork in most mildly affected patients early in the course of the disease.

Reduced perception of pinprick or temperature sensation is less frequently seen. It, too, has a variable pattern of distribution, but it may show a spinal cord level. A picture resembling Brown-Séquard's syndrome is occasionally seen (40).

A fairly specific sensory symptom of MS is Lhermitte's sign (a misnomer, since this is a subjective complaint) (41,42). Patients complain of sudden electric-like sensations radiating down the spine or extremities for a brief moment. This typically occurs when the neck is flexed.

Several distinct pain syndromes may occur in MS patients. Some experience severe, lancinating neuralgic pains in the limbs or elsewhere; others complain of more persistent, intolerable dysesthesias, frequently with a burning quality (36,37). Patients with spasticity often report painful spasms or cramping sensations in the legs.

Although low back pain is a very common ailment among the general population, it is perhaps even more so among persons with MS. This may be related to abnormal postures and gaits associated with weakness and spasticity. Radicular pain may occur on occasion in the absence of compressive pathology and, in a recent report, was the presenting complaint in 3.9% of patients with newly diagnosed MS (43).

Another concern for patients with multiple sclerosis, and another source of pain, is the risk of osteoporosis. Cosman et al. reported a history of fractures in the absence of major trauma in 22% of MS patients, compared with only 2% of controls ($p < 0.002$) (44). Determining bone mass by dual x-ray absortiometry, the authors observed that, over 2 years of prospective follow-up, both women and men with MS lost substantially more bone than controls. There was a trend, which did not reach statistical significance, for diminished ambulatory status and long duration of steroid therapy to predict higher bone loss. In another study, however, this group noted that "after controlling for age, cumulative steroid use was not a determinant of bone mineral density" (45), a finding also of Schwid et al. (46). However, low vitamin D intake and diminished exposure to sunlight appear to be major contributors to the problem.

Although headache has not been particularly associated with MS, a recent report cited a patient with severe acute headache associated with a solitary new lesion in the periaqueductal gray region (47). This unusual case supports recent observations in patients with implanted electrodes that perturbation in this area can produce headache.

In another unusual case, headache mimicking subarachnoid hemorrhage, occurred. A patient with a history of facial myokymia developed apoplectic headache and a third-nerve palsy. Investigations revealed no evidence of subarachnoid hemorrhage or aneurysm, but MRI showed more than 30 white matter lesions, and CSF examination revealed oligoclonal bands (48).

C. Brainstem Symptoms

Although protean manifestations of abnormal brainstem function appear in MS, impairments of ocular motility are most frequently encountered. Nystagmus, most often horizontal, occurs extremely commonly, with a frequency as high as 40 to 70% in some series (30,31). Other forms of nystagmus—including rotatory, upbeating, and downbeating—occur less often. In most patients the nystagmus is asymptomatic, but other patients may complain of blurred vision, images jumping (oscillopsia), or sometimes double vision.

Internuclear ophthalmoplegia, either unilateral or bilateral, is a common manifestation of MS, resulting from lesion(s) of the median longitudinal fasciculus (49,50). In young adults, this sign, in fully developed form, consists of failure of the eye ipsilateral to the lesion to adduct, whereas the contralateral eye abducts fully, but with horizontal nystagmus ("dissociated nystagmus" (50). The eyes are orthophoric at rest and patients do not usually complain of visual symptoms. Incomplete forms are common (51,52).

Other abnormalities of extraocular motility—including horizontal (sometimes bilateral) (53) and vertical gaze paresis (54,55), the one-and-a-half syndrome (56,57), dysfunction of individual nerves to the extraocular muscles (30), and skew deviation (58)—may occur. Transient or sustained diplopia is a common complaint (30–33). Alternatively, patients with prominent nystagmus may report that images are jumpy or jittery, a symptom known as oscillopsia.

Dysarthria is frequent in MS, especially in chronic, more advanced cases. A particular type of speech disturbance, known as *scanning speech*, has long been considered most typical of MS. However, impaired articulatory agility is much more common (59). The term *scanning speech* refers to a particular rhythm and cadence in which each word or syllable is given emphasis. "There is a pause after every syllable and the syllables themselves are pronounced slowly" (3). However, scanning speech seldom interferes with communication.

Other types of dysarthria occur less frequently. Nasal speech may result from involvement of cranial nerves IX and X. Bilateral involvement of corticobulbar tracts may lead to the explosive, poorly modulated speech characteristic of pseudobulbar palsy (59). Two patients have been reported in whom a lifelong problem with stuttering disappeared with the onset of signs of MS (60).

Although facial paresis is usually of the central type and is seen with other motor signs, occasionally a facial palsy of peripheral type develops (61). This presumably results from demyelination of the facial nerve within the brainstem itself.

Blepharospasm, generally in association with other brainstem signs, has been described (62). Facial myokymia an "undulating, wavelike fascicular twitching," usually beginning in the orbicularis oculi, occurs occasionally (63,64).

Auditory disturbance is uncommon in MS, although hearing loss, either unilateral or bilateral, sometimes occurs (65). It is generally caused by lesions in the brainstem (66,67), but an unusual case of deafness due to cerebral disease has been reported (68). Among patients presenting with isolated hearing loss, MRI not infrequently reveals unexpected evidence of MS (65). Tinnitus is experienced occasionally. Vertigo is a frequent complaint of MS patients, usually as part of an acute exacerbation and associated with other signs of brainstem dysfunction. Intractable hiccups have been reported as an unusual manifestation of MS (70,71).

D. Visual Pathway Symptoms

Optic neuritis is one of the most common presenting manifestations of MS, occurring in 14 to 23% of cases (30–33). Patients usually complain of dimming of vision unilaterally, generally accompanied by photophobia and pain aggravated by eye movement. Examination reveals diminished visual acuity of varying severity, and detailed visual field evaluation usually shows a central scotoma (72). Visual loss is seldom total, and good recovery of vision usually occurs, even when the initial visual loss is extremely severe (73). Fundoscopy may show a swollen optic nerve head with hemorrhages or exudates (papillitis), or a normal optic disk (retrobulbar neuritis).

Even in the absence of acute optic neuritis, many patients demonstrate clinical abnormalities of optic neuropathy. This may be manifest by diminished visual acuity, impairment of color vision as detected with Ishihara plates (74), abnormal visual field examination, or a positive "swinging flashlight test" (75), indicative of an afferent pupillary defect (Marcus Gunn pupil). Fundoscopy may reveal optic atrophy. Visual-evoked responses will often be abnormal in patients who never had clinical evidence of optic nerve disease (76,77). Many patients experience bilateral optic nerve dysfunction, but blindness is relatively uncommon.

Virtually any type of visual field defect may occur in MS, depending on the site of the inflammatory-demyelinating lesions. For example, recent reports have cited the presentation of the disease with bilateral homonymous visual field defects (78,79) and acute quadrantic field loss (80). Others have reported similar deficits occurring in the course of MS and, as in the former reports, associated with anatomically appropriate lesions demonstrated by MRI.

E. Olfaction and Gustation

Although spontaneous complaints about abnormalities in the senses of smell and taste are infrequent (81,82), recent reports have demonstrated that disturbances of olfaction are relatively common. Two studies employing the University of Pennsylvania Smell Identification Test (UPSIT) reported abnormalities in 15 and 38.5% respectively. In the latter study of 26 patients, Doty et al. found 7.7% with severe impairment, 19.3%, moderate, and 11.5%, mild (83). They noted a strong negative correlation between a high UPSIT score (normal olfaction) and the number of lesions within the inferior frontal and temporal lobe regions, which are involved with olfaction. Hawkes et al. further demonstrated involvement of olfactory systems by noting abnormalities to hydrogen sulfide evoked responses (H_2S-ER) in MS patients (84). A group with the disease had statistically increased latency and decreased amplitude in the H_2S-ER compared to controls. In general, results on the UPSIT correlated well with the evoked response, although an abnormality on one test did not always indicate an abnormality on the other.

Patients with MS rarely complain of disturbances in taste (85). However, a case has been reported in which hemiageusia was the presenting manifestation of the disorder, preceding other signs of trigeminal and brainstem involvement by more than a week (86). A lesion in the right medulla in the floor of the fourth ventricle was observed on MRI. A previous report had noted the occurrence of hemiageusia in a patient with simultaneous right facial numbness (87).

F. Cerebellar Manifestations

Disturbances resulting from both vermian and hemispheric cerebellar lesions are common in MS. Gait ataxia was an initial complaint in 13% in one series (30). Although common in patients with chronic disease, its incidence is difficult to discern from published series because many patients are included under vague categories, such as balance. Examination may show appendicular ataxia, dysmetria, intention tremor on finger-nose-finger test, or dysdiadochokinesia when the patient tries to perform rapid alternating movements. Dysmetria on the heel-knee-shin test is also frequently present. At times the tremors, present even at rest, may assume violent proportions with attempted movement (so-called rubral tremor). Limb ataxia or intention tremor has been reported in 45 to 50% of patients with chronic disease (31,33).

G. Cognitive and Psychiatric Disturbances

Awareness of cognitive dysfunction in MS patients has increased in recent years, although abnormalities have been variably reported in 0 to 90% of cases (88). Clearly, severe dementia is unusual in MS, but more subtle abnormalities of cognitive function are common. These are often unnoticed by patients, families, or physicians, but they may be detected on more formal neuropsychiatric evaluation. The most frequently encountered difficulties are with memory, attention-concentration, and conceptual reasoning–problem solving (88–91). Although cognitive impairments are variable, they most typically follow patterns usually associated with subcortical lesions. Thus far, correlation or cognitive status with either duration or severity of illness has been poor. Dementia did not correlate with number of distribution of lesions on MRI scans in one study (92), but a more recent study did find such a correlation (93). More focal cognitive abnormalities, such as aphasia (94–96) and neglect (97), have been reported, but they are very unusual.

Earlier literature described euphoria as a feature of MS (98). However, depression is now recognized much more commonly, with as many as 75% of patients experiencing this affective disturbance in some form during the course of the illness (99,100). Although this is usually relatively mild, major depression can occur (101). The so-called euphoria is often actually the inability to inhibit emotional expression, which occurs with subcortical forebrain lesions (102). With this condition, "inappropriate" laughing and crying both occur in MS. Other instances of apparent euphoria seem to be associated with evidence of significant cognitive decline. Euphoria is rarely if ever seen as an early sign in patients with mild symptoms (35).

On rare occasions, other psychotic states, mimicking schizophrenia or other delusional syndromes, may occur in MS. Limited data suggest that the patient with these symptoms may have more disease in the temporal lobe periventricular area (103,104). Also, one must always consider the possibility of iatrogenic symptomatology in patients being treated with a variety of the medications used in MS.

H. Fatigue and Sleep

Fatigue is one of the three most frequently disabling symptoms of MS (105) and may be considered abnormal in as many as 78% of patients (106). A particular feeling of enervation, severe enough to prevent a patient from carrying out duties and responsibilities or to interfere with work, family, or social life, occurs (107). This specific but poorly understood type of fatigue in MS must be distinguished from symptoms of depression, medication side effects, or the physical tiredness.

The prevalence of sleep complaints was three times greater in a group of MS patients than in controls. Sleep complaints were associated with greater levels of depression. In addition, several lesion sites subserving supplementary motor areas were related to the sleep complaints. The authors speculated that such lesions might be related to the production of sleep-disturbing nocturnal spasms (108).

I. Bladder, Bowel, and Sexual Disturbances

Disturbances of defecation and especially of micturition are among the most disabling features of MS, occurring in up to 78% of patients during the course of the illness (109). Patients may complain of urinary frequency, urgency, and incontinence. Alternatively, the urge to urinate may be accompanied by an inability to initiate urine flow voluntarily. History alone is an unreliable indicator of the physiological status of micturition and must be supplemented by further investigation (110,111). This will usually require only a determination of voided volume followed by measurement of residual urine volume, either by direct catheterization or by some other method for estimation, such as ultrasonography or radionuclide study (112). Disturbances of micturition may be divided into failure to store urine, failure to empty the bladder adequately, or a combination of both (110,111). In some patients, good contraction of the bladder detrusor is inappropriately associated with contraction of the external urethral sphincter rather with than relaxation. This condition, known as detrusor–external sphincter dyssynergia, may then lead to retention of urine and, particularly in males, to vesicoureteral reflux, with the threat of hydronephrosis and progressive renal failure (113). Retention of urine also increases the risk of urinary tract infection, which, in turn, may suddenly precipitate urinary symptoms.

Bowel dysfunction in MS has received much less attention than disturbances of micturition. However, studies have shown a prevalence rate of constipation ranging from

39 to 53% (114–116). Suggested causes include slow colonic transit due to autonomic dysfunction, abnormal rectal function, and intussuception (116–118). The problem is often compounded by a tendency of patients to reduce fluid intake in an attempt to decrease urinary frequency and urgency. In a recent survey of unselected outpatients, Hinds et al. found that 51% of patients had experienced bowel incontinence at least once in the preceding 3 months, whereas 25% had experienced the symptom at least weekly (114). Fecal incontinence appeared to correlate with degree of disability, duration of disease, and the presence of urological symptoms.

Sexual symptoms are also common among MS patients. Men most often experience erectile dysfunction but may also suffer from problems with ejaculation (109,119). These symptoms typically accompany abnormal micturition. Women most typically experience difficulty achieving orgasm but may also complain of problems with lubrication (120). Both men and women may also complain of diminished libido.

J. Paroxysmal Symptoms

Many MS patients with stereotyped, repetitive paroxysmal symptoms and signs have been described. Tonic ''seizures'' have been reported most often (40,121–125). Patients suddenly experience dystonic posturing of part of the body, most typically the hand or arm, lasting 30 s to 2 min. Sometimes the attack is painful. Episodes may occur infrequently or many times a day and tend to cluster for periods of weeks to months. The anatomical lesions apparently responsible for the dystonia have been found in a variety of sites, including the basal ganglia, internal capsule, thalamus, cerebral peduncle, the cervical cord (126–129).

Episodes of paroxysmal dysarthria with or without other brainstem dysfunction have also been reported (130,131). The author has encountered a patient with episodic aphasia. Some patients experience paroxysms of itching, and this has been reported as the initial symptom of MS (132). Hemifacial spasm may occur and may be associated with lesions in or near the facial nucleus, as identified by MRI (133).

Trigeminal neuralgia is the most common paroxysmal disturbance. The clinical syndrome is usually indistinguishable from that in non-MS patients except that onset tends to occur at an earlier age and symptoms are more frequently bilateral (134). Occasionally, the usual feature of excruciating, lancinating pain is associated with objective sensory disturbance in the MS patient.

K. Movement Disorders

A variety of other movement disorders occasionally occur in MS. An unusual case of hemiballismus in a convincing case of infantile MS has been reported (18). Kinesigenic dystonia (135) and paroxysmal kinesigenic choreoathetosis (136) have each marked the onset of MS. Segmental myoclonus of spinal origin has been noted (137), and a rare case of trismus has been reported (138). Micrographia, a sign more typically associated with Parkinson's disease, was reported in association with an enhancing lesion in the dominant parietal white matter (139).

L. Autonomic Disturbance

Although not commonly reported, autonomic dysfunction (other than disturbances of bowel and bladder) may be noted. Abnormal sweating has been described, and some patients have coldness or discoloration of the legs or feet (140,141). Autonomous respiration, a syndrome in which the patient loses voluntary control of breathing, has been described (142). Respiratory failure may rarely occur as a result of bilateral diaphragmatic paralysis with or even without significant quadriparesis (143,144).

Recently several cases in which patients experienced acute relapses associated with hypothermia were reported (145). Most of the patients were severely disabled and all displayed signs during relapse of other brainstem lesions, suggesting that the hypothermia may be secondary to brainstem rather than hypothalamic involvement. Thrombocytopenia commonly accompanied the disturbed temperature regulation.

V. COURSE

The course of MS is highly variable. Lublin and Reingold, after polling many MS experts, have defined four temporal patterns (146). In most patients (80 to 85%), the disease initially follows a relapsing pattern of acute exacerbations (attacks) punctuated, usually after some improvement, by periods of stability (remissions). This form of disease, in which the baseline is stationary between attacks, is referred to as *relapsing-remitting MS*. Approximately 10 to 15% of patients never manifest acute attacks. Rather, from the onset they follow a course of steady worsening, perhaps with occasional plateaus. This type is referred to as *primary progressive MS*. A very small proportion of patients (probably fewer than 5%) start off as if they are going to have primary progressive disease. However, the course is then interrupted by discrete exacerbations. This form is thus referred to as *progressive-relapsing MS*. Of those patients presenting initially with the relapsing-remitting form of the disease, many (probably 50 to 60%), after some years, begin to steadily worsen between attacks. Some of them do continue to have discernible exacerbations, but the hallmark of this form of the disease, which is referred to as *secondary progressive MS*, is that the baseline does not remain stable, as the patient gradually deteriorates.

In usual cases, the initial attack of MS resolves completely or nearly so and the patient remains entirely well until the next discrete episode. In 1 series, more than 25% of patients relapsed within 1 year and more than 50% within 3 years (30). However, Muller found a latent phase of at least 15 years in 6% of patients followed for that period (31). According to several series, the attack rate varies from 0.1 to 0.85 per year in the early stages of the illness (30,147–151). In several recent clinical trials that selected patients experiencing recently active disease, attack rates in placebo-treated groups ranged from 0.87 to 1.3 annually (152–154). However, in most studies, the frequency of identifiable attacks appears to diminish with increasing duration of illness (30,147,155,156).

Exacerbations most often develop over hours to days. However, the onset may at times be abrupt (strokelike) and in other cases more indolent. Remission of symptoms tends to occur within weeks to a few months. Muller reported that up to 85% of patients seen within 2 months of relapse remitted completely, but the rate fell to 30% at 3 months and 10% at 6 months (31). Recent MRI studies indicate that gadolinium enhancement, currently the best imaging marker of new activity, usually disappears within 4 to 6 weeks (157). Once progression has begun, it generally continues, but at a relatively slow rate. Natural history studies by Weinshenker et al. (159) found that 50% of patients required assistance to walk by 15 years after the onset of symptoms. In one series of patients scored with the widely used Kurtzke Expanded Disability Status Scale (EDSS), those who were ambulatory when first examined worsened by 1.0 to 1.5 steps over the next 5 years (160).

Those who required assistance to walk or were wheelchair-dependent worsened 0.3 to 0.7 steps over that period. Even in progressing patients, the disease course may appear to stabilize for long periods. In one clinical trial, approximately 20% of patients selected because of their progressive course showed little or no worsening during serial examinations over the next 12 months (161). Wynn et al. (162) reported a 74% survival rate at 25 years, compared with an expected 86%, and Kurtzke et al. (163) similarly found about 75% of normal survival in that interval.

At times MS follows an extremely benign course. The patient experiences two or more attacks with complete remissions and no cumulative disability over many years (30). In Weinshenker's cohort, 10 to 20% of MS patients remained mildly affected after 25 years (159). However, most studies show only 11 to 34% of patients able to work within 15 years (30,150,164).

Unfortunately, predicting the course of MS in an individual patient is virtually impossible. Generally, patients whose initial attacks are marked by sensory symptoms have a better prognosis than those who early manifest corticospinal tract or cerebellar dysfunction (30,165,166). The course of the disease over the first 5 years provides a clue, on a statistical basis, to the subsequent progression. Thus, in a group of U.S. servicemen, nearly 90% of those with minimal disability at 5 years after onset continue to be ambulatory at 15 years. Of those with moderate disability but walking unaided at 5 years, 60% were walking independently at 15 years (167). Age of onset also influences prognosis, with patients experiencing their first symptoms after age 40 tending to follow a more rapidly progressive course.

No factors have been clearly recognized to alter the long-term course of MS. However, certain conditions may tend to precipitate acute exacerbations. Viral infection seems to trigger attacks (168,169). This may occur by stimulation of interferon gamma which, in turn, leads to increased antigen presentation precipitating the episode (169).

The role of stress, both physical and psychological, in precipitating exacerbations of MS has been controversial (170). Early reports suggested that physical trauma may lead to worsening, but in a detailed controlled study, no significant associations were found between any form of trauma and an increased frequency of attacks (171). Similarly, surgery and anaesthesia do not appear to aggravate the condition, despite earlier suggestions to the contrary (170,172). A recent review by a committee of the American Academy of Neurology concluded that physical trauma was not associated with MS exacerbation (173). However, the group found that evidence about the relationship to psychological stress was inconclusive.

Measurement of psychological stress and its role in worsening of MS has been extremely difficult. Methodological problems have included retrospective study design, which is subject to recall bias; small or highly selected samples; and inadequate psychological tests (174–177). This issue remains unresolved, although recent studies suggest that psychological stress may influence the course of MS (177). This could result from changes in the immune system associated with psychological factors. Interestingly, however, attack rate declined among Israeli MS patients during the period of SCUD missile attacks on the country in the Gulf War (178).

Sudden and transient neurological deterioration often results from situations that elevate body temperature (179). Such worsening is most often associated with febrile illness but may also occur with physical exertion. Even moderate exercise may be associated with an aggravation or precipitation of neurological symptoms, with blurring of vision most frequently reported (Uhthoff's phenomenon) (180,181). Provocation of neurological signs by raised body temperature has been the basis of a clinical tool, the "hot-bath test" (182). Although seldom performed today, this technique can be used to uncover additional anatomical lesions in monosymptomatic patients. However, a reported patient developed a persistent neurological deficit following the test (183). The basis for the neurological worsening seems to be the development of conduction block in partially demyelinated axons with elevated temperature (184).

VI. PREGNANCY

For many years pregnancy was considered to have an adverse effect on the course of MS (185). Several modern studies have reexamined this question both retrospectively (147,186–190) and prospectively (191–192). Pregnancy itself appears to be associated with a lower exacerbation rate than that in age-matched controls. However, the postpartum period, particularly the first 3 months after delivery, is accompanied by an increase in the frequency of attacks, according to most but not all reports (147,186,188,190–192). In the largest study, Confavreux et al. (193) followed 254 women with MS through 269 pregnancies in 12 European countries. Relapse rates were lower during pregnancy, most strikingly in the third trimester, when the attack rate dropped to 0.2 ± 1.0 compared with 0.7 ± 0.9 during the year before pregnancy ($p < 0.001$). However, during the first 3 months postpartum, the rate increased to 1.2 ± 2.0, significantly greater than that during the year before pregnancy ($p < 0.001$). The rate then returned to baseline. Breast-feeding did not have an adverse effect on relapse rate. These data are consistent with most but not all earlier reports. Whether the increased postpartum frequency is related to change in immunological status after pregnancy, hormonal alteration, the stress of caring for a newborn, or other factors is unknown (190,193).

No current evidence suggests a long-term negative influence of pregnancy on the disease. In fact, recent reports suggest it may convey a better prognosis (194,195).

REFERENCES

1. Acheson ED. Epidemiology of multiple sclerosis. Br Med Bull 1977; 33;9–14.
2. Kurtzke JF, Beebe GW, Norman JE. Epidemiology of multiple sclerosis in US veterans: 1. Race, sex, and geographical distribution. Neurology 1979; 29:1228–1235.
3. Charcot JM. Lectures on the Disease of the Nervous System, vol 1. London: New Sydenham Society, 1877.
4. Schumacher GA, Beebe G, Kubler RF, et al. Problems of experimental trials of therapy in multiple sclerosis: Report by the panel on the evaluation of experimental trials of therapy in multiple sclerosis. Ann NY Acad Sci 1965; 122:522–568.
5. Miller DH. Magnetic resonance in monitoring the treatment of multiple sclerosis. Ann Neurol 1994; 36(suppl):S91–S94.
6. Yahr MD, Goldensohn SS, Kabat EA. Further studies on the gamma globulin content of cerebrospinal fluid in multiple sclerosis and other neurological diseases. Ann NY Acad Sci 1954; 58:613–624.
7. Lumsden CE. The proteins of cerebrospinal fluid (continued). In: McAlpine D, Lumsden CE, Acheson ED, eds. Multiple Sclerosis: A Re-appraisal. Edinburgh: Churchill Livingstone, 1972, pp 543–548.
8. Olsson JE, Peterson B. A comparison between agar gel electrophoresis and CSF serum quotients of IgG and albumin in neurological disease. Acta Neurol Scand 1976; 53:308–322.

9. Tourtellotte WW, Ma BI. Multiple sclerosis: the blood-brain barrier and measurement of de novo central system IgG synthesis. Neurology 1978; 28:76–83.

10. Link H. Muller R. Immunoglobulins in multiple sclerosis and infections of the nervous system Arch Neurol 1971; 25:326–344.

11. Schmidt RM, Neumann V. CSF-oligoclonal bands in multiple sclerosis, In: Bauer HJ, Poser S, Ritter G, eds. Progress in Multiple Sclerosis Research. Berlin: Springer-Verlag, 1980, pp 123–128.

12. Kostulas VK, Link H. Agarose isoelectric focusing of unconcentrated CSF and radioimmunofixation for detection of oligoclonal bands in patients with multiple sclerosis and other neurological diseases. J Neurol Sci 1982; 54:117–127.

13. Ebers GC, Paty DW. CSF electrophoresis in one thousand patients. Can J Neurol Sci 1980; 7:275–280.

14. Poser CM, Paty DW, Scheinberg L, et al. New diagnostic criteria for multiple sclerosis: Guidelines for research protocols. Ann Neurol 1983; 13:227–231.

15. Filippi M, Horsefield MA, Morrissey SP, et al. Quantitative brain MRI lesion load predicts the cours of clinically isolated syndromes suggestive of multiple sclerosis. Neurology 1994; 44:635–641.

16. Paty DW, Oger JJF, Kastrukoff LF, et al. MRI in the diagnosis of MS: A prospective study with comparison of clinical evaluation, evoked potentials, oligoclonal banding, and CT. Neurology 1988; 38:180–185.

17. Offenbacher H, Fazekas F, Schmidt R, Freidl W, Flooh E, Payer F, Lechner H. Assessment of MRI criteria for a diagnosis of MS. Neurology 1993; 43:905–909.

18. Giroud M. Semama D. Pradrans L. Gouyon JB, Dumas R, Nivelon JL. Hemiballismus revealing multiple sclerosis in an infant. Childs Nerv Syst 1990; 6:236–238.

19. Brandt S. Gyldensted C, Offner H, Melchior JC. Multiple sclerosis with onset in a two-year old boy. Neuropediatrics 1981; 12:75–82.

20. Hauser SL, Bresman MJ, Reinherz EL, Weiner HL. Childhood multiple sclerosis: Clinical features and demonstration of changes in T cell subsets with disease activity. Ann Neurol 1982; 11:463–468.

21. Muller R. Course and prognosis of disseminated sclerosis in relation to age of onset. Arch Neurol Psychiatry 1951; 66:561–570.

22. Allison RS, Millar JHD. Prevalence and familiar incidence of disseminated sclerosis in Northern Island. Ulster Med 1954; 23(2):1–92.

23. Poskanzer DC, Schapira K, Miller H. Epidemiology of multiple sclerosis in the counties of Northumberland and Durham. J Neurol Neurosurg Psychiatry 1963; 26:368–376.

24. Duquette P, Murray TJ, Pleines J, et al. Multple sclerosis in childhood: clinical profile in 125 patients. J Pediatr 1987; 111:359–363.

25. Noseworthy J, Paty D, Wonnacott T, Feasby T, Ebers G. Multiple sclerosis after age 50. Neurology 1983; 33:37–44.

26. Cazzulo GL, Ghezzi A, Marforio S, Caputo D. Clinical picture of multiple sclerosis with late onset. Acta Neurol Scand 1978; 58:190–196.

27. Leibowitz U, Alter M, Halper L. Clinical studies of multiple sclerosis in Israel: III. Clinical course and prognosis related to age. Neurology 1964; 14:926–932.

28. Shepherd DI. Clinical features of multiple sclerosis in north-east Scotland. Acta Neurol Scand 1979; 60:218–230.

29. Friedman AP, Davison C. Multiple sclerosis with late onset of symptoms. Arch Neurol Psychiatry 1945; 54:348–360.

30. McAlpine D. Symptoms and signs. In: McAlpine D, Lumsden CE, Acheson Ed, eds. Multiple Sclerosis: A Reappraisal. Baltimore: Williams & Wilkins, 1972, pp 132–196.

31. Muller R. Studies on disseminated sclerosis with special reference to symptomatology, course and prognosis. Acta Med Scand Suppl 1949; 222:1–214.

32. Adams DK, Sutherland JM. Early clinical manifestations of disseminated sclerosis. BMJ 1950; 2:431–436.

33. Kurtzke JF. Clinical manifestations of multiple sclerosis. In: Vinken PJ, Bruyn GW, eds. Handbook of Clinical Neurology, vol 9. Multiple Sclerosis and Other Demylinating Diseases. Amsterdam: North Holland, 1970, pp 161–216.

34. Scheinberg LC, Geisser BS. Drug therapy in multiple sclerosis. In: Scheinberg LC, Holland NJ, eds. Multiple Sclerosis: A Guide for Patients and Their Families, 2nd ed. New York: Raven Press, 1987, pp 53–66.

35. Matthews WP. Symptoms and signs. In: Matthews WB, Acheson ED, Bachelor JR, Weller RO, eds. McAlpine's Multiple Sclerosis. Edinburgh: Churchill Livingstone, 1985, pp 98–116.

36. Clifford DB, Trotter JL. Pain in multiple sclerosis. Arch Neurol 1984; 41:1270–1272.

37. Moulin DE, Foley KM, Ebers GC. Pain syndromes in multiple sclerosis. Neurology 1988; 38:1830–1834.

38. Lumsden CE. The neuropathology of multiple sclerosis. In: Vinken PJ, Bruyn GW, eds. Handbook of Clinical Neurology, vol 9. Multiple sclerosis and other demyelinating diseases. Amsterdam: North Holland, 1970, pp 217–309.

39. Cowan J. Ormerod IE, Rudge P. Hemiparetic multiple sclerosis. J Neurol Neurosurg Psychiatry 1990; 53:675–680.

40. Mathews WB. Tonic seizures in disseminated sclerosis. Brain 1958; 81:193–206.

41. Lhermitte J, Bollak P, Nichas M. Les douleurs a type de decharge electrique consecutives a la fexion cephalique dans la sclerose en plaques. Rev Neurol 1924; 42:56–62.

42. Kanchandani R, Howe JG. Lhermitte's sign in multiple sclerosis: A clinical survey and review of the literature. J Neurol Neurosurg Psychiatry 1982; 45:308–312.

43. Ramirez-Lassepas M. Tullock JW, Quinones MR, Snyder BJ. Acute radicular pain as a presenting symptom in multiple sclerosis. Arch Neurol 1992; 49:255–258.

44. Cosman F, Nieves J, Komar L, Ferrer G, Herbert J, Formica C, Shen V, Lindsay R. Fracture history and bone loss in patients with multiple sclerosis. Neurology 1998; 51:1161–1165.

45. Nieves J, Cosman F, Herbert J, Shen V, Lindsay R. High prevalence of vitamin D deficiency and reduced bone mass in multiple sclerosis. Neurology 1994; 44:1687–1692.

46. Schwid SR, Goodman AD, Puzas JE, McDermott MP, Mattson DH. Sporadic corticosteroid pulses and osteoporosis in multiple sclerosis. Arch Neurol 1996; 53:753–757.

47. Haas DC, Kent PF, Freidman DL. Headache caused by a single lesion of multiple sclerosis in the periaqueductal gray area. Headache 1993; 33:452–455.

48. Galer BS, Lipton RB, Weinstein S, Bello L., Solomon S. Apoplectic headache and oculomotor palsy: an unusual presentation of multiple sclerosis. Neurology 1990: 40:1465–1455.

49. Wilson SAK. Case of disseminated sclerosis with weakness of each internal rectus and nystagmus on lateral deviation limited to the outer eye. Brain 1906; 29:298.

50. Bender MB, Weinstein EA. Dissociated monocular nystagmus with paresis of horizontal ocular movements. Arch Ophthalmol 1939; 21:266–272.

51. Cogan DG. Internuclear ophthalmopegia, typical and atypical. Arch Ophthalmol 1970; 84:583–589.

52. Muri R, Meienberg O. The clinical spectrum of internuclear ophthalmoplegia in multiple sclerosis. Arch Neurol 1985; 42:851–855.

53. Joseph R, Pullicino P, Goldberg CDS, Rose FC. Bilateral pontine gaze palsy. Arch Neurol 1985; 42:93–94.

54. Slyman JF, Kline LB. Dorsal midbrain syndrome in multiple sclerosis. Neurology 1981; 31:196–198.

55. Quint DJ, Cornblath WT, Trobe JD. Multiple sclerosis presenting as Parinaud syndrome. Am J Neuroradiol 1993; 14:1200–1202.

56. Fisher CM. Some neuro-ophthalmological observations. J Neurol Neurosurg Psychiatry 1967; 30:383–392.

57. Wall M, Wray SH. The one-and-a-half syndrome—A unilateral disorder of the pontine tegmentum: A study of 20 cases and review of the literature. Neurology 1983; 33:971–980.

58. Keane JR. Alternating skew deviation: 47 patients. Neurology 1985; 35:725–728.

59. Dailey FL, Brown JR, Goldstein FJ. Dysarthria in multiple sclerosis. Speech Hear Res 1972; 15:229–245.

60. Miller AE. Cessation of stuttering with progressive multiple sclerosis. Neurology 1985; 35: 1341–1343.

61. Ivers RR, Goldstein NP. Multiple sclerosis: a current appraisal of symptoms and signs. Mayo Clin Proc 1963; 338:457–466.

62. Jankovic J. Patel SC. Blepharospasm associated with brainstem lesions. Neurology 1983; 33:1237–1240.

63. Andermann F, Cosgrove JBR, Lloyd-Smith DL, Gloor P, McNaughton FL. Facial myokymia in multiple sclerosis Brain 1961; 84:31–44.

64. Matthews WB. Facial myokymia. J Neurol Neurosurg Psychiatry 1966; 29:35–39.

65. Daugherty WT, Lederman RJ, Nodar RH, Conomy JP. Hearing loss in multiple sclerosis. Arch Neurol 1983: 40:33–35.

66. Drulovic B, Ribaric-Jankes K, Kostic V, Sternic N. Sudden hearing loss as the initial mon- symptom of multiple sclerosis. Neurology 1993; 43:2703–2705.

67. Sasaki O, Ootsuka K, Taguchi K, Kikukawa M. Multiple sclerosis presented acute hearing loss and vertigo. J Otorhinolaryngol Rel Spec 1994; 56:55–59.

68. Tabira T, Tsuji S, Nagashima T, Nakajima T, Kuroiwa Y. Cortical deafness in multiple sclerosis. J Neurol Neurosurg Psychiatry 1981; 44:433–436.

69. Cure JK, Cromwell D, Case JL, Johnson GD, Musiek FE. Auditory dysfunction caused by multiple sclerosis: Detection with MR imaging. Am J Neuroradiol 1990; 11:817–820.

70. Birkhead R, Friedman HJ. Hiccups and vomiting as initial manifestations of multiple sclero- sis. J Neurol Neurosurg Psychiatry 1987; 50:232–233.

71. McFarlin DA, Susac JO. Hoquet diabolique: intractable hiccups as a manifestation of multiple sclerosis. Neurology 1979; 29:797–801.

72. Perkin GD, Rose FC. Optic Neuritis and Its Differential Diagnosis. Oxford: Oxford Univer- sity Press, 1979.

73. Slamovits TL, Rosen CE, Cheng KP, Striph GG. Visual recovery in patients with optic neuri- tis and visual loss to no light perception. Am J Ophthalmol 1991; 111:209–214.

74. Steinmetz R, Kearns TP, H-R-R pseudoisochromatic plates as a diagnostic aid in retrobulbar neuritis of multiple sclerosis. Am J Ophthalmol 1956; 41:833–837.

75. Stanley JA, Baise G. The swinging flashlight test to detect minimal optic neuropathy. Arch Ophthalmol 1968; 80:769–771.

76. Halliday AM, McDonald WI, Mushin J. Delayed visual evoked response in optic neuritis. Lancet 1972; 1:982–985.

77. Lowitzsch K. Pattern-evoked visual potentials in 251 multiple sclerosis patients in relation to ophthalmological findings and diagnostic classification. In: Bauer HJ, Poser S, Ritter G, eds. Progress in Multiple Sclerosis Research. Berlin: Springer Verlag, 1980, pp. 571–577.

78. Sanchez-Dalmau B, Goni FJ, Gurro M, Ruig C, Duch-Bordas F. Bilateral homonymous visual field defects as initial manifestation of multiple sclerosis. Br J Ophthalmol 1991; 75: 185–187.

79. Slavin ML. Acute homonymous field loss: Really a diagnostic dilemma Surv Ophthalmol 1990; 34:399–407.

80. Frederiksen JL, Larsson HB, Nordenho AM, Seedorff HH. Plaques causing hemianopsia or quadrantanopsia in multiple sclerosis identified by MRI and VEP. Acta Ophthalmol 1991; 69:169–177.

81. Wender M. Szmeja Z. Examination of vestibular system function, taste and olfactory systems in patients with disseminated sclerosis. Neurol Neurochir Pol 1971; 21:179–184.

82. Matthews WB. Symptoms and signs. In: Matthews WB, Acheson ED, Batchelor JR, Weller RO, eds. McAlpine's Multiple Sclerosis. Edinburgh: Churchill Livingstone, 1985:119–145.

83. Doty RL, Li C, Mannon LJ, Youssam DM. Olfactory dysfunction in multiple sclerosis. N Engl J Med 1997; 336:1918–1919.

84. Hawkes CM, Shephard BC, Kobal G. Assessment of olfaction in multiple sclerosis: Evidence of dysfunction by olfactory evoked response and identification tests. J Neurol Neurosurg Psychiatry 1997; 63:145–151.

85. Cohen L. Disturbance of taste as a symptom of multiple sclerosis. Br J Oral Surg 1965; 2: 184–185.

86. Pascual-Leone A, Altafullah I, Dhura A. Hemiageusia: An unusual presentation of multiple sclerosis. J Neurol Neurosurg Psychiatry 1991; 54:657.

87. Harris W. Rare forms of paroxysmal trigeminal neuralgia, and their relation to disseminated sclerosis. BMJ 1950; 2:1015.

88. Rao SM, Hammeke TA, McQuillen MP, Khatri BO, Lloyd D. Memory disturbance in chronic progressive multiple sclerosis. Arch Neurol 1984; 41:625–631.

89. Peyser JM, Edward KR, Poser CM, Filskov SB. Cognitive function in patients with multiple sclerosis. Arch Neurol 1980; 37:577–579.

90. Beatty WW. Cognitive and emotional disturbances in multiple sclerosis. Neurol Clin 1993; 11:189–204.

91. Hamalainen P, Ruutiainen J. Cognitive decline in multiple sclerosis. Int Mult Scler J 1999; 6:51–57.

92. Huber SJ, Paulson GW, Shuttleworth EC, et al. Magnetic resonance imaging correlates of dementia in multiple sclerosis. Arch Neurol 1987; 44:732–736.

93. Franklin GM, Heaton RK, Nelson LM, Filley CM, Seibert C. Correlation of neuropsychological and MRI findings in chronic/progressive multiple sclerosis. Neurology 1988; 38:1826–1829.

94. Olmos-Lau N, Ginsberg MD, Geller JB. Aphasia in multiple sclerosis. Neurology 1977; 27: 623–626.

95. Friedman JH, Brem H, Mayeux R. Global aphasia in multiple sclerosis. Ann Neurol 1983; 13:222–223.

96. Achiron A, Ziv I, Djaldetti R, Goldberg H, Kuritzky A, Melamed E. Aphasia in multiple sclerosis: Clinical and radiologic correlations. Neurology 1992; 42:2195–2197.

97. Graff-Radford NR, Rizzo M. Neglect in a patient with multiple sclerosis. Eur Neurol 1987; 26:100–103.

98. Cottrell SS, Wilson SAK. The affective symptomatology of disseminated sclerosis. J Neurol Psychopathol 1926; 7:1–30.

99. Whitlock FA. Siskind MM. Depression as a major symptom of multiple sclerosis. J Neurol Neurosurg Psychiatry 1980; 43:861–865.

100. Baretz RM, Stephenson GR. Emotional responses to multiple sclerosis. Psychosomatics 1981; 22:117–127.

101. Schiffer RB. The spectrum of depression in multiple sclerosis: an approach for clinical management. Arch Neurol 1987; 44:596–599.

102. Schiffer RB, Herndon RM, Rudick RA. Treatment of pathologic laughing and weeping with amitriptyline. N Engl J Med 1985; 312:1480–1482.

103. Honer WG, Hurwitz, Li DKB, et al. Temporal lobe involvement in multiple sclerosis patients with psychiatric disorders. Arch Neurol 1987; 44:187–190.

104. Feinstein A, duBoulay G, Ron MA. Psychotic illness in multiple sclerosis: A clinical and magnetic resonance imaging study. Br J Psychiatry 1992; 161:680–685.

105. Murray TJ. Amantadine therapy for fatigue in multiple sclerosis. Can J Neurol Sci 1985; 12:251–254.

106. Freal JE, Kraft GH, Coryell SK. Symptomatic fatigue in multiple sclerosis. Arch Phy Med Rehabil 1984; 65:135–138.

107. Krupp L, La Rocca NG, Muir-Nash J, Steinberg AD. Fatigue severity scale. Neurology 1988; 38(1):99–100.

108. Clark CM, Fleming JA, Li D, Oger J, Klonoff H, Paty D. Sleep disturbances, depression, and lesion site in patients with multiple sclerosis. Arch Neurol 1992; 49:641–643.

109. Miller H. Simpson CA, Yeates WK. Bladder dysfunction in multiple sclerosis. BMJ 1965; 1:1265–1269.

110. Blaivas JG. Management of bladder dysfunction in multiple sclerosis. Neurology 1980; 30: 12–18.

111. Blaivas JG. Holland NJ, Geisser B, LaRocca N, Madonna M, Scheinberg L. Multiple sclerosis bladder: Studies and care. Ann NY Acad Sci 1984; 436:328–346.

112. Strauss BS, Blaufox MD. Estimation of residual urine and urine flow rate without urethral catheterization. J Nucl Med 1970; 11:81–85.

113. Blaivas JG, Barbalias GA. Detrusor-external sphincter dyssynergia in men with multiple sclerosis: An ominous urologic condition. J Urol 1984; 131:91–94.

114. Hinds JP, Eidelman BH, Wald A. Prevalence of bowel dysfunction in multiple sclerosis: a population survey. Gastroenterology 1990; 98:1538–1542.

115. Sullivan SN, Ebers GC. Gastrointestinal dysfunction in multiple sclerosis (letter). Gastroenterology 1982; 84:1640.

116. Fowler CJ, Henry MM. Gastrointestinal dysfunction in multiple sclerosis. Int Mult Scler J 1999; 6:59–61.

117. Chia YW, Fowler C, Kamm M et al. Prevalence of bowel dysfunction in patients with multiple sclerosis and bladder dysfunction. J Neurol 1995; 242:105–108.

118. Nordenbo A, Andersen J, Andersen J. Disturbances of ano-rectal function in multiple sclerosis. J Neurol 1996; 243:445–451.

119. Vas CJ. Sexual impotence and some autonomic disturbances in men with multiple sclerosis. Acta Neurol Scand 1969; 45:166–183.

120. Lundberg PO. Sexual dysfunction in female patients with multiple sclerosis. Int Rehabil Med 1981; 3:32–34.

121. Joynt RJ. Green D. Tonic seizures as a manifestation of multiple sclerosis. Arch Neurol 1962; 6:293–299.

122. Twomey JA, Espir MLE. Paroxysmal symptoms as the first manifestations of multiple sclerosis. J Neurol Neurosurg Psychiatry 1980; 43:296–304.

123. Heath PD, Nightingale S. Clusters of tonic spasms as an initial manifestation of multiple sclerosis. Ann Neurol 1986; 12:494–495.

124. Berger JR, Sheremata WA, Melamed E. Paroxysmal dystonia as the initial manifestation of multiple sclerosis. Arch Neurol 1984; 41:747–750.

125. Osterman PO, Westerberg CE. Paroxysmal attacks in multiple sclerosis. Brain 1975; 98: 189–202.

126. Maimone D, Reder AT, Finocchiaro F, Recuper E. Internal capsule plaque and tonic spasms in multiple sclerosis. Arch Neurol 1991; 48:427–429.

127. Burguera JA, Catala J, Casanova B. Thalamic demyelination and paroxysmal dystonia in multiple sclerosis. Mov Disord 1991; 6:379–381.

128. Rose MR, Ball JA, Thompson PD. Magnetic resonance imaging in tonic spasms of multiple sclerosis. J Neurol 1993; 241:115–117.

129. Uncini A, DiMuzio A, Thomas A, Lugaresi A, Gambi D. Hand dystonia secondary to cervical demyelinating lesion. Acta Neurol Scand 1994; 90:51–55.

130. Espir MLE, Watkins MS, Smith HV. Paroxysmal dysarthria and other transient neurological disturbances in disseminated sclerosis. J Neurol Neurosurg Psychiatry 1966; 29:323–330.

131. Anderman F, Cosgrove JBR, Lloyd-Smith D, Walters AM. Paroxysmal dysarthria and ataxia in multiple sclerosis. Neurology 1959; 9:211–215.

132. Yamamoto M, Yabuki SK, Hayabara T, Otsuki S. Paroxysmal itching in multiple sclerosis: A report of three cases. J Neurol Neurosurg Psychiatry 1981; 44:19–22.

133. Telischi FF, Grobman LR, Sheremata WA, Apple M, Ayyar R. Hemifacial spasm occurring in multiple sclerosis. Arch Otolaryngol Head Neck Surg 1991; 117:554–556.

134. Brisman R. Trigeminal neuralgia in multiple sclerosis. Arch Neurol 1987; 44:379–381.

135. Rozza L, Bortolotti P, Sica A, Wereonig S, Orrico D. Kinesigenic dystonia as the first mani-

festation of multiple sclerosis with cervical and brainstem lesions. Eur Neurol 1993; 34:331–332.

136. Roos RA, Wintzen AR, Vielvoye G, Polder TW. Paroxysmal kinesigenic choreoathetosis as presenting symptom of multiple sclerosis. J Neurol Neurosurg Psychiatry 1991; 54:657–658.

137. Kapoor R, Brown P, Thompson PD, Miller DH. Propriospinal myoclonus in multiple sclerosis. J Neurol Neurosurg Psychiatry 1992; 55:1086–1088.

138. D'Costa DF, Vania AK, Millac Pa. Multiple sclerosis associated with trismus. Postgrad Med J 1990; 66:853–854.

139. Scolding NJ, Lees AJ. Micrographia associated with a parietal lobe lesion in multiple sclerosis. J Neurol Neurosurg Psychiatry 1994; 57:739–741.

140. Noronha MJ, Vas CJ, Aziz H. Autonomic dysfunction (sweating responses) in multiple sclerosis. J Neurol Neurosurg Psychiatry 1968; 31:19–22.

141. Cartlidge NEF. Autonomic function in multiple sclerosis. Brain 1972; 95:661–664.

142. Newsom-Davis J. Autonomous breathing. Arch Neurol 1974; 30:480–483.

143. Kuwahira I, Kondo T, Ohta Y, Yamabayashi H. Acute respiratory failure in multiple sclerosis. Chest 1990; 97:246–248.

144. Aisen M, Arlt G, Foster S. Diaphragmatic paralysis without bulbar or limb paralysis in multiple sclerosis. Chest 1990; 98:499–501.

145. White KD, Scoones DJ, Newman PK. Hypothermia in multiple sclerosis. J Neurol Neurosurg Psychiatry 1996; 61:369–375.

146. Lublin FD, Reingold SC. Defining the clinical course of multiple sclerosis: Results of an international survey. Neurology 1996; 46:907–911.

147. Millar JHD, Allison RS, Cheeseman EA, Merrett JD. Pregnancy as a factor influencing relapse in disseminated sclerosis. Brain 1959; 82:417–426.

148. Gudmundsson KR. Clinical studies of multiple sclerosis in Iceland. Acta Neurol Scand Suppl 1971; 48:1–78.

149. Leibowitz U, Alter M. Multiple Sclerosis: Clues to Its Cause. Amsterdam: North Holland, 1973.

150. Confavreux C, Aimard G, Devic M. Course and prognosis of multiple sclerosis assessed by the computerized data processing of 349 patients. Brain 1980; 103:281–300.

151. Alexander L. Berkeley AW, Alexander AM. Prognosis and treatment of multiple sclerosis: Quantitative nosometric study JAMA 1958; 166:1943–1949.

152. Interferon beta-1b Multiple Sclerosis Study Group. Interferon beta 1b is effective in relapsing-remitting multiple sclerosis: I. Clinical results of a multicenter, randomized, double-blind, placebo-controlled trial. Neurology 1993; 43:655–661.

153. Jacobs LD, Cookfair DL, Rudick RA, et al. Intramuscular interferon beta-1a for disease progression in relapsing multiple sclerosis. Ann Neurol 1996; 39:285–294.

154. Johnson KP, Brooks BR, Cohen JA, et al. Copolymer 1 reduces the relapse rate and improves disability in relapsing-remitting multiple sclerosis: Results of phase III multicenter, double-bind, placebo-controlled trial. Neurology 1995; 445:1268–1276.

155. Broman T, Anderson O, Bergmann L. Clinical studies on multiple sclerosis: I. Presentation of an incidence material from Gothenberg. Acta Neurol Scand 1981; 63:6–33.

156. Lhermitte F, Marteau RK, Gazengel J, Dordain G, Deloche G. The frequency of relapse in multiple sclerosis: A study based on 245 cases. J Neurol 1973; 205:47–59.

157. Smith ME, Stone LA, Albert PS, et al. Clinical worsening in multiple sclerosis is associated with increased frequency and area of gadopentetate dimeglumine-enhancing magnetic resonance lesions. Ann Neurol 1993; 33:480–489.

158. Panelius M. Studies on epidemiological, clinical and etiological aspects of multiple sclerosis. Acta Neurol Scand Suppl 1969; 39:1–82.

159. Weinshenker BG, Bass B, Rice GPB, et al. The natural history of multiple sclerosis: a geographically-based study. 1. Clinical course and disability. Brain 1989; 112:133–146.

160. Sibley WA. Therapeutic Claims in Multiple Sclerosis 2nd ed. New York: Demos, 1988.

161. Miller A, Drexler E, Keilson M, et al. Spontaneous stabilization in patients with chronic progressive MS. Neurology 1988; 38(supp 1):194.

162. Wynn DR, Rodriquez M, O'Fallon WM, Kurland LT. A reappraisal of the epidemiology of multiple sclerosis in Olmsted County, Minnesota. Neurology 1990; 40:780–786.

163. Kurtzke JF, Beebe GW, Nagler B, Nefzger MD, Auth TL, Kurland LT. Studies on the natural history of multiple sclerosis: 5. Long-term survival in young men. Arch Neurol 1970; 22: 215–225.

164. Bauer HJ, Firnhaber W. Zur leistungsprofnose Multiple Sklerose-kranker. Dtsch Med Wochenschr 1963; 88:1357–1364.

165. Kraft GH, Freal JE, Coryell JK, Hanana CL, Chitnis N. Multiple sclerosis: Early prognostic guideline. Arch Phys Med Rehabil 1981; 62:54–58.

166. Bonduelle M. Les formes benignes de la sclerose en plaques. Presse Med 1967; 75:2023–2026.

167. Kurtzke JF, Beebe GW, Nagler B, Kurland LT, Auth TL. Studies on the natural history of multiple sclerosis: 8. Early prognostic features of the later course of the illness. J Chronic Dis 1977; 30:819–830.

168. Sibley WA, Bamford CR, Clark K. Clinical viral infections in multiple sclerosis. Lancet 1985; 1:313–315.

169. Panitch HS. Influence of infection on exacerbations of multiple sclerosis. Ann Neurol 1994; 36:S25–S28.

170. McAlpine D, Compston ND. Some aspects of the natural history of disseminated sclerosis. Q J Med 1952; 21:135–167.

171. Banford CR, Sibley WA, Thies C, Laguna JF, Smith MS, Clark K. Trauma as an etiologic and aggravating factor in multiple sclerosis. Neurology 1981; 31:1229–1234.

172. Ridley A, Schapira K. Influence of surgical procedures on the course of multiple sclerosis. Neurology 1961; 11:81–82.

173. Goodin DS, Ebers GC, Johnson KP, Rodriguez M, Sibley WA, Wolinsky JS. The relationship of MS to physical trauma and psychological stress: Report of the Therapeutics and Technology Assessment Subcommittee of the American Academy of Neurology. Neurology 1999; 52:1737–1745.

174. Braceland FJ, Griffin ME. The mental changes associated with multiple sclerosis (an interim report). Res Publ Assoc Res Nerv Ment Dis 1950; 28:450–455.

175. Pratt RTC. An investigation of the psychiatric aspects of disseminated sclerosis. J Neurol Neurosurg Psychiatry 1951; 14:326–332.

176. Alter M. Antonovsky AK, Leibowitz U. Epidemiology of multiple sclerosis in Israel. In: Alter M, Kurtzke J, eds. The Epidemiology of Multiple Sclerosis. Springfield IL: Charles C Thomas 1968, pp 83–109.

177. Franklin GM, Nelson LM, Heaton RK, Burks JS, Thompson DS. Stress and its relationship to acute exacerbations in multiple sclerosis. J Neurol Rehabil 1988; 2:7–11.

178. Nispeanu P, Korczyn A. psychological stress as risk factor for exacerbations in multiple sclerosis. Neurology 1993; 43:1311–1312.

179. Nelson DA, McDowell F. The effects of induced hyperthermia on patients with multiple sclerosis. J. Neurol Neurosurg Psychiatry 1959; 22:113–116.

180. Uhthoff W. Untersuchungen uber die bei der multiplen Herdsklerose vorkommenden Augenstorungen. Arch Psychiatr Nevenkr 1889; 20:55.

181. Goldstein JE, Cogan DG. Exercise and the optic neuropathy of multiple sclerosis. Arch Ophthalmol 1964; 72:168–170.

182. Nelson DA, Jeffreys WH, McDowell F. Effects of induced hyperthermia on some neurological diseases. Arch Neurol Psychiatry 1958; 79:31–39.

183. Berger JR, Sheremata WA. Persistent neurological deficits precipitated by the hot bath test in multiple sclerosis. JAMA 1983; 249:1751–1753.

184. Rasminsky M. The effects of temperature on conduction in demyelinated single nerve fibers. Arch Neurol 1973; 28:287–292.

185. Tilman JB. The effect of pregnancy on multiple sclerosis and its management. Res Publ Assoc Res Nerv Ment Dis 1950; 28:548–582.

186. Korn-Lubetzki I, Kahana E, Cooper G, Abramsky O. Activity of multiple sclerosis during pregnancy and puerperium. Ann Neurol 1984; 15:229–231.

187. Thomason DS, Nelson LM, Burns A, Burks JS, Franklin GM. The effects of pregnancy in multiple sclerosis: A retrospective study. Neurology 1986; 36:1097–1099.

188. Frith JA, McLeod JG. Pregnancy and multiple sclerosis. J. Neurol Neurosurg Psychiatry 1988; 51:495–498.

189. Leibowitz U, Antonovsky A, Kats R, Alter M. Does pregnancy increase the risk of multiple sclerosis? J Neurol Neurosurg Psychiatry 1967; 30:354–357.

190. Birk K, Rudick R. Pregnancy and multiple sclerosis. Arch Neurol 1986; 43:719–725.

191. Birk K, Smeltzer SK, Ford C, Miller R, Rudick R. The effect of pregnancy in multiple sclerosis. Neurology 1988; 38(suppl 1):237.

192. Sadovnick AD, Eisen K, Hashimoto SA, et al. Pregnancy and multiple sclerosis: A prospective study. Arch Neurol 1994; 51:1120–1124.

193. Confavreux C, Hutchinson M, Hours MM, Cortinovis-Tourniaire P, Moreau T, and the Pregnancy in Multiple Sclerosis Group: Rate of pregnancy-related relapse in multiple sclerosis. N Engl J Med 1998; 339:285–291.

194. Runmarker B, Anderson O. Pregnancy is associated with a lower risk of onset and a better prognosis in multiple sclerosis. Brain 1995; 118:253–261.

195. Berdru P, Theys P, D'Hooghe MB et al. Pregnancy in multiple sclerosis: The influence on long-term disability. Clin Neurol Neurosurg 1994; 96:38–41.

10

Cognitive Impairment in Multiple Sclerosis

JILL S. FISCHER

Mellen Center for MS Treatment and Research, Cleveland Clinic Foundation, Cleveland, Ohio

I. INTRODUCTION

During the last decade, clinicians have become increasingly aware of the prevalence of MS-related cognitive impairment and its potentially devastating impact on patients' everyday function. In previous editions of this handbook, cognitive manifestations of MS were briefly covered in the chapter on clinical features. Due to the burgeoning literature on cognitive impairment in MS, it now merits a chapter of its own. This chapter covers the characteristics and course of MS-related cognitive impairment, its clinical and neuroradiological correlates, treatments for MS-related cognitive impairment, and management of cognitively impaired MS patients in clinical practice.

II. PREVALENCE

Historically, clinicians have underestimated the prevalence of MS-related cognitive impairment (1). Two related factors may account for this: (a) MS-related cognitive impairment is often difficult to detect in brief office visits and (b) the prevailing belief for years was that cognitive impairment occurred rarely in MS, and then only in advanced disease. However, data from two large-scale controlled studies challenge this belief (2,3). Nearly half of all MS patients perform more poorly on neuropsychological (NP) testing than do demographically matched healthy controls [43% of a community-based sample (3) and 44% of a clinic-based sample (2) after adjusting for impairment rates in controls]. The similarity in these two prevalence estimates is striking given the differences in patient mix, measures administered, and methods used to define cognitive impairment between

233

the studies. Clearly, cognitive impairment is one of the more common disease manifestations in MS.

III. FUNCTIONAL IMPACT

MS-related cognitive impairment can have striking effects on patients' everyday functioning. For example, cognitive impairment significantly affects the ability to maintain employment (4,5): in one study, cognitively impaired MS patients were three times less likely to be employed than cognitively intact patients with comparable physical disability (6). Cognitive impairment also influences a patient's independence in carrying out daily activities, potentially compounding the limitations imposed by physical impairment (4,7,8). For example, cognitively impaired patients need more assistance than cognitively intact patients to carry out basic activities of daily living as well as to perform more complex household tasks, such as cooking (4). Clinical experience suggests that cognitively impaired MS patients have difficulty following complex multistep procedures (including treatment regimens), are more accident-prone (both at home and while driving), and often need assistance in making sound decisions and managing their finances. Cognitive impairment can also limit a patient's capacity to benefit from inpatient rehabilitation (9). Finally, cognitive impairment can disrupt interpersonal relationships. Cognitively impaired MS patients are perceived by others as more confused and less emotionally stable, and they tend to engage in fewer social activities than cognitively intact patients (4). Thus, cognitive impairment is a significant, although underrecognized, contributor to functional disability in MS.

IV. CHARACTERISTICS AND PATTERNS

The nature of MS-related cognitive impairment can make it difficult for the clinician to detect. It is typically circumscribed (i.e., confined to specific cognitive domains) rather than global. Furthermore, pronounced deficits in language and visual perception that might be readily apparent during an office visit occur rarely. Table 1 gives an overview of the frequency of significant impairment in different domains of cognitive function. Pertinent research in each of these domains is summarized below.

A. Impact of MS on Specific Cognitive Domains

Memory

MS patients often complain of memory problems. Consequently, it is not surprising that memory impairment has been the most thoroughly investigated cognitive deficit in MS. *Memory* is a very broad term that is often used imprecisely. For example, patients may refer to problems with ''short-term memory,'' by which they mean memory for recent events and conversations as opposed to memory for the more distant past. However, the term *short-term memory* has quite a different meaning in memory research. Consequently, it is preferable in speaking with patients to refer to difficulty remembering recent events and conversations as problems with *recent memory* and to difficulty remembering information and events from the distant past as *remote memory*.

Most studies of MS-related memory impairment have used standard clinical measures, on which the patient is asked to learn new verbal or visual material and then recall or recognize it after a delay. These measures assess *explicit memory* (i.e., memory for

Table 1 Features of MS-Related Cognitive Impairment

Domain of cognitive function	Prevalence of severe impairment[a]
Most commonly impaired	
Episodic memory	22–31%
Complex attention/processing speed	22–25%
Verbal fluency	22%
Impaired moderately often	
Executive functions	13–19%
Visual perception	12–19%
Less frequently impaired	
Language/semantic memory	8–10%
Attention span	7–8%

[a] Severe impairment = performance below the fifth percentile of demographically matched healthy controls. Ranges reflect the prevalence of severe impairment across multiple measures within a domain. These values do not include patients with milder forms of impairment.
Source: From Ref. 3.

material that a person is explicitly instructed to learn), specifically a form of explicit memory known as *episodic memory* (i.e., memory for events and conversations). As a group, MS patients are impaired in their ability to explicitly learn and subsequently recall new material, regardless of whether the material is verbal or visual (7,10–19). Recognition memory may also be impaired, but these deficits are typically less pronounced than deficits in free and cued recall (20–22)

Some investigators have suggested that MS preferentially disrupts retrieval as opposed to encoding and storage processes (15,23). The "retrieval hypothesis" has been challenged by several recent observations, however: (a) delayed recall is intact if MS patients are allowed additional trials to learn material to a level comparable to that of controls (24,25); (b) MS patients are less likely than controls to spontaneously apply systematic learning strategies, such as semantic clustering (26) or visual imagery (27); and (c) MS patients' performance across trials on multitrial learning tasks is less consistent than that of controls (28,29). Thus, MS can disrupt both acquisition (i.e., encoding and storage) and retrieval processes.

Another aspect of explicit memory involves remembering previously acquired knowledge, such as words or facts (*semantic memory*). MS patients often complain bitterly about word-finding problems. Deficits in the recall of names of objects (*confrontation naming*) (12,30), famous people and events (12,31), facts learned through formal education (3), and even personal facts (31) have all been reported, but these are rare in patients with relapsing disease (14,18). Phonemic cuing often facilitates retrieval in MS patients, suggesting that the structure of semantic knowledge is preserved (unlike the case in Alzheimer's disease). In contrast, *semantic fluency* (i.e., rapid generation of words that fit into a specific category) and *phonemic fluency* (i.e., speeded production of words beginning with a specific letter) are often impaired in MS, regardless of disease course (12,14,15,18). However, successful performance on verbal fluency tasks requires not only efficient access to semantic memory but also rapid information processing, which is often impaired in MS (see "Attention/Information Processing," below).

Unlike explicit memory, implicit memory is relatively spared in MS. *Implicit memory* refers to learning and remembering without conscious awareness and is demonstrated through a change in task performance or behavior. Thus, MS patients perform comparably to controls on lexical, semantic, and perceptual *priming* tasks, which assess memory for words encountered during the performance of other tasks (23,32,33). *Skill learning* (also termed *procedural memory*) is also reasonably intact in MS patients, as evidenced by performance comparable to that of controls on pursuit rotor (33), serial visual reaction time (23), and mirror-reading tasks (23). Thus, exclusive reliance on traditional clinical measures of memory, which tap explicit memory, may lead to underestimation of an MS patient's ability to acquire knowledge and skills via an intact implicit memory system. Table 2 summarizes how MS affects these various memory processes.

Attention/Information Processing

Many MS patients report that they feel "slowed down" mentally, noting that they have difficulty thinking quickly or keeping up with conversations. Deficits in information processing speed are well documented in studies of MS patients (12,14,19,24,25,34–39) and have been observed in patients with clinically isolated lesions as well (40). Impaired transfer of information between cerebral hemispheres has also been documented, using a variety of specialized interhemispheric transfer tasks (41–44). Some investigators have likened the generalized slowing of information processing speed in MS to that seen in normal aging, conceptualizing it in terms of a reduced "signal-to-noise" ratio resulting from a weakened neural signal, more background noise, or both (45).

In addition to feeling slowed down, MS patients often describe problems related to attention. For example, they report that they must exert more mental effort on tasks that

Table 2 Overview of Intact and Impaired Processes in MS Within Key Cognitive Domains

Domain	Often impaired	Usually intact
Memory	Episodic memory	
		Semantic memory[a]
		Autobiographical memory (events)
		Implicit memory
		Priming
		Skill learning
Attention/ Information processing	Processing speed	
		Attention span[a]
	Selective attention[b]	
	Alternating attention	
	Divided attention	
Executive functions	Abstract reasoning	
	Problem-solving	
	Planning/sequencing	
	Temporal ordering	
	Frequency monitoring	
	Cognitive estimation	

[a] Depends on patient sample.
[b] Depends on task demands.

they previously performed automatically, have difficulty "filtering out" distractions, and can no longer do two things concurrently. Like memory, *attention* is a very broad term, which is used to refer to anything from simple attention span (i.e., focusing attention for a few seconds) to divided attention (i.e., processing and responding simultaneously to multiple stimuli). To complicate matters further, the research literature often refers to attention span as *primary memory* and to complex attentional processes as *working memory*. Attention can be conceptualized as a hierarchy of processes ranging from *attention span* to *selective attention* (i.e., focusing on one stimulus while ignoring others) to *alternating attention* (i.e., rapidly shifting attention from one stimulus to another) and *divided attention*.

Attention span, the simplest form of attention, is often reported to be intact in MS (2,7,15,18,35). Impairment of auditory attention span (and, less commonly, visuospatial span) has been observed in samples with larger proportions of patients with progressive MS, however (13,24,25,39,46). Selective attention may or may not be impaired in MS, depending on task demands. MS patients often perform comparably to controls on selective attention tasks that are self-paced (ones that allow a person to slow down to maintain accuracy) and ones that have few stimulus or response choices (3,34,38,39,47). In contrast, they are typically impaired on speeded tasks involving more complex stimulus or response choices (12,19,34,36,38,39,48–50) or on tasks that require inhibition of a previously correct response (3,46,48). There have been conflicting findings with some tasks (e.g., Brown-Peterson), with deficits being observed in some samples, typically those with larger proportions of active or progressive patients (10,12,51), but not in others (3,14,23,52).

Attentional processes at higher levels of the hierarchy, namely alternating attention and divided attention, are frequently impaired in MS. MS patients as a group perform more poorly than controls on tasks requiring them to shift attention back and forth from one stimulus to another (2,3,10,18,19,24,25,34,39). Similarly, they exhibit deficits when required to perform two tasks simultaneously, with the absolute magnitude of their impairment depending on the extent to which the tasks compete for the same limited set of cognitive resources (49). A summary of the effects of MS on information processing speed and attentional processes can be found in Table 2.

Complex attentional processes (i.e., selective attention, alternating attention, and divided attention) overlap with the construct of *working memory*, a hypothesized limited capacity system responsible for the temporary storage of information (*phonological loop* and *visuospatial sketchpad*) and its controlled processing (*central executive*). The construct of working memory is a useful one. It may explain why selective attention is impaired under some conditions (i.e., on tasks that place greater demands on working memory) but not others and in some patient samples (i.e., those whose working memory system is compromised) but not others. MS patients exhibit deficits on a variety of auditory and visuospatial tasks specifically developed to tax the resources of the working memory system (23,39,46,50,52,53). There is converging evidence (both performance-based and electrophysiological) to suggest that auditory verbal working memory may be preferentially disrupted in MS, at least in relapsing remitting patients (53). Not surprisingly, working memory is emerging as a strong determinant of everyday function in MS (5,8).

Executive Functions

Deficits in executive functions are often more apparent to clinicians and family members than they are to patients themselves. Family members and friends may observe that an MS patient has difficulty grasping complex concepts, stubbornly pursues an ineffective course of action, or has difficulty planning and sticking to a schedule. *Executive functions* comprise a variety of higher-level cognitive functions (including abstract reasoning, problem solving, planning, and self monitoring), which are often impaired in MS. As a group, MS patients have an impaired ability to identify features common to a set of objects (*concept formation*) and to deduce rules that link items in a series (*abstract reasoning*) (2,46,54,55). Their performance on these tasks is often characterized by perseverative responding (2,3,14,16,49). However, some investigators (55,56) have observed that if MS patients are presented with several options, they can indeed shift conceptual frameworks, suggesting that their set-shifting difficulty stems from a primary deficit in concept formation.

MS patients have deficits in other executive functions as well. On tasks requiring patients to plan and carry out a sequence of actions (*planning/sequencing*), MS patients as a group are less efficient and make more errors than controls (26,46,57). In addition, they may have difficulty placing events in the correct temporal sequence (*temporal ordering*) (58), keeping track of how often or in what form items are presented (*frequency monitoring* and *stimulus modality monitoring*) (17), and making many types of estimates (*cognitive estimation*) (46). MS patients may also have difficulty monitoring and regulating their own behavior (59). Thus, most executive functions are affected by MS.

Executive dysfunction clearly affects performance on other cognitive and motor tasks. It has been specifically associated with impaired recall (60) and recognition (26) on explicit memory tasks, as well as with failure to spontaneously apply systematic strategies to facilitate learning and subsequent recall (26,27). Performance on measures of executive function also predicted the magnitude of benefit that patients obtained from learning imagery-based mnemonic techniques (27). Thus, accurate information about a patient's executive functions may facilitate prediction of potential benefit from various rehabilitation programs.

Visual Perception

Impairment of visual perception is nearly as common as executive dysfunction in MS (3), yet it has received little systematic study. Patients rarely complain about problems with visual perception per se, although they may report problems with "vision." However, family members may express concern about a patient who drives too close to a lane line, or one who has had some "near misses" on the highway. Deficits in the perception of faces (*facial perception*, or "knowing who") (3,12,14) and of pictures or geometric figures (*visual form perception*, or "knowing what") (18,48,50) are reasonably common in MS. Visual agnosias are rare in MS, although one case has been reported (61).

Deficits in the perception of spatial relationships among objects (*visuospatial perception*, or "knowing where") may be slightly less common than other visual perceptual disorders in MS. Visuospatial deficits have been observed in samples with large proportions of chronic progressive MS patients (12,34) but not in samples with large proportions of relapsing remitting patients (49,50,53) unless the sample size was quite large (3,18). Some investigators (62) have observed that visuospatial deficits in MS patients are associated with substantial cerebral atrophy or unusually large lesions. Further study of visual perception in MS is clearly warranted.

Language

Language has also received little systematic investigation in MS. Frank abnormalities of language are rare, although a handful of patients presenting with aphasia syndromes have been described [e.g., global aphasia (63), nonfluent aphasia (64), conduction aphasia (65), and alexia with impaired auditory comprehension (66)]. In MS patients, deficient performance on measures of ''language'' usually stems from impairment in other cognitive domains. Thus, poor performance on a confrontation naming task typically reflects deficient retrieval from semantic memory rather than a breakdown in the fundamental structure of semantic knowledge. Similarly, impaired sentence repetition in an MS patient usually signals attentional problems, and difficulty following commands can result from impairment of attention and/or difficulties with sequencing.

Recent work suggests that subtle abnormalities of receptive and expressive language may be present in MS, however. For example, patients in one recent study were impaired in their comprehension of concept meanings and attributes, suggesting a degradation of semantic knowledge; these patients had deficits in other cognitive domains as well (67). In a different study, MS patients were impaired in their ability to decode the meaning of complex or ambiguous grammatical structures (68). Finally, the verbal output of MS patients has been described as ''empty,'' characterized by fewer complete and grammatically correct sentences and fewer information units per sentence (69). Thus, language impairment may be more common in MS than initially thought, albeit fairly subtle. Even subtle language difficulties are likely to have important functional consequences, however, disrupting interpersonal relationships and affecting work performance in occupations that are heavily verbal in nature and depend on in-depth, specialized knowledge.

B. Patterns of MS-Related Cognitive Dysfunction

Some investigators (70) have suggested that the pattern of cognitive deficits observed in MS resembles that seen in other diseases involving subcortical structures (e.g., Huntington's disease, Parkinson's disease, and HIV encephalopathy). However, the concept of *subcortical dementia* has been a controversial one (71,72). Not only does it presume that there is a distinct and homogeneous set of cognitive deficits common to disorders with subcortical pathology, but it also implies that patients with a given disease (i.e., MS) have a single homogeneous pattern of impairment that meets criteria for dementia. This is simply not the case.

Just as the clinical features of MS can vary from patient to patient, there is considerable cognitive heterogeneity among MS patients. In studies of patterns of memory impairment, three distinct subgroups of MS patients were identified (11,13,28): (a) those whose memory is intact, or even slightly better than that of demographically comparable healthy controls (24 to 36%); (b) patients whose scores on memory measures are technically ''within normal limits'' but whose performance is characterized by inconsistent recall across trials or mild impairment of delayed recall (43 to 56%); and (c) patients with flattened learning curves and severe memory deficits (20 to 22%). The concordance in the results of these three studies is striking in light of substantial differences in sample composition and memory measures administered.

Patterns of cognitive impairment across different domains have been examined in two studies (18,73), both of which involved large samples of patients with relapsing remitting MS. The concordance in the results of these studies is again impressive, given differences in the choice of NP measures and approaches to statistical analysis. Six distinct subgroups were identified: a cognitively intact subgroup (34 to 46%); three subgroups with relatively isolated deficits (totaling 37 to 49%); and two subgroups with deficits in multiple domains that differed in severity (each totaling 17%). Two important conclusions can be drawn from these studies: (a) MS-related cognitive impairment is clearly heterogeneous and frequently involves circumscribed deficits in only one or two cognitive domains and (b) only a small proportion of MS patients would meet criteria for dementia.

V. NATURAL HISTORY

Few controlled longitudinal studies of MS-related cognitive dysfunction have been published. Consequently, its evolution and course are not well understood. Early studies of MS patients with varied disease characteristics suggested that cognitive function (or dysfunction) was reasonably stable in most MS patients, at least over 3- to 4-year periods (74,75). However, a subset of patients did deteriorate markedly during this interval [6 to 12% in the Dutch study (74) and 20% in the United States study (SM Rao, personal communication)]. A subsequent 4 1/2-year follow-up of recent-onset patients, most of whom had relapsing remitting MS, not only confirmed the persistence of cognitive deficits (i.e., learning/memory and abstract reasoning) over time but also revealed that new deficits (e.g., information processing) emerged within this time frame (7). Furthermore, the performance of the MS group (but not the control group) became more variable over time, suggesting the existence of subgroups of intact and impaired patients within this sample.

The heterogeneous course of MS-related cognitive dysfunction was further illustrated in a sample composed largely of chronic progressive patients (76). Most patients who were cognitively intact at baseline remained so, but a sizable proportion (35%) deteriorated slightly over the 2- to 4-year follow-up period. Meanwhile, the majority of patients who were cognitively impaired at baseline continued to deteriorate, particularly on measures of attention/information processing and learning/recent memory; only a small proportion of this group (23%) remained stable or improved. Thus, it appears that once cognitive impairment is present, it rarely remits. It is difficult to predict the rate of progression or the specific pattern of deficits that will develop in a given patient, however.

VI. CLINICAL CORRELATES

Efforts to identify clinical variables predictive of MS-related cognitive impairment have been disappointing. Performance on most NP measures is only weakly related to disease duration (3,77), although the relationship between disease duration and complex attentional (i.e., working memory) performance may be stronger (20). It should not be surprising that disease duration is a poor predictor of cognitive function in MS: not only do recent studies of axonal transection (78) and brain atrophy (79) suggest that conventional methods of establishing disease duration (from clinical symptom onset or diagnosis) may be flawed but only about half of all MS patients develop measurable cognitive impairment at any point in the disease.

Clinicians consistently overestimate the magnitude of the relationship between physical disability and cognitive impairment in MS patients (1). Two factors may account for this: (a) clinical rating scales, such as the Expanded Disability Status Scale (EDSS) (80), were designed to capture abnormalities observable during the neurological examination, and not sensitive to the cognitive deficits typical of MS and (b) patients with only spinal cord involvement can have substantial physical disability while remaining cognitively intact. In fact, the EDSS is only a modest predictor of overall cognitive function (2,3,77).

Like disease duration, however, it may be better at predicting the integrity of complex attentional processes than it is at predicting other cognitive functions (20). Specific neurologic signs such as cerebellar or brainstem findings may also have slightly better predictive value than the overall EDSS (4).

In contrast, disease course clearly influences the likelihood of developing MS-related cognitive impairment. Patients characterized as having a chronic progressive course consistently perform more poorly as a group on NP testing than relapsing remitting MS patients do (2,13,16,81), although relapsing remitting patients also exhibit deficits when compared with matched controls (7,12,18,81). However, disease course is a surprisingly weak predictor of performance on individual NP measures (77). Two factors may explain this: (a) there is considerable cognitive heterogeneity among MS patients who have the same disease course and (b) the chronic progressive group in the early studies included both primary progressive and secondary progressive patients. Subsequent research has revealed that secondary progressive MS patients perform considerably worse on NP testing than either relapsing remitting or primary progressive patients do (82), consistent with observations that they have the greatest T2 lesion burden on magnetic resonance imaging (MRI) (83,84). Cognitive impairment in primary progressive MS may not be as rare as initially thought, however (19).

Clinical observations suggest that disease activity also affects cognitive function, although the empirical evidence for this is currently limited. In one recent study (85), attentional processes (attention span and selective attention) and episodic memory were impaired during acute relapse, and attention (but not memory) was significantly better when assessed 6 weeks later, during remission. In another study (86), changes in NP test performance were moderately to strongly correlated with changes in cerebrospinal fluid (CSF) somatostatin levels, which are known to fluctuate during MS relapses and remissions and to decrease over time in progressive patients. Thus, cognitive function appears to fluctuate in conjunction with disease fluctuations, although these changes may not be uniform across all cognitive domains.

The relationship between cognitive dysfunction and fatigue is not yet clear. Experimentally induced fatigue does not adversely affect NP test performance (48,74). However, a recent positive emission tomography (PET) study of patients with documented fatigue revealed abnormal patterns of resting cerebral glucose metabolism (CMRGlu) involving many regions known to be involved in key cognitive functions (87). This observation, together with subsequent PET studies documenting a moderate to strong correlation between global CMRGlu and NP test performance (88,89), raises the intriguing possibility that fatigue and cognitive dysfunction in MS may share a common substrate (disrupted frontal cortico-subcortical circuits secondary to demyelination). Self-reported depression in MS patients is only weakly related to overall cognitive function (12,14,16,90). However, depressed mood does appear to be associated with poorer performance on attentional-capacity demanding (working memory) tasks (20,91,92), in effect compounding the impairment of working memory that is directly related to the disease itself. Finally, NP test performance does not appear to be adversely affected by most medications (2,3,14,18), although few systematic studies of medication effects have been conducted. In summary, certain clinical features (i.e., presence of cerebellar or brainstem findings, secondary progressive course, acute relapse or observable disease progression, or significant fatigue) should prompt the clinician to probe carefully for evidence of cognitive impairment, although the absence of these features does not imply that a patient is cognitively intact.

VII. NEURORADIOLOGICAL CORRELATES

Cognitive impairment in MS is much more strongly associated with magnetic resonance imaging (MRI) parameters than it is with clinical characteristics. Contrary to early assertions that the vast majority of T2 lesions are "clinically silent" (93), it is now abundantly clear that these lesions can have substantial effects on cognitive function. Cognitively impaired MS patients consistently have a larger T2 lesion burden than those who remain cognitively intact (6,34). In one study (6), a total lesion area of 30 cm² or greater was an almost certain indicator of significant cognitive dysfunction. The converse was not true, however: nearly half of the cognitively impaired group had lesion areas less than 30 cm². The 30 cm² threshold may be more sensitive, albeit less specific, in detecting cognitive impairment in patients with more acute disease (94). Correlations between T2 lesion burden and NP test performance in early studies were generally moderate to strong ($|r| = 0.29$ to 0.54) (6,34), with the magnitude of these correlations increasing in subsequent studies as MRI image acquisition and quantitation methods improved ($|r| = 0.43$ to 0.82) (95–97). Changes in NP test performance (e.g., Paced Auditory Serial Addition Test, or PASAT) are also strongly associated with changes in total lesion volume over 1-year intervals (96).

Initially, it was hoped that specific cognitive deficits in MS could be associated with lesions in a given region. For example, executive function has been reported to be specifically associated with frontal-lobe lesion burden (94,100). Subsequent investigations have indicated that performance on measures of executive functions is equally well explained by overall lesion burden, however (46,97,99). The presence of subcortical lesions may have better predictive value: patients with lesions in the subcortical region (including U fibers) are more likely to have deficits in selected cognitive functions (e.g., auditory selective attention, memory) than patients with a comparable lesion load but no subcortical lesions (100,101). Several factors may account for the difficulty in establishing precise relationships between NP and MRI variables in MS: (a) it is difficult to attribute specific cognitive abnormalities to focal brain lesions when there is widespread disease; (b) T2 lesions are nonspecific, reflecting several different pathological processes (e.g., edema, inflammation, demyelination, and axonal loss), not all of which may have an impact on cognitive function; and (c) performance on many NP tasks is most likely subserved by distributed cognitive networks, rather than a specific brain region.

Cognitive dysfunction in MS has also been associated with several indicators of brain atrophy. Patients with extensive periventricular involvement do considerably worse on NP testing than patients with less periventricular involvement (6,102–104), confirming the findings of an early computed tomography (CT) study with chronic progressive MS patients (105). Patients with prominent confluent lesions perform particularly poorly (104,106,107). Third-ventricle size is the linear measurement most strongly associated with learning/memory performance (105,107,108). Cognitively impaired patients also have more callosal atrophy (6,43,109). Callosal size has been specifically associated with performance on information processing tasks (6,43,94), verbal fluency (6,94,110), and various interhemispheric transfer tasks (43,111). Name-face learning is strongly correlated with the size of the splenium (i.e., the most caudal section of the corpus callosum) (112). Finally, patients with greater overall cerebral atrophy do more poorly on a variety of NP measures, including measures of general intellectual functioning (19,62,98,113).

Pathology visible on T2 images is not the only pathology in MS, however. Although NP test performance correlates more strongly with T2 lesion burden than it does with T1 lesion burden (97) or NAA/Cr ratios obtained through MR spectroscopy (114), magnetization transfer imaging (MTI) is at least as sensitive to MS-related cognitive dysfunction as T2 imaging. Not only are the correlations between NP test performance and the magnetization transfer ratio (MTR) generally of the same magnitude as those reported for NP-T2 correlations ($|r| = 0.45$ to 0.59) (97) but certain cognitive functions (e.g., information processing) appear to be more strongly related to MT parameters than to T2 (97,113). MTI, which is sensitive to demyelination and axonal damage, may be particularly useful in identifying abnormalities in normal-appearing brain tissue that can impair cognitive function (115).

VIII. TREATMENT AND REHABILITATION

The treatment of cognitive impairment in MS is in its infancy. Assessment of NP outcomes in trials of disease-modifying medications is a recent phenomenon, and few symptomatic treatments for MS-related cognitive impairment (either pharmacological agents or cognitive rehabilitation) have been systematically evaluated (116). None of the trials of disease-modifying medications and few trials of symptomatic medications to date have featured cognitive impairment as an explicit selection criterion. Furthermore, sample sizes in studies of symptomatic treatments have been small. Nonetheless, encouraging results have been obtained in trials of both symptomatic and disease-modifying treatments.

A. Symptomatic Treatments (Including Cognitive Rehabilitation)

Intravenous physostigmine had a beneficial effect on verbal learning in an early pilot study of MS patients with documented memory impairment (117). This benefit failed to generalize to other memory measures in a subsequent study of oral physostigmine, however (118). Newer cholinesterase inhibitors such as donepezil (Aricept) have shown promise in uncontrolled studies of patients with documented memory deficits (119,120), but these results await confirmation in controlled clinical trials. In two trials with cognitively heterogeneous samples, amantadine (Symmetrel) had a mild beneficial effect on selective attention/processing speed (but not other cognitive functions) in patients with documented fatigue (121,122). In addition, a trend toward improved information processing and visuospatial memory was observed in a trial of 4-aminopyridine (4-AP) with cognitively heterogeneous MS patients (123). However, no NP benefits were observed in a trial of a related agent (3,4 diaminopyridine) in patients with documented leg weakness (124). Thus, it appears that symptomatic treatments may exert specific, rather than general, effects on MS-related cognitive deficits. Clearly, additional studies of symptomatic medications with the potential to improve cognitive function in MS patients need to be performed.

Promising results have been obtained in two controlled trials of cognitive rehabilitation. Both process-specific and general beneficial effects were observed in MS patients with documented attentional impairment who underwent 18 weeks of process-specific attentional retraining; these gains were maintained over a 9-week follow-up period (125). A 6-week cognitive rehabilitation program improved selected cognitive functions (visual perception, and to a lesser extent visuospatial memory) in inpatients, whose gains were also maintained over a 6-month follow-up (126). In contrast, the limited gains observed in the nonspecific treatment (control) group did not persist over the follow-up period. Finally, a 24-week group psychotherapy program also had beneficial effects on selected cognitive functions (verbal learning and abstract reasoning), although maintenance of gains was not assessed in this study (127). Thus, cognitive rehabilitation programs specifically designed to improve attention and visual perception appear to have beneficial and potentially long-lasting effects in MS patients.

B. Disease-Modifying Medications

There is every reason to expect that disease-modifying medications with a beneficial effect on traditional clinical or MRI measures would also benefit cognitive function in MS patients. NP outcomes have been systematically assessed and reported in five clinical trials of disease-modifying medications, two in chronic progressive MS and three in relapsing remitting MS. In an early chronic progressive trial, cyclosporine did not have any demonstrable effect on information processing speed (the only NP outcome assessed in this trial); however, its effects on the primary outcome measures were mixed (128) (Syndulko, personal communication). In a small trial, low-dose oral methotrexate had a beneficial effect on selective attention/processing speed, an effect that was evident early in the trial and persisted throughout 2 years of treatment; effects on other cognitive functions were limited, however (129).

In relapsing remitting MS, visual memory (and to a lesser extent, complex attentional processes) improved during IFN-β-1b (Betaseron) treatment (130). However, the sample was small and no pre-treatment assessment of cognitive function was obtained, so these results are difficult to evaluate. In a large trial, IFN-β-1a (Avonex) had a significant beneficial effect on complex attentional processes and memory, with a trend toward benefits on visuospatial abilities and executive functions as well (131). No NP effects, either beneficial or adverse, were observed in a similarly large trial of glatiramer acetate (Copaxone), however (132). One additional study worth noting is a small trial of IV methylprednisolone, which had a transient adverse effect on explicit memory but not other cognitive functions (133). This effect was apparent 1 week after initiation of treatment but had resolved 2 months later. Taken together, the results of these disease-modifying medication trials suggest that (a) information about the benefits (or potentially, adverse effects) associated with disease-modifying medications can assist the clinician and patient in making informed treatment decisions and (b) clinicians should consider monitoring cognitive function in patients undergoing disease-modifying treatment, particularly those patients with objective evidence of cognitive impairment.

IX. ASSESSMENT AND MANAGEMENT IN CLINICAL SETTINGS

A. Neuropsychological Evaluation

Objective NP assessment is the ''gold standard'' for determining whether MS has affected a patient's cognitive function. Comprehensive NP evaluation of the MS patient consists of a diagnostic interview with the patient (and if available, a family member), detailed testing of cognitive functions often impaired in MS (attention/information processing, learning/memory, executive functions, and visual perception), and briefer assessment of domains less often impaired in MS. The choice of specific NP tests may vary, depending on the referral question, the clinical neuropsychologist's training, and the patient's tolerance for NP testing. Self-report measures of emotional status, perceived cognitive function, and quality of life may also be administered. Ideally, the neuropsychologist will review the principal findings of the NP evaluation with the patient and family, and will also provide a report to the referring clinician. Graphs can simplify the presentation of complex test findings. Many MS comprehensive care centers have an identified clinical neuropsychologist to whom they refer patients. In addition, most major medical centers also have clinical neuropsychologists on their staffs.

B. Subjective Ratings of Cognitive Function

It is difficult to accurately gauge the cognitive status of an MS patient without formal NP assessment. In one early study, neurologists identified only 21% of patients who were objectively impaired on NP testing; neurologists were rarely inaccurate if they thought that a patient was cognitively impaired, however (134). MS patients' subjective ratings of their memory function correlate only weakly with their performance on objective memory measures (135–137). Two types of inaccuracies can occur: some patients greatly underestimate their memory performance, whereas others overestimate their performance. MS patients who underestimate their performance are often emotionally distressed: patients' subjective ratings of memory function correlate moderately with self-reported depression (135,137). Overestimation of objective memory function is often associated with executive dysfunction [including impaired concept formation (136,138) and poor self-monitoring (136)] or with significant memory impairment (138); subjective ratings of memory function are the least accurate when both types of deficits are present (138).

C. Screening for MS-Related Cognitive Impairment

It is impractical to refer all MS patients seen in clinical practice for a comprehensive NP evaluation. However, clinicians should have a systematic approach for identifying patients in need of NP referral. Ideally, the clinician would have at his or her disposal a brief, cost-effective, and reliable NP screening measure that would accurately identify patients whose impairment would be confirmed on comprehensive NP testing ("true positives"), while minimizing the number of identified patients who would not have any deficits on comprehensive NP testing ("false positives").

The utility of several NP screening measures has been evaluated in MS (see Table 3). The most well-known of these is the Mini-Mental State Examination (MMSE) (139). The MMSE has repeatedly been shown to be insensitive to MS-related cognitive impairment except in the most severely compromised patients (3,94,140,141). This should not be surprising, considering the disparities between the circumscribed impairment usually observed in MS and the global impairment that the MMSE was designed to detect. Other variants on the mental status exam either have similarly high false-negative rates (142) or they have not yet been adequately validated (140,143).

Another approach to screening MS patients neuropsychologically has been to construct a brief battery of NP measures covering functions commonly impaired in MS. Four such batteries have been proposed, each with sensitivities considerably higher than those of mental status exam-based measures, but slightly lower specificities (see Table 3). These NP screening batteries can be administered by nondoctoral personnel who have been trained in NP test administration and scoring. Either the Screening Examination for Cognitive Impairment (SEFCI) (144) or the Brief NP Battery proposed by Rao (3) (or a variant of this battery proposed by the National MS Society's Cognitive Functions Study Group) would appear to be a reasonable means of obtaining a "ballpark" estimate of a patient's cognitive function to determine if further testing is appropriate. Screening batteries are not a substitute for comprehensive NP evaluation, however: by design, these batteries only assess a limited range of cognitive functions, and consequently, do not cover some domains critical to everyday function (e.g., executive functions).

Table 3 Overview of NP Screening Measures Used in MS

Measure	Description	Estimated administration time	Sensitivity	Specificity
Mental status examinations				
Mini-Mental State Examination (MMSE) (139)	30-item global screening measure	5–10 min	36% [34] 21% [140] 23% [3] 28% [141]	94% [34] 100% [140] 98% [3] 89% [141]
Cognitive Capacity Status Examination (CCSE) (142)	30-item global screening measure	5–10 min	41% [34]	94% [34]
Quantitative Mental Status Examination (QMSE) (143)	Expanded mental status exam, assessing Orientation + letter span +10-word list × 4 trials (+ delay) + abstract reasoning + arithmetic + language (incl. semantic fluency and naming) +visual construction	20 min	Not given	Not given
Screening Examination for Cognitive Impairment in MS (SECIMS) (140)	Modified MMSE (including 15-item BNT + 7-word list) + Oral SDMT	15 min	Not given	Not given
NP screening batteries				
Neuropsychological Screening Battery (34)	SDMT + Trails A, B + Numerical Attention Test + WMS Story Memory (× 3 trials) + WMS Figure Memory (× 3 trials) and copy + selected Multilingual Aphasia Examination subtests + Western Aphasia Battery Commands with Auditory Sequencing + phonemic fluency	30–45 min	55%	94%
Screening Examination for Cognitive Impairment (SEFCI) (144)	10-item word-list × 3 trials (with delay) + Shipley Institute of Living Scale + Oral SDMT	25–30 min	74–86%	90–91%

Table 3   Continued

Measure	Description	Estimated administration time	Sensitivity	Specificity
Brief NP Battery (3)	Buschke Selective Reminding Test (12 items × 12 trials, with delay) + 7/24 Spatial Recall Test + PASAT + COWAT	30–35 min	68%	85%
Basso Screening Battery (145)	WMS-R Logical Memory + COWAT + Seashore Rhythm Test + graphesthesia + stereognosis	15–25 min	100%*	80%*

Note: *Sensitivity* and *specificity* refer to prediction of cognitive impairment on measures from a comprehensive NP battery with minimal sensory and motor demands. Values marked with an asterisk (*) are artificially elevated due to overlap between predictor and criterion measures.

Key: BNT, Boston Naming Test; SDMT, Symbol-Digit Modalities Test; PASAT, Paced Auditory Serial Addition Test; COWAT, Controlled Oral Word Association Test; WMS, Wechsler Memory Scale; WMS-R, Wechsler Memory Scale-Revised.

An alternative method for identifying patients appropriate for NP referral is to apply a clinical algorithm similar to the one shown in Table 4. Asking a series of general screening questions, and probing further as needed, is less time consuming than administering an objective NP screening battery. It also has the advantage of allowing the clinician to probe for behavioral evidence of deficits in executive functions not covered by a screening battery. Finally, it increases the likelihood that patients whose subjective memory complaints stem from an underlying depression are evaluated and referred for psychological or psychiatric services. This informal NP screening method does run the risk of missing patients who may be unaware of subtle cognitive deficits, however.

D.   Clinical Management of Cognitively Impaired MS Patients

The presence of cognitive dysfunction has important implications for the clinical care of MS patients. There is accumulating evidence that cognitive impairment (particularly worsening cognitive impairment) should be considered an independent indicator for initiating treatment with disease-modifying medications, regardless of a patient's physical disability. Comprehensive NP evaluation early in the disease course can not only facilitate clinical decision making but can also provide a baseline with which to compare subsequent assessments.

Patients with moderate to severe MS-related cognitive impairment may have difficulty weighing the advantages and disadvantages of various treatment options (disease-modifying or symptomatic), however. Patient education sessions should be supplemented

Table 4   Clinical Algorithm for Identifying MS Patients Appropriate for NP Referral

Sample screening questions (to ask all patients)
Do you have trouble remembering appointments or remembering to take medication?
Is it hard for you to hold your train of thought or to do two things at once?
Is it hard for you to follow what you're reading or what people are saying to you?
Do you have trouble concentrating while you're driving?
Do you feel disorganized and have trouble planning activities?
Do you have trouble coming up with good solutions to problems when they arise?
(If working) Are you having any cognitive problems at work that you think might be related to
    your MS?

Heightened suspicion (if any of these are present, query further re: cognitive difficulties)
    Recent relapse or observable disease progression
    Secondary progressive course
    ?Cerebellar signs
    ?Brainstem signs
    Significant fatigue
    "Red flags" on MRI (total lesion area >30 cm^2 or significant atrophy)

Automatic referral for NP evaluation
    1. Early disease/baseline for treatment planning
    2. Patient or family member complains of patient's cognitive problems OR
       Clinician suspects patient's cognitive impairment
           AND
       Diagnostic uncertainty OR
       Employment/disability retirement decisions OR
       Treatment planning/monitoring OR
       Competency determination

with written materials summarizing key points and listing specific treatment recommendations. Patients with moderate to severe cognitive impairment may also have difficulty following complex treatment regimens (or rehabilitation programs) and managing any treatment-related problems that may arise. External aids (e.g., calendars, reminders from a family member or friend to exercise or to take medication, and pill cases) can promote adherence in patients with memory deficits. A checklist of steps to follow can help patients with impaired executive function follow complex treatment and rehabilitation programs and take appropriate action if treatment-related problems arise. Finally, if specific problems related to cognitive impairment are encountered with an individual patient, consultation with health care professionals accustomed to managing cognitive impairment (e.g., clinical neuropsychologists, occupational therapists, speech pathologists) is strongly recommended.

REFERENCES

1. Fischer JS, Foley FW, Aikens JA, et al. What do we really know about cognitive dysfunction, affective disorders, and stress in multiple sclerosis? A practitioner's guide. J Neurol Rehab 1994; 8:151–164.
2. Heaton RK, Nelson LM, Thompson DS, Burks JS, Franklin GM. Neuropsychological findings in relapsing-remitting and chronic-progressive multiple sclerosis. J Consult Clin Psychol 1985; 53:103–110.

3. Rao SM, Leo GJ, Bernardin L, Unverzagt F. Cognitive dysfunction in multiple sclerosis: I. Frequency, patterns, and prediction. Neurology 1991; 41:685–691.

4. Rao SM, Leo GJ, Ellington L, Nauertz T, Bernardin L, Unverzagt F. Cognitive dysfunction in multiple sclerosis: II. impact on employment and social functioning. Neurology 1991; 41: 692–696.

5. Beatty WW, Blanco CR, Wilbanks SL, Paul RH, Hames KA. Demographic, clinical, and cognitive characteristics of multiple sclerosis patients who continue to work. J Neurol Rehab 1995; 9:167–173.

6. Rao SM, Leo GJ, Haughton VM, St. Aubin-Faubert P, Bernardin L. Correlation of magnetic resonance imaging with neuropsychological testing in multiple sclerosis. Neurology 1989; 39:161–166.

7. Amato MP, Ponziani G, Pracucci G, Bracco L, Siracusa G, Amaducci L. Cognitive impairment in early-onset multiple sclerosis: Pattern, predictors, and impact on everyday life in a 4-year follow-up. Arch Neurol 1995; 52:168–172.

8. Higginson CI, Arnett PA, Voss WD. The ecological validity of clinical tests of memory and attention in multiple sclerosis. Arch Clin Neuropsychol 2000; 3:185–204.

9. Langdon DW, Thompson AJ. Multiple sclerosis: A preliminary study of selected variables affecting rehabilitation outcome. Mult Scler 1999; 5:94–100.

10. Grant I, McDonald WI, Trimble MR, Smith E, Reed R. Deficient learning and memory in early and middle phases of multiple sclerosis. J Neurol Neurosurg Psychiatry 1984; 47:250–255.

11. Rao SM, Hammeke TA, McQuillen MP, Khatri BO, Lloyd D. Memory disturbance in chronic progressive multiple sclerosis. Arch Neurol 1984; 41:625–631.

12. Beatty WW, Goodkin DE, Monson N, Beatty PA, Hertsgaard D. Anterograde and retrograde amnesia in patients with chronic progressive multiple sclerosis. Arch Neurol 1988; 45:611–619.

13. Fischer JS. Using the Wechsler Memory Scale-Revised to detect and characterize memory deficits in multiple sclerosis. Clin Neuropsychol 1988; 2:149–172.

14. Beatty WW, Goodkin, Monson N, Beatty PA. Cognitive disturbances in patients with relapsing remitting multiple sclerosis. Arch Neurol 1989; 46:1113–1119.

15. Rao SM, Leo GJ, St. Aubin-Faubert P. On the nature of memory disturbance in multiple sclerosis. J Clin Exp Neuropsychol 1989; 11:699–712.

16. Minden SL, Moes EJ, Orav J, Kaplan E, Reich P. Memory impairment in multiple sclerosis. J Clin Exp Neuropsychol 1990; 11:566–586.

17. Grafman J, Rao S, Bernardin L, Leo GJ. Automatic memory processes in patients with multiple sclerosis. Arch Neurol 1991; 48:1072–1075.

18. Ryan L, Clark CM, Klonoff H, Li D, Paty D. Patterns of cognitive impairment in relapsing-remitting multiple sclerosis and their relationship to neuropathology on magnetic resonance images. Neuropsychology 1996; 2:176–193.

19. Camp SJ, Stevenson VL, Thompson AJ, et al. Cognitive function in primary progressive and transitional progressive multiple sclerosis: A controlled study with MRI correlates. Brain 1999; 122:1341–1348.

20. Thornton AE, Raz N. Memory impairment in multiple sclerosis: A quantitative review. Neuropsychology 1997; 3:357–366.

21. Wishart H, Sharpe D. Neuropsychological aspects of multiple sclerosis: A quantitative review. J Clin Exp Neuropsychol 1997; 6:810–824.

22. Zakzanis KK. Distinct neurocognitive profiles in multiple sclerosis subtypes. Arch Clin Neuropsychol 2000; 15:115–136.

23. Rao SM, Grafman J, DiGuilio D, et al. Memory dysfunction in multiple sclerosis: Its relation to working memory, semantic encoding, and implicit learning. Neuropsychology 1993; 7: 364–374.

24. DeLuca J, Barbieri-Berger S, Johnson S. The nature of memory impairments in multiple sclerosis: Acquisition versus retrieval. J Clin Exp Neuropsychol 1994; 16:183–189.

25. DeLuca J, Gaudino EA, Diamond BJ, Christodoulou C, Engel RA. Acquisition and storage deficits in multiple sclerosis. J Clin Exp Neurospychol 1998; 20:376–390.

26. Arnett PA, Rao SM, Grafman, et al. Executive functions in multiple sclerosis: An analysis of temporal ordering, semantic encoding, and planning abilities. Neuropsychology 1997; 11: 535–544.

27. Canellopoulou M, Richardson JTE. The role of executive function in imagery mnemonics: Evidence from multiple sclerosis. Neuropsychologia 1998; 36:1181–1188.

28. Beatty WW, Wilbanks SL, Blanco CR, Hames KA, Tivis R, Paul RH. Memory disturbance in multiple sclerosis: Reconsideration of patterns of performance on the Selective Reminding Test. J Clin Exp Neuropsychol 1996; 18:56–62.

29. Coolidge FL, Middleton PA, Griego JA, Schmidt MM. The effects of interference on verbal learning in multiple sclerosis. Arch Clin Neuropsychol 1996; 11:605–611.

30. Beatty WW, Monson N. Lexical processing in Parkinson's disease and multiple sclerosis. J Geriatric Psychiatry Neurol 1989; 2:151–158.

31. Paul RH, Blanco CR, Hames KA, Beatty WW. Autobiographical memory in multiple sclerosis. J Int Neuropsychol Soc 1997; 3:246–251.

32. Beatty WW, Monson N. Semantic priming in multiple sclerosis. Bull Psychonom Soc 1990; 28:397–400.

33. Beatty WW, Goodkin DE, Monson N, Beatty PA. Implicit learning in patients with chronic progressive multiple sclerosis. Intl J Clin Neuropsychol 1990; 12:166–172.

34. Franklin GM, Heaton RK, Nelson LM, Filley CM, Seibert C. Correlation of neuropsychological and MRI findings in chronic/progressive multiple sclerosis. Neurology 1988; 38:1826–1829.

35. Litvan I, Grafman J, Vendrell P, Martinez JM. Slowed information processing in multiple sclerosis. Arch Neurol 1988; 45:281–285.

36. Rao SM, St. Aubin-Faubert P, Leo GJ. Information processing speed in patients with multiple sclerosis. J Clin Exp Neuropsychol 1989; 11:471–477.

37. DeLuca J, Johnson SK, Natelson BH. Information processing efficiency in chronic fatigue syndrome and multiple sclerosis. Arch Neurol 1993; 50:301–304.

38. Kujala P, Portin R, Revonsuo A, Ruutiainen J. Automatic and controlled information processing in multiple sclerosis. Brain 1994; 117:1115–1126.

39. Paul RH, Beatty WW, Schneider R, Blanco C, Hames K. Impairments of attention in individuals with multiple sclerosis. Mult Scler 1998; 4:433–439.

40. Callanan MM, Logsdail SJ, Ron MA, Warrington EK. Cognitive impairment in patients with clinically isolated lesions of the type seen in multiple sclerosis: A psychometric and MRI study. Brain 1989; 112:361–374.

41. Rubens AB, Froehling BS, Slater G, Anderson D. Left ear suppression on verbal dichotic test in patients with multiple sclerosis. Ann Neurol 1985; 18:459–463.

42. Lindeboom J, ter Horst RT. Interhemispheric disconnection effects in multiple sclerosis. J Neurol Neurosurg Psychiatry 1988; 51:1445–1447.

43. Rao SM, Bernardin L, Leo GJ, Ellington L, Ryan SB, Burg LS. Cerebral disconnection in multiple sclerosis. Arch Neurol 1989; 46:918–920.

44. Wishart HA, Strauss E, Hunter M, Moll A. Interhemispheric transfer in multiple sclerosis. J Clin Exp Neuropsychol 1995; 17:937–940.

45. Kail R. Speed of information processing in patients with multiple sclerosis. J Clin Exp Neuropsychol 1998; 20:98–106.

46. Foong J, Rozewicz L, Quaghebeur G et al. Executive function in multiple sclerosis: The role of frontal lobe pathology. Brain 1997; 120:15–26.

47. Jennekens-Schinkel A, Sanders CM, Lanser JBK, van der Velde EA. Reaction time in ambulant multiple sclerosis patients: Part II. Influence of task complexity. J Neurol Sci 1988; 85: 187–196.

48. van den Burg W, van Zomeren AH, Minderhoud JM, Prange AJA, Meijer NSA. Cognitive

impairment in patients with multiple sclerosis and mild physical disability. Arch Neurol 1987; 44:494–501.

49. D'Esposite M, Onishi K, Thompson H, Robinson K, Armstrong C, Grossman M. Working memory impairments in multiple sclerosis: Evidence from a dual task paradigm. Neuropsychology 1996; 10:51–56.

50. Pelosi L, Geesken JM, Holly M, Hayward M, Blumhardt LD. Working memory impairment in early multiple sclerosis: Evidence from an event-related potential study of patients with clinically isolated myelopathy. Brain 1997; 120:2039–2058.

51. Grigsby J, Ayarbe SD, Kravcisin N, Busenbark D. Working memory impairment among persons with chronic progressive multiple sclerosis. J Neurol 1994; 241:125–131.

52. Litvan I, Grafman J, Vendrell P, et al. Multiple memory deficits in patients with multiple sclerosis: Exploring the working memory system. Arch Neurol 1988; 45:607–610.

53. Ruchkin DS, Grafman J, Krauss GL, Johnson R, Canoune H, Ritter W. Event-related brain potential evidence for a verbal working memory deficit in multiple sclerosis. Brain 1994; 117:289–305.

54. Beatty PA, Gange JJ. Neuropsychological aspects of multiple sclerosis. J Nerv Ment Dis 1977; 164:42–50.

55. Beatty WW, Hames KA, Blanco CR, Paul RH, Wilbanks SL. Verbal abstraction deficit in multiple sclerosis. Neuropsychology 1995; 2:198–205.

56. Beatty WW, Monson N. Problem solving by patients with multiple sclerosis: Comparison of performance on the Wisconsin and California Card Sorting Tests. J Int Neuropsychol Soc 1996; 2:134–140.

57. Beatty WW, Monson N. Picture and motor sequencing in multiple sclerosis. J Clin Exp Neuropsychol 1994; 16:165–172.

58. Beatty WW, Monson N. Memory for temporal order in multiple sclerosis. Bull Psychonom Soc 1991; 29:10–12.

59. Grigsby J, Kravcisin, Ayarbe SD, Busenbark D. Prediction of deficits in behavioral self-regulation among persons with multiple sclerosis. Arch Phys Med Rehabil 1993; 74:1350–1353.

60. Troyer AK, Fisk JD, Archibald CJ, Ritvo PG, Murray TJ. Conceptual reasonging as a mediator of verbal recall in patients with multiple sclerosis. J Clin Exp Neuropsychol 1996; 18:211–219.

61. Okuda B, Tanaka H, Tachibana H, et al. Visual form agnosia in multiple sclerosis. Acta Neurol Scand 1996; 94:38–44.

62. Pugnetti L, Mendozzi L, Mott A, et al. MRI and cognitive patterns in relapsing-remitting multiple sclerosis. J Neurol Sci 115:S59–S65.

63. Friedman JH, Brem H, Mayeux R. Global aphasia in multiple sclerosis. Ann Neurol 1983; 13:222–223.

64. Achiron A, Ziv I, Djaldetti R, Goldberg H, Kuritzky A, Melamed E. Aphasia in multiple sclerosis: Clinical and radiologic correlations. Neurology 1992; 42:2195–2197.

65. Arnett PA, Rao SM, Hussain M, Swanson SJ, Hammeke TA. Conduction aphasia in multiple sclerosis: A case report with MRI findings. Neurology 1996; 47:576–578.

66. Jonsdottir MK, Magnusson T, Kjartansson O. Pure alexia and word-meaning deafness in a patient with multiple sclerosis. Arch Neurol 1998; 55:1473–1474.

67. Laatu S, Hamalainen P, Revonsuo A, Portin R, Ruutiainen J. Semantic memory deficit in multiple sclerosis; Impaired understanding of conceptual meanings. J Neurol Sci 1999; 162:152–161.

68. Grossman M, Robinson KM, Onishi K, Thompson H, Cohen J, D'Esposito M. Sentence comprehension in multiple sclerosis. Acta Neurol Scand 1995; 92:324–331.

69. Wallace GL, Holmes S. Cognitive-linguistic assessment of individuals with multiple sclerosis. Arch Phys Med Rehabil 1993; 74:637–643.

70. Rao SM. Neuropsychology of multiple sclerosis: A critical review. J Clin Exp Neuropsychol 1986; 8:503–542.

71. Mayeux R, Stern Y, Rosen J, Benson DF. Is ''subcortical dementia'' a recognizable clinical entity? Ann Neurol 1983; 14:278–283.

72. Brown RG, Marsden CD. ''Subcortical dementia'': The neuropsychological evidence. Neuroscience 1988; 25:363–387.

73. Fischer JS, Jacobs LD, Cookfair DL et al. Heterogeneity of cognitive dysfunction in multiple sclerosis. Clin Neuropsychol 1998; 12:286.

74. Jennekens-Schinkel A, Laboyrie PM, Lanser JBK, van der Velde EA. Cognition in patients with multiple sclerosis: After four years. J Neurol Sci 1990; 99:229–247.

75. Bernardin L, Rao SM, Luchetta TL, et al. A prospective, long-term, longitudinal study of cognitive dysfunction in multiple sclerosis. J Clin Exp Neuropsychol 1993; 15:17.

76. Kujala P, Portin R, Ruutiainen J. The progress of cognitive decline in multiple sclerosis: A controlled 3-year follow-up. Brain 1997; 120:289–297.

77. Beatty WW, Goodkin DE, Hertsgaard D, Monson N. Clinical and demographic predictors of cognitive performance in multiple sclerosis: Do diagnostic type, disease duration, and disability matter? Arch Neurol 1990; 47:305–308.

78. Trapp BD, Peterson J, Ransohoff RM, Rudick R, Mork S, Bo L. Axonal transection in the lesions of multiple sclerosis. N Engl J Med 1998; 338:278–285.

79. Rudick RA, Fisher E, Lee J-C, et al. Use of the brain parenchymal fraction to measure whole brain atrophy in relapsing-remitting MS. Neurology 1999; 53:1698–1704.

80. Kurtzke JF. Rating neurologic impairment in multiple sclerosis: An expanded disability status scale (EDSS). Neurology 1983; 33:444–452.

81. Grossman M, Armstrong C, Onishi K, et al. Patterns of cognitive impairment in relapsing-remitting and chronic progressive multiple sclerosis. Neuropsychiatry Neuropsychol Behav Neurol 1994; 7:194–210.

82. Filippi M, Alberoni M, Martinelli V. et al. Influence of clinical variables on neuropsychological performance in multiple sclerosis. Eur Neurol 1994; 34:324–328.

83. Gonzalez CF, Swirsky-Sacchetti T, Mitchell D, Lublin FD, Knobler RL, Ehrlich SM. Distributional patterns of multiple sclerosis brain lesions: Magnetic resonance imaging-clinical correlation. J Neuroimaging 1994; 4:188–195.

84. Comi G, Filippi M, Martinelli V, et al. Brain MRI correlates of cognitive impairment in primary and secondary progressive multiple sclerosis. J Neurol Sci 1995; 132:222–227.

85. Foong J, Rozewicz, Quaghebeur, Thompson AJ, Miller DH, Ron MA. Neuropsychological deficits in multiple sclerosis after acute relapse. J Neurol Neurosurg Psychiatry 1998; 64: 529–532.

86. Roca CA, Su T-P, Elpern S, McFarland H, Rubinow DR. Cerebrospinal fluid somatostatin, mood, and cognition in multiple sclerosis. Biol Psychiatry 1999; 46:551–556.

87. Roelcke U, Kappos L, Lechner-Scott J, et al. Reduced glucose metabolism in the frontal cortex and basal ganglia of multiple sclerosis patients with fatigue: A ^{18}F-fluorodeoxyglucose positron emission tomography study. Neurology 1997; 48:1566–1571.

88. Blinkenberg M, Rune K, Jensen CV, et al. Cortical cerebral metabolism correlates with MRI lesion load and cognitive dysfunction in MS. Neurology 2000; 54:558–564.

89. Paulesu, E, Perani D, Fazio F, et al. Functional basis of memory impairment in multiple sclerosis: A ^{18}F-FDG PET study. Neuroimage 1996; 4:87–96.

90. McIntosh-Michaelis SA, Roberts MH, Wilkinson SM, et al. The prevalence of cognitive impairment in a community survey of multiple sclerosis. Br J Clin Psychol 1991; 30:333–348.

91. Arnett PA, Higginson CI, Voss WD, et al. Depressed mood in multiple sclerosis: relationship to capacity-demanding memory and attentional functioning. Neuropsychology 1999; 13: 434–446.

92. Arnett PA, Higginson CI, Voss WD, Bender WI, Wurst JM, Tippin JM. Depression in multiple sclerosis: Relationship to working memory capacity. Neuropsychology 1999; 13:546–556.

93. Jacobs L, Kinkel WR, Polachini I, et al. Correlations of nuclear magnetic resonance imaging, computerized tomography, and clinical profiles in multiple sclerosis. Neurology 1986; 36: 27–34.

94. Swirsky-Sacchetti T, Mitchell DR, Sward J, et al. Neuropsychological and structural brain lesions in multiple sclerosis: A regional analysis. Neurology 1992; 42:1291–1295.

95. Huber SJ, Bornstein RA, Rammohan KW, Christy JA, Chakeres DW, McGhee RB. Magnetic resonance imaging correlates of neuropsychological impairment in multiple sclerosis. J Neuropsychiatry Clin Neurosci 1992; 4:152–158.

96. Hohol MJ, Guttmann CRG, Orav J, et al. Serial neuropsychological assessment and magnetic resonance imaging analysis in multiple sclerosis. Arch Neurol 1997; 54:1018–1025.

97. Rovaris M, Filippi M, Falautano M, et al. Relation between MR abnormalities and patterns of cognitive impairment in multiple sclerosis. Neurology 1998; 50:1601–1608.

98. Arnett PA, Rao SM, Bernardin L, Grafman J, Yetkin FZ, Lobeck L. Relationship between frontal lobe lesions and Wisconsin Card Sorting Test performance in patients with multiple sclerosis. Neurology 1994; 44:420–425.

99. Huber SJ, Bornstein RA, Rammohan KW, Christy JA, Chakeres DW, McGhee RB. Magnetic resonance imaging correlates of executive function impairments in multiple sclerosis. Neuropsychol Behav Neurol 1992; 5:33–36.

100. Damian MS, Schilling G, Bachmann G, Simon C, Stöppler S, Dorndorf W. White matter lesions and cognitive deficits: Relevance of lesion pattern? Acta Neurol Scand 1994; 90: 430–436.

101. Miki Y, Grossman RI, Udupa JK, et al. Isolated U-fiber involvement in MS: Preliminary observations. Neurology 1998; 50:1301–1306.

102. Anzola GP, Bevilacqua L, Cappa SF, et al. Neuropsychological assessment in patients with relapsing-remitting multiple sclerosis and mild functional impairment: Correlation with magnetic resonance imaging. J Neurol Neurosurg Psychiatry 1990; 53:142 145.

103. Maurelli M, Marchioni E, Cerretano R, et al. Neuropsychological assessment in MS: Clinical, neurophysiological and neuroradiological relationships. Acta Neurol Scand 1992; 86:124–128.

104. Comi G, Filippi M, Martinelli V, et al. Brain magnetic resonance imaging correlates of cognitive impairment in multiple sclerosis. J Neurol Sci 1993; 115:S66–S73.

105. Rao SM, Glatt S, Hammeke TA, et al. Chronic progressive multiple sclerosis: Relationship between cerebral ventricular size and neuropsychological impairment. Arch Neurol 1985; 42:678–682.

106. Medaer R, Nelissen E, Appel B, Swerts M, Geutjens J, Callaert H. Magnetic resonance imaging and cognitive functioning in multiple sclerosis. J Neurol 1987; 235:86–89.

107. Pozzilli C, Passafiume D, Bernardi S, et al. SPECT, MRI and cognitive functions in multiple sclerosis. J Neurol Neurosurg Psychiatry 1991; 54:110–115.

108. Izquierdo G, Campoy F, Mir J, Gonzalez M, Martinez-Parra C. Memory and learning disturbances in multiple sclerosis: MRI lesions and neuropsychological correlation. Eur J Radiol 1991; 13:220–224.

109. Huber SJ, Paulson GW, Shuttleworth EC, et al. Magnetic resonance imaging correlates of dementia in multiple sclerosis. Arch Neurol 1987; 44:732–736.

110. Pozzilli C, Bastianello S, Padovani A, et al. Anterior corpus callosum atrophy and verbal fluency in multiple sclerosis. Cortex 1991; 27:441–445.

111. Pelletier J, Habib M, Lyon-Caen O, et al. Functional and magnetic resonance imaging correlates of callosal involvement in multiple sclerosis. Arch Neurol 1993; 50:1077–1082.

112. Barkhof F, Elton M, Lindeboom J, et al. Functional correlates of callosal atrophy in relapsing-remitting multiple sclerosis patients: A preliminary MRI study. J Neurol 1998; 245:153–158.

113. van Buchem MA, Grossman RI, Armstrong C, et al. Correlation of volumetric magnetization transfer imaging with clinical data in MS. Neurology 1998; 50:1609–1617.

114. Foong J, Rozewicz L, Davie CA, Thompson AJ, Miller DH, Ron MA. Correlates of executive function in multiple sclerosis: The use of magnetic resonance spectroscopy as an index of focal pathology. J Neuropsychiatry Clin Neurosci 1999; 11:45–50.

115. Filippi M, Tortorella C, Rovaris M, et al. Changes in the normal appearing brain tissue and cognitive impairment in multiple sclerosis. J Neurol Neurosurg Psychiatry 2000; 68:157–161.

116. Fischer, JS. Assessment of neuropsychological function. In: Rudick RA, Goodkin DE, eds. Multiple Sclerosis Therapeutics. London: Martin Dunitz, 1999, pp 31–47.

117. Leo GJ, Rao SM. Effects of intravenous physostigmine and lecithin on memory loss in multiple sclerosis: Report of a pilot study. J Neurol Rehab 1988; 2:123–129.

118. Unverzagt FW, Rao SM, Antuono P. Oral physostigmine in the treatment of memory loss in multiple sclerosis. J Clin Exp Neuropsychol 1991; 13:74.

119. Krupp LB, Elkins LE, Scott SR, Smiroldo J, Coyle PK. Donepezil for the treatment of memory impairment in multiple sclerosis. Neurology 1999; 52:A137.

120. Green YM, Tariot PN, Wishart H, et al. A 12-week, open trial of donepezil hydrochloride in multiple sclerosis patients with associated cognitive impairments. J Clin Psychopharmacol 2000; 20:350–356.

121. Cohen RA, Fisher M. Amantadine treatment of fatigue associated with multiple sclerosis. Arch Neurol 1989; 46:676–680.

122. Geisler MW, Sliwinski, Coyle PK, Masur DM, Doscher C, Krupp LB. The effects of amantadine and pemoline on cognitive functioning in multiple sclerosis. Arch Neurol 1996; 53: 185–188.

123. Smits RCF, Emmen HH, Bertelsmann FW, Kulig BM, van Loenen AC, Polman CH. The effects of 4-aminopyridine on cognitive function in patients with multiple sclerosis: A pilot study. Neurology 1994; 44:1701–1705.

124. Bever CT, Anderson PA, Leslie J, et al. Treatment with oral 3,4 diaminopyridine improves leg strength in multiple sclerosis patients: Results of a randomized, double-blind, placebo-controlled, crossover trial. Neurology 1996; 47:1457–1462.

125. Plohmann AM, Kappos L, Ammann W, et al. Computer assisted retraining of attentional impairments in patients with multiple sclerosis. J Neurol Neurosurg Psychiatry 1998; 64: 455–462.

126. Jønsson A, Korfitzen EM, Heltberg A, Ravnborg MH, Byskov-Ottosen E. Effects of neuropsychological treatment in patients with multiple sclerosis. Acta Neurol Scand 1993; 88: 394–400.

127. Rodgers D, Khoo K, MacEachen M, Oven M, Beatty WW. Cognitive therapy for multiple sclerosis: A preliminary study. Altern Ther Health Med 1996; 2:70–74.

128. Multiple Sclerosis Study Group. Efficacy and toxicity of cyclosporine in chronic progressive multiple sclerosis: A randomized, double-blinded, placebo-controlled clinical trial. Ann Neurol 1990; 27:591–605.

129. Goodkin DE, Fischer JS. Treatment of multiple sclerosis with methotrexate. In: Goodkin DE, Rudick RA, eds. Treatment of Multiple Sclerosis: Advances in Trial Design, Results, and Future Perspectives. Springer: London, 1996, pp 251–287.

130. Pliskin NH, Hamer DP, Goldstein DS, et al. Improved delayed visual reproduction test performance in multiple sclerosis patients receiving interferon β-1b. Neurology 1996; 47:1463–1468.

131. Fischer JS, Priore RL, Jacobs LD, et al. Neuropsychological effects of interferon beta-1a in relapsing multiple sclerosis. Ann Neurol. In press.

132. Weinstein A, Schwid SR, Schiffer RB, McDermott MP, Giang DW, Goodman AD. Neuropsychological status in multiple sclerosis after treatment with glatiramer acetate (Copaxone). Arch Neurol 1999; 56:319–324.

133. Oliveri RL, Sibilia G, Valentino P, Russo C, Romeo N, Quattrone A. Pulsed methylprednisolone induces a reversible impairment of memory in patient with relapsing-remitting multiple sclerosis. Acta Neurol Scand 1998; 97:366–369.

134. Peyser JM, Edwards KR, Poser CM, Filskov SB. Cognitive function in patient with multiple sclerosis. Arch Neurol 1980; 37:577–579.

135. Fischer JS. Objective memory testing in multiple sclerosis. In: Jensen K, Knudsen L, Stenager E, Grant I, eds. Current Problems in Neurology: 10. Mental disorders and Cognitive Deficits in Multiple Sclerosis. London: Libbey, 1989, pp. 39–49.

136. Taylor R. Relationships between cognitive test performance and everyday cognitive difficulties in multiple sclerosis. Br J Clin Psychol 1990; 29:251–252.

137. Landro NI, Sletvold H, Celius EG. Memory functioning and emotional changes in early phase multiple sclerosis. Arch Clin Neuropsychol 2000; 15:37–46.

138. Beatty WW, Monson N. Metamemory in multiple sclerosis. J Clin Exp Neuropsychol 1991; 13:309–327.

139. Folstein MF, Folstein SE, McHugh PR. "Mini-Mental State": a practical method for grading the cognitive state of patients for the clinician. J Psychiatr Res 1975; 12:189–198.

140. Beatty WW, Goodkin DE. Screening for cognitive impairment in multiple sclerosis: An evaluation of the Mini-Mental State Examination. Arch Neurol 1990; 47:297–301.

141. Swirsky-Sacchetti T, Field HL, Mitchell DR, et al. The sensitivity of the Mini-Mental State Exam in the white matter dementia of multiple sclerosis. J Clin Psychol 1992; 48:779–786.

142. Jacobs JW, Bernhard MR, Delgado A, Strain JJ. Screening for organic mental syndromes in the medically ill. Ann Intern Med 1977; 86:40–46.

143. Mahler ME, Davis RJ, Benson DF. Screening multiple sclerosis patients for cognitive impairment. In: Jensen K, Knudsen L, Stenager E, Grant I, eds. Current Problems in Neurology: 10. Mental Disorders and Cognitive Deficits in Multiple Sclerosis. London: Libbey, 1989, pp 11–14.

144. Beatty WW, Paul RH, Wilbanks SL, Hames KA, Blanco CR, Goodkin DE. Identifying multiple sclerosis patients with mild or global cognitive impairment using the Screening Examination for Cognitive Impairment (SEFCI). Neurology 1995; 45:718–723.

145. Basso MR, Beason-Hazen S, Lynn J, Rammohan K, Bornstein RA. Screening for cognitive dysfunction in multiple sclerosis. Arch Neurol 1996; 53:980–984.

11

Loss and Restoration of Impulse Conduction in Disorders of Myelin

STEPHEN G. WAXMAN

Yale University School of Medicine, New Haven, and Rehabilitation Research Center, VA Connecticut, West Haven, Connecticut

I. INTRODUCTION

Multiple sclerosis (MS) exhibits a spectrum of clinical courses, including subclinical disease, progressive MS, relapsing-remitting MS, and stable MS. Demyelination, the presence of which can be inferred noninvasively in MS patients by neuroimaging and clinical electrophysiological methods, has classically been considered to be a hallmark of the lesions that occur in the brain and spinal cord in this disorder. Thus it is not surprising that many clinical signs and symptoms in MS reflect the abnormal behavior of demyelinated axons.

This chapter examines the pathophysiology of demyelinated axons in which impulse conduction is impaired. Abnormal conduction in these fibers is due not only to changes in passive electrical properties due to the loss of myelin insulation but also to alterations in active electrogenic properties which reflect the molecular structure of the axon itself. The role of demyelination in symptom production and the roles of neuronal and glial plasticity (not only at the cellular level but also at the ion channel—i.e., molecular, level) in the remission of clinical deficits are reviewed in the context of the physiology of impulse conduction. While most discussions of the pathophysiology of MS have focused on demyelinated axons within the center of plaques, we also examine the physiological implications of changes in the axon and myelin at the edges of these lesions, which—in addition to providing a border zone that may "confine" demyelination to the plaque—can play a critical physiological role in determining whether impulses will invade and propagate through demyelinated axons. Axonal injury also occurs in MS and probably contributes to the acquisition of irreversible deficits (1) but is discussed elsewhere in this volume.

Because C fibers in humans and nonmyelinated axons in many lower species function adequately without myelin, a theory of the pathophysiology of MS must explain why demyelination produces clinical deficits. A theory of the pathophysiology of demyelination must also explain the basis for the remissions that occur in many patients and for asymptomatic demyelinated plaques as well as the mechanisms that underlie liability of signs and symptoms and clinical remissions. Finally, a theory of pathophysiology should also suggest strategies for the development of new therapeutic interventions. Current knowledge of the pathophysiology of demyelination, as reviewed in this chapter, does, in fact, provide plausible explanations for these observations and, in addition, has provided clues that may open up new approaches to therapy.

II. FUNCTIONAL ORGANIZATION OF CENTRAL MYELINATED FIBERS

The myelinated fiber consists of an axon and its insulating myelin sheath. Myelin sheaths within the CNS are produced by oligodendrocytes (2,3). In contrast to Schwann cells, which myelinate single axons, each oligodendrocyte produces myelin sheaths around a family of axons in its vicinity, with estimates ranging from 1 or 2 to nearly 100 axons per family. The oligodendrocyte cell body usually does not surround or hug its myelin sheaths as a Schwann cell does but, on the contrary, is connected to its myelin sheaths by thin cytoplasmic bridges, a fact that has been interpreted as suggesting a tenuous connection between the genomic and biosynthetic machinery in the oligodendrocyte cell body and the myelin that might explain the paucity of remyelination within the central nervous system (CNS). There is considerable evidence, however, for local synthesis of myelin membrane in distal parts of oligodendroglial processes close to the myelin sheaths (4,5), where polyribosomes are present (4) and focal axon–oligodendrocyte interactions appear

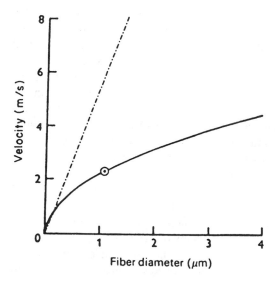

Figure 1 Relation between conduction velocity (*y* axis) and diameter (*x* axis), shown for both myelinated (*solid line*) and nonmyelinated (*dashed line*) axons. Note that, above a diameter of 0.2 μm, at which the two relationships cross, myelinated axons conduct more rapidly than nonmyelinated axons of the same size. (Modified from Ref. 8.)

to regulate properties of the myelin sheath such as its thickness and internode distance (4,5).

The myelin sheath consists of a compact spiral of glial membranes. The compact layered structure of the myelin endows it with electrical properties (a high electrical resistance and a low capacitance) which permit it to function as an electrical insulator surrounding the axon. Periodic interruptions (*nodes of Ranvier*) are present in the myelin sheath, at distances ranging from less than 100 μm (small-diameter fibers) to slightly over 1 mm (larger-diameter fibers). The regions between the nodes are termed the *internodes*. In contrast to nonmyelinated fibers, which usually conduct impulses in a continuous manner, myelinated fibers conduct action potentials in a discontinuous, or *saltatory*, manner (6,7). In nonmyelinated fibers, conduction velocity is proportional to the square root of the diameter, whereas in myelinated fibers, conduction velocity is approximately proportional to fiber diameter (8). Thus, above a critical diameter at which the conduction velocity–diameter relationships for nonmyelinated and myelinated fibers intersect, myelinated fibers conduct impulses more rapidly than nonmyelinated fibers of the same diameter; this critical diameter is approximately 0.2μm (8) (Fig. 1).

III. MEMBRANE ARCHITECTURE OF THE MYELINATED AXON

In contrast with most nonmyelinated axons, which conduct action potentials in a continuous manner and have membranes with uniform properties along their length, myelinated fibers support saltatory conduction and are constructed of axon membranes that express several types of voltage-sensitive ion channels in a spatially heterogeneous manner (Fig. 2). Sodium (Na$^+$) channels cluster in high density (approximately 1000/μm^2) in the axon membrane at the node of Ranvier, where action potential electrogenesis takes place in normal myelinated axons (9,10). In the internodal axon membrane under the myelin sheath, the density of Na$^+$ channels is much lower (<25/μm^2) (9–11), too low to support conduction under most circumstances.

As discussed later in this chapter, multiple sodium channels are encoded by different genes. They display distinct molecular differences superimposed on an invariant overall motif (four similar domains, each containing six membrane-spanning segments). The types of sodium channels that are present in myelinated axons are currently under study.

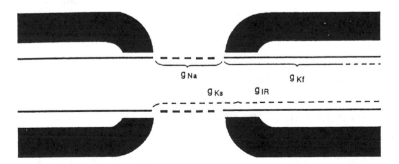

Figure 2 Working model of ion channel organization of the myelinated fiber. g$_{Na}$, sodium channels; g$_{Kf}$, fast potassium channels; g$_{Ks}$, slow potassium channels; g$_{IR}$, inward rectifier channels. Sodium channels are clustered at the node of Ranvier. In contrast, fast potassium channels, responsible for repolarization of the action potential, are present in the internodal axon membrane.

At least three types of potassium K^+ channels are expressed in myelinated fibers: a "fast" K^+ channel, a "slow" K^+ channel, and an inward rectifier that is permeable to both K^+ and Na^+ (see Ref. 12). Fast K^+ channels, which can be blocked by externally applied 4-aminopyridine (A-AP) if it is given access to these channels, are distributed in a pattern that is complementary to that of the Na^+ channels that are clustered in the nodal axon membrane. Fast K^+ channels are expressed in relatively low densities in the nodal axon membrane and are present in higher density in the axon membrane under the myelin (13–18). Voltage-clamp experiments demonstrate a density of fast K^+ channels that is highest in the paranode, decreasing to one-sixth of the paranodal density in the node and internode (19).

The clustering of Na^+ channels at high density in the nodal axon membrane and the paucity of these channels in the axon membrane under the myelin, together with the expression of fast K^+ channels in the paranodal axon membrane under the myelin, have important implications for axonal pathophysiology:

1. The low density of Na^+ channels in the demyelinated axon membrane, following acute damage to the myelin, results in a low density of inward Na^+ current that is inadequate for action potential electrogenesis, and this interferes with the conduction of action potentials.
2. Following demyelination, fast K^+ channels in the paranodal axon membrane are unmasked, and tend to clamp the demyelinated axon membrane close to the K^+ equilibrium potential E_K, further impeding action potential conduction.

Na^+, K^+-ATPase molecules are also present in the axon membrane at the node (20,21), where they maintain ionic homeostasis and produce electrogenic hyperpolarization (22). Intra-axonal recordings (23) demonstrate that experimentally demyelinated peripheral nervous system (PNS) axons are hyperpolarized as a result of Na^+, K^+-ATPase activity. Ouabain, an inhibitor of Na^+, K^+-ATPase, reduces the hyperpolarization and can lead to restoration of conduction. On the basis of these findings Bostock and Grafe (23) suggested that pharmacological blockade of Na^+, K^+-ATPase activity might improve conduction of high-frequency impulse trains in demyelinated axons. Experimental results have provided some observations that tend to confirm this suggestion.

The molecular architecture of the axon membrane also has important implications for recovery of conduction following demyelination. Recent studies, discussed later in this chapter, have demonstrated a molecular reorganization of the demyelinated axon membrane, with acquisition of a higher-than-normal density of Na^+ channels in some demyelinated (former internodal) regions, which develop the capability to support action potential conduction. The membrane structure of the myelinated fiber also suggests the possibility of pharmacologically blocking the fast K^+ channels that are unmasked by demyelination, thereby increasing the safety factor for conduction in demyelinated axons.

IV. IMPAIRED ACTION POTENTIAL CONDUCTION IN DEMYELINATED AXONS

The high-resistance, low-capacitance myelin functions as an insulator in normal myelinated fibers, shunting the action current from each active node of Ranvier, though the relatively low-resistance axoplasm, to the subsequent node (Fig. 3A). The threshold for excitation at the next node is reached in mammalian myelinated axons at 37°C after a brief interval (termed the *internodal conduction time*) of approximately 20 μs (24), and

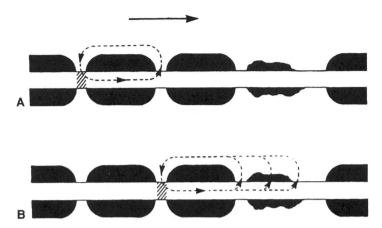

Figure 3 Diagrammatic representation of current flow associated with conduction through normally (A) myelinated and (B) demyelinated regions of an axon. The action potential is conducted from left to right (*arrow*). This idealized diagram represents the myelin as a perfect insulation. Dashed arrows illustrate current flow resulting from an action potential that is located at the crosshatched node. Current is lost in demyelinated regions as a result of capacitative and resistive shunting.

the impulse travels along the fiber by jumping sequentially from node to node in a saltatory manner with a high conduction velocity. A measure of the reliability of conduction is provided by the *safety factor* (ratio between the current available to stimulate a node of Ranvier and the current required to stimulate the node). The safety factor is 5 to 7 in normal myelinated fibers, so that there is a high degree of reliability for impulse conduction (6).

When the myelin is damaged, the density of action current is reduced as a result of capacitative and resistive shunting (see Fig. 3B). The safety factor is thus decreased because the transmembrane current density is low. If the safety factor is reduced but still is greater than 1.0, the charging time for the nodal membrane may be increased, so that it will take longer than normal for the axon to reach threshold and conduction velocity will be reduced. In more severely demyelinated axons, the safety factor can be reduced to values less than 1, and threshold will not be reached; hence conduction will fail (25).

From a phenomenological point of view, demyelinated axons display a spectrum of conduction abnormalities (Fig. 4). Signs and symptoms that are negative in the jacksonian sense can reflect slowed, desynchronized, or blocked conduction (see Fig. 4B to E). As discussed below, slowed conduction is less important than conduction block in producing clinical deficits. Clinical abnormalities that are *positive* in the jacksonian sense are presumably the result of ectopic impulse generation or abnormal cross talk between demyelinated axons (see Fig. 4F to I).

Early electrophysiological studies in demyelinated axons showed that demyelination can result in *decreased conduction velocity, failure to transmit high-frequency trains of action potentials*, or *total conduction block* (26,27). These conduction abnormalities are confined to the zone of demyelination in focally demyelinated fibers, with apparently normal conduction in regions proximal and distal to the site of demyelination (Fig. 5). Resistive and capacitative shunting across the (former internodal) demyelinated axon membrane contributes to these conduction abnormalities. In ventral root fibers demyelin-

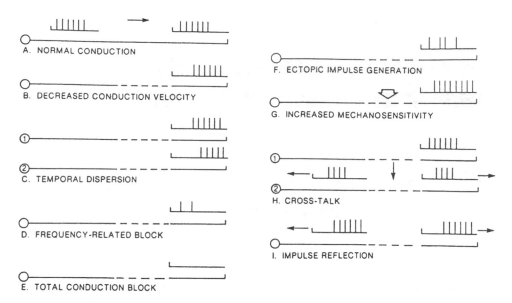

Figure 4 Conduction abnormalities in demyelinated axons. Demyelinated regions of the axon are diagrammatically shown as dashed lines. Cell bodies are located to the left, and axon terminals to the right. The direction of normal conduction is indicated by the arrow; see text for further explanation.

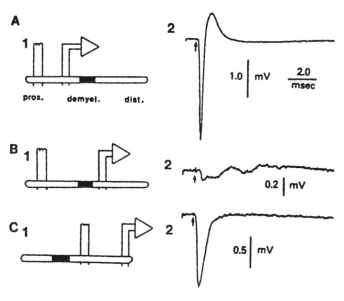

Figure 5 Recording obtained proximal to (A) across (B) and distal (C) to a focally demyelinated region (injected with lysophosphatidylcholine) from rat sciatic nerve. Conduction is relatively normal in proximal and distal nerve segments (A2,C2). However, conduction slowing, block, and temporal dispersion (B2) are present when action potentials are conducted through the lesion site. (Modified from Ref. 168.)

ated with diphtheria toxin, internodal conduction time can be increased to nearly 500 μs compared with approximately 20μs in normal fibers (24). Thus, the impulse takes longer to travel along the fiber; hence, conduction velocity is reduced (see Fig. 4B).

As a result of varying degrees of damage to the myelin, internodal conduction time can vary between individual demyelinated internodes along single fibers or between neighboring demyelinated fibers in a nerve or CNS tract. *Temporal dispersion*, or loss of synchrony in CNS tracts in which different fibers exhibit different degrees of conduction slowing, is a corollary of decreased conduction velocity and reflects the variability in internodal conduction times seen in demyelinated axons (see Fig. 4C). Temporal dispersion can produce clinical abnormalities by interfering with functions that require synchronous discharge.

Conduction block also occurs in demyelinated fibers (24,27). Both passive and active characteristics of the demyelinated fiber contribute to conduction block. Failure of conduction in focally demyelinated axons is partly due to impedance mismatch, which results in decreased current density and thereby decreases the safety factor at sites of demyelination (28,29). The paucity of Na^+ channels in the demyelinated axon membrane also contributes to conduction block (9,10). Moreover, fast K^+ channels (normally covered by the myelin in the paranode and internode) are unmasked in demyelinated axons, and this impedes action potential electrogenesis because they tend to clamp the demyelinated membrane close to the potassium equilibrium potential E_K (30,31).

Conduction block can be frequency-related, with high-frequency impulse trains failing to propagate while low-frequency trains conduct reliably (see Fig. 4D); or conduction failure can be complete, with single action potentials failing to propagate beyond the zone of demyelination (see Fig. 4E). Hyperpolarization of the axon membrane, due to electrogenic pump (Na^+, K^+-ATPase) activity, can contribute to conduction block of high-frequency impulse trains (23). Increased intracellular Na^+ concentration at the "driving node" (24) and depolarization of demyelinated axons due to increases in extracellular K^+ concentration (32) may also contribute to block of high-frequency impulse trains.

Positive conduction abnormalities are illustrated in Fig. 4F to I. *Ectopic action potential generation* (see Fig. 4F) has been observed, for example, in demyelinated axons in cat dorsal columns (33). Differences in the accommodative properties of demyelinated sensory versus motor axons (34) are consistent with the more frequent occurrence of paresthesia (a positive sensory abnormality), compared with extraneous motor activity, in MS patients. *Increased mechanosensitivity* (33) has also been observed in CNS demyelinated fibers (see Fig. 4G) and probably accounts for clinical phenomena such as Lhermitte's symptom (35). In addition, *abnormal fiber–fiber excitation* (cross talk) may occur between abnormally myelinated axons (see Fig. 4H). This cross talk, which is also termed *ephaptic transmission*, occurs at frequencies up to 70 Hz in the dysmyelinated spinal cord axons of the dy-dy mouse but appears to occur preferentially in a unidirectional manner in this model system, from bare fibers to myelinated fibers (36).

Impulse reflection also occurs in demyelinated fibers (37) and may result in extraneous sensory or motor activity (e.g., paresthesia, pain, or tonic spasms); because the reflected (antidromic) impulses can collide with and abolish orthodromic impulses, impulse reflection can interfere with normal impulse traffic. Positive conduction abnormalities probably interact by positive feedback, with ectopic activity being amplified by, for example, impulse reflection or cross talk (36). The high packing density of demyelinated axons in some plaques, with no or few intervening glial elements, may contribute to cross talk and abnormal discharge.

V. RELATION BETWEEN CONDUCTION ABNORMALITIES AND CLINICAL STATUS

Clinicopathological and neuroimaging studies show that demyelinated plaques can be present in MS patients without necessarily producing clinical deficits. Useful visual acuity is retained, for example, in some MS patients with demyelination of the total cross section of the optic nerves for more than 1 cm (38,39). Evoked potential studies indicate that demyelinating lesions can produce slowed conduction without necessarily leading to clinical deficit. For example, visual-evoked responses may be delayed by more than 40 ms in MS patients who have never experienced visual difficulties or after recovery from optic neuritis (40). Recovery from acute optic neuritis usually includes parallel improvements in visual acuity and amplitude of the visual evoked response, but recovery of the prolonged evoked response latency usually does not accompany clinical recovery. Serial recordings show that somatosensory evoked response latencies can lag behind clinical improvement of sensory symptoms in MS patients; in some cases, resolution of clinical abnormalities antedates the recovery of evoked response latencies by months. Thus clinical recovery does not depend on a return of conduction velocities to normal.

Subclinical slowing of conduction along demyelinated axons is not a rare phenomenon. A study on evoked potentials (42) in MS suspects who subsequently developed definite MS (McAlpine criteria) showed that a significant proportion of evoked potential abnormalities (59% of the visual evoked potential abnormalities that were observed; 41%

Table 1 Evoked Potential Abnormalities at Time of Referral in MS Suspects Who Subsequently Developed Definite MS[a]

Initial diagnosis[b]	Follow-up diagnosis	N	Follow-up (mo)	Unexpected abnormal/expected abnormal/ number tested[c]			
				PVEP	SEP	BAEP	At least one abnormal EP
Probable MS	Definite MS	19	23	6/12/19	4/6/19	0/3/19	9/9/19
Possible MS	Definite MS	15	32	9/1/14	8/4/14	2/2/14	12/1/15
Myelopathy	Definite MS	4	25	4/0/4	0/4/4	2/0/4	4/0/4
AND	Definite MS	10	28	6/1/10	0/3/9	2/1/10	6/2/10
ON	Definite MS	3	39	0/3/3	0/0/3	0/0/3	0/3/3
CND	Definite MS	1	36	0/0/1	0/0/1	0/0/1	0/0/1
Total		52		25/17/51	12/17/50	6/6/51	31/15/52
Unexpected abnormalities/EPs performed				49.0%	24.0%	11.8%	59.6%
Unexpected abnormalities/total abnormalities (expected and unexpected)				59.5%	41.4%	50.0%	

[a] Includes 52 patients in whom diagnosis of definite MS was made at follow-up, from a series of 269 patients between the ages of 15 and 60 who were referred for evaluation of suspected MS.

[b] AND, acute neurological disease initially undiagnosed (single episode of symptoms, duration <3 mo); ON, optic neuritis; CND, chronic neurological disease (neurological symptoms without remission) >3-mo duration; EP, evoked potential.

[c] PVEP, pattern visual-evoked potential; SEP, somatosensory-evoked potential; BAEP, brain stem auditory-evoked potential.

Source: Modified from Ref. 42.

somatosensory; 50% auditory) were clinically silent (i.e., they were not accompanied by evidence, on history and physical examination, of pathology in the pathway under study; Table 1). The observations that asymptomatic demyelinated plaques are not uncommon in MS patients and that increases in conduction latency do not necessarily produce clinical abnormalities are not entirely unexpected, since the input-output functions of some neural systems are relatively robust, even in the face of changes in latency that can be measured in milliseconds. Significant changes in conduction velocity occur with physiological changes in body temperature (Fig. 6A), since the Q_{10} for conduction velocity is greater than 1.5 in CNS axons (43–45). Even though conduction velocity—and thus conduction time—is dependent on temperature, most neural systems continue to function efficiently, even in poikilothermic species, as temperature changes within the physiological range.

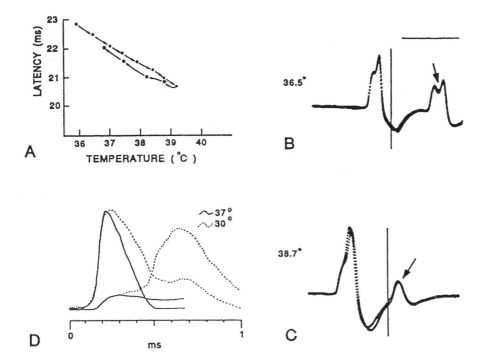

Figure 6 Temperature effects on axonal impulse conduction. A. Relation between brain temperature and antidromic latency for axon in corpus callosum of the rabbit. There is a reduction in latency (i.e., an increase in conduction velocity) when temperature increases. B and C. Antidromic impulse conduction in a callosal projection neuron at (B) 36.5°C and (C) 38.7°C. The vertical line marks the tracings 16.8 ms after stimulation. Latency is decreased, owing to *increased conduction velocity*, at higher temperatures (compare first spike in panel C with that in panel B). For the second action potential evoked at high frequency, safety factor is reduced, resulting in an inflection (*arrow in panel B*) between the initial segment spike and the somadendritic spike at 36.5°C. At increased temperature, the action potential fails to invade the soma (*arrow in panel C*), as a result of *decreased safety factor*. Calibration = 2.0 ms. (Modified from Ref. 44.) D. Temperature effect on conduction in demyelinated axons. Action potentials at two adjacent nodes of fiber demyelinated with diptheria toxin are shown. At 37°C (*solid lines*) conduction is blocked. At 30°C (*dashed lines*) the action potential at first node is prolonged and a second node is excited after more than 300 μs. (From Ref. 52.)

Conduction block prevents the transmission of action potentials that encode information and is correlated with clinical abnormalities. A somatosensory evoked potential study showed that impaired frequency-following in MS patients was qualitatively correlated with degree of clinical involvement (41). Because neural information can be encoded by the pattern or frequency of impulses transmitted along axons in some CNS tracts, the ability of myelinated axons to carry trains of impulses at specific frequencies or in specific patterns may be an important determinant of clinical status. Loss of even a fraction of impulses within a train, as a result of frequency-related conduction block, can degrade neural messages. Total conduction block produces significant loss of function unless alternative conduction pathways are available.

MS patients are often sensitive to temperature, with symptoms becoming more pronounced as body temperature increases (46–49). Increased temperature is correlated both with increased conduction velocity (see above) and with decreased safety factor in CNS axons in situ. Worsening of clinical status in MS patients as temperature increases implies that, in human subjects with MS, conduction block is a more important determinant of clinical status than decreased conduction velocity.

VI. LABILITY OF ACTION POTENTIAL CONDUCTION IN DEMYELINATED AXONS

Patients with MS often note a lability in their clinical status, i.e. changes that can occur on an hour-to-hour basis. While incompletely understood, this lability appears to have a basis in the pathophysiology of demyelinated axons. Numerous studies have confirmed that there can be a striking thermosensitivity in MS patients, with clinical status worsening as temperature increases (46,47,49). Increased susceptibility to thermally induced, reversible conduction block has been demonstrated in microelectrode studies on demyelinated axons (50) and at other sites of reduced safety factor such as the axon initial segment–soma junction (see Fig. 6B and C) (44). The mechanism underlying the conduction block in experimentally demyelinated fibers includes a reduced time integral of inward (depolarizing) nodal current that occurs because ion channels open and close more quickly at higher temperatures as a result the temperature-dependence of channel kinetics (51). Even small increases in temperature (0.5°C) can reversibly block conduction in some fibers. Figure 6D (52) shows that conduction block can be temporarily overcome and the action potential prolonged as temperature is lowered in demyelinated axons.

In an analysis of thermal sensitivity in demyelinated axons, Schauf and Davis (53) concluded that, as the safety factor is decreased from its normal value of 5 to 6 (6), conduction should become increasingly labile. For axons with safety factor only slightly greater than 1.0, conditions that marginally decrease it (i.e., conditions that might have little, if any, effect on conduction in normal fibers) would be expected to lead to transient conduction failure. Conversely, in demyelinated axons with safety factor slightly less than 1.0, conditions that increase safety factor would be expected to restore conduction. Changes in metabolic status as well as alterations in temperature, therefore, would be expected to transiently alter the conduction properties of demyelinated fibers. This has, in fact, been demonstrated in human subjects with MS. For example, changes in acid-base balance, which can be produced by oral phosphate or intravenous bicarbonate administration or by hyperventilation, can produce reversible alterations in neurological status in MS patients (54,55). These observations in humans illustrate the sensitivity of demyelinated fibers to changes in metabolic status.

Superimposed on baseline conduction abnormalities caused by demyelination, labile conduction in demyelinated axons, resulting from their increased sensitivity to temperature and metabolic changes, may produce periodic fluctuations in clinical status. The lability of action potential conduction in demyelinated axons suggests that pharmacological modification in channel kinetics or in other membrane properties may enhance action potential conduction. This provides part of the rationale for the development of drugs that improve safety factor in demyelinated axons.

VII. SODIUM CHANNEL–BLOCKING FACTORS?

It is possible—although not yet proven—that antibody- or lymphokine-mediated effects on Na^+ channels also participate in the pathophysiology of MS and related disorders (56). Patients with MS commonly report evanescent, rapidly fluctuating symptoms, and these may appear to be unaccompanied by changes in temperature or metabolic status sufficient to interfere with the conduction of action potentials. Moreover, abnormalities of neuromuscular transmission (57) and in the electroretinogram [reflecting physiological abnormalities within the retina where there is no myelin (58,59)] have been observed in MS.

The hypothesis of "neuroelectric" blocking factors that interfere with axonal conduction or synaptic transmission in demyelinating disorders has been the subject of controversy (see, e.g., Ref. 60). Recent results have renewed interest in this area. It is known that block of Na^+ channels without demyelination can produce decreases in axonal conduction velocity (61,62). Recent results have been interpreted as suggesting that acute paralysis in Guillain-Barré syndrome is due to a Na^+ channel–blocking factor in the cerebrospinal fluid (63) and that the cerebrospinal fluid of MS patients contains factors that can impair the function of Na^+ channels (64). In addition, Brinkmeier et al. (65) reported that interleukin-2 (IL-2), which is present at elevated levels in MS (66,67), can block Na^+ channels. There have been several reports indicating that nitric oxide (NO) can produce conduction block in axons (68,69), possibly with a preferential blocking action on demyelinated axons (69). This may be a result of the blocking action of NO and Na^+ channels (70). Since levels of NO and its synthesizing enzymes are increased in MS (71,72) and in animal models such as experimental allergic encephalomyelitis (73,74), this may be relevant to the pathophysiology of MS. Takigawa et al. (75) showed that antibodies against GM1 gangliosides can attenuate voltage-sensitive Na^+ currents in a complement-dependent manner, suggesting that these antibodies can block Na^+ channels. The suppression of Na^+ current was sufficient to retard action potential electrogenesis as measured by voltage clamp, prompting the authors to suggest that these antibodies might play a role in the pathophysiology of some neurological disorders.

Although these results are provocative, the existence of blocking factors still requires confirmation. Moreover, little information is available about the biochemical or immunological mechanisms involved in the generation of antibodies or other factors that interfere with Na^+ channels, about the epitopes or target areas within the channel that are involved (channel protein? glycosylated dome of the channel? associated extracellular molecules in the nodal gap?), or about the details of the mechanisms that interfere with channel function. More research on Na^+ channel blocking factors is needed.

VIII. PHARMACOLOGICAL RESTORATION OF CONDUCTION IN DEMYELINATED AXONS

The hyperpolarizing effects of fast K^+ channels and Na^+, K^+-ATPase in demyelinated axons suggest the therapeutic strategy of using pharmacological agents to improve the safety factor and thereby overcome conduction block. Increased inward transmembrane current, associated with prolonged action potential duration after blockade of fast K^+ channels, would be expected to produce greater depolarization of the axon membrane at sites of demyelination. Inhibition of Na^+, K^+-ATPase would be expected to attenuate the pump-mediated hyperpolarization, bringing the membrane closer to threshold.

Action potential prolongation and reversal of conduction block have, in fact, been observed following application of drugs that block fast K^+ channels [such as 4-aminipyridine (4-AP)] in demyelinated spinal roots (30), sciatic nerve (76,77), and posterior column axons in a spinal cord contusion model (78). Because fast K^+ channels that are sensitive to 4-AP tend to be localized under the myelin in normal axons, 4-AP has a relatively specific effect, increasing the duration of the action potential in demyelinated but not in normal axons, where the 4-AP-sensitive K^+ channels are covered by the myelin.

Reversal of conduction block in an experimentally demyelinated axon following focal application of 4-AP is shown in Fig. 7 (76). Stimulating electrodes were located on both ends of a focally demyelinated nerve, and recordings from single axons were obtained with a microelectrode on one side of the lesion (Fig. 7A). Under control conditions (no drugs), in response to stimulation of the axon proximal to the lesion (so that the conduction path did not include the demyelinated zone), a propagated action potential could be recorded; in contrast, following stimulation on the contralateral side of the lesion (so that conduction had to cross the zone of demyelination), conduction failed at the site of demye-

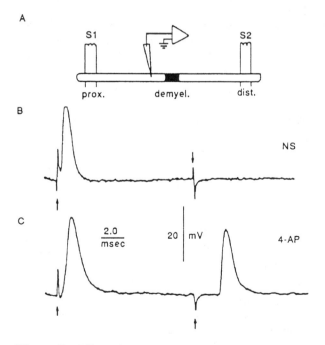

Figure 7   Effect of 4-AP on conduction block in a demyelinated fiber. A. Experimental design permits examination of conduction through normal (stimulation at S_1) or demyelinated (stimulation at S_2) regions. B. Stimulation of S_1 leads to an action potential, but conduction block occurs following S_2 stimulation, when the demyelinated zone is interposed between the stimulation and recording site. C. Application of 4-AP leads to overcoming of the conduction block. NS, normal solution. (Modified from Ref. 77.)

lination so that an action potential could not be recorded (Fig. 7B). To block fast K^+ channels, the nerve was then exposed to 4-AP (1.0 mM). Following exposure to 4-AP, conduction proceeded with a high safety factor, so that the action potential traveled successfully (but with an increased latency reflecting decreased conduction velocity) through the demyelinated zone (Fig. 7C).

Clinical studies with 4-AP and with the related drug 3,4 diaminopyridine (3,4-DAP) have documented transient improvement in motor function, reduction in scotomata, and improved critical flicker fusion in MS patients (79,80). Although additional clinical studies will be necessary to more fully assess the therapeutic potential and the short- and long-term side effects of 4-AP and related drugs in MS, these results demonstrate, at a minimum, that it is possible to rationally design pharmacological approaches that reverse conduction block in demyelinated axons.

Pharmacological inhibition of Na^+, K^+-ATPase has also been studied as a potential means of overcoming conduction block in demyelinated axons. Kaji and Sumner (81) observed that systemic digitalis can reverse the latency increase and improve frequency-following, as studied by somatosensory evoked potentials in rats with focal demyelinated lesions of the spinal cord. They also observed improved conduction velocity and reversal of conduction block in demyelinated axons following exposure to ouabain (82). Small degrees of clinical improvement were reported concurrent with changes in evoked potentials following treatment of MS patients with intravenous digoxin (0.22 mg/kg body weight) (83). These studies suggest that inhibition of Na^+, K^+-ATPase activity may provide an alternative approach to restoring conduction in patients with demyelinating disorders; inhibition of Na^+, K^+-ATPase could possibly be used in parallel with blockade of fast K^+ channels. Basic and clinical studies on these alternative approaches to pharmacological restoration of conduction are currently under way.

IX. RECOVERY OF IMPULSE TRANSMISSION DEMYELINATED AXONS: CONTINUOUS CONDUCTION

Clinical remissions, at least in some patients, appear to have a basis in the restoration (or maintenance) of impulse conduction along demyelinated axons. Clinicopathological observations provide inferential evidence for the recovery, in some chronically demyelinmated axons, of secure conduction. Useful visual acuity is retained or recovered in some MS patients with extensive (>1 cm) demyelination of the total cross section of the optic nerves (38,39). In cases such as these, mechanisms such as synaptic plasticity, utilization of alternative conduction pathways, or remyelination cannot account for recovery. Action potential conduction must have been retained or recovered in at least a subpopulation of the demyelinated axons.

The slow conduction velocity (similar to those of nonmyelinated axons) seen in early electrophysiological studies of demyelinated axons (84,85) was interpreted as suggesting that action potentials might be conducted in a continuous manner (similar to propagation in nonmyelinated axons) in demyelinated axon regions. Longitudinal current analysis in single, undissected normal nerve fibers confirms saltatory conduction, with excitability apparently confined to the nodes of Ranvier (24). In contrast, a continuous mode of action potential conduction has been observed in some chronically demyelinated axons. In rat ventral root fibers exposed to diphtheria toxin, the inward membrane current traveled continuously along demyelinated axons segments, where it could proceed for as far as 1.5 times the average internode distance, suggesting that action potentials could propagate continuously along extensive regions of the demyelinated axons (86,87). Continuous conduction was observed beginning 4 to 6 days after demyelination, and had a velocity of 1/20 to 1/40 of the normal (saltatory) conduction velocity for these fibers. An example of continuous conduction is shown in Fig. 8. These results suggested that the demyelinated internodal axon membrane, at least in some regions, can develop widespread excitability that supports continuous conduction. Felts et al. (88) recorded from axons within experimental demyelinating lesions in the spinal cord and subsequently examined them by serial-section ultrastructural analysis; they confirmed that some axons can conduct over continuous lengths of demyelination exceeding 2 mm (several internodes) in length.

Given what we know about the molecular architecture of axons, how can continuous conduction occur following demyelination? Computer simulations suggest that, in some small-caliber demyelinated axons, the density of preexisting Na^+ channels in the demyelinated (formerly internodal) region may be large enough to support conduction of at least single action potentials (28,89). In fact, in some small-diameter (<0.5 μm) axons that lack myelin, action potential conduction can be supported by low Na^+ channel densities (<40/μm^2) (90–92), at least if temperature is lowered. In the smallest axons (<0.25 μm), the conduction of action potentials (at low frequencies) can be supported by Na^+ channel densities of <10/μm^2 (93). These results may be relevant to small-diameter axons that have been demyelinated or to axons in which diameter has decreased following demyelination. Diameter of some demyelinated axons is, in fact, reduced in regions where myelin is

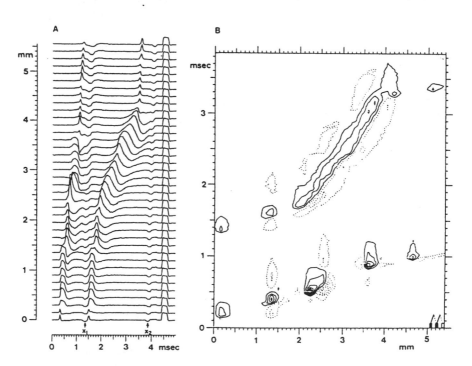

Figure 8 Continuous conduction and internodal electrogenesis in a demyelinated ventral root axon 14 days after experimental demyelination produced by injection of diphtheria toxin. Two fibers were recorded simultaneously at 30°C. A. Longitudinal current averages ($n = 1024$; current calibration 2.2 nA; X1 and X2, conduction time indications). B. Membrane current contours (contour interval: 0.5nA/150 μm). (From Ref. 87.)

lost (94,95), possibly as a result of decreased neurofilament phosphorylation and increased neurofilament packing density in demyelinated regions (96,97). However these results are probably not applicable to larger axons, because the input resistance of cylindrical axons is proportional to (diameter)$^{-3/2}$. Given the relatively small input impedance of larger myelinated axons, they probably require reorganization of the axon membrane, with development of a higher-than-normal Na$^+$ channel density following demyelination, for restoration of conduction. Experimental evidence indicates that this membrane reorganization does take place.

The early observation of continuous conduction in experimentally demyelinated axons were paralleled by electron microscopic studies that demonstrated, along these axons, the development of regions of axon membrane with cytochemical (98) and freeze-fracture (99) properties similar to those of nodal membrane. Additional evidence for the acquisition of high Na$^+$-channel densities in the demyelinated axon membrane has been provided by immunocytochemical studies. In studies on fish lateral line nerves (100), relatively high densities of Na$^+$ channels were observed in previously internodal axon regions by 14 to 21 days following injection of the demyelinating toxin doxorubicin; immunocytochemical observations suggest the induction of sodium channels at newly formed nodes along remyelinated axons (101).

The development of Na$^+$-channel densities that are higher than normal in persistently demyelinated regions may represent a dedifferentiation of the axon membrane (102). Although the mature internodal membrane appears to be inexcitable (9,10), the premyelinated axon membrane (including regions destined to develop into internodal membrane) is electrically excitable (17,93). Studies on the developing internodal axon during normal ontogenesis suggest that suppression of Na$^+$ channel expression reduces excitability after axons are covered by myelin. The downregulation of Na$^+$ channels in the presumptive internodal axon membrane does not occur during normal development until myelination has begun (103). This might be expected from a teleological point of view because, if the axon membrane were preprogrammed to lose excitability at a predetermined time, even small delays in myelination would be accompanied by conduction block; which could be lethal. The maintenance of Na$^+$-channel density in the internodal axon membrane, until there is a suppression of Na$^+$-channel expression by the overlying myelin or glial cell, appears to provide a mechanism that ensures that conduction is not lost during development. Although the factor(s) responsible for attenuation of sodium channel expression in the internodal membrane are unknown, their identification might permit the development of manipulations that would facilitate a reexpression of Na$^+$ channels in the denuded axon membrane.

X. NONUNIFORM CONDUCTION FOLLOWING DEMYELINATION

A different mode of impulse propagation—nonuniform—may also subserve recovery of conduction in some demyelinated axons. In this type of conduction, the action potential propagates between isolated foci of inward current generation (termed ''phi nodes''), which appear to be scattered aggregations of Na$^+$ channels, established before remyelination. These hot spots may represent the precursors of nodes in fibers that are about to remyelinate. Smith et al. (104) noted that phi nodes develop several days before remyelination in ventral root axons demyelinated with lysophosphatidylcholine (Fig. 9). Phi nodes were initially observed as isolated foci of inward current spaced at 100 to 200 μm (i.e., the distance between the nodes that will form during remyelination). In some fibers studied

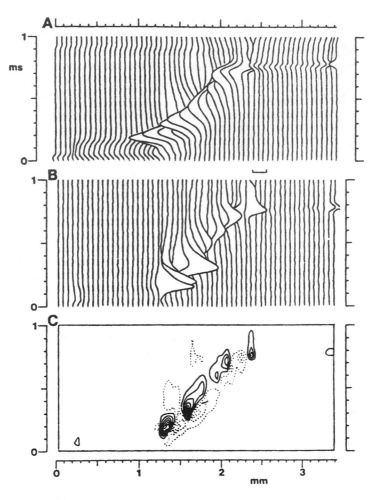

Figure 9 phi-Nodes demonstrated by electrophysiological recording in rat ventral root axon demyelinated with lysophosphatidylcholine. A. Longitudinal currents. B. Membrane currents. C. Membrane current contour map showing conduction that propagates through the lesion, 6 days following lysophosphatidylcholine injection. (A,B: Calibration bar = 10 nA, C: Contour intervals 3.5 nA/60 μm.) (From Ref. 104.)

several days before remyelination, phi nodes appeared to support conduction through the lesion.

Electron microscopy demonstrates an ultrastructural correlate of phi nodes (i.e., focal regions of axon membrane specialization characterized by a dense cytoplasmic undercoating similar to that at normal nodes of Ranvier) (105). These specialized regions of the axon membrane extend for only several micrometers along each axon, a length similar to (although not identical with) that of the node of Ranvier. Freeze-fracture demonstrates a counterpart for these axon membrane specialization. Patches of E-face intramembranous particles, of a size similar to those in the nodal axon, are present along axons permanently demyelinated with ethidium bromide, and may represent cluster of Na$^+$ channels (106). Intramembranous particle patches with similar properties are observed along axons that have been deprived of myelination by irradiation during gliogenesis (107). The number of intramembranous particles in each patch is approximately the same as at a mature node, consistent with the idea that each patch is the precursor of a node of Ranvier.

XI. MOLECULAR BASIS FOR MEMBRANE REORGANIZATION IN DEMYELINATED AXONS

Increased densities of Na^+ channels in the demyelinated axon membrane could reflect the redistribution of Na^+ channels into the demyelinated (previously internodal) membrane. It has been argued (89), however, that the spread of Na^+ channels by diffusion is not sufficient to support action potential conduction through demyelinated regions. At former nodes of Ranvier in demyelinated axons studied by patch-clamp recording, sharp gradients in channel density have been observed, and have been interpreted as suggesting that Na^+ channels do not diffuse away from the node in large numbers following demyelination (11). Radioimmunoassay studies show a significant increase in Na^+ channel concentration per wet weight of tissue (approximately threefold at 21 to 28 days after demyelination), thereby providing some evidence for the insertion of new Na^+ channels into the demyelinated axon membrane, in the fish lateral line nerve (108). Quantitative autoradiography with [^{3}H]saxitoxin (STX) in demyelinated white matter in MS patients reveals a fourfold increase in STX binding sites, compared with normal white matter, consistent with insertion of new Na^+ channels into the demyelinated axon membrane (109).

The source of the Na^+ channels destined for the demyelinated axon membrane has not yet been identified. Channel synthesis in the neuronal cell body, with movement by axonal transport, is one possibility. Electrophysiological experiments show the deployment of new Na^+ channels by neurons after axonal transection (110–112). Axonal transport of Na^+ channels has been demonstrated in peripheral nerves (113).

Increased synthesis and deployment of sodium channels in demyelinated neurons does not necessarily imply that the appropriate types of sodium channels are added to the neuronal nerve. It is now clear that there are nearly a dozen genes, each encoding a sodium channel with the same overall structure (about 1800 amino acid residues organized into four homologous domains, each containing six membrane-spanning segments). The amino acid sequences of the different sodium channels vary somewhat and, as a result, the different channels have different kinetics, voltage dependencies, and pharmacological profiles. At least eight different sodium-channel genes are expressed in the CNS (114). Following axonal transection, there are changes in the pattern of sodium-channel gene actuation in the affected neurons that express abnormal combinations of sodium channel mRNA (115–117) which are associated with abnormal patterns of sodium current expression (118,119). Abnormal patterns of sodium-channel expression have also been observed in several models of demyelination (120,121) and more recently the abnormal expression of the sensory neuron-specific (SNS) sodium channel (which is not present in the normal brain) has been observed in Purkinje cells from patients with MS (121a). MS thus appears to include a channelopathy. This may be functionally significant because the abnormal mixtures of sodium channels would be expected to result in mistuning of the affected neurons, producing hyperexcitability, which could lead to positive clinical symptoms such as paraesthesia or pain, (119,122,123) or to negative symptoms due to problems in impulse conduction as a result of abnormal background traffic.

A second possible source of new sodium channels is synthesis in glial cells, with subsequent transfer to the axon (124,125). Perinodal astrocyte processes and Schwann cell microvilli contact the Na$^+$ channel–rich axon membrane at the node in highly specific manner (126–128). Glial cell processes are apposed to demyelinated axons at sites of Na$^+$-channel clustering (106,107,129–131), and the two specializations (glial contact and Na$^+$-channel clustering) usually are precisely juxtaposed, suggesting that glial cell contact may be necessary for Na$^+$-channel clustering in the axon membrane. Moreover, it has been demonstrated that astrocytes express voltage-sensitive Na$^+$ channels (124,132–136) as well as the mRNAs for neuronal-type Na$^+$-channel α and β subunits (137–139). However, even in this context, transfer of channels from glial cells to axons has not been demonstrated. Increased numbers of Na$^+$ channels have been observed along demyelinated axons in fish lateral line nerves after injection of doxorubicin; because Schwann cells are killed by this drug, it has been argued that glial synthesis of Na$^+$ channels is unlikely (108). Other functions have been proposed for astrocyte Na$^+$ channels [e.g., providing a return pathway for Na$^+$ ions that maintains and modulates astrocyte Na$^+$, K$^+$-ATPase activity (140)]. Alternatively, it has been suggested (141) that astrocytes may secrete extracellular molecules that participate in the targeting or anchoring of Na$^+$ channels at sites of aggregation.

XII. IMPEDANCE MATCHING IN DEMYELINATED AXONS

As described above, restoration of conduction in chronically demyelinated axons is associated with the development of higher-than-normal Na$^+$-channel density in the banned axon membrane. Yet the development of high Na$^+$-channel density in demyelinated axon regions does not, in itself, ensure reliable impulse conduction. *Impedance mismatch* reflects the passive properties of the nerve fiber and is due to the electrical loading that occurs (largely as a result of increased membrane capacitance) at sites of axonal inhomogeneity, such as the transition between myelinated and demyelinated regions. At these sites, impendance mismatch can increase the total charge movement (and thus the charging time) needed for action potential propagation (142). Impedance mismatch can prevent the action potential from invading a demyelinated region and thus be a significant factor causing conduction failure, even if there is a very high density of Na$^+$ channels.

If action potentials are to successfully invade the demyelinated zone, impedance mismatch must be overcome; this is termed *impedance matching*. Mechanisms of impedance matching include the development of relatively short myelinated segments proximal to the demyelinated area (28), decrease in axon diameter of the demyelinated region relative to the proximal myelinated segment (52), the development of an increased Na$^+$-channel density at the node proximal to the demyelinated area, or the development of a specialized transition zone (with relatively high Na$^+$-channel densities or relatively low K$^+$-channel densities) at the border of the region of demyelination (143). Figure 10 shows computer-simulated action potentials (28) in a fiber in which one internode (between nodes D_1 and D_4) has been totally demyelinated, under the assumption that the demyelinated axon membrane has developed a high Na$^+$-channel density (similar to that at nodes). Conduction failure occurs at the junction between normal and demyelinated axon regions (D_1), despite the high Na$^+$ channel density in the demyelinated area, because impedance mismatch prevents threshold from being reached. Figure 11 shows a similar fiber, with two short internodes (A-B; B-D$_1$) interposed just before the demyelinated zone. The membrane properties or the axon are the same as in Fig. 10 except for the introduction of these short myelinated segments and the intervening nodes of Ranvier, which have normal properties. The short internodes (and the extra nodes) provide a mechanism for impedance matching

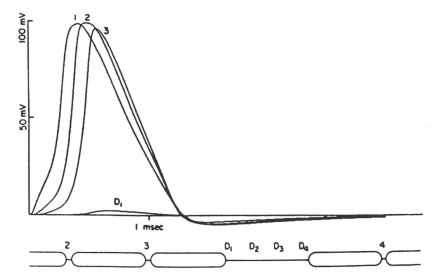

Figure 10 Computer simulations showing conduction through a focally demyelinated axon. Even in the presence of an adequate density of sodium channels in the demyelinated zone (D_1-D_4), conduction fails as a result of impedance mismatch. (Modified from Ref. 28.)

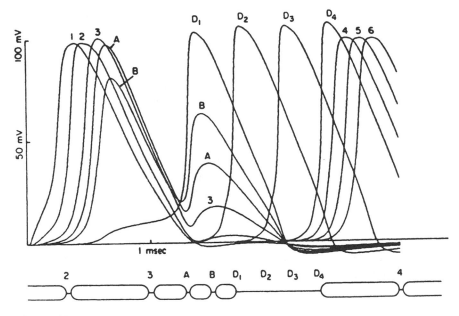

Figure 11 Interposition of short internodes (A–B; B–D_1), proximal to the demyelinated zone, facilitates invasion of action potentials. (Modified from Ref. 28.)

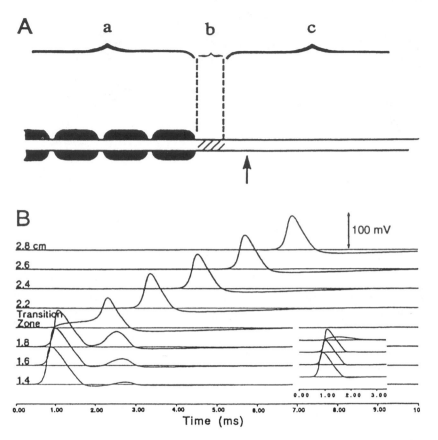

Figure 12 A. Interposition of a transition region (b) with increased Na$^+$ channel density or decreased K$^+$ conductance at the junction between myelinated (a) and demyelinated (c) regions facilitates impulse invasion of the demyelinated zone. B. Action potentials measured at 2-mm intervals along a demyelinated fiber that contains a 50-μm transition zone in which Na$^+$ conductance is increased by 50%. G$_{Na}$ = 0.12 mho/cm^2 in the demyelinated region. Although conduction failure occurs when Na$^+$ conductance is not increased in the transition zone (*inset*), insertion of Na$^+$ channels into this small region facilitates invasion. (Modified from Ref. 143.)

that permits the action potential to successfully invade the demyelinated axon region so that it can propagate through the demyelinated zone. An alternative mechanism for overcoming impedance mismatch (Fig. 12) is the development of a transition zone, at which the axon membrane has a high Na$^+$-channel density, or a low K$^+$-channel density, at the border between myelinated and demyelinated area (143). The number of Na$^+$ channels in the transition zone and their spatial distribution are both important determinants of whether impedance mismatch will be overcome (143).

Short myelinated internodes (144) and transitional "heminodes" at which the axon membrane displays a structure similar to that at the nodes (99) have both been observed along experimentally demyelinated fibers and are present at the periphery of demyelinated plaques in MS (145–147). These specializations may play an adaptive role by facilitating invasion of demyelinated axon regions in a manner similar to that of short internodes located proximal to nonmyelinated preterminal axon arborizations (28,148). Even small degrees of remyelination or axon membrane remodeling at the periphery of plaquest in MS may serve to facilitate conduction in demyelinated axons. Reductions in axon diameter, which have been observed in demyelinated regions (96), may also contribute to impedance matching.

Because impedance mismatch is most pronounced at the border of the demyelinated zone, even relatively subtle changes in the structure of axons and myelin in region may rapidly alter conduction in demyelinated axons. MS plaques grow circumferentially as a result of new or ongoing centrifugal myelin damage (149) implying that there may be some instability of the transitional internodes at the border between myelinated and demyelinated areas. Increased numbers of cytotoxic-suppresser and helper-inducer T cells have been observed at the edges of active and inactive plaques in MS (150). Given the pivotal role of the transition zone in determining whether secure conduction will occur, even minor changes in internodal or nodal structure at the edge of the plaque might be expected to have significant physiological effects.

XIII. REMYELINATION

Computer modeling suggests that remyelination with even thin or short myelin segments should promote conduction through previously demyelinated fibers—assuming that remyelinated nodes of Ranvier develop membrane properties similar to those in normal fiber (28,151,152). Conduction in remyelinated peripheral nervous system (PNS) fibers occurs at velocities close to those predicted from their internode distances, suggesting the development of near-normal Na^+ channel densities at the newly formed nodes (153). In fact, cytochemical studies show that newly formed nodes along remyelinated axons develop normal properties (154). In experimentally demyelinated-remyelinated axons in sciatic nerve, there is an increase in STX binding that is proportional to the increase in nodal membrane area imposed by the shorter spacing between remyelinated nodes (15). Thus, newly formed nodes along remyelinated axons appear to develop a high density of Na^+ channels.

Even thin remyelinated sheaths provide a shield against capacitative and resistive current loss and should support action potential conduction (151,152). The reduced internode distances in remyelinated fibers result in conduction velocities that are higher than in demyelinated axons but lower than in normally myelinated axons (153). However, decreased conduction velocity does not necessarily, of itself, produce clinical deficits; hence, restoration of conduction as a result of remyelination would still be expected to lead to clinical improvement. In peripheral nerves demyelinated with lysophosphatidylcholine, conduction velocity approaches normal values and the ability to conduct high-frequency impulse trains is improved by remyelination (155). Conduction is restored following remyelination of experimentally demyelinated CNS axons in dorsal columns of the cat. The refractory period for transmission returns to normal following remyelination, even though the remyelinated fibers are surrounded by abnormally thin and short internodes (156,157). Clinical recovery in rats with experimental allergic encephalomyelitis is correlated with remyelination in both the PNS and CNS (largely initiated by Schwann cells and oligodendrocytes), and restoration of conduction associated with remyelination appears to provide a physiological basis for this clinical improvement (158).

Oligodendrocytes and Schwann cells can each remyelinate CNS axons, and both oligodendrocyte and Schwann cell-mediated remyelination can enhance conduction. Remyelination of dorsal column axons by Schwann cells, for example, appears to be effective in restoring secure action potential conduction, characterized by a normal refractory period of transmission in these fibers (159,160).

XIV.   TRANSPLANTATION OF MYELIN-FORMING CELLS

The strategy of improving conduction in demyelinated axons by transplantation of exogenous myelin-forming cells or their precursors is under active study in several laboratories. It is clear from morphological studies that transplanted Schwann cells and oligodendrocytes can form myelin with a relatively normal compact structure around demyelinated axons with the CSN (161–163). Transplanted 02-A glial progenitor cells can also differentiate and form myelin in the CNS (164). Until recently, however, the primary assay for the outcome of transplantation was structural (i.e., a determination of whether or not morphologically normal myelin was formed). As should be clear from the foregoing discussion, the formation of compact myelin by transplanted cells does not, in itself, ensure improved conduction, since impedance mismatch, incomplete or patchy myelination, of failure to form nodes with an adequate Na^+ channel density can lower safety factor.

A study of the conduction properties of myelin-deficient axons in the *md* rat spinal cord (165) demonstrated a marked increase in conduction velocity which approached myelinated control values after formation of myelin by transplanted glial cells from unaffected littermates (Fig. 13). The three- to fourfold increase in conduction velocity could not have been produced by an increase in size of the demyelinated axons, because this would have required a nearly tenfold increase in axon diameter. Ability to follow high-frequency stimulation was restored almost to normal in axons myelinated by these transplanted cells. Moreover, action potentials could be initiated outside the transplant region, could invade and propagate into the region of demyelination, and could then propagate beyond the

Figure 13   Increased conduction velocity in dorsal column axons on the spinal cord of myelin-deficient (*md*) rat 16 days following transplantation of myelin-forming cells. Field potentials from control (nontransplant) and transplant regions of dorsal columns are shown. A. Schematic showing the transplant region (~3 mm in this animal) and two stimulation sites (S_1 and S_2) that provide recording tracks with recording intervals of 0.5 mm within and outside the transplant region. B. Field potentials outside the transplant region typically show a single main negativity, with occasional components either before or after the main negativity (fifth trace from top). C. Field potentials from transplant region show two distinct negativities (N_1 and N_2) with increasingly distinct latencies as the recording electrode is positioned farther away from the stimulus site. Conduction velocity for the N_1 component is increased. Stimulation site for these records is outside the transplant region, indicating propagation of the impulse across the junction between myelin deficient and myelinated regions. D. Aggregate conduction latencies in nontransplant (*upper graph*) and transplant regions (*lower graph*) of *md* dorsal columns. The top graph shows the latency of the main N negativity from 100 recording sites from 17 recording tracks *outside the transplant region* of the dorsal columns. Latency from the closest recording site in each track has been set at 0 ms. The linear regression slope indicates an average conduction velocity of 0.9 ± 0.03 m/s. In the bottom graph, recordings *from the transplant region* show a significantly smaller increase in latency with increasing conduction distance. Average conduction velocity in the transplant region is increased to 3.2 ± 0.23 m/s. (Modified from Ref 165).

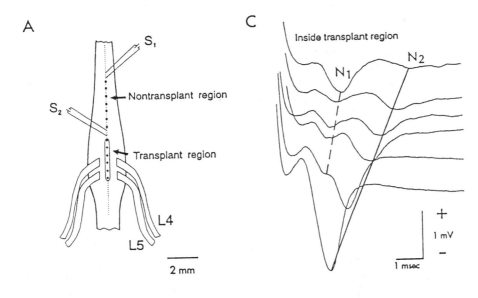

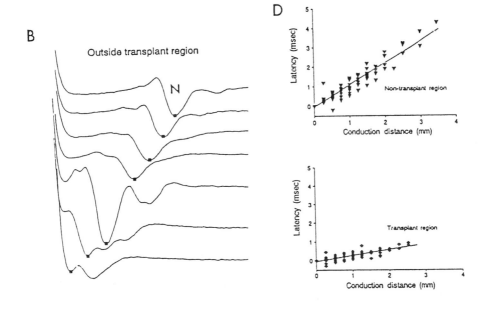

demyelinated region. Similar improvements in action potential conduction have been observed following transplantation of Schwann cells (166) and olfactory ensheathing cells (167) to demyelinating lesions within the spinal cords of adult rats. These results demonstrate that action potential conduction in myelin-deficient axons can be enhanced following myelination by exogenous, transplanted cells. Further studies (e.g., 169) are under way that will examine the effects of glial cell transplantation in other models and the long-term results of transplantation.

XV. OVERVIEW

As summarized in this chapter, a multiplicity of mechanisms contributes to disturbed action potential conduction and to restoration of conduction in CNS axons following demyelination. Passive and active properties interact to shape the conduction properties of these demyelinated axons, and a variety of cellular and molecular mechanisms contribute to these properties. The multifactorial determinants of altered axonal conduction after demyelination have made it more difficult to study but also have provided multiple options for the development of therapeutic strategies that may enhance the function of demyelinated axons. These include the pharmacological manipulation of K^+ channels, the promotion of Na^+ channel expression in demyelinated axons, the manipulation of cellular characteristics at the edge of the plaque, and the transplantation of myelin-forming cells so that they can restore conduction in demyelinated axons.

ACKNOWLEDGMENTS

Research in the author's laboratory has been supported in part by grants from the National Multiple Sclerosis Society, the Medical Research Service and Rehabilitation Research Service of the Veterans Administration, the EPVA, and the PVA.

REFERENCES

1. Waxman SG. Multiple sclerosis as a neuronal disease. Arch Neurol 2000; 57:22–24.
2. Bunge MB, Bunge RP, Pappas GD. Electron microscopic demonstration of connections between glia and myelin sheaths in the developing mammalian central nervous system. J Cell Biol 1961; 12:448–453.
3. Hirano A. A confirmation of the oligodendroglial origin of myelin in the adult rat. J Cell Biol 1968; 38:637–340.
4. Waxman SG, Sims TJ. Specificity in central myelination: Evidence for local regulation of myelin thickness. Brain Res 1984; 292:179–185.
5. Waxman SG, Sims TJ, Gilmore SA. Cytoplasmic membrane elaborations in oligodendrocytes during myelination of spinal motoneuron axons. Glia 1988; 1:286–291.
6. Tasaki I. Conduction of the nerve impulse: In: American Physiological Society. Handbook of Physiology: Sect. 1 Neurophysiology 1959; Bethesda MD: American Physiological Society, 1959.
7. Huxley AF, Stampfli R. Evidence for saltatory conduction in peripheral myelinated nerve fibres. J Physiol (Lond) 1949; 108:315–339.
8. Waxman SG, Bennett MVL. Relative conduction velocities of small myelinated and nonmyelinated fibers in the central nervous system. Nature 1972; 238:217–219.
9. Ritchie JM, Rogart RB. The density of sodium channels in mammalian myelinated nerve fibers and the nature of the axonal membrane under the myelin sheath. Proc Natl Acad Sci USA 1977; 74:211–215.

10. Waxman SG. Conduction in myelinated, unmyelinated, and demyelinated fibers. Arch Neurol 1977; 34:585–590.

11. Shrager P. Sodium channels in single demyelinated mammalian axons. Brain Res 1989; 483: 149–154.

12. Waxman SG, Ritchie JM. Molecular dissection of the myelinated axon. Ann Neurol 1993; 33:121–136.

13. Chiu SY, Ritchie JM. Potassium channels in nodal and internodal axonal membrane in mammalian myelinated fibers. Nature 1980; 284:170–171.

14. Chiu SY, Ritchie JM. Evidence for the presence of potassium channels in the paranodal region of acutely demyelinated mammalian nerve fibres. J Physiol (Lond) 1981; 313:415–437.

15. Ritchie JM. Sodium and potassium channels in regenerating and developing mammalian myelinated nerves. Proc R Soc Lond Biol Sci 1982; 215:273–287.

16. Kocsis JD, Waxman SG, Hildebrand C, Ruiz JA. Regenerating mammalian nerve fibres: Changes in action potential waveform and firing characteristics following blockage of potassium conductance. Proc R Soc Lond Biol Sci 1982; 217:277–287.

17. Foster RE, Connors BW, Waxman SG. Rat optic nerve: Electrophysiological, pharmacological, and anatomical studies during development. Dev Brain Res 1982; 3:361–376.

18. Eng DL, Gordon TR, Kocsis JD, Waxman SG. Development of 4-AP and TEA sensitivities in mammalian myelinated nerve fibers. J Neurophysiol 1988; 60:2168–2179.

19. Roper J, Schwarz JR. Heterogeneous distribution of fast and slow potassium channels in myelinated rat nerve fibers. J Physiol (Lond) 1989; 416:93–110.

20. Wood JG, Dou HJ, Whitaker JN, et al. Immunocytochemical localization of the sodium, potassium activated ATPase in knifefish brain. J Neurocytol 1977; 6:571–581.

21. Ariyasu RG, Ellisman MN. The distribution of $(NA^+/K^+)ATPase$ is continuous along the axolemma of unensheathed axons from spinal roots of "dystrophic" mice. J Neurocytol 1987; 16:239–248.

22. Gordon TR, Kocsis JD, Waxman SG. Electrogenic pump $(Na^+/K^+\text{-}ATPase)$ activity in rat optic nerve. Neuroscience 1990; 37:829–837.

23. Bostock H, Grafe P. Activity-dependent excitability changes in normal and demyelinated rat spinal root axons. J Physiol (Lond) 1985; 365:239–257.

24. Rasminsky M, Sears TA. Internodal conduction in undissected demyelinated nerve fibers. J Physiol (Lond) 1972; 227:323–350.

25. Waxman SG. Membranes, myelin and the pathophysiology of multiple sclerosis. N Engl J Med 1982; 306:1529–1533.

26. McDonald WI. The effects of experimental demyelination on conduction in peripheral nerve: A histological and electrophysiological study. Electrophysiological observations. Brain 1963; 86:501–524.

27. McDonald WI, Sears TA. The effects of experimental demyelination on conduction in the central nervous system. Brain 1970; 93:583–598.

28. Waxman SG, Brill MH. Conduction through demyelinated plaques in multiple sclerosis: Computer simulations of facilitation by short internodes. J Neurol Neurosurg Psychiatry 1978; 41:408–417.

29. Sears TA, Bostock H, Sherratt M. The pathophysiology of demyelination and its implications for the symptomatic treatment of multiple sclerosis. Neurology 1978; 28:21–26.

30. Bostock H, Sears TA, Sherratt RM. The effects of 4-aminopyridine and tetraethyl-ammonium ions on normal and demyelinated mammalian nerve fibers. J Physiol (Lond) 1981; 313:301–315.

31. Ritchie JM, Chiu SY. Distribution of sodium and potassium channels in mammalian myelinated nerve. In: Waxman SG, Ritchie JM, eds. Demyelinating Diseases, Basic and Clinical Electrophysiology. New York: Raven Press, 1981, pp 329–342.

32. Brismar T. Specific permeability properties of demyelinated rat nerve fibers. Acta Physiol Scand 1981; 113:167–176.

33. Smith KJ, McDonald WI. Spontaneous and mechanically evoked activity due to central demyelinating lesions. Nature 1980; 286:154–155.

34. Bowe CM, Kocsis JD, Targ EF, Waxman SG. Physiological effects of 4-aminopyridine on demyelinated mammalian motor and sensory fibers. Ann Neurol 1987; 22:264–268.

35. Vollmer TL, Brass LM, Waxman SG. Lhermitte's sign in a patient with herpes zoster. J Neurol Sci 1991; 106:153–157.

36. Rasminsky M. Hyperexcitability of pathologically myelinated axons and positive symptoms in multiple sclerosis. In: Waxman SG, Ritchie JM, eds. Demyelinating Diseases: Basic and Clinical Electrophysiology. New York: Raven Press, 1981, pp 289–297.

37. Burchiel K. Abnormal impulse generation in focally demyelinated trigeminal roots. J Neurosurg 1980; 53:674–683.

38. Wisniewski HM, Oppenheimer D, McDonald WE. Relation between myelination and function in MS and EAE. J. Neuropathol Exp Neurol 1976; 35:327.

39. Ulrich J, Groebke-Lorenz W. The optic nerve in multiple sclerosis: A morphological study with retrospective clinicopathological correlation. Neurol Ophthalmol 1983; 3:149–159.

40. Halliday AM, McDonald WI, Mushin J. The visual evoked response in the diagnosis of multiple sclerosis. BMJ 1973; 4:661–664.

41. Namerow NS. Somatosensory evoked responses in multiple sclerosis patients with varying sensory loss. Neurology 1968; 18:1197–1204.

42. Hume AL, Waxman SG. Evoked potentials in suspected multiple sclerosis: Diagnostic value and prediction of clinical course. J Neurol Sci 1988; 83:191–210.

43. Moore JW, Moyner RW, Brill MH, et al. Simulations of conduction in uniform myelinated fibres: Relative sensitivity to changes in nodal and internodal parameters. Biophys J 1978; 21:147–161.

44. Swadlow HA, Waxman SG, Weyand TG. Effects of variations in temperature on impulse conduction along nonmyelinated axons in the mammalian brain. Exp Neurol 1981; 71:383–389.

45. Stys PK, Waxman SG, Ransom BR. Effects of temperature on evoked electrical activity and anoxic injury in CNS white matter. J Cereb Blood Flow Metab 1992; 12:977–986.

46. Guthrie TC. Visual and motor changes in patients with multiple sclerosis Arch Neurol Psychiatry 1951; 65:437.

47. Watson CW. Effects of lowering body temperature on the symptoms and signs of multiple sclerosis. N Engl J Med 1959; 261:1252–1259.

48. Namerow NS. Circadian temperature rhythm and vision in multiple sclerosis. Neurology 1968; 18:417–422.

49. Waxman SG, Geschwind N. Major morbidity related to hyperthermia in multiple sclerosis. Ann Neurol 1983; 13:348.

50. Davis FA, Jacobson S. Altered thermal sensitivity of injured cat demyelinated nerve. J Neurol Neurosurg Psychiatry 1971; 34:551–561.

51. Rasminsky M. The effects of temperature on conduction in demyelinated single nerve fibers. Arch Neurol 1973; 28:287–292.

52. Sears TA, Bostock H. Conduction failure in demyelination: is it inevitable? In: Waxman SG, Ritchie JM, eds. Demyelinating Diseases: Basic and Clinical Electrophysiology. New York: Raven Press, 1981;357–375.

53. Schauf CL, Davis FA. Impulse conduction in multiple sclerosis: A theoretical basis for modification by temperature and pharmacological agents. J Neurol Neurosurg Psychiatry 1974; 37:152–161.

54. Davis FA, Becker FO, Michael JA, Sorensen E. Effect of intravenous sodium bicarbonate, disodium edetate, and hyperventilation on visual and oculomotor signs in multiple sclerosis. J Neurol Neurosurg Psychiatry 1970; 33:723–732.

55. Becker FO, Michael JA, Davis FA. Acute effects of oral phosphate on visual function in multiple sclerosis. Neurology 1974; 24:601–607.

56. Waxman SG. Sodium channel blockade by antibodies: A new mechanism of neurological disease? Ann Neurol 1995; 37:421–423.

57. Eisen A. Yufe R, Trop D, Campbell I. Reduced neuromuscular transmission safety factor in multiple sclerosis. Neurology 1978; 28:498–602.

58. Papakostopoulos D, Fotiou F, Dean Hart JD, Banerji NK. The electroretinogram in multiple sclerosis and demyelinating optic neuritis. Electroencephalogr Clin Neurophysiol 1989; 74:1–10.

59. Ikeda H, Tremain K, Sanders MD. Neurophysiological investigation in optic nerve disease: Combined assessment of the visual evoked response and electroretinogram. Br J Ophthalmol 1978; 62:227–239.

60. Schauf CL, Davis FA. Circulating toxic factors in multiple sclerosis: a perspective. Adv Neurol 1981; 31:267–280.

61. Stys PK, Ransom BR, Waxman SG. Tertiary and quaternary local anesthetics protect CNS white matter from anoxic injury at concentrations that do not block excitability. J Neurophysiol 1992; 67:236–240.

62. Yokota T, Saito Y, Miyatake T. Conduction slowing without conduction block of compound muscle and nerve action potentials due to sodium channel block. J Neurol Sci 1994; 124:220–224.

63. Brinkmeier H, Wollinsky KH, Hulser P-J, et al. The acute paralysis in Guillain-Barré syndrome is related to a Na^+ channel blocking factor in the cerebrospinal fluid. Pflugers Arch 1992; 421:552–557.

64. Brinkmeier H, Wollinsky KH, Seewald MJ, et al. Factors in the cerebrospinal fluid of multiple sclerosis patients interfering with voltage-dependent sodium channels Neurosci Lett 1993; 156:172–175.

65. Brinkmeier H, Kaspar A, Wietholter H, Rudel R. Interleukin-2 inhibits sodium currents in human muscle cells Pflugers Arch 1992; 173:621–623.

66. Trotter JL, Clifford DB, Anderson CB, et al. Elevated serum interleukin-2 levels in chronic progressive multiple sclerosis. N Engl J Med 1988; 318:1206.

67. Hauser SL, Doolittle TH, Lincoln R, et al. Cytokine accumulations in CSF of multiple sclerosis patients. Neurology 1990; 40:1735–1739.

68. Shrager P, Custer AW, Kazarinoa K, Rasband MN, Mattson D. Nerve conduction block by nitric oxide that is mediated by the axonal environment. J Neurophysiol 1998; 79:529–536.

69. Redford EJ, Kapoor R, Smith KJ. Nitric oxide donors reversibly block axonal conduction: Demyelinated axons are especially susceptible. Brain 1997; 120:2149–2157.

70. Renganathan M, Cummins TR, Hormuzdiar WN, Black JA, Waxman SG. Nitric oxide is an autocrine regulator of Na^+ currents in axotomized DRG neuron. J Neurophysiol 1999; 83:2431–2443.

71. Bagasra O, Michaels FH, Zheng YM, Bobroski LE, Spitsin SV, Fu ZF, et al. Activation of the inducible form of nitric oxide synthase in the brains of patients with multiple sclerosis. Proc Natl Acad Sci USA 1995; 92:12041–12045.

72. Johnson AW, Land JM, Thompson EJ, Bolanos JP, Clark JB, Heales SJ. Evidence for increased nitric oxide production in multiple sclerosis. J Neurol Nurosurg Psychiatry 1995; 58:107.

73. Hooper DC, Ohnishi ST, Kean R, Numagami Y, Dietzschold B, Koprowski H. Local nitric oxide production in viral and autoimmune diseases of the central nervous system. Proc Natl Acad Sci USA 1995; 92:5312–5316.

74. Cross AH, Keeling RM, Goorha S, San M, Rodi C, Wyatt PS, et al. Inducible nitric oxide synthase gene expression and enzyme activity correlate with disease activity in murine experimental autoimmune encephalomyelitis. J Neuroimmunol 1996; 71:145–153.

75. Takigawa T, Yasuda H, Kikkawa R, et al. Antibodies against GM1 ganglioside affect K+ and Na+ currents in isolated rat myelinated nerve fibers. Ann Neurol 1995; 57:436–442.

76. Targ EF, Kocsis JD. 4-Aminopyridine leads to restoration of conduction in demyelinated rat sciatic nerve. Brain Res 1985; 328:358–361.

77. Targ EF, Kocsis JD. Action potential characteristics of demyelinated rat sciatic nerve following application of 4-aminopyridine. Brain Res 1986; 363:1–9.

78. Blight AR. Effect of 4-AP on axonal conduction block in chronic spinal cord injury. Brain Res Bull 1989; 22:47–52.

79. Stefoski D, Davis FA, Faut M, Schauf CL. 4-Aminopyridine improves clinical signs in multiple sclerosis. Ann Neurol 1987; 21:71–77.

80. Davis FA, Stefoski D, Rush J. Orally administered 4-aminopyridine improves clinical signs in multiple sclerosis. Ann Neurol 1990; 27:186–192.

81. Kaji R, Sumner AJ. Effects of digitalis on CNS demyelinative conduction block. Ann Neurol 1989; 25:159–166.

82. Kaji R, Sumner AJ. Ouabain reverses conduction disturbances in single demyelinated nerve fibers. Neurology 1989; 39:1364–1368.

83. Kaji R, Happel L, Sumner AJ. Effect of digitalis on clinical symptoms and conduction variables in patients with multiple sclerosis. Ann Neurol 1990; 28:582–584.

84. Lehmann HJ, Ule G. Electrophysiological findings and structural changes in circumscript inflammation of peripheral nerves. Prog Brain Res 1964; 6:169–173.

85. Cragg BG, Thomas PK. Changes in nerve conduction in experimental allergic neuritis. J Neurol Neurosurg Psychiatry 1964; 27:106–115.

86. Bostock H, Sears TA. Continuous conduction in demyelinated mammalian nerve fibres. Nature 1976; 263:786–787.

87. Bostock H, Sears TA. The internodal axon membrane: electrical excitability and continuous conduction in segmental demyelination. J Physiol (Lond) 1978; 280:273–301.

88. Felts, PA, Baker TA, Smith KJ. Conduction in segmentally demyelinated mammalian central axons. J Neurosci 1997; 17:7267–7277.

89. Hines M, Shrager P. A computational test of the requirements for conduction in demyelinated axons. Restor Neurol Neurosci 1991; 3:81–93.

90. Ritchie JM, Rogart RB, Strichartz G. A new method for labeling saxitoxin and its binding to non-myelinated fibres of the rabbit vagus, lobster walking, and garfish olfactory nerves. J Physiol (Lond) 1976; 261:477–494.

91. Tang CM, Strichartz GR, Orkand RK. Sodium channels in axons and glial cells of the optic nerve of *Necturus maculosa*. J Gen Physiol 1979; 74:629–642.

92. Strichartz GR, Small RK, Pfenninger KH. Components of the plasma membrane of growing axons: III. Saxitoxin binding to sodium channels. J Cell Biol 1984; 98:1444–1452.

93. Waxman SG, Black JA, Kocsis JD, Ritchie JM. Low density of sodium channels supports action potential conduction in axons of neonatal rat optic nerve. Proc Natl Acad Sci USA 1989; 86:1406–1410.

94. Prineas J, Connell F. The fine structure of chronically active multiple sclerosis plaques. Neurology 1978; 28:68–75.

95. Smith ME, Kocsis JD, Waxman SG. Myelin protein metabolism in demyelination and remyelination in the sciatic nerve. Brain Res 1983; 270:37–44.

96. De Waegh SM, Lee VM, Brady ST. Local modulation of neurofilament phosphorylation, axonal caliber, and slow axonal transport by myelinating Schwann cells. Cell 1992; 68:451–463.

97. Brady ST. Axonal dynamics and regeneration. In: Gorio A, ed. Neuroregeneration. New York: Raven Press, 1993, pp. 7–36.

98. Foster RE, Whalen CC, Waxman SG. Reorganization of the axonal membrane of demyelinated nerve fibers: Morphological evidence. Science 1980; 210:661–663.

99. Black JA, Waxman SG, Smith ME. Macromolecular structure of axonal membrane during acute experimental allergic encephalomyelitis in rat and guinea pig spinal cord. J Neuropathol Exp Neurol 1987; 46:167–184.

100. England JD, Gamboni F, Levinson SR, Finger TE. Changed distribution of sodium channels along demyelinated axons. Proc Natl Acad Sci USA 1990; 87:6777–6786.

101. Dugandzija-Novakovic S, Koszowski AG, Levinson SR, Shrager P. Clustering of Na⁺ chan-

nels and node of Ranvier formation in remyelinating axons. J Neurosci 1995; 15:492–503.

102. Waxman SG. Molecular organization of the cell membrane in normal and pathological axons: Relation to glial contact. In: Althaus H, Siefert W, eds. Glial-Neuronal Communication in Development and Regeneration. Berlin: Springer-Verlag, 1987, pp. 711–736.

103. Black JA, Waxman SG, Sims TJ, Gilmore SA. Effects of delayed myelination by oligodendrocytes and Schwann cells on the macromolecular structure of axonal membrane in rat spinal cord. J Neurocytol 1986; 15:745–762.

104. Smith KJ, Bostock H, Hall SM. Saltatory conduction precedes remyelination in axons demyelinated with lysophosphatidyl choline. J Neurol Sci 1982; 54:12–31.

105. Blakemore WF, Smith KJ. Node-like axonal specializations along demyelinated central nerve fibers: Ultrastructural observations. Acta Neuropathol 1983; 60:291–296.

106. Rosenbluth J, Blakemore WF. Structural specializations in cat of chronically demyelinated spinal cord axons as seen in freeze-fracture replicas. Neurosci Lett 1984; 48:171–177.

107. Black JA, Sims TJ, Waxman SG, Gilmore SA. Membrane ultrastructure of developing axons in glial cell deficient rat spinal cord. J Neurocytol 1985; 14:79–104.

108. England JD, Gamboni F, Levinson SR. Increased numbers of sodium channels form along demyelinated axons. Brain Res 1991; 548:334–337.

109. Moll C, Mourre C, Lazdunski M, Ulrich J. Increase of sodium channels in demyelinated lesions of multiple sclerosis. Brain Res 1991; 556:311–316.

110. Kuno M, Llinas R. Enhancement of synaptic transmission by dendritic potentials in chromatolysed motoneurones of the cat. J Physiol (Lond) 1970; 210:807–821.

111. Dodge FA, Cooley JW. Action potential of the motorneuron. IBM J Res Dev 1973; 17:219–229.

112. Titmus MJ, Faber DS. Altered excitability of goldfish Mauthner cell following axotomy: II. Localization and ionic basis. J Neurophysiol 1986; 55:1440–1454.

113. Lombet A, Laduron P, Mourre C, et al. Axonal transport of the voltage-dependent Na channel protein identified by its tetrodotoxin-binding site in rat sciatic nerves. Brain Res 1985; 345:153–158.

114. Black JA, Dib-Hajj S, McNabola K, Jeste S, Rizzo MA, Kocsis JD, Waxman SG. Spinal sensory neurons express multiple sodium channel α-submit mRNAs. Mol Brain Res 1996; 43:117–132.

115. Waxman SG, Kocsis JD, Black JA. Type III sodium channel mRNA is expressed in embryonic but not adult spinal sensory neurons, and is re-expressed following axotomy. J Neurophysiol 1994; 72:466–470.

116. Dib-Hajj S, Black JA, Felts P, Waxman SG. Down-regulation of transcripts for Na channel α-SNS in spinal sensory neurons following axotomy. Proc Natl Acad Sci USA 1996; 93:14950–14954.

117. Dib-Hajj SD, Tyrrell L, Black JA, Waxman SG. NaN, a novel voltage-gated Na channel preferentially expressed in peripheral sensory neurons and down-regulated following axotomy. Proc Natl Acad Sci USA 1998; 95:8963–8968.

118. Rizzo MA, Kocsis JD, Waxman SG. Selective loss of slow and enhancement of fast Na^+ currents in cutaneous afferent DRG neurons following axotomy. Neurobiol Dis 1995; 2:87–96.

119. Cummins TR, Waxman SG. Down-regulation of tetrodotoxin-resistant sodium currents and up-regulation of a rapidly repriming tetrodotoxin-sensitive sodium current in small spinal sensory neurons following nerve injury. J Neurosci 1997; 17:3503–3514.

120. Westenbroek RE, Noebels JL, Catteral WA. Elevated expression of type II Na^- channels in hypomyelinated axons to shiverer mouse brain. J Neurosci 1992; 12:2259–2267.

121. Black JA, Fjell J, Dib-Hajj S, Duncan ID, O'Connor LT, Fried K, Gladwell Z, Tate S, Waxman SG. Abnormal expression of SNS/PN3 sodium channel in cerebellar Purkinje cells following loss of myelin in the taiep rat. Neuroreport 1998; 10:913–918.

121a. Black JA, Dib-Hajj S, Baker D, Newcombe J, Luzner ML, Waxman SG. Sensory neuron-specific solution channel SNS is abnormally expressed in the brain of mice with experimental allergic encephalomyelits and humans with multiple sclerosis. Proc Natl Acad Sci USA. In press.

122. Rizzo MA, Kocsis JD, Waxman SG. Mechanisms of paresthesiae, dysesthesiae, and hyperesthesiae: Role of Na^+ channel heterogeneity. Eur Neurol 1996; 36:3–12.

123. Kapoor R, Li YG, Smith KJ. Slow sodium-dependent potential oscillations contribute to ectopic firing in mammalian demyelinated axons. Brain 1997; 120:647–652.

124. Bevan S, Chiu SY, Gray PTA, Ritchie JM. The presence of voltage-gated sodium potassium and chloride channels in rat cultured astrocytes. Proc R Soc Lond Biol Sci 1985; 225:229–313.

125. Gray PT, Ritchie JM. Ion channels in Schwann and glial cells. Trends Neurosci 1985; 8: 411–415.

126. Hildebrand C. Ultrastructural and light-microscopic studies of the nodal region in large myelinated fibers of the adult feline spinal cord white matter. Acta Physiol Scand Suppl 1971; 364:43–71.

127. Waxman SG, Black JA. Freeze-fracture ultrastructure of the perinodal astrocyte and associated glial junctions. Brain Res 1984; 308:77–87.

128. Raine CS. On the association between perinodal astrocytic processes and the nodes of Ranvier in the CNS. J Neurocytol 1984; 13:21–27.

129. Bray GM, Cullen MJ, Aguayo AJ, Rasminsky M. Node-like areas of intramembranous particles in the unensheathed axons of dystrophic mice. Neurosci Lett 1979; 13:203–208.

130. Rosenbluth J. Aberrant axon-Schwann cell junctions in dystrophic mouse nerves. J Neurocytol 1979; 8:655–672.

131. Rosenbluth J. Intramembranous particle patches in myelin-deficient rat mutant. Neurosci Lett 1985; 62:19–24.

132. Nowak L, Ascher P, Berwald-Netter Y. Ionic channels in mouse astrocytes in culture. J Neurosci 1987; 7:101–109.

133. Barres BA, Chun LLY, Corey DP. Glial and neuronal forms of the voltage-dependent sodium channels: Characteristics and cell-type distribution. Neuron 1989; 2:1375–1388.

134. Sontheimer H, Ransom BR, Cornell-Bell AH, et al. Na^+-current expression in rat hippocampal astrocytes in vitro: Alternations during development. J Neurophysiol 1991; 65:3–19.

135. Sontheimer H, Black JA, Ransom BR, Waxman SG. Ion channels in spinal cord astrocytes in vitro: I. Transient expression of high levels of Na^+ and K^+ channels. J Neurophysiol 1992; 68:985–999.

136. Black JA, Westenbroek R, Ransom BR, et al. Type II sodium channels in spinal cord astrocytes: Immunocytochemical observations. Glia 1994; 12:219–227.

137. Oh Y, Black JA, Waxman SG. The expression of rat brain voltage-sensitive Na^+ channel mRNAs in astrocytes. Mol Brain Res 1994; 23:57–65.

138. Oh Y, Waxman SG. The β_1 subunit mRNA for rat brain Na^+ channels is expressed in glial cells. Proc Natl Acad Sci USA 1994; 91:9985–9989.

139. Black JA, Yokoyama S, Waxman SG, et al. Sodium channel mRNAs in cultured spinal cord astrocytes: in situ hybridization in identified cell types. Mol Brain Res 1994; 23:235–245.

140. Sontheimer H, Fernandez-Marques E, Ullrich N, et al. Astrocyte Na^+ channels are required for maintenance of Na^+/K^+-ATPase activity. J Neurosci 1994; 14:2464–2476.

141. Waxman SG. The perinodal astrocyte: functional and developmental considerations. In: Fedoroff S, Doucette R, Juurlink BH, eds. Biology and Pathobiology of Astrocyte-neuron Interactions. New York: Plenum, 1993; 15–29.

142. Waxman SG. Prerequisites for conduction in demyelinated fibers. Neurology 1978; 28:27–34.

143. Waxman SG, Wood SL. Impulse conduction in inhomogeneous axons: Effects of variation in voltage-sensitive ionic conductances on invasion of demyelinated axon segments and preterminal fibers. Brain Res 1984; 294:111–122.

144. Gledhill RF, Harrison B, McDonald WI. Demyelination and remyelination after acute spinal cord compression. Exp Neurol 1973; 38:472–487.

145. Prineas J, Connell F. Remyelination in multiple sclerosis. Ann Neurol 1979; 5:22–31.

146. Suzuki K, Andrews JM, Waltz JJ, Terry RD. Ultrastructural studies of multiple sclerosis. Lab Invest 1969; 20:444–451.

147. Andrews JM, ed. The Ultrastructural Neuropathology of Multiple Sclerosis. New York: Academic Press, 1972.

148. Quick DC, Kennedy WR, Donaldson L. Dimensions of myelinated nerve fibers near the motor and sensory fibers of cat tenuissimus muscles. Neuroscience 1979; 4:1089–1096.

149. Lumsden CE. The neuropathology of multiple sclerosis. In: Vinken PJ, Bruyn GW, eds. Handbook of Clinical Neurology, vol 9: Multiple sclerosis and other demyelinating diseases. New York: Elsevier, 1970, pp 217–309.

150. McCallum K, Esiri MM. Tourtellotte W, Booss J. T-cell subsets in multiple sclerosis: Gradients at plaque borders and differences in non-plaque regions. Brain 1987; 110:1297–1308.

151. Koles ZJ, Rasminsky M. A computer simulation of conduction in demyelinated nerve fibres. J Physiol (Lond) 1972; 227:351–364.

152. Funch PG, Faber DS. Measurement of myelin sheath resistances: Implications for axonal conduction and pathophysiology. Science 1984; 224:538–540.

153. Brill MH, Waxman SG, Moore JW, Joyner RW. Conduction velocity and spike configuration in myelinated fibers: Computed dependence on internode distance. J. Neurol Neurosurg Psychiatry 1977; 40:769–774.

154. Weiner LP, Waxman SG, Stohlman SA, Kwan A. Remyelination following viral-induced demyelination: Ferric ion-ferrocyanide staining of nodes of Ranvier within the CNS. Ann Neurol 1980; 8:580–583.

155. Smith KJ, Hall SM. Nerve conduction during peripheral demyclination and remyelination. J Neurol Sci 1980; 48:201–219.

156. Smith KJ, Blakemore WF, McDonald WI. The restoration of conduction by central remyelination. Brain 1981; 104:383–404.

157. Smith KJ, Blakemore WF, McDonald WI. Central remyelination restores secure conduction. Nature 1983; 280:395–396.

158. Stanley GP, Pender MP. Pathophysiology of chronic relapsing experimental allergic encephalomyelitis. Brain 1991; 114:1827–1853.

159. Blight AR, Young W. Central axons in injured cat spinal cord recover electrophysiological function following remyelination by Schwann cells. J Neurol Sci 1989; 91:15–34.

160. Felts PA, Smith KJ. Conduction properties of central nerve fibers remyelinated by Schwann cells. Brain Res 1991; 574:178–192.

161. Duncan ID, Hammang JP, Jackson KF, et al. Transplantation of oligodendrocytes and Schwann cells into the spinal cord of the myelin-deficient rat. J Neurocytol 1988; 17:351–360.

162. Gout O, Gansmuller A, Baumann N, Gumpel M. Remyelination by transplanted oligodendrocytes of a demyelinated lesion in the spinal cord of the adult shiverer mouse. Neurosci Lett 1988; 87:195–199.

163. Rosenbluth J, Hasegawa M, Shirasaki N, et al. Myelin formation following transplantation of normal fetal glia into myelin-deficient rat spinal cord. J Neurocytol 1990; 19:718–730.

164. Groves AK, Barnett SC, Franklin RJM, et al. Repair of demyelinated lesions by transplantation of purified 0-2A progenitor cells. Nature 1993; 362:453–456.

165. Utzschneider DA, Archer DR, Kocsis JD, et al. Transplantation of glial cells enhances action potential conduction of amyelinated spinal cord axons in the myelin deficient rat. Proc Natl Acad Sci USA 1994; 91:53–57.

166. Honmou O, Felts PA, Waxman SG, Kocsis JD. Restoration of normal conduction properties in demyelinated spinal cord axons in the adult rat by transplantation of exogenous Schwann cells. J Neurosci. 1996; 16:3199–3208.

167. Imaizumi T, Lankford KL, Waxman SG, Green CA, Kocsis JD. Transplanted olfactory en-

sheathing cells remyelinate and enhance axonal conduction in the demyelinated dorsal columns of the rat spinal cord. J Neurosci 1998; 18:6176–6185.

168. Kocsis JD, Waxman SG. Demyelination: Causes and mechanisms of clinical abnormality and functional recovery. In: Koetsier JC, ed. Handbook of Clinical Neurology, vol 3: The Demyelinating Diseases. Amsterdam: Elsevier, 1985, pp. 29–47.

169. Kato T, Honmou D, Verde T, Hoshi K, Kocsis JD. Transplantation of human olfactory ensheathing cells elicits remyelination in demyelinated rat spinal cord. Glia 2000. In press.

12

Pathology of Multiple Sclerosis

JOHN W. PRINEAS

*Veterans Administration Medical Center, East Orange, New Jersey,
and University of Sydney, Sydney, Australia*

I. INTRODUCTION

The pathological changes that serve to define multiple sclerosis (MS) in its various clinical forms, which range from rapidly fatal acute MS to lifelong subclinical MS, are, first, the focal nature of the lesions—i.e., the occurrence of discrete, circumscribed lesions located in normal central nervous tissue; second, the relatively large size of the lesions; third, their perivenous location; and finally, the histological finding within lesions of extensive myelin and oligodendrocyte loss without concomitant destruction of nerve cells and axons. These features—which signal the activity of a highly selective, destructive process that eventually results in a complete and permanent loss of oligodendrocytes and myelin from circumscribed regions of tissue—distinguish MS from other focal and diffuse white matter diseases associated with primary demyelination, that is, myelin loss with axonal preservation, such as progressive multifocal leukoencephalopathy, subacute sclerosing panencephalitis, inherited leukodystrophies, and central pontine myelinolysis.

The conditions that show the closest morphological resemblance to MS are the perivenous encephalomyelitides, a group of spontaneous and experimental central nervous system (CNS) disorders which, like MS, are characterized by the presence of perivenous demyelination. This group includes the experimental diseases acute and chronic experimental allergic encephalomyelitis (EAE). It is chiefly this morphological evidence linking MS and EAE that is responsible for the current view that MS is an autoimmune disease in which lesion formation is the result of an immune response directed against an unidentified myelin and/or oligodendrocyte antigen.

II. GROSS PATHOLOGY AND ASSOCIATED DISEASES

In patients with typical long-standing disease, the changes found outside the CNS are limited to unrelated diseases and to nonspecific complications associated with any long-standing paralytic illness, including emaciation, pressure sores, flexion contractures in the arms and legs, renal calculi, chronic renal tract infections, and pulmonary infections (8).

Morphological changes of uncertain significance (reduced myelin thickness at some internodes) have been detected in the peripheral nerves in some MS patients in whom poor nutrition and pressure palsies could be discounted as causes of the peripheral nerve changes (9). Arguing against significant peripheral nerve involvement in multiple sclerosis is the common observation that subpial plaques in the spinal cord and brainstem do not extend into spinal nerve roots or cranial nerves myelinated by Schwann cells. Although peripheral nervous system (PNS) and CNS myelin share a number of antigens—including myelin associated glycoprotein (MAG), galactocerebroside (GalC), and sulfatide—it is remarkable that the several diseases of humans believed to be autoimmune diseases targeting myelin almost never involve both CNS and PNS myelin in the same patient. Of the reported few cases of proven MS associated with acute inflammatory demyelinating polyneuropathy (AIDP) (158) or chronic inflammatory demyelinating polyneuropathy (CIDP) (11), it is uncertain whether this is a chance association or represents an overlapping immune response as seen in some models of EAE and in rabies postvaccination encephalomyelitis (66). Subtle, usually asymptomatic peripheral nerve electrophysiological abnormalities present in MS patients, some of which can be accounted for by demyelination or interruption within the spinal cord of anterior horn cell axons or centrally projecting axons of dorsal root ganglion cells, are reviewed by Waxman (160).

The meninges and external surfaces of the brain and spinal cord may reveal no abnormality on direct inspection. However, mild cortical atrophy with widening of cerebral sulci may be present, and the brainstem and spinal cord may appear shrunken. Irregularly shaped, depressed gray areas, firm to the touch in unfixed tissue, may be present on the surface of the pons, medulla, corpus callosum, optic nerves, optic chiasm, or scattered along the length of the spinal cord. In severe cases, where virtually all myelin has disappeared from the spinal cord, the whole cord appears atrophic and gray.

Coronal slices of the fixed brain often show some ventricular enlargement, which may be marked (13,149), and plaques straddling subependymal veins may be visible through the ependymal lining of the lateral and fourth ventricles. On cut surfaces the plaques appear as scattered, irregularly shaped, usually circumscribed, translucent gray areas 1 to 15 mm in diameter (Fig. 1). It is unusual to find a white matter lesion on later microscopic examination that was not apparent on naked-eye examination. Lesions not easily detected macroscopically are plaques located wholly within the cerebral cortex, and some resolving lesions, in which the color and texture of the affected tissue may appear and feel normal. Plaques containing large numbers of foamy macrophages have a characteristic chalky (opaque) white appearance, present throughout the plaque in the case of fresh lesions or restricted to a fine white line outlying the perimeter of the plaque in chronic active lesions.

Although plaques may occur anywhere in the CNS, they tend to occur more frequently in some areas than others, and their shape and size are partly dependent on their location. Sites of predilection in the brain include tissue bordering the lateral and fourth ventricles, periaqueductal tissue, corpus callosum, the optic nerves (14), chiasma and

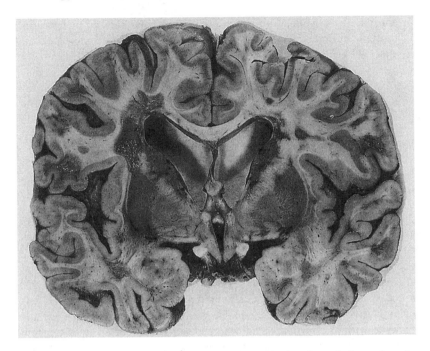

Figure 1   Coronal slice of fixed brain showing typical periventricular and corticomedullary junction MS plaques.

tracts, the corticomedullary junction (15), and subpially in the brainstem. In the spinal cord, lesions are especially common in the anterior columns on either site of the median fissure, subpially, and centrally located in the dorsal columns. In both brain and spinal cord, lesions commonly extend into or are restricted to gray matter, and cases have been described in which plaques located in the cerebral cortical gray matter have outnumbered hemispheric white matter lesions (2). Symmetrical lesions occurring in the same anatomical location on either side of the midline are seen occasionally in the cerebrum, brainstem, and spinal cord in relation to matching blood vessels.

Viewed in three dimensions, lesions located away from surfaces are basically ellipsoidal in shape with the long axis of the ellipsoid centered on a vein. Plaques situated close to pial and ependymal surfaces tend to broaden out as they approach the surface, becoming wedge-shaped with the base of the wedge located at the surface. The vast majority of periventricular lesions are centered on veins (151), frequently with extension into the surrounding white matter along blood vessels crossing the plaque margin ["Dawson's fingers" (16)]. Hemispheric plaques enlarging toward the cerebral cortex tend to stop short of subcortical U fibers. Except for the latter example, the rate and direction of expansion of chronic active lesions seem to occur without regard to the direction of nerve fiber bundles or the presence of gray matter. Other factors that contribute to the final shape of long-standing lesions are recurrent edge activity leading to fusion with contiguous lesions, remyelination of a portion of the lesion, and the superimposition of fresh lesions. Serial gadolinium-diethylenetriamine pentaacetic acid (DTPA)-enhanced MRI studies (146) and recent pathological studies (18) indicate that many chronic lesions are the outcome not of a single earlier episode of demyelination, which is the traditional view of their origin, but the residua of multiple episodes of acute angiocentric demyelination centered on the same segment or adjacent segments of the same blood vessel or group of blood vessels.

Why plaques tend to occur in particular locations is uncertain. However, there may be a relationship between plaque distribution and the system of perivascular (Virchow-Robin) spaces, which is strongly developed in white matter but not gray matter (19) and which, by virtue of its normal complement of lymphocytes and macrophages expressing MHC class II molecules (20,128), probably functions as the major constitutive antigen-presenting site in the normal CNS (21).

III. HISTOLOGY

In keeping with the overall progressive course of the disease, in most long-standing cases it is usual to find at autopsy a mixture of old inactive lesions together with chronic lesions showing evidence of recent edge activity. In very severe cases, extensive confluent demyelination of both cerebral hemispheres may be present together with widespread axonal loss, gliosis, and some remyelination—a condition termed "diffuse MS" by Jellinger (149). Newly formed lesions located in previously unaffected white matter are rarely encountered in patients with long-standing disease. The greatest variation in plaque pathology is seen in patients with severe disease in whom death has occurred within a few months to a year or two following the onset of symptoms. Here it is common to find a mixture of new lesions located in regions of previously unaffected white matter, remyelinating shadow plaques, inactive demyelinated plaques, and remyelinating lesions exhibiting fresh demyelinative activity.

A. Old Lesions

Old, inactive plaques consist of fields of demyelinated axons embedded in a feltwork of fibrous astroglial processes, inconspicuous inflammatory cell infiltration and with few or no lipid-filled (foamy) macrophages present (Figs. 2 to 4). Where gray matter is involved, nerve cell bodies in the demyelinated area appear normal (all gray matter normally contains some myelinated axons). The number of axons present may appear almost normal or there may be a pronounced loss of axons, especially in old lesions exhibiting an expanded extracellular space (22). In patients with extensive disease, wallerian degeneration of axons destroyed in plaques results in atrophy of the corpus callosum and central white matter and some loss of fibers from long tracts in the spinal cord and brainstem. Recent magnetic resonance imaging (MRI) and magnetic resonance spectroscopy (MRS) evidence implicating axonal loss as the likely cause of irreversible functional deficits in MS (161) is supported by quantitative pathological studies that show axon densities reduced on average by 82% in chronic spinal cord lesions and by 60 to 64% in brain lesions (152,167). Axon numbers may also be markedly reduced in normal-appearing white matter, especially in the presence of large lesion loads (139,150). Regarding the timing and nature of axon injury and loss, several studies suggest that this occurs chiefly in actively demyelinating and recently active lesions, as it is in such lesions that the most florid signs of axon injury occur—namely, axonal swelling, transection with end-bulb formation, and amyloid precursor protein accumulation within axons (31,86). Experimental studies indicate that extensive destruction of axons may occur as an incidental nonspecific "bystander" effect of inflammatory mediators acting on demyelinated axons (148), which may explain axonal

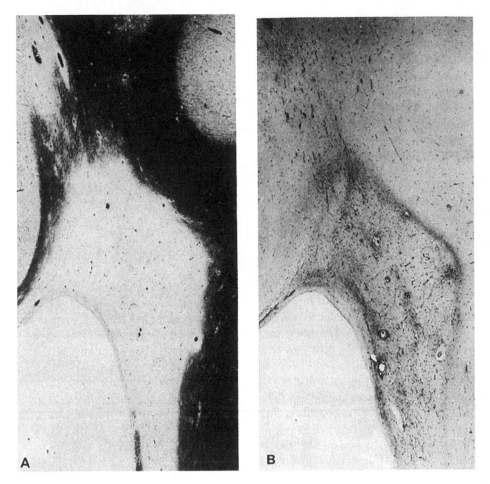

Figure 2 An old, inactive periventricular plaque stained for myelin (A) and immunostained by the PAP method for IgG (B). Moderate reactivity for IgG is present throughout the demyelinated zone and especially at the lesion edge. At greater magnification, it was apparent that this IgG was located chiefly within plasma cells and astrocytes and on the surface of scattered foamy macrophages.

loss in MS. Evidence of axonal regeneration in old lesions has been observed—namely, the presence of very thin axons irregularly disposed in the lesion, and axons that react with antineurofilament antibodies specific for regenerating axons (170). Demyelinated axons within plaques may contact each other (23) (Fig. 4), but usually they are separated by investing astroglial processes that attach themselves via desmosomes and gap junctions to the surface of demyelinated axons (24) and occupy to a variable extent the space originally occupied by myelin sheaths. Oligodendrocytes are sparse or absent (167), with the few present exhibiting a variety of morphological abnormalities, including an unusually small cell body, the formation of abnormal junctions with demyelinated axons (25), and myelin formation around and within the cell perikaryon (26). A narrow fringe of thinly myelinated axons is sometimes seen bordering old lesions. These thin sheaths consist of a mixture of remyelinating internodes (thin short internodes) similar to those seen in

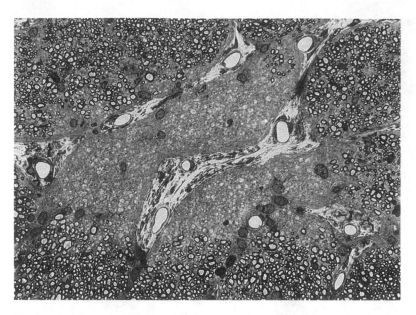

Figure 3 A small optic nerve lesion in a patient with long-standing MS. There is no evidence of remyelination or of oligodendrocytes in the demyelinated zone. Toluidine blue-stained 1-μm epoxy section. (From Ref. 23.)

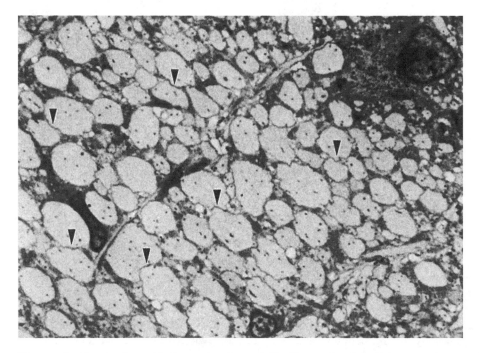

Figure 4 Center of an old plaque showing a field of large, demyelinated axons. Arrow points indicate close apposition of adjacent demyelinated axons. Toluidine blue stained 1-μm epoxy section. (From Ref. 23.)

remyelinating shadow plaques together with unusual internodes in which myelin sheaths of normal thickness exhibit progressive attenuation, the latter probably representing damaged internodes (25) (Fig. 5). Extensive remyelination of demyelinated axons by Schwann cells that have migrated into the lesion from nearby spinal nerve roots is a not uncommon finding in subacute and chronic spinal cord lesions (30) (Fig. 6).

In the absence of evidence of recent myelin breakdown, inflammatory cell infiltrates in old plaques appear, in routine paraffin sections, as small perivascular collections of lymphocytes, plasma cells, and macrophages. Cell counts utilizing semithin sections of optimally fixed lesions, however, show that the total number of lymphocytes and plasma cells present in small perivascular spaces throughout the demyelinated tissue and in the surrounding white matter may be large (19).

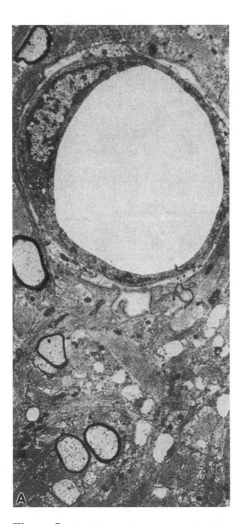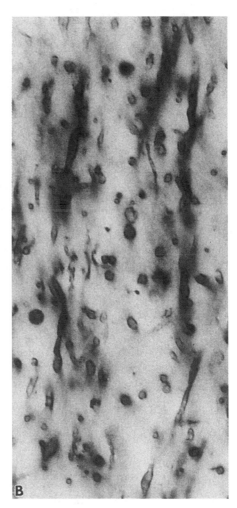

Figure 5 A. An electron micrograph of the edge of an old plaque showing several thinly myelinated axons separated by astroglial processes filled with bundles of glial filaments. B. Center of a shadow plaque in a case of acute MS showing numerous thinly remyelinated axons. Paraffin section stained for myelin. (From Ref. 25.)

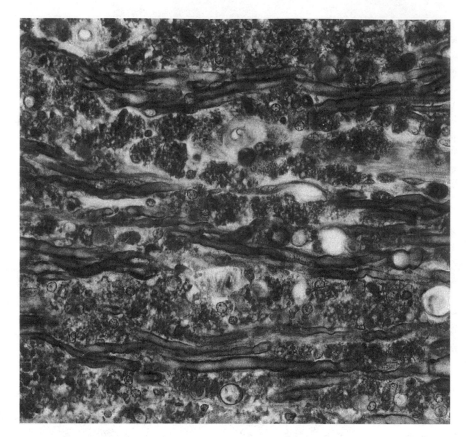

Figure 6   A longitudinally sectioned spinal cord lesion showing axons remyelinated by Schwann cells traversing an area filled with macrophages containing myelin breakdown products. The new myelin sheaths in this lesion were shown to be peripheral in type by electron microscopy and by specific immunostaining. Epoxy section 6-μm thick of osmicated tissue.

B.   Chronic Active Lesions

Serial MRI studies show that ongoing disease activity—i.e., the appearance of new areas of enhancement—frequently occurs in relation to preexisting lesions. The pathological correlate of this is the rare finding at autopsy of a zone of active demyelination located at the edge of an established demyelinated lesion or surrounding a blood vessel close to a plaque. Phagocytosed myelin retains some of its normal staining characteristics and immunoreactivity for several days or weeks following ingestion by macrophages, and the presence of macrophages containing Luxol fast blue (LFB)–positive particles or particles immunoreactive for certain myelin-specific determinants [myelin basic protein (MBP), MAG, 2′3′ cyclic nucleotide 3′-phosphodiesterase (CNP)] at the plaque margin is the most reliable light microscopical indicator of active demyelination. Foamy macrophages filled with neutral lipids and variable amounts of periodic acid Schiff (PAS)–positive material but which are LFB- and MBP-negative remain in the tissue for many months following cessation of active myelin destruction. As in newly forming lesions, oligodendrocytes are depleted in number in the usually narrow zone of ongoing myelin breakdown associated with infiltrating LFB-positive macrophages, with recruitment of new oligodendrocytes and limited remyelination restricted to recently demyelinated tissue (18,29,85). Although oligodendrocytes exhibiting evidence of DNA fragmentation (85,123,165), lymphocyte-mediated lysis (5), morphological apoptosis, and complement-mediated lysis (85) have all been observed in chronic active lesions, the changes that most myelinating oligodendrocytes undergo as they degenerate and disappear together with myelin in such lesions remain unknown.

A second type of chronically active lesion, somewhat more common than the above, is characterized by the presence of lipid macrophages at the edge of the lesion and infiltrating periplaque white matter (12,23,29) with knots of HLA-DR–positive microglial cells (83) clustered along short segments of disrupted myelin that are immunoreactive for C3d, the opsonic component of activated complement (109).

The chief histological changes found in intact tissue bordering plaques are nonspecific reactive changes in astrocytes, including an increase in their number, size, glial fibrillary acidic protein reactivity, and lysosomal enzyme content (33), some reduction in intensity of staining using myelin stains, increased numbers of microglia, and increased numbers of lymphocytes and plasma cells in surrounding perivascular spaces and in the meninges. The recent finding by Evangelou and Esiri (139,150) that myelinated axons are sometimes markedly depleted in distant white matter in chronic MS is consistent with MR studies that have detected evidence of reduced neuronal integrity in white matter distant from plaques (142).

C. Formation of a New Lesion

The histological changes that accompany the formation of a new plaque and its transformation into an old lesion have been worked out by studying lesions of different histological age in patients with a short clinical illness and in whom new lesions have continued to appear up until the time of death.

The earliest structural changes presaging myelin breakdown remain uncertain. Classic accounts of the evolution of new lesions provide two very different pictures of myelin destruction in the acute plaque. According to some authors, myelin fragmentation and the formation of extracellular myelin debris precedes by days or weeks the appearance in the tissue of activated microglia and myelin phagocytes (2). Other authors have been unable to detect any morphological changes in myelin before the appearance of macrophages in the tissue (34) and have suggested that these infiltrating cells may play a more direct role in myelin destruction. Recent immunohistochemical and ultrastructural studies strongly support the latter view, providing direct evidence that fragmentation and disappearance of myelin sheaths from axons in acute lesions is effected by macrophages which phagocytose myelin in situ without the formation of extracellular myelin debris (23,36–38) (Figs. 7 and 8). This transfer of myelin from nerve fibers to macrophages—which is probably completed in areas of fresh activity within 2 or 3 weeks and which coincides with the appearance of infiltrating lymphocytes, vasogenic edema, and a substantial loss of oligodendrocytes (39–42,134)—leaves the affected area totally demyelinated and packed with lipid-laden foamy macrophages containing myelin breakdown products that no longer stain with Luxol fast blue and are unreactive for MBP. Although oligodendrocytes exhibiting evidence of DNA fragmentation or morphological apoptosis have been identified in acute lesions, as in chronic active lesions, the manner in which the bulk of oligodendrocytes are destroyed in acute lesions is unknown. During these initial few weeks, axons traversing the lesion may show pronounced irregular beading, plump astrocytes appear throughout

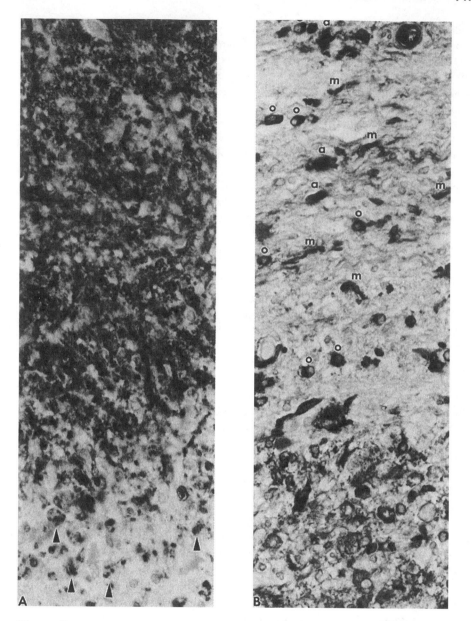

Figure 7   Edge of a fresh lesion in a case of acute MS showing infiltrating IgG+ macrophages (m) in bordering white matter in which myelin density appears normal. a = IgG + astrocytes; o = IgG + oligodendrocytes. Arrows indicate macrophages containing MBP + myelin debris in the demyelinated zone. A. Immunostained for MBP. B. Immunostained for IgG. (From Ref. 71.)

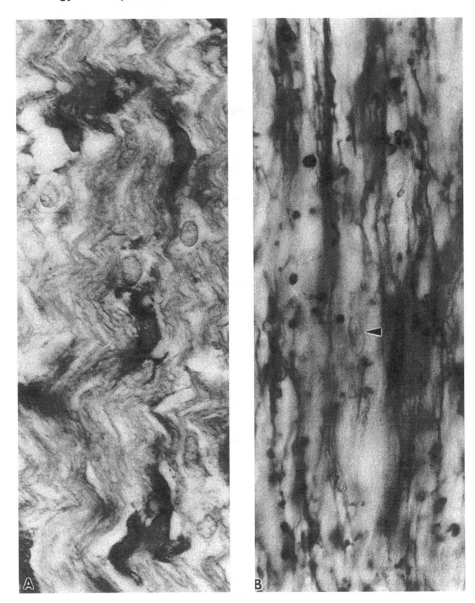

Figure 8   Areas of commencing myelin destruction in an acute lesion. A. Paraffin section immunostained for IgG shows IgG + macrophages infiltrating the affected tissue. B. Comparable field
stained for myelin shows commencing disintegration of myelin sheaths and the formation of myelin
balls in tissue infiltrated by macrophages (arrowhead indicates nucleus of a macrophage). Electron
microscopical studies of similar lesions show that the myelin balls are located within macrophage
cytoplasm. (From Ref. 37.)

the hypercellular demyelinated tissue, and perivascular cuffs of lymphocytes, plasma cells, and lipid-laden macrophages become increasingly prominent. Lymphocytes and plasma cells are also present outside the perivascular compartment among demyelinated axons and at the margin of the lesion.

D. Oligodendrocyte Regeneration and Remyelination

The subsequent organization of a fresh lesion and its conversion into a typical old plaque have been viewed traditionally as a process akin to scar formation, with increasing fibrillary gliosis, a decrease in the size of astrocytes and a slow disappearance of fatty macrophages and inflammatory cells from the demyelinated tissue and perivascular spaces (2). However, more recent studies of rare, severe cases, where death occurred within a few weeks or months of clinical onset, indicate that early lesions frequently exhibit evidence of extensive new myelin formation resulting in large "shadow plaques" composed of fields of thinly remyelinated axons (6,29,40,43) (Figs. 5B and 9). This vigorous regenerative activity commences in plaques that still contain large numbers of foamy macrophages (6,29) and is an indication that within a few weeks the environment within some fresh lesions is no longer hostile toward oligodendrocytes and myelin. Regarding the source of oligodendrocytes responsible for new myelin formation in fresh lesions, Brück et al. (41), Ozawa et al. (42), Raine (102,118), and others have reported findings originally interpreted as indicating that the capacity of a plaque to remyelinate depended upon large numbers of mature albeit truncated oligodendrocytes surviving within the lesion. However, in an autopsy study of a large number of exceptionally early MS cases (90 plaques analyzed in 18 patients, 7 of whom had died within 10 weeks of onset) and in which oligodendrocytes were immunostained for the markers MBP, CNP, MAG, carbonic anhydrase, and GalC, it was observed that in actively demyelinating areas (partially myelinated tissue infiltrated by macrophages containing MBP-positive myelin fragments) oligodendrocytes were markedly reduced in number, while in slightly older lesions (totally demyelinated areas packed with MBP-negative lipid macrophages), oligodendrocytes were often present in large numbers (5,39), with new myelin beginning to appear in such lesions within a few weeks (40). This observation, that oligodendrocytes are lost then reappear in most acute MS lesions, has been confirmed in a recent study by Lucchinetti et al. (134) and is consistent with other evidence of oligodendrocyte proliferation in early MS (44). The new oligodendrocytes that repopulate acute lesions within a few weeks express heat shock protein (HSP) 60 (102) and react intensely for the L2/HNK-1 epitope (39), a carbohydrate epitope associated with a family of cell adhesion molecules that includes MAG and myelin oligodendrocyte glycoprotein (MOG) (45). With the commencement of axon ensheathment and expression of MBP and other late differentiation antigens, L2/HNK-1 immunoreactivity of oligodendrocyte perikarya diminishes. The same sequence of oligodendrocyte loss followed by oligodendrocyte recruitment and remyelination has been observed in numerous models of experimental demyelination [reviewed by Wolswijk (173)]. There is good evidence that in these models, new oligodendrocytes derive from highly motile oligodendrocyte precursor cells (OPCs) that are immunoreactive for the marker NG2 chondroitin sulfate proteoglycan and that divide, migrate into the lesion, and differentiate into immobile GalC-positive oligodendrocytes (178,179,184). OPCs have been identified in MS tissue and in normal adult human nervous tissue (173). The origin of newly generated oligodendrocytes in acute MS lesions has been traced back to an unusual-looking GFAP-negative glial cell with a large round nucleus and relatively abundant cytoplasm

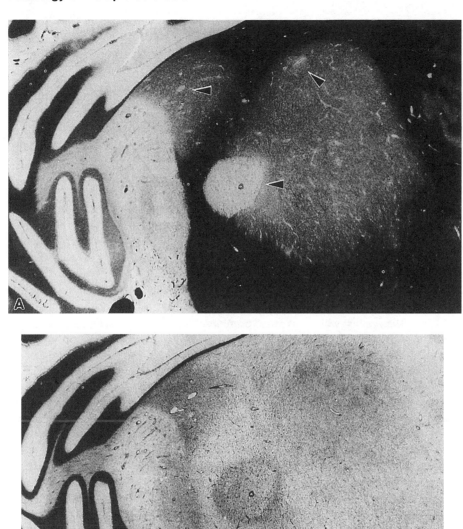

Figure 9 Cerebellar white matter with two remyelinating shadow plaques, the one on the left contiguous with an old demyelinated plaque. Fresh activity, as evidenced by hypercellularity and commencing myelin loss (*arrow points*), is present in each remyelinating lesion. A. Heidenhain's stain for myelin; B. Nissl stain for cell density. (From Ref. 18.)

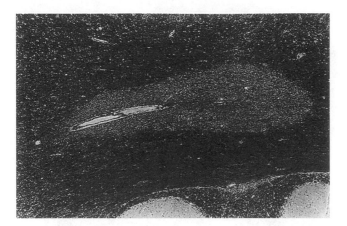

Figure 10   A Remyelinated shadow plaque in a patient with longstanding MS. Paraffin section stained for myelin.

that reacts intensely for the HNK-1 epitope and with variable, usually faint, immunoreactivity for CNP. These cells, which have also been observed in experimental remyelinating lesions (183), appear very early in evolving MS lesions, both within and close to areas of active demyelination and in white matter bordering recently demyelinated tissue (39). That these cells are the immediate source of new oligodendrocytes in MS has now been shown by Maeda et al. (108) using triple immunostaining and confocal laser scanning microscopy to analysis cells of this phenotype in early MS cases. Consistent, intense immunoreactivity for platelet-derived growth factor α receptor (PDGF-αR) identified them as OPCs, they were variably positive for the early oligodendrocyte differentiation antigen CNP, and, most importantly, they formed the majority of the usually small number of cells present that were positive for the cell proliferation marker Ki 67. These findings also explain the presence of HNK-1–positive oligodendrocytes within reactive astrocytes in subacute MS lesions prior to the onset of new myelin formation (80). It is likely that this phenomenon results from emperipolesis (migration of one cell into another) (169), which is consistent with the above evidence that acute lesions are repopulated by migrating OPCs that remain highly mobile until differentiating into immobile oligodendrocytes.

Although some shadow plaques become sites of fresh demyelinative activity, either by superimposition of new lesions or by spread from adjacent lesions (18), other shadow plaques remyelinate permanently, appearing in long-standing cases of the disease as plaque-like areas of gliosis filled with nerve fibers with myelin sheaths only slightly less thick than normal (6) (Fig. 10).

IV.   VARIANTS OF MULTIPLE SCLEROSIS

Isolated optic neuritis, subclinical MS, benign MS, and the Marburg type of acute MS (46) differ from the ordinary relapsing and remitting form of the disease in the number and location of plaques and the timing of their appearance rather than in any recognized qualitative differences in the lesions. Other variants—such as Baló's concentric sclerosis (47), Dévic's disease (48), the Schilder type of MS (49), and MS associated with acute necrotizing myelopathy (50)—are distinguished not only by an unusual clinical course but also by the presence of tissue changes that are not seen in the common form of the disease.

A. Benign and Subclinical Multiple Sclerosis

Plaques discovered unexpectedly at autopsy in older individuals with no history of neurological disease (subclinical MS) or in patients in whom the disease remitted apparently permanently following one or two brief clinical episodes in early adult life (benign or arrested MS) do not differ grossly or microscopically from old lesions found in patients with more typical long-standing disease (51). The lesions are usually few in number and in some cases only a single lesion has been present. In a series of 11 clinically silent cases reported by Mews et al. (167), 45 of 54 plaques examined were demyelinated lesions, 9 revealed advanced remyelination, no active lesions were present, and inflammatory cells were sparse. The incidence of subclinical disease based on autopsy series is estimated to be between 5 and 20% of all MS cases (54). In view of recent evidence mentioned earlier that plaques may remyelinate permanently, the true incidence of subclinical disease may be greater than this.

B. Acute Severe Multiple Sclerosis

Multiple sclerosis sometimes pursues a rapidly downhill course, which may be interrupted by brief remissions, leading to severe disability or death within a few months of onset. In its most malignant form, death may occur within days or weeks of the first symptom (55). The postmortem diagnosis of MS in such clinically atypical cases is based on finding one or more lesions that resemble fresh lesions seen in typical cases of somewhat longer duration.

Several forms of the acute disease have been defined pathologically. In the type described by Marburg, there are usually numerous lesions present in the brain and spinal cord. Some variation in the histological age of the lesions is usually apparent, even in the most acute cases, with fresh hypercellular lesions in which demyelinative activity has ceased intermixed with remyelinating lesions and actively demyelinating lesions. In the Baló form of acute MS (154,187), some or all of the newly formed lesions, which range in size from 0.5 to 4 cm in diameter, are surrounded by multiple concentric bands of preserved myelin (57). A third pathological variant, which may be rapidly fatal, was described by Schilder in 1912 (49); it is characterized by the presence of giant plaques in one or both cerebral hemispheres occurring together with more typical lesions (58). Lesions may be single or multiple, sometimes with mass effect, and they may have a cystic or necrotic center. They tend to spare the cortex and usually show ring enhancement on MRI. The spinal fluid may or may not show oligoclonal bands or an increase in IgG content (156). The course may be monophasic or relapsing and remitting (163,164).

C. Dévic's Disease

The term *Dévic's disease* (neuromyelitis optica) refers to cases of MS in which visual failure and spinal cord signs dominate the clinical picture. The visual loss and spinal cord involvement tend to occur within a relatively short interval and are often severe. Autopsy usually reveals a preponderance of lesions in the optic nerves and upper thoracic cord. Lesions may be necrotic, with destruction of all tissue elements including axons and nerve cells, together with cavitation and cyst formation. It is thought that necrosis results from ischemia caused by containment of the swollen tissue by the unyielding pia mater. Necrosis of the spinal cord associated with inflammatory demyelination also occurs in the unrelated disease acute disseminated encephalomyelitis (ADEM). Clinically typical cases of Dévic's disease with elevated anticardiolipin antibody titers have been described (166). Autopsy studies, however, will be required to determine whether such cases have Dévic's disease or some unrelated condition.

In Japan, the Dévic form of MS ("Asian-type MS") is relatively more common than in the West. Among Japanese MS patients, significant differences in HLA-DR2 haplotypes have been found between this form of the disease and western-type MS, a finding that suggests that Dévic's disease may be an immunogenetically distinct variant of MS (188).

D. Primary Progressive Multiple Sclerosis

Plaques in the spinal cord, brainstem, and cerebrum in patients in whom the disease is progressive from the beginning, without periods of remission, exhibit significantly less inflammation than similarly located lesions in patients with secondary progressive MS (59). This is in keeping with MRI evidence that lesions less frequently enhance in the primary progressive group (60). Also, there are reports that significantly fewer cases of primary progressive MS compared to cases of secondary progressive MS have MBP-like material in their spinal fluid (153) or show increased reactivity of peripheral blood mononuclear cells to proteolipid protein (177). On the other hand, no evidence of genetic heterogeneity was observed in an extensive study of HLA-DR and other candidate susceptibility genes in patients with primary progressive, secondary progressive, and relapsing-remitting MS (143). What underlying pathogenetic mechanism distinguishes primary progressive MS from the more common forms of the disease remains unknown.

E. Multiple Sclerosis Diagnosed by Biopsy

Zagzag et al. (61), Kepes (62), and others have reported numerous patients presenting with epilepsy, hemiplegia, confusion, or symptoms of a mass lesion and with MRI evidence of solitary or multiple ring-enhancing lesions in whom a diagnosis of MS was based on biopsy findings. The histological features observed in virtually every case have comprised hypercellularity due largely to the presence of lipid macrophages, areas of complete myelin loss with relative preservation of axons, and perivascular cuffs of lymphocytes. Astrocytes may be inconspicuous, or swollen-bodied astrocytes, some with multiple nuclei or mitotic figures, may be prominent. While some biopsied cases have involved acute, severe disease of Marburg, Schilder, or Baló type, most patients have survived the initial illness. The subsequent course may be relapsing and remitting or progressive, or there may be no clinical or radiological evidence of further activity for several years. The spinal fluid frequently shows no increase in IgG content or the presence of oligoclonal bands (156). Although it is not unusual for ADEM to be considered in the differential diagnoses in such cases prior to biopsy (155), it is interesting how few cases of ADEM diagnosed by biopsy have been reported. The histological findings in MS are quite unlike those observed in ADEM, and a tissue diagnosis of MS in these circumstances reliably excludes ADEM.

V. PATHOGENESIS

Indirect evidence suggests that MS is an organ-specific autoimmune disease in which there is a loss of tolerance to an unidentified oligodendrocyte and/or myelin antigen, that this loss of tolerance is in part genetically determined, and that it is related in some way to an environmental event, possibly a viral infection, early in the person's life (35). Facts that support this hypothesis are, first, no microbial or other foreign antigen has been consistently identified in affected tissue; second, the disease closely resembles in some of its most important pathological features chronic relapsing EAE produced by immunizing susceptible strains of animals with components of normal myelin (Fig. 11); third, evolving lesions exhibit a highly selective, apparently targeted destruction of oligodendrocytes and myelin; and fourth, the disease is strongly linked to MHC class II genes, as occurs in EAE and also in other human diseases thought to be autoimmune in nature such as type I diabetes and rheumatoid arthritis.

The main argument against autoimmunity in MS is the fact that although levels of T-cell and antibody immunoreactivity against myelin determinants are sometimes raised in MS patients compared to normal subjects and patients with other neurological diseases (67), the differences are not clear-cut or consistent. Also, it is uncertain whether antimyelin immunoreactivity detected in MS is a result rather than the cause of tissue breakdown (92). There are two recent reports, however, of a highly significant increase in T-cell and antibody reactivity to an immunodominant MBP epitope in MS patients compared to patients with other neurological diseases (133,136).

In individuals of European descent, MS is strongly associated with immunoregulatory genes of the HLA-class II complex. That this genetic predisposition is not by itself sufficient to cause the disease is shown by the low concordance rate of 20 to 30% in identical twins and by epidemiological evidence that exposure to some unknown environmental factor early in life is critical in determining who will develop the disease later in life.

T Lymphocytes

T cells specific for CNS peptides—including MBP, CNP, MAG, PLP (proteolipid protein), and MOG—are normally present in peripheral lymphoid organs and in the blood. There is evidence that unstimulated T cells are normally excluded from the CNS but that

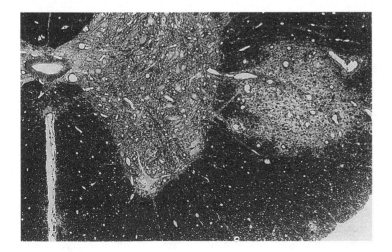

Figure 11 Experimental allergic encephalomyelitis. Juvenile Hartley guinea pig 10 weeks postsensitization with guinea pig central white matter showing large MS-like spinal cord plaque of demyelinated axons. Toluidine blue. (Courtesy of Dr. Y. Maeda and Dr. R. Maeda.)

activated T cells of any specificity cross the blood-brain barrier to patrol the CNS (130). The initiation of a T cell–mediated inflammatory reaction by a CD4 T cell requires the lymphocyte to contact peptide in the context of MHC class II molecules together with costimulatory molecules on the surface of an antigen-presenting cell. In the normal CNS, constitutive expression of MHC class II molecules is restricted largely to macrophages located in perivascular spaces and the subarachnoid space (128). It is likely that in EAE and in MS, this is the location where activated antigen-specific T cells that have entered the CNS first encounter processed antigen. In EAE, the CD4 T cells that proliferate and initiate lesion formation following contact with processed antigen, the latter presumably derived from physiological turnover, are of the T-helper 1 phenotype (129,138). CD4 T cells of this phenotype promote cellular immune reactions by releasing proinflammatory cytokines that include interferon γ (INF-γ), interleukin-2 (IL-2), and tumor necrosis factor α and β (TNF-α and TNF-β). These cytokines orchestrate an inflammatory cascade that begins with opening of the blood-brain barrier, vasogenic edema, and recruitment into the CNS of T cells, monocytes, and B lymphocytes following upregulation of adhesion molecules on these cells and the corresponding ligands on vascular endothelial cells. The same cytokines induce production of cytotoxic cytokines, enzymes, and other toxic molecules by T cells, macrophages, and glia; they also upregulate MHC class II molecule expression on microglia and vascular endothelial cells (121), cause B-cell differentiation toward IgG isotypes that fix complement, mediate antigen-specific cytotoxic CD8 T-cell functions via IL-2, and activate secretory and phagocytic functions of macrophages and microglia. Immunohistochemical studies of early-evolving lesions in MS suggest that a similar Th1-type cellular immune response is responsible for tissue damage in this disease [reviewed by Esiri and Gay (27)]. In actively demyelinating MS lesions, both CD4 and CD8 T cells are present, together with infiltrating macrophages and microglia displaying enhanced expression of MHC class II antigens (87,120), Fc and complement receptors (74,113), and Fas ligand (1,117). The endothelium of venules and capillaries associated with such lesions show upregulation of MHC class II antigens and the adhesion molecules ICAM-1 and VCAM-1 (94,97). Th1-type cytokines IL-1, IL-2, TNF-α and INF-γ as well as Th2-type anti-inflammatory cytokines IL-4, IL-10, and transforming growth factor β(TGF-β) have been detected in plaques of different ages (91,97,124). Reports that treatment of MS patients with INF-γ exacerbates the disease (101) and that peripheral blood lymphocytes in MS show more Th1-type cytokines than lymphocytes from patients with other neurological disease (144) also point to Th1-type cellular immunity in MS.

Activation of autoaggressive T cells in EAE occurs in peripheral lymphoid organs following immunization with antigen plus adjuvants. In MS, as in most other naturally occurring autoimmune diseases, the trigger that activates specific T cells is unknown. Exposure to microbial antigens that cross react with self antigens is one possibility, as it has been shown that a number of viral and bacterial antigens can activate MBP-specific T cells (106). Other possible triggers include antigen-independent activation of encephalitogenic clones by cytokines or by bacterial or viral superantigens that activate large numbers of T-cell clones (35).

Oligodendrocytes and Myelin

As noted above, several patterns of oligodendrocyte destruction have been observed in MS, namely apoptosis defined morphologically or by the presence of DNA fragmentation shown by in situ end-labeling (ISEL) and lysis (117). These patterns have been reproduced experimentally by exposing oligodendrocytes in vitro to toxic factors known to be present in MS plaques (27,137). These studies show that TNF-α (104), TNF-β (105), and INF-γ (123) cause oligodendrocyte apoptosis, while INF-γ-activated macrophages and microglia (145), CD4 T cells (via a non-MHC-dependent mechanism) (119), γδ T cells (141), reactive oxygen species (117), nitric oxide metabolites (117), and Fas-Fas ligand interactions (117) result in oligodendrocyte lysis. Fas, a member of the TNF-receptor superfamily, when expressed on a cell surface and ligated by Fas ligand produced by macrophages and T cells, usually results in apoptotic cell death. However, there is a report that Fas-Fas ligand interactions involving cultured oligodendrocytes causes cell lysis (117). In MS tissue, both Fas-positive (117) and Fas ligand–positive oligodendrocytes, the latter colocalizing with cells exhibiting DNA fragmentation (122), have been observed. Antigen-specific CD8 cytotoxic lymphocytes, which destroy target cells either by perforin-based or Fas-Fas ligand interactions, recognize peptides only in association with MHC class 1 molecules. As MHC class 1 molecules are not expressed by normal oligodendrocytes or by oligodendrocytes in acute MS lesions (63,98), it is unlikely that specific CD8 T cells contribute in this way to oligodendrocyte loss in MS.

Regarding myelin breakdown, that this could be secondary to oligodendrocyte destruction remains an uncertain issue in MS pathology, although, as described earlier, there are no reports that convincingly demonstrate oligodendrocyte loss or injury occurring prior to commencing myelin breakdown. There is good evidence, however, that whatever it is that directs activated macrophages in MS to attack myelin, these cells, which are the major effectors of tissue damage in Th1-type cell-mediated immune reactions, are largely responsible for disrupting and removing myelin from nerve fibers in areas of active myelin breakdown. In addition to peeling myelin directly off affected nerve fibers by receptor-mediated phagocytosis (5), they secrete all of the toxic cytokines and metabolites listed above (27,126,137) as well as matrix metalloproteinases (70,91) and other neutral proteases (10,65) that have been shown to damage myelin in vitro (125).

The view has been expressed that injury to oligodendrocytes and myelin in MS may be a nonspecific bystander effect of an inflammatory lesion located in myelinated tissue. It is difficult to reconcile this with the highly selective destruction of myelin and oligodendrocytes often seen in early MS lesions in the absence of any hint of irreversible injury to other CNS components. Also the rapid, extensive, and almost always complete loss of myelin seen in newly forming lesions points to myelin being targeted in a way not seen in most other chronic inflammatory diseases of the CNS, such as subacute sclerosing panencephalitis, herpes simplex encephalitis, and tropical spastic paraplegia, all conditions that have cellular infiltrates and cytokine profiles not too dissimilar to those found in MS (27). Exceptions to this are that there may be more γδ T cells (95) and fewer CD45R-positive T cells (96) in MS lesions than in lesions in other neurological diseases.

Antibodies and Complement

Experimental evidence is lacking that activated T cells alone can induce demyelination. In EAE induced, for example, using astrocyte-associated proteins (157) or activated anti-MBP lymphocytes (100), perivascular inflammatory lesions in the CNS are not associated with significant demyelination. To obtain demyelination in EAE, evidence indicates that antibodies need to be present that react with determinants exposed on the outer surface of oligodendrocytes and myelin. The possibility that antimyelin antibodies might be involved in lesion pathogenesis in MS was raised more than 30 years ago in a series of studies showing that there are factors present in MS and EAE serum that demyelinate organotypic cultures of CNS myelin (78). This possibility has been reinforced by recent findings in MOG-EAE (115). MOG is a minor myelin protein present on the exposed surface of CNS myelin. Induction of MOG-EAE in Brown Norway rats, marmosets, and other susceptible animals results in a progressive or relapsing and remitting disease in which the inflammatory demyelinating and remyelinating lesions in the CNS resemble somewhat more closely than those in other types of EAE the lesions seen in early MS (77,114), although changes more typical of ADEM—i.e., the presence of numerous small perivenous lesions—may also be prominent (77). The immune response is complex, with Th1-type CD4 T cells initiating inflammatory lesions and Th2-type CD4 T cells driving the production of anti-MOG antibodies that cross the blood-brain barrier to mediate myelin breakdown (110,115,116). Affected fibers show evidence of IgG and complement deposition (68) and, on electron microscopy, appear swollen and vesiculated (77), an ultrastructural pattern of myelin disruption also seen in other experimental autoimmune demyelinating diseases (168) and in some cases of acute MS (52,56,64). Comparable immunohistochemical studies in MS aimed at identifying antibody by determining the location of tissue bound IgG in active lesions have for the most part been unrewarding. In frozen section, most of the IgG present disappears after washing (32), and in paraffin sections the distribution of most of the large amount of IgG present in the tissue is similar to that seen in other inflammatory neurological diseases. In optimally fixed tissue from subacute MS cases, however, IgG has been observed, not on myelin sheaths but colocalizing with fragments of myelin on the surface of macrophages (37,71) (Fig. 12) and, in acute cases, again not on myelin sheaths but associated with myelin debris located within macrophages (32). The latter observations suggest that if the IgG in plaques is antibody, it is directed at hidden myelin epitopes rather than epitopes exposed on the surface of myelin sheaths. Other recent studies, however, report evidence of IgG deposition on myelin sheaths in active lesions in acute MS (77) and of IgG and membrane attack complex (MAC) on disrupted myelin sheaths in active lesions in a patient with chronic MS (85). A report that IgG-positive disrupted myelin sheaths in acute MS bind gold-labeled encephalitogenic peptides of MOG and MBP may indicate that the deposited IgG is antimyelin antibody and not IgG bound nonspecifically via Fc receptors as reported to occur with isolated myelin (171). Reports that anti-MOG antibodies are present somewhat more often and at higher titers in serum and CSF in MS than in other neurological diseases is seen as supporting a possible pathogenetic role for anti-MOG antibody in MS (132). If exposure of intact myelin sheaths to complement-fixing antimyelin antibodies is the cause of myelin destruction in MS, it is difficult to understand why there is frequently no evidence of ongoing myelin breakdown in long-standing lesions, where persistent defects in the blood-brain barrier allow serum proteins to permeate through the tissue (82), especially as it has been shown that injection of anti-MOG antibody directly into CNS tissue causes immediate and extensive demyelination (131).

Several lines of evidence suggest that complement plays an important role in myelin recognition and uptake by macrophages in MS. In vitro studies using isolated myelin show that activated complement degrades myelin and augments myelin phagocytosis (90,186,189), and it greatly enhances antibody-mediated phagocytosis (17,73,89). In addition, ligation of microglial complement receptor (CR)3 by C3d causes the release of the proinflammatory cytokines IL-2 and TNF-α as well as nitric oxide and reactive oxygen species (89). In vivo studies also show that recognition and uptake of altered myelin is largely dependent on myelin being opsonized by activated C3 (3,4). In MS, components of activated complement are present in CSF (79,84), with levels increasing during disease activity (72). In plaques, activated complement has been detected in blood vessel walls

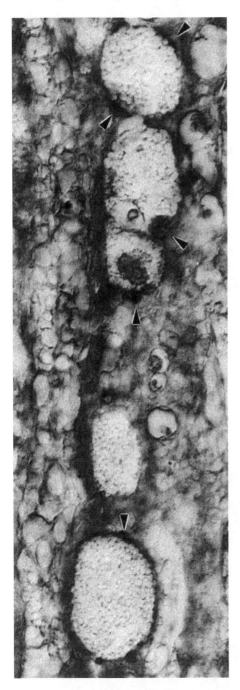

Figure 12 Macrophages engaged in active myelin destruction at the edge of an old plaque exhibit a restricted distribution (capping) of surface IgG (*arrowheads*). This appearance can be accounted for by the presence of a multivalent particulate antigen close to the cell surface. (From Ref. 71.)

(7), in macrophages containing IgG and myelin (32), and most recently on myelin in areas of active myelin breakdown in a terminally fulminant case of chronic MS (85) and in patients with severe secondary progressive MS (109). In the latter study, a majority of the numerous plaques present in each of two cases studied revealed C3d, the opsonic component of activated complement, deposited on short segments of disrupted myelin located within knots of microglia in periplaque white matter, the latter corresponding to the knots of microglia observed electron microscopically to engage myelin via clathrin-coated pits in white matter bordering plaques (23) (Figs. 13 and 14). As C3d is internalized via clathrin-coated pits following attachment to CR3 (76), the major receptor utilized by

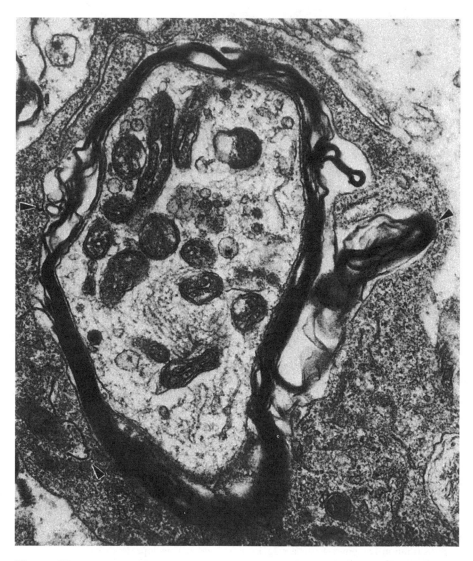

Figure 13 Pattern of active myelin destruction at the edge of an expanding chronic plaque. A partially demyelinated nerve fiber is surrounded by macrophage processes. Superficial myelin lamellae in contact with the macrophage are loosened and can be seen entering the macrophage in the form of fingerlike processes attached to clathrin-coated pits on the macrophage surface (*arrowheads*).

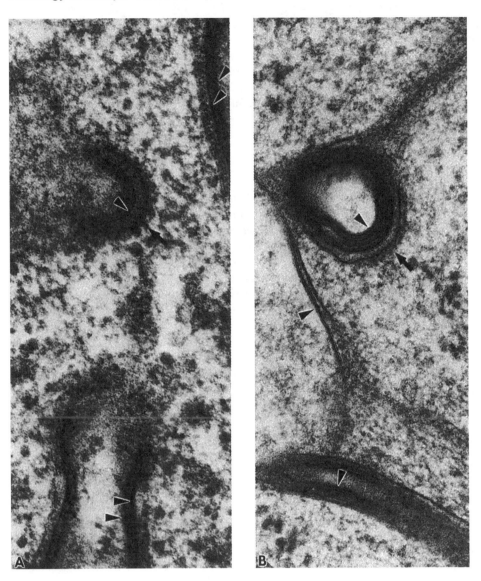

Figure 14 Attachment of myelin lamellae to clathrin-coated pits on the surface of macrophages engaged in myelin destruction. A. Edge of an active chronic MS plaque. B. Acute EAE. Arrowheads indicate myelin lamellae and arrows indicate the clathrin undercoat. There is evidence that the ligand occupying the space between the two membranes is C3d, the opsonic component of activated complement. (From Ref. 23.)

macrophages for phagocytosis, and which is upregulated on activated microglia in MS plaques (88,113), these findings are strong evidence that myelin recognition and uptake by macrophages in chronic active lesions is complement-mediated. The fact that C3d deposition was observed in the latter study only on disrupted segments of myelin and not on intact sheaths again suggests that the putative MS antigen may be a hidden myelin epitope, especially as it is known that attachment of C3d greatly augments the immunogenicity of antigens exposed to B-cell receptors, even to the point of breaking tolerance to a self antigen (28).

The mechanism underlying complement activation associated with myelin breakdown in MS is uncertain. In the patient described by Storch et al. (85) but not in the other two cases referred to above, affected myelin sheaths also exhibited evidence of IgG deposition, suggesting antibody-dependent complement activation in that case. Alternatively, colocalization of IgG and complement on affected myelin could be explained by the fact that physically altered myelin by itself can activate complement (190) and also bind IgG (171).

Chronicity

It is a feature of many newly forming MS lesions that within a few weeks of their appearance there are signs of a robust downregulation in inflammatory activity, manifest as cessation of active demyelination at the plaque margin, reappearance of oligodendrocytes among the still numerous lipid macrophages present throughout the lesion, and commencing formation of new myelin. In MBP-induced EAE there is evidence that cessation of local disease activity is related to selective elimination by apoptosis of autoreactive T cells (191), resulting in a switch from a Th1-type proinflammatory to a Th2-type anti-inflammatory response, the latter dominated by cytokines that inhibit INF-γ–induced macrophage activation (140). The only evidence at present of a similar mechanism occurring in MS is the finding that the production by blood and CSF mononuclear cells of transforming growth factorβ (TGF-β) and IL-10, the two best-defined anti-inflammatory cytokines known to cause activated macrophages to return to their resting state, coincides with clinical recovery and the recovery phase of MRI activity (103,127,159). Reactivation may be related to "epitope spreading." In experimental autoimmune diabetes and in type 1 diabetes in humans, immunoreactivity of T cells and antibody spreads during the course of the disease to target-cell antigens not initially involved in the disease. Similarly in EAE induced by a single PLP peptide, immunoreactivity has been observed to spread to MBP (107).

Disease Heterogeneity

There is new evidence that the diversity of disease expression in MS may reflect major differences in underlying pathogenetic mechanisms (Fig. 15). In a series of immunohistochemical studies of plaques from patients with acute and chronic forms of the disease biopsied or examined at autopsy early in the course of the disease, Ozawa, Lucchinetti, Lassman, Brück, Rodriguez, and others initially reported that there appeared to be two main types of MS based on oligodendrocyte pathology. In one type, observed in autopsied cases of early fatal MS, there was a dramatic loss of oligodendrocytes, apoptotic oligodendrocytes were numerous, and oligodendrocyte recruitment and remyelination was scant or absent. In the second type, observed in biopsies from patients with early classic MS, there was little or no oligodendrocyte loss, few apoptotic oligodendrocytes were seen, and remyelination was present (42,69). In subsequent studies of additional cases, however, substantial oligodendrocyte loss was observed in active lesions both in Marburg-type cases (i.e., early fatal cases) as well as patients with typical long-standing disease biopsied early in the course of the disease (134). This evidence of pathogenetic heterogeneity in early and malignant forms of MS has been revised somewhat in several recent reports from the same group of investigators. In approximately 70% of patients biopsied or autopsied early in the course of malignant or classic MS, a substantial loss of oligodendrocytes (more than

60% loss), accompanied active myelin loss at the plaque margin, with oligodendrocyte recruitment and variable remyelination present at the plaque center. In approximately 30% of cases, the one or more actively demyelinating lesions examined in each case showed the same severe loss of oligodendrocytes, but no evidence of oligodendrocyte recruitment or remyelination (134). In a further study it was observed that in cases characterized by conspicuous oligodendrocyte apoptosis and loss and no remyelination, there was a preferential loss of MAG in white matter bordering active lesions, suggesting that some form of oligodendrocyte injury or dysfunction precedes myelin breakdown in such cases. In contrast, in cases typified by active lesions in which oligodendrocyte loss was followed by oligodendrocyte proliferation and remyelination (50% of all cases studied), deposits of IgG and membrane attack complex were present at sites of active demyelination (112,162). The authors suggest that early in the course of both acute and chronic forms of multiple sclerosis, in about one-third of patients, some unknown form of oligodendrocyte injury or dysfunction precedes tissue breakdown, while in about 50% of cases, myelin destruction is mediated by complement activating antimyelin antibody. These findings need to be confirmed as others have been unable to detect, in equally large series of comparable cases, evidence of IgG deposition on myelin sheaths in evolving early lesions (32). Also, a similar preferential loss of MAG has been observed around some fresh ischemic infarcts, suggesting that this may be a nonspecific reaction to white matter injury (71).

Differences in the clinical and pathological expression of EAE in different animals, such as differences in disease susceptibility, whether the illness is acute or chronic, the size and distribution of demyelinating lesions within the CNS, and the extent of axonal damage are determined largely by genetic factors. This is evident not only between species but also between different strains of the same species (114,147), which, it is important to remember, represent different individuals in the larger population (35). Attempts to link differences in the expression of MS in different patients to genetic factors have so far been unrewarding, although differences between western-type and Asian-type MS are thought to be hereditary in origin. Disease diversity in MS may be related to factors other than genetic makeup that have been shown to affect disease expression in EAE. Such factors include the particular myelin component used to induce the experimental disease (93), the timing and route of administration of the immunogen, and what adjuvants are present.

Why remyelination ultimately fails in subacute and long-standing MS lesions, in contrast to newly formed lesions located in previously unaffected white matter, is an important but unsettled issue (174). Possible mechanisms suggested by pathological and experimental studies of failed central remyelination include recurrent or protracted demyelination (18,75,111), the presence of myelination-inhibiting antibodies (78,181) or T cells or antibody reactive against oligodendrocyte differentiation antigens (53), endocytosis of oligodendrocytes by astrocytes (Fig. 16) (80), persistent exposure of demyelinated tissue to normal plasma constituents (81,82), gliosis (180), large lesion size (175), and increasing age (176). While remyelination failure in MS has been viewed as a failure of oligodendrocyte precursor cells to repopulate affected lesions, there is now evidence that persistently demyelinated plaques do, in fact, contain OPCs, albeit in small numbers, and that remyelination failure in MS is due, at least in part, to failure of OPCs located inside old plaques to proliferate and differentiate (135,172). Methods used successfully to reverse remyelination block in experimental animals are reviewed by Rodriguez and Lennon (182), Duncan et al. (99), and Franklin and Blakemore (185).

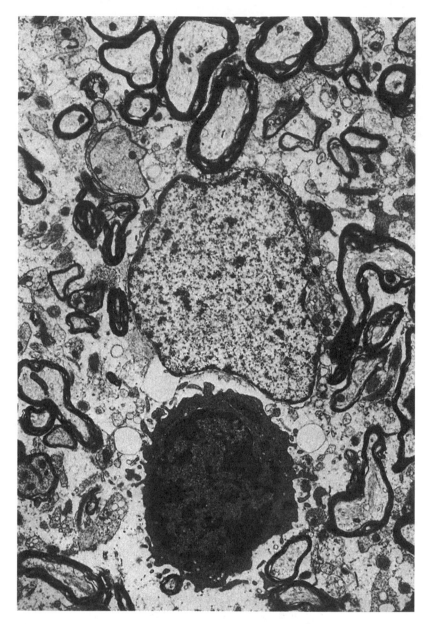

Figure 15 Edge of an active chronic MS plaque showing a degenerating oligodendrocyte with an enlarged watery nucleus and lysed cytoplasm—suggestive of osmotic lysis—in contact with a lymphocyte. This finding suggests cell-mediated destruction of oligodendrocytes in expanding lesions. (From Ref. 5.)

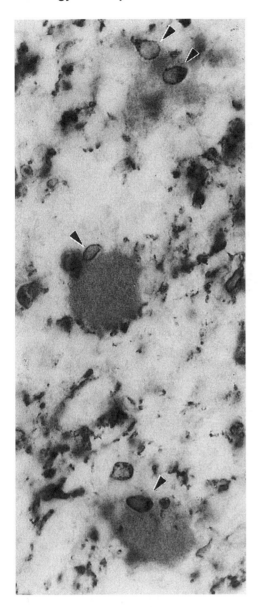

Figure 16 Paraffin section of a plaque immunostained for a carbohydrate-containing epitope (HNK-1) expressed by developing oligodendrocytes. Positively stained oligodendrocytes (*arrow points*) can be seen located within or close to astrocytes. (From Ref. 80.)

ACKNOWLEDGMENTS

This work was supported by the Veterans Affairs Medical Center Research Service, the National Multiple Sclerosis Society, and the Nerve Research Foundation of the University of Sydney.

REFERENCES

1. Brosnan CF, Raine CS. Mechanisms of immune injury in multiple sclerosis. Brain Pathology 1996; 6:243–257.
2. Lumsden CE. The neuropathology of multiple sclerosis. In: Vinken PJ, Bruyn GW, eds. Handbook of Clinical Neurology, vol 9. Amsterdam: North Holland, 1970, pp 217–309.
3. Brück W, Friede RL. Anti-macrophage CR3 antibody blocks myelin phagocytosis by macrophages in vitro. Acta Neuropathol 1990; 80:415–418.
4. Brück W, Brück Y, Diederich U, Piddlesden SJ. The membrane attack complex of complement mediates peripheral nervous system demyelination in vitro. Acta Neuropathol 1995; 90:601–607.
5. Prineas JW. The neuropathology of multiple sclerosis. In: Vinken PJ, Bruyn GW, Klawans GW, Koetsier JC, eds. Demyelinating Diseases: Handbook of Clinical Neurology, vol 47. Amsterdam: Elsevier, 1985, pp 213–257.
6. Lassmann H. Comparative Neuropathology of Chronic Experimental Allergic Encephalomyelitis and Multiple Sclerosis. Berlin: Springer-Verlag, 1983.
7. Compston DAS, Morgan BP, Campbell AK, Wilkins P, Cole G, Thomas ND, Jasani B. Immunocytochemical localization of the terminal complement complex in multiple sclerosis. Neuropathol Appl Neurobiol 1989; 15:307–317.
8. Allen IV, Millar JHD, Hutchinson MJ. General disease in 120 necropsy-proven cases of multiple sclerosis. Neuropathol Appl Neurobiol 1978; 4:279–284.
9. Pollock M, Calder C, Allpress S. Peripheral nerve abnormality in multiple sclerosis. Ann Neurol 1977; 2:41–48.
10. Cuzner ML, Norton WT. Biochemistry of demyelination. Brain Pathol 1996; 6:231–242.
11. Schoene WC, Carpenter S, Behan PO, Geschwind N. Onion bulb formations in the central and peripheral nervous system in association with multiple sclerosis and hypertrophic polyneuropathy. Brain 1977; 100:755–773.
12. Cuzner ML, Gveric D, Strand C, Loughlin AJ, Paemen L, Opdenakker G, Newcombe J. The expression of tissue-type plasminogen activator, matrix metalloproteases and endogenous inhibitors in the central nervous system in multiple sclerosis: Comparison of stages in lesion evolution. J Neuropathol Exp Neurol 1996; 55:1194–1204.
13. Barnard RO, Triggs M. Corpus callosum in multiple sclerosis. J Neurol Neurosurg Psychiatry 1974; 37:1259–1264.
14. Ulrich J, Groebke-Lorenz W. The optic nerve in multiple sclerosis: A morphological study with retrospective clinicopathological correlations. Neuroophthalmology 1983; 3:149–159.
15. Brownell B, Hughes JT. The distribution of plaques in the cerebrum in multiple sclerosis. J Neurol Neurosurg Psychiatry 1962; 25:315–320.
16. Dawson JW. The histology of multiple sclerosis. Trans R Soc Edinb 1916; 50:517–740. (With plates; reproduced by the Montreal Neurological Institute, Montreal, 1973.)
17. De Jong BA, Smith ME. A role for complement in phagocytosis of myelin. Neurochem Res 1997; 22:491–498.
18. Prineas JW, Barnard RO, Revesz T, Kwon EE, Sharer L, Cho E-S. Multiple sclerosis: Pathology of recurrent lesions. Brain 1993; 116:681–693.
19. Prineas JW, Wright RG. Macrophages, lymphocytes and plasma cells in the perivascular compartment in chronic multiple sclerosis. Lab Invest 1978; 38:409–421.

20. Esiri MM, Reading MC. Macrophage populations associated with multiple sclerosis plaques. Neuropathol Appl Neurobiol 1987; 13:451–465.

21. Prineas JW. Multiple sclerosis: Presence of lymphatic capillaries and lymphoid tissue in the brain and spinal cord. Science 1979; 203:1123–1125.

22. Barnes D, Munro PMG, Youl BD, Prineas JW, McDonald WI. The longstanding MS lesion: A quantitative MRI and electron microscopic study. Brain 1991; 114:1271–1280.

23. Prineas JW, Connell F. The fine structure of chronically active multiple sclerosis plaques. Neurology 1978; 28(9, part 2):68–75.

24. Raine CS. Membrane specializations between demyelinated axons and astroglia in chronic EAE lesions and multiple sclerosis plaques. Nature 1978; 275:326–327.

25. Prineas JW, Connell F. Remyelination in multiple sclerosis. Ann Neurol 1979; 5:22–31.

26. Suzuki K, Andrews JM. Waltz JM, Terry RD. Ultrastructural studies of multiple sclerosis. Lab Invest 1969; 20:444–454.

27. Esiri MM, Gay D. The immunocytochemistry of multiple sclerosis plaques. In: Raine CS, McFarland HF, Tourtellotte WW, eds. Multiple Sclerosis: Clinical and Pathological Basis. London, Weinheim, New York, Tokyo, Melbourne, Madras: Chapman and Hall Medical, 1997, pp 173–186.

28. Fearon DT, Locksley RM. The instructive role of innate immunity in the acquired immune response. Science 1996; 272:50–54.

29. Prineas JW, Kwon EE, Cho E-S, Sharer LR. Continual breakdown and regeneration of myelin in progressive multiple sclerosis plaques. In: Scheinberg L, Raine CS, eds. Multiple sclerosis: experimental and clinical aspects. Ann NY Acad Sci 1984; 436:11–32.

30. Itoyama Y, Webster H de F, Richardson EP Jr, Trapp BD. Schwann cell remyelination of demyelinated axons in spinal cord multiple sclerosis lesions. Ann Neurol 1983; 14:339–346.

31. Ferguson B, Matyszak MK, Esiri MM, Perry VH. Axonal damage in acute multiple sclerosis lesions. Brain 1997; 120:393–399.

32. Gay FW, Drye TJ, Dick GWA, Esiri MM. The application of multifactorial cluster analysis in the staging of plaques in early multiple sclerosis: Identification and characterization of the primary demyelinating lesion. Brain 1997; 120:1461–1483.

33. Allen IV, McKeown SR. A histological, histochemical and biochemical study of the macroscopically normal white matter in multiple sclerosis. J Neurol Sci 1979; 41:81–91.

34. Adams RD, Kubik CS. The morbid anatomy of the demyelinative diseases. Am J Med 1952; 12:510–546.

35. Hohlfeld R. Biotechnological agents for the immunotherapy of multiple sclerosis: Principles, problems and perspectives. Brain 1997; 120:865–916.

36. Prineas JW, Raine CS. Electron microscopy and immunoperoxidase studies of early multiple sclerosis lesions. Neurology 1976; 26(6, part 2):29–32.

37. Prineas JW, Graham JS. Multiple sclerosis: Capping of surface immunoglobulin G on macrophages engaged in myelin breakdown. Ann Neurol 1981; 10:149–158.

38. Woodroofe MN, Bellamy AS, Feldmann M, Davison AN, Cuzner ML. Immunocytochemical characterization of the immune reaction in the central nervous system in multiple sclerosis: Possible role for microglia in lesion growth. J Neurol Sci 1986; 74:135–152.

39. Prineas JW, Kwon EE, Goldenberg PZ, et al. Multiple sclerosis: Oligodendrocyte proliferation and differentiation in fresh lesions. Lab Invest 1989; 61:489–503.

40. Prineas JW, Barnard RO, Kwon EE, Sharer LR, Cho E-S. Multiple sclerosis: Remyelination of nascent lesions. Ann Neurology 1993; 33:137–151.

41. Brück W, Schmied M, Suchanek G, et al. Oligodendrocytes in the early course of multiple sclerosis. Ann Neurol 1994; 35:65–73.

42. Ozawa K, Suchanek G, Breitschope H, Brück W, Budka H, Jellinger K, Lassmann H. Patterns of oligodendroglia pathology in multiple sclerosis. Brain 1994; 117:1311–1322.

43. Moore GRW, Neumann PE, Suzuki K, Lijtmaer HN, Traugott U, Raine CS. Baló's concentric sclerosis: New observations on lesion development. Ann Neurol 1985; 17:604–611.

44. Morris CS, Esiri MM, Sprinkle TJ, Gregson N. Oligodendrocyte reactions and cell proliferation markers in human demyelinating diseases. Neurolopath Appl Neurobiol 1994; 20:272–281.

45. Burger D, Steck AJ, Bernard CCA, Kerlero de Rosbon. Human myelin/oligodendrocyte glycoprotein: A new member of the L2/HNK-1 family. J Neurochem 1993; 61:1822–1827.

46. Marburg O. Die sogenannte "akute multiple Sklerose" (encephalomyelitis periaxialis scleroticans). Jahrb Psychiatr Neurol (Leipzig) 1906; 27:213–311.

47. Baló J. Leucoencephalitis periaxialis concentrica. Magy Novosi Arch 1927; 28:108–124.

48. Dévic E. Myélite subaigüe compliquée de nérvite optique (abstr). Bull Méd (Paris) 1894; 8: 1033–1034.

49. Schilder P. Zur kenntnis der sogenannte diffusen sklerose. Z Neurol Psychiatr 1912; 10:1–60.

50. Hughes JT. Pathology of the Spinal Cord. London: Lloyd-Luke, 1966, pp 146–159.

51. Phadke JG, Best PV. Atypical and clinically silent multiple sclerosis: A report of 12 cases discovered unexpectedly at necropsy. J Neurol Neurosurg Psychiatry 1983; 46:414–420.

52. Kirk J, The fine structure of the CNS in multiple sclerosis: II. Vesicular demyelination in the acute case. Neuropathol Appl Neurobiol 1979; 5:289–294.

53. Voskuhl RR, McFarlin DE, Rhame L, Deibler G, Stone R, Maloni H, McFarland HF. A novel candidate autoantigen in a multiplex family with multiple sclerosis: T-lymphocytes specific for an MBP epitope unique to myelination are as prevalent as epitopes within 18.5 kd MBP. J Neuroimmunol 1993; 46:137–144.

54. Morariu M, Klutzow WF. Subclinical multiple sclerosis. J Neurol 1976; 213:71–76.

55. Harper CG. Acute central nervous system disorder mimicking stroke. Med J Aust 1981; 1: 136–138.

56. Lassmann H. Comparative Neuropathology of Chronic Experimental Allergic Encephalomyelitis and Multiple Sclerosis. Berlin-Heidelberg, New York, Tokyo: Springer, 1983.

57. Yao D-L, Webster H de F, Hudson LD et al. Concentric sclerosis (Baló): Morphometric and in situ hybridization study of lesions in six patients. Ann Neurol 1994; 35:18–30.

58. Poser CM. Myelinoclastic diffuse and transitional sclerosis. In: Vinken PJ, Bruyn GW, eds. Handbook of Clinical Neurology, vol. 9: Multiple Sclerosis and Other Demyelinating Disease. Amsterdam: North Holland, 1970, pp. 469–484.

59. Revesz T, Kidd D, Thompson AJ, Barnard RO, McDonald WI. A comparison of the pathology of primary and secondary progressive multiple sclerosis. Brain 1994; 117:759–765.

60. Thompson AJ, Kermode AG, Wicks D, et al. Major differences in the dynamics of primary and secondary progressive multiple sclerosis. Ann Neurol 1991; 29:53–62.

61. Zagzag D, Miller DC, Kleinman GM, Abati A, Donnenfeld H. Budzilovich GN. Demyelinating disease versus tremor in surgical neuropathology: Clues to a correct pathological diagnosis. Am J Surg Pathol 1993; 17:537–545.

62. Kepes JJ. Large focal tumor-like demyelinating lesions of the brain: Intermediate entity between multiple sclerosis and acute disseminated encephalomyelitis? A study of 31 patients. Ann Neurol 1993; 33:182–127.

63. Lee SC, Raine CS. Multiple sclerosis: Oligodendrocytes in active lesions do not express class II major histocompatability complex molecules. J Neuroimmunol 1989; 25:261–266.

64. Lee SC, Moore GRW, Golenwsky G, Raine CS. Multiple sclerosis: A role for astroglia in active demyelination suggested by class II MHC expression and ultrastructural study. J Neuropathol Exp Neurology 1990; 49:122–136.

65. Li H, Newcombe J, Groome NP, Cuzner ML. Characterization and distribution of phagocytic macrophages in multiple sclerosis plaques. Neuropathol Appl Neurobiol 1993; 19:214–223.

66. Uchimura I. Shiraki H. A contribution to the classification and the pathogenesis of demyelinating encephalomyelitis: With special reference to the central nervous system lesions caused by preventive inoculation against rabies. J Neuropathol Exp Neurol 1957; 16:139–208.

67. Link H. B cells and autoimmunity. In: Russell WC, ed. Molecular Biology of Multiple Sclerosis. New York: Wiley 1997, pp 161–190.
68. Piddlesden SJ, Lassmann H, Zimprich F, Morgan BP, Linington C. The demyelinating potential of antibodies to myelin oligodendrocyte glycoprotein is related to their ability to fix complement. Am J Pathol 1993; 143:555–564.
69. Lucchinetti CF, Brück W, Rodriguez M, Lassmann H. Distinct patterns of multiple sclerosis pathology indicates heterogeneity in pathogenesis (review). Brain Pathol 1996; 6:259–274.
70. Maeda A, Sobel RA. Matrix metalloproteinases in the normal human central nervous system, microglial nodules and multiple sclerosis lesions. J Neuropathol Exp Pathol 1996; 55:300–309.
71. Prineas JW, Kwon EE, Sternberger NH, Lennon VA. The distribution of myelin associated glycoprotein and myelin basic protein in actively demyelinating multiple sclerosis lesions. J Neuroimmunol 1984; 6:251–264.
72. Morgan BP, Campbell AK, Compston DA. Terminal component of complement (C9) in cerebrospinal fluid of patients with multiple sclerosis. Lancet 1984; 2:251–254.
73. Mosley K, Cuzner ML. Receptor-mediated phagocytes of myelin by macrophages and microglia: Effect of opsonization and receptor blocking agents. Neurochemistry 1996; 21:481–487.
74. Nyland H, Matre R, Mork S. Fc receptors on microglial lipophages in multiple sclerosis. N Engl J Med 1980; 302(2):120–121.
75. Johnson ES, Ludwin SK. The demonstration of recurrent demyelination and remyelination of axons in the central nervous system. Acta Neuropathol 1981; 53:93–98.
76. Rabb H, Michishita M, Sharma CP, Brown D, Arnaout MA. Cytoplasmic tails of human complement receptor type 3 (CR3, CD11b/CD18) regulate ligand avidity and the internalization of occupied receptors. J Immunol 1993; 151:990–1002.
77. Raine CS, Cannella B, Hauser SL, Genain CP. Demyelination in primate autoimmune encephalomyelitis and acute multiple sclerosis lesions: A case study for antigen-specific antibody mediation. Ann Neurol 1999; 46:144–160.
78. Bornstein, MB, Raine CS. Experimental allergic encephalomyelitis: Antiserum inhibition of myelination in vitro. Lab Invest 1970; 23:536–542.
79. Sanders ME, Alexander EL, Koski CL, Shin ML, Sano Y, Frank MM, Joiner KA. Terminal complement complexes (SC5b-9) in cerebrospinal fluid in autoimmune nervous system diseases. Ann NY Acad Sci 1988; 540:387.
80. Prineas JW, Kwon EE, Goldenberg PZ, Cho E-S, Sharer LR. Interaction of astrocytes and newly formed oligodendrocytes in resolving multiple sclerosis lesions. Lab Invest 1990; 63:624–636.
81. Perry VH, Lund RD. Evidence that the lamina cribrosa prevents intraretinal myelination of retinal ganglion cell axons. J Neurocytol 1990; 19:265–272.
82. Kwon EE, Prineas JW. Blood-brain barrier abnormalities in longstanding multiple sclerosis lesions: An immunohistochemical study. J Neuropathol Exp Neurol 1994; 53:625–636.
83. Sanders V, Conrad AJ, Tourtellotte WW. On classification of post-mortem multiple sclerosis plaques for neuroscientists. J Neuroimmunol 1993; 46:207–216.
84. Sellebjerg F, Christiansen M, Garred P. MBP, anti-MBP and anti-PLP antibodies, and intrathecal complement activation in multiple sclerosis. Mult Scler 1998; 4:127–131.
85. Storch MK, Piddlesden S, Haltia M, Iivanainen M, Morgan P, Lassmann H. Multiple sclerosis: In situ evidence for antibody- and complement-mediated demyelination. Ann Neurol 1998; 43:465–471.
86. Trapp BD, Peterson J, Ransohoff RM, Rudick R, Mörk S, Bö L. Axonal transection in the lesions of multiple sclerosis. N Engl J Med 1998; 338:278–285.
87. Traugott U, Reinherz EL, Raine CS. Multiple sclerosis: Distribution of T cells, T cell subsets, and Ia-positive macrophages in lesions of different ages. J Neuroimmunol 1983; 4:201–221.
88. Ulvestad E, Williams K, Mörk S, Antel J, Nyland H. Phenotypic differences between human

monocyte/macrophage and microglial cells studied in vitro. J Neuopathol Exp Neurol 1994; 53:492–501.

89.   van der Laan LJW, Ruucs SR, Weber KS, Lodder J, Dopp EA, Dijkstra CD. Macrophage phagocytosis of myelin in vitro determined by flow cytometry: Phagocytosis is mediated by CR3 and induces production of tumor necrosis factor-α and nitric oxide. J Neuroimmunol 1996; 70:145–152.

90.   Vanguri P, Shin ML. Hydrolysis of myelin basic protein in human myelin by terminal complement complexes. J Biol Chem 1988; 263:7228–7234.

91.   Woodroofe MN, Cuzner ML. Cytokine mRNA expression in inflammatory multiple sclerosis lesions: Detection by non-radioactive in situ hybridisation. Cytokine 1993; 5:583–588.

92.   Schmidt S. Candidate autoantigens in multiple sclerosis. Mult Scler 1999; 5:147–160.

93.   Lassmann H, Vass K. Are current immunological concepts of multiple sclerosis reflected by the immunopathology of its lesions? Springer Semin Immunopathol 1995; 17:77–87.

94.   Sobel RA, Mitchell M, Fondren G. Intercellular adhesion molecule-1 (ICAM-1) in cellular immune reactions in the human central nervous system. Am J Pathol 1990; 136:1309–1316.

95.   Selmaj K, Brosnan CF, Raine CS. Colocalisation of TCR gamma/delta lymphocytes and hsp$^+$ oligodendrocytes in multiple sclerosis. Proc Natl Acad Sci USA 1991; 88:6452–6456.

96.   Sobel RA, Hafler DA, Castro EE, Morimoto C, Weiner HL. The 2H4 (CD45R) antigen is selectively decreased in multiple sclerosis lesions. J Immunol 1988; 140:2210–2214.

97.   Cannella B, Raine CS. The adhesion molecule and cytokine profile of multiple sclerosis lesions. Ann Neurol 1995; 37:424–435.

98.   Hayashi T, Morimoto C, Burks JS, Kerr C, Hauser SL. Dual-label immunocytochemistry of the active multiple sclerosis lesion: Major histocompatability complex and activation antigens. Ann Neurol 1988; 24:523–531.

99.   Duncan ID. Glial cell transplantation and remyelination of the central nervous system (review). Neuropathol Appl Neurobiol 1996; 22:87–100.

100. Linington C, Bradl M, Lassmann H, Brunner C, Vass K. Augmentation of demyelination in rat acute allergic encephalomyelitis by circulating mouse monoclonal antibodies directed against myelin/oligodendrocyte glycoprotein. Am J Pathol 1988; 130:443–454.

101. Panitch HS, Hirsch RL, Schindler J, Johnson KP. Treatment of multiple sclerosis with gamma interferon: Exacerbations associated with activation of the immune system. Neurology 1987; 37:1097–1102.

102. Raine CS, Wu E, Ivanyi J, Katz D, Brosnan CF. Multiple sclerosis: A protective or a pathogenic role for heat shock protein 60 in the central nervous system? Lab Invest 1996; 75: 109–123.

103. Rieckmann P, Albrecht M, Kitze B, Weber T, Tumani H, Broocks A, et al. Cytokine mRNA levels in mononuclear blood cells from patients with multiple sclerosis. Neurology 1994; 44:1523–1526.

104. Selmaj KW, Raines CS. Tumour necrosis factor mediates myelin and oligodendrocyte damage in vitro. Ann Neurol 1988; 23:339–346.

105. Selmaj K, Raine CS, Farooq M, Norton WT, Brosnan CF. Cytokine cytotoxicity against oligodendrocytes: Apoptosis induced by lymphotoxin. J Immunol 1991; 147:1522–1529.

106. Wucherpfennig KW, Strominger JL. Molecular mimicry in T cell–mediated autoimmunity: Viral peptides activate human T cell clones specific for myelin basic protein. Cell 1995; 80: 695–705.

107. Yu M, Johnson JM, Tuohy VK. A predictable sequential determinant spreading cascade invariably accompanies progression of experimental autoimmune encephalomyelitis: A basis for peptide-specific therapy after onset of clinical disease. J Exp Med 1996; 183:1777–1788.

108. Maeda Y, Solanky M, Mennona J, Dowling P. Platelet derived growth factor receptor–positive oligodendroglia are frequent in multiple sclerosis lesions. Neurology 2000; 54:124.

109. Cho ES, Sharer LR, Prineas JW. Deposition of activated complement on myelin engaged by macrophages in evolving MS lesions. J Neuropathol Exp Neurol 2000; 59:431.

110. Schluesener HJ, Sobel RA, Linington C, Weiner HL. A monoclonal antibody against a myelin oligodendrocyte glycoprotein induces relapses and demyelination in central nervous system autoimmune disease. J Immunol 1987; 139:4016–4021.

111. Ludwin SK. Chronic demyelination inhibits remyelination in the central nervous system: An analysis of contributing factors. Lab Invest 1980; 43:382–387.

112. Lucchinetti C, Brück W, Parisi J, Scheithauer B, Rodriguez M, Lassmann H. Heterogeneity of multiple sclerosis lesions: Implications for the pathogenesis of demyelination. Ann Neurol 2000; 47:707–717.

113. Ulvestad E, Williams K, Vedeler C, Antel J, Nyland H, Mörk S, Matre R. Reactive microglia in multiple sclerosis lesions have an increased expression of receptors for the Fc part of IgG. J Neurol Sci 1994; 121:125–131.

114. Storch MK, Stefferl A, Brehm U, Weissert R, Wallström E, Kerschensteiner M, Olsson T, Linington C, Lassmann H. Autoimmunity to myelin oligodendrocyte glycoprotein in rats mimics the spectrum of multiple sclerosis pathology. Brain Pathol 1998; 8:681–694.

115. Bernard CCA, Johns TG, Slavin A, Ichikawa M, Ewing C, Liu J, Bettadapura J. Myelin oligodendrocyte glycoprotein: A novel candidate autoantigen in multiple sclerosis. J Mol Med 1997; 75:77–88.

116. Linington C, Lassmann H. Antibody responses in chronic relapsing experimental allergic encephalomyelitis: Correlation of serum demyelinating activity with antibody titre to MOG. J Neuroimmunol 1987; 17:61–69.

117. D'Souza SD, Bonetti B, Balasingam V, Cashman NR, Barker PA, Troutt AB, Raine CS, Antel JP. Multiple sclerosis: Fas signalling in oligodendrocyte cell death. J Exp Med 1996; 184:2361–2370.

118. Raine CS. The Dale E McFarlin Memorial Lecture: The immunology of the multiple sclerosis lesion. Ann Neurol 1994; 36:561–572.

119. Antel JP, Williams K, Blain M, McRea E, McLaurin J. Oligodendrocyte lysis by CD4$^+$ T cells independent of tumour necrosis factor. Ann Neurol 1994; 341–348.

120. van der Maesen K, Hinojoza JR, Sobel BS. Endothelial cell class II major histocompatability complex molecule expression in stereotactic brain biopsies of patients with acute inflammatory/demyelinating conditions. J Neuropathol Exp Neurol 1999; 58(4):346–358.

121. Sobel RA, Blanchette BW, Bhan AK, Colvin RB. The immunopathology of acute experimental allergic encephalomyelitis: II. Endothelial cell Ia expression increases prior to inflammatory cell infiltration. J Immunol 1984; 132:2402–2406.

122. Dowling P, Shang G, Raval S, Menonna J, Cook S, Husar W. Involvement of CD95 the (APO-1/Fas) receptor/ligand system in multiple sclerosis brain. J Exp Med 1996; 184:1513–1518.

123. Vartanian T, Li Y, Zhao M, Stefansson K. Interferon-γ–induced oligodendrocyte cell death: implications for the pathogenesis of multiple sclerosis. Mol Med 1995; 1(7):732–743.

124. Traugott U, Lebon J. Interferon-γ and Ia antigen are present on astrocytes in active chronic multiple sclerosis lesions. Neurol Sci 1988; 84:257–264.

125. Cammer W, Bloom BR, Norton WT, Gordon S. Degradation of basic protein in myelin by neutral proteases secreted by stimulated macrophages: A possible mechanism of inflammatory demyelination. Proc Natl Acad Sci USA 1978; 75:1554–1558.

126. Hartung H-P, Rieckmann P. Pathogenesis of immune-mediated demyelination in the CNS. In: Riederer P et al, eds. Springer Medicine, vol 5. Wien, New York: Springer, 1997, pp 173–181.

127. Link J, Söderström M, Olsson T, Bo H, Ljungdahl A, Link H. Increased transforming growth factor-β, interleukin-4, and interferon-τ in multiple sclerosis. Ann Neurol 1994; 36:379–386.

128. Hickey WF, Kimura H. Perivascular microglia cells of the CNS are bone marrow derived and present antigen in vivo. Science 1988; 239:290–292.

129. Olsson T. Role of cytokines in multiple sclerosis and experimental autoimmune encephalomyelitis. Eur J Neurol 1994; 1:7–9.

130. Wekerle H, Linington C, Lassmann H, Meyermann R. Cellular immune reactivity within the CNS. Trends Neurosci 1986; 9:271–277.

131. Westland KW, Pollard JD, Sander S, Bonner JG, Linington C, McLeod JG. Activated non-neural specific T cells open the blood-brain barrier to circulating antibodies. Brain 1999; 122:1283–1291.

132. Karni A, Bakimer-Kleiner R, Abramsky O, Ben-Nuan A. Elevated levels of antibody to myelin oligodendrocyte glycoprotein is not specific for patients with multiple sclerosis. Arch Neurol 1999; 56(3)311–315.

133. Wucherpfennig KW, Catz I, Hausmann S, et al. Recognition of the immunodominant myelin basic protein peptide by autoantibodies and HLA-DR2–restricted T cell clones from multiple sclerosis patients: Identity of key contact residues by the B-cell and T-cell epitopes. J Clin Invest 1997; 100:1114–1122.

134. Lucchinetti C, Brück W, Parisi J, Scheithauer B, Rodriguez M, Lassmann H. A quantitative analysis of oligodendrocytes in multiple sclerosis lesions: A study of 113 cases. Brain 1999; 122:2279–2295.

135. Wolswijk G. Oligodendrocyte survival, loss and birth in lesions of chronic-stage multiple sclerosis. Brain 2000; 123:105–115.

136. LaGanke CC, Freeman DW, Whitaker JN. Cross-reactive idiotypy in cerebrospinal fluid immunoglobulins in multiple sclerosis. Ann Neurol 2000; 47:87–92.

137. Merrill JE, Benveniste EN. Cytokines in inflammatory brain lesions: Helpful and harmful. Trends Neurosci 1996; 19:331–338.

138. Benveniste EN. In Aggarawal B, Puri R eds. Human Cytokines: Their Role in Research and Therapy. Oxford, UK: Blackwell, 1995, pp 195–216.

139. Evangelou N, Konz D, Palace J, Esiri MM, Mathews PM. Relating regional axonal loss in the normal appearing white matter to distant lesions: A pathological study in multiple sclerosis. Mult Scler 1999; 5(suppl 2):S2.

140. Jensen MA, Dayal AS, Arnason BGW. Immune deviation from a TH1 toward a TH2-type T-cell response occurs during recovery from monophasic experimental autoimmune encephalomyelitis. Ann Neurol 1996; 40:552.

141. Zeine R, Freedman MS, Pon R, Nguyen V. Mechanism of gamma-delta T-cell cytotoxicity in multiple sclerosis. Ann Neurol 1996; 40:555.

142. Fu I, et al. Imaging axonal damage of normal-appearing white matter in multiple sclerosis. Brain 1998; 121:103–113.

143. McDonnell GV, Graham CA, McMillan SA, Middleton D, Hawkins SA. Primary progressive multiple sclerosis (PPMS) as a discrete disease. Mult Scler 1998; 4:356.

144. Ozenci MV, Kouwenhoven MCM, Huang YM, Kivisakk P, Link H. The proinflammatory cytokines TNF-α and IL-6 in MS. Mult Scler 1998; 4:345.

145. Nicholas RS, Compston DAS, Wing MG. Microglia support the survival of ''stressed'' oligodendrocytes. Mult Scler 1998; 4:346.

146. Tortorella C, Rocca MA, Codella M, Gasperini C, Capra R, Pozzilli C, Filippi M. Disease activity in multiple sclerosis studied with weekly triple dose magnetic resonance imaging. Mult Scler 1998; 4:303.

147. Weissert R, Wallström E, Storch MK, Stefferl A, Lorentzen J, Lassmann H, Linington C, Olsson T. MHC haplotype-dependent regulation of the clinical profile and lesional pathology of myelin-oligodendrocyte-glycoprotein-induced experimental autoimmune encephalomyelitis in rats. Mult Scler 1998; 4:277.

148. Perry VH. Axonal damage in a model of an MS lesion. Mult Scler 1998; 4:278.

149. Jellinger K, Boltzman L. Neuropathology of ''MS'' encephalopathy. Mult Scler 1998; 4:287.

150. Evangelou N, Esiri M, Palace J, Mathews PM. A quantitative pathological study of axonal loss in the corpus callosum in multiple sclerosis. Mult Scler 1998; 4:287.

151. Tan IL, Barkhof F, Hoogenraad FGC, Hofman MBM, Reichenbach JR, Manoliu RA. MR venography in multiple sclerosis. Mult Scler 1998; 4:302.

152. van Waesberghe JHTM, Kamphorst W, De Groot CJA, van Walderveen MAA, Castelijns JA, Ravid R, et al. Axonal loss in multiple sclerosis lesions: Magnetic resonance imaging insights into substrates of disability. Ann Neurol 1999; 46:747–754.

153. Bashir K, Layton B, Whatley W, Whitaker JN. Clinical and laboratory features of primary progressive and secondary progressive multiple sclerosis. Ann Neurol 1998; 44:466.

154. Chen C-J, Chu N-S, Lu C-S, Sung C-Y. Serial magnetic resonance imaging in patients with Balòs concentric sclerosis: natural history of lesion development. Ann Neurol 1999; 46:651–656.

155. Kesselring J, Miller DH, Robb SA, Kendall BE, Moseley IF, Kingsley D, du Boulay EP, McDonald WI. Acute disseminated encephalomyelitis: MRI findings and the distinction from multiple sclerosis. Brain 1990; 113:291–302.

156. Eblen F, Poremba M, Grodd W, Optiz H, Roggendorf W, Dichgans J. Myelinclastic diffuse sclerosis (Schilders disease): Cliniconeuroradiologic correlations. Neurology 1991; 41:589–591.

157. Wekerle H, Kojima K, Lannes-Vieira J, Lassmann H, Linington C. Animal models. Ann Neurol 1994; 36:547–553.

158. Best PV. Acute polyradiculoneuritis associated with demyelinated plaques in the central nervous system: Report of a case. Acta Neuropathol (Berl) 1985; 67:230–234.

159. Söderström M, Hillert J, Link J, Navikas H, Frederiksen S, Link H. Expression of IFN-γ, IL-4 and TGF-α in multiple sclerosis in relation to HLA-Dw2 phenotype an stage of disease. Mult Scler 1995; 1:173–180.

160. Waxman SG. Editorial: Peripheral nerve abnormalities in multiple sclerosis. Muscle Nerve 1993; 16:1–5.

161. De Stefano N, Matthews PM, Fu L, Narayanan S, Stanley J, Francis GS, Antel JP, et al. Axonal damage correlates with disability in patients with relapsing-remitting multiple sclerosis. Results of a longitudinal magnetic resonance spectroscopy study. Brain 1998; 121:1469–1477.

162. Lassmann H. Mechanisms of demyelination in multiple sclerosis. Mult Scler 1999; 5:51.

163. Youl BD, Kermode AG, Thompson AJ, et al. Destructive lesions in demyelinating disease. J Neurol Neurosurg Psychiatry 1991; 54:288–292.

164. Harpey JP, Renault F, Foncin JF, Gardeur D, Horn YE, Roy C. Démyélinisation aiguë pseudotumorale à poussées régressives. Arch Fr Pédiatr 1983; 40:407–409.

165. Dowling P, Husar W, Menonna J, Donnenfeld H, Cook S, Sidhu M. Cell death and birth in multiple sclerosis brain. J Neurol Sci 1997; 149:1–11.

166. Karussis D, Leker RR, Ashkenazi A, Abramsky O. A subgroup of multiple sclerosis patients with anticardiolipin antibodies and unusual clinical manifestations: Do they represent a new nosological entity? Ann Neurol 1998; 44:629–634.

167. Mews I, Bergmann M, Bunkowski S, Gullotta F, Brück W. Oligodendrocyte and axon pathology in clinically silent multiple sclerosis lesions. Mult Scler 1998; 4:55–62.

168. Dal Canto MC, Wiśniewski HM, Johnson AB, Brostoff SW, Raine CS. Vesicular disruption of myelin in autoimmune demyelination. J Neurol Sci 1975; 24:313–319.

169. Ghatak NR. Occurrence of oligodendrocytes within astrocytes: A form of emperipolesis. J Neuropathol Exp Neurol 1990; 49:285.

170. Dahl D, Perides G, Bignami A. Axonal regeneration in old multiple sclerosis plaques: Immunohistochemical study with monoclonal antibodies to phosphorylated and non-phosphorylated neurofilament proteins. Acta Neuropathol 1989; 79:154–159.

171. Aarli JA, Aparicio SR, Lumsden CE, Tönder O. Binding of normal human IgG to myelin sheaths, glia and neurons. Immunology 1975; 28:171–186.

172. Wolswijk G. Chronic stage multiple sclerosis lesions contain a relatively quiescent population of oligodendrocyte precursor cells. J Neurosci 1998; 18:601–609.

173. Wolswijk G. Oligodendrocyte regeneration in the adult rodent CNS and the failure of this process in multiple sclerosis (review). Prog Brain Res 1998; 117:233–247.

174. Compston A. Remyelination in multiple sclerosis: A challenge for therapy. The 1996 European Charcot Foundation Lecture. Mult Scler 1997; 3:51–70.

175. Franklin RJM, Blakemore WF. To what extent is oligodendrocyte progenitor migration a limiting factor in the remyelination of multiple sclerosis lesions? Mult Scler 1997; 3:84–87.

176. Gilson J, Blakemore WF. Failure of remyelination in areas of demyelination in the spinal cords of old rats. Neuropathol Appl Neurobiol 1993; 19:173–181.

177. Greer JM, Csurhes PA, Cameron KD, McCombe PA, Good MF, Pender MP. Increased immunoreactivity to two overlapping peptides of myelin proteolipid protein in multiple sclerosis. Brain 1997; 120:1447–1460.

178. Franklin RJM, Bayley SA, Blakemore WF. Transplanted CG4 cells (an oligodendrocyte progenitor cell line) survive, migrate and contribute to repair of areas of demyelination in x-irradiated and damaged spinal cord, but not in normal spinal cord. Exp Neurol 1996; 137: 263–276.

179. Scolding NJ, Rayner PJ, Susman J, Shaw C, Compston DAS. A proliferative adult human oligodendrocyte progenitor. Neuroreport 1995; 6:441–445.

180. Ishikawa M, Tsukamoto T, Yamamoto T. Long-term cultured astrocytes inhibit myelin formation, but not axonal growth in the co-cultured nerve tissue. Mult Scler 1996; 2:91–95.

181. Rosenbluth J. Glial transplantation in the treatment of myelin loss or deficiency. In: Bostock H, Kirkwood PA, Pullen AH eds. The Neurobiology of Disease: Contributions from Neuroscience to Clinical Neurology. Cambridge, UK: Cambridge University Press, 1996, pp. 124–148.

182. Rodriguez M, Miller DJ, Lennon VA. Immunoglobulins reactive with myelin basic protein promote CNS remyelination. Neurology 1996; 46:538–545.

183. Carroll WM, Jennings AR. In vivo CNS remyelination: HNK-1 labels newly differentiated oligodendrocytes but not precursors. J Neurocytol 1993; 22:583–589.

184. Carroll WM, Jennings AR, Mastaglia FL. The origin of remyelinating oligodendrocytes in antiserum-mediated demyelinative optic neuropathy. Brain 1990; 113:953–957.

185. Franklin RJM, Blakemore WF. Transplanting oligodendrocyte progenitors into the adult CNS. J Anat 1997; 190:23–33.

186. Vanguri P, Koski CL, Silverman B, Shin ML. Complement activation by isolated myelin: Activation of classical pathway in the absence of myelin specific antibodies. Proc Natl Acad Sci USA 1982; 79:3290–3294.

187. Moore GRW, Berry K, Oger JJF, Nugent RA, Graeb DA, Mackay AL. Balo's concentric sclerosis with bands of normal myelin in a patient with an eight year history of multiple sclerosis. J Neuropathol Exp Neurol 1996; 55:657.

188. Kira J, Kanai T, Nishimura Y, Yamasaki K, Matsushita S, Kawano Y, Hasuo K, Tobimatsu S, Kobayashi T. Western versus Asian types of multiple sclerosis: Immunogenetically and clinically distinct disorders. Ann Neurol 1996; 40:569–574.

189. Cammer W, Brosnan CF, Basile C, Bloom BR, Norton WT. Complement potentiates the degradation of myelin proteins by plasmin: Implications for a mechanism of inflammatory demyelination. Brain Res 1986; 364:91–101.

190. Tabi Z, McCombe PA, Pender MP, Cyong JC, Witkins S, Rieger B, Barbarese E, Good RA, Day NK. Antibody-independent complement activation by myelin via classical pathway. J Exp Med 1982; 155:587–598.

191. Tabi Z, McCombe PA, Pender MP. Apoptotic elimination of $V\beta 8.2^+$ cells from the central nervous system during recovery from experimental autoimmune encephalomyelitis induced by passive transfer of $V\beta 8.2^+$ encephalitogenic T cells. Eur J Immunol 1994; 24:2609–2617.

13

Axonal Injury in Multiple Sclerosis

CARL BJARTMAR and BRUCE D. TRAPP

Lerner Research Institute, Cleveland Clinic Foundation, Cleveland, Ohio

I. INTRODUCTION

The histopathological hallmarks of MS are focal inflammation, demyelination, loss of oligodendrocytes, reactive astrogliosis, and axonal pathology. Of these characteristics, myelin loss has attracted most interest, and MS research has traditionally focused on mechanisms associated with inflammatory demyelination and remyelination. Although MS is regarded as a primarily demyelinating disease, a number of reports describe axonal injury in MS (1–9). The view that axons degenerate in MS is not new. In fact, axonal pathology in MS lesions has been addressed in the literature for more than a century (10). Charcot (1868), for example, described MS lesions in terms of demyelination and astrogliosis, but he also indicated axonal loss (11). Increased knowledge about interactions between myelin-forming cells and myelinated axons as well as insights regarding the functional consequences of axonal loss in demyelinating diseases, have drawn new attention to the issue.

Current data on axonal pathology in MS has been provided through a variety of methodological approaches. Studies using both magnetic resonance imaging (MRI) and magnetic resonance spectroscopy (MRS) (2,3,5,12–17) as well as combined MRI and morphological studies (1,8,18) have suggested axonal loss during the course of MS. Recent immunohistochemical studies have emphasized the correlation between inflammation and axonal damage early in the disease course (4,7). In addition, axonal pathology has been described in animal models of inflammatory demyelinating central nervous system (CNS) disease (19–21), and a number of myelin protein gene knockout and transgene models indicate that lack of myelin-related molecules can result in axonal pathology. Together, these data suggest that cumulative axonal degeneration constitutes a significant component

325

of the pathogenesis in MS and indicate that loss of axons may be a main determinant of the progressive neurological disability seen in these patients (7,9,22–24).

There has been a significant progress in MS research in recent years, which has increased our understanding of the disease. Insights regarding the role of axon pathology in MS is one such example. This implies new challenges for those working on MS but also novel therapeutic possibilities for MS patients. This chapter reviews current data on axonal pathology associated with MS. Mechanisms of axonal degeneration in MS as well as functional consequences and clinical implications are discussed.

II. AXONAL PATHOLOGY IN MS LESIONS

According to the prevailing concept on the pathogenesis of acute MS, neurological disability during relapsing-remitting MS (RR-MS) is caused by focal inflammation and demyelination, which causes conduction block. Three mechanisms are considered to contribute to clinical remission: resolution of the inflammation, redistribution of axolemmal sodium channels, and remyelination (9,25) (Fig. 1). Although demyelination itself may cause neurological deficits during RR-MS, it does not convincingly explain the irreversible functional impairment seen during secondary progressive (SP-MS) stages of the disease. For example, demyelinated axons can conduct impulses relatively well after initial compensatory remodeling of axolemmal ion channels (26–28). However, a number of early as well as more recent reports describe substantial axonal injury in MS lesions, which may provide the pathological substrate for irreversible disability in SP-MS patients.

A. Early Reports

Although it is a somewhat controversial subject, axonal pathology was mentioned in the early literature on MS. These reports include descriptions of axonal swellings, axonal

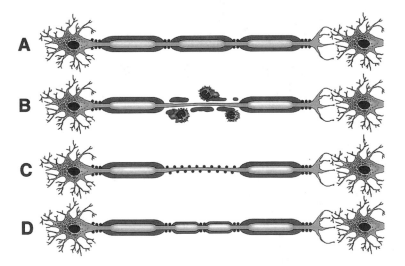

Figure 1   Pathogenesis of neurological disability during RR-MS. Normal myelinated axon (A). Inflammatory demyelination causes conduction block (B). Resolution of the inflammation, redistribution of axolemmal Na$^+$ channels (*dots*) (C), and remyelination (D) restores conduction and contributes to remission.

transection, and Wallerian degeneration as well as discussions regarding the functional consequences of such pathology (10). In their classic works, both Charcot and Marburg described MS pathology in terms of demyelination and reactive gliosis. However, they also emphasized the relative sparing of axons in the lesions (11,29). In 1936, Putnam reported a 50% loss of axons in MS lesions from 11 patients (30). In contrast, Greenfield and King reported normal axon densities in more than 90% of MS lesions from 13 patients the same year (31). The differences between these works were suggested to result from more sensitive axon staining in the latter. Subsequently, the axonal component of MS pathogenesis received less attention, and the question regarding axonal damage in MS remained unclear for a long time.

B. Current Evidence

Axonal Transection During Early Stages of MS

Amyloid precursor protein (APP), which is present in neurons at levels not normally detected by immunohistochemistry, is transported by fast axonal transport (32). Immunohistochemical detection of axonal APP indicates functional impairment of the labeled axons. Ferguson *et al.* described APP accumulation in axons located in active MS lesions and at the border of chronic active MS lesions (4). Some APP immunoreactive structures exhibited the morphology of terminal axonal swellings, suggesting axonal transection. The number of APP-labeled axonal swellings correlated with the degree of inflammation in the lesions (4). Using confocal microscopy and computer-based three-dimensional reconstruction, extensive axonal transection was demonstrated in cerebral MS lesions from 11 patients with disease duration ranging from 2 weeks to 27 years (7) (Fig. 2). Axonal ovoids were identified as terminal ends of transected axons in the confocal microscope, and the degree of inflammation in the lesions was characterized by the presence of activated macrophages and microglia. Active lesions contained over 11,000 terminal ends per cubic millimeter, the edge of chronic active lesions contained over 3000 terminal ends per cubic millimeter and the core of chronic active lesions contained on average 875 terminal ends per cubic millimeter. In contrast, less than 1 transected axon was found per cubic millimeter in control white matter. Together, these data demonstrate a positive correlation between axonal transection and degree of inflammation in cerebral MS lesions undergoing demyelination. The presence of terminal ends in patients with short disease duration suggests that axonal transection begins at an early stage of MS (7).

Axonal Loss in Spinal Cord MS Lesions

Terminal axonal ovoids appear transiently after transection, and are therefore considered to represent relatively recent axonal injury. The significant presence (875/cubic millimeter) of ovoids in the hypocellular center of chronic active brain lesions, indicate that a proportion of axonal degeneration in MS results from transection of chronically demyelinated axons (see below). This hypothesis is supported by the fact that functional impairment proceeds in some patients with SP-MS that do not display clinical, laboratory or MRI evidence for inflammatory attacks, and who respond marginally to anti-inflammatory or immunosupressive drugs. The continuous progressive, irreversible, neurological decline in many of these SP-MS patients raises quantitative questions regarding the role of axonal loss in chronic MS. Quantification of axon loss in sections from brain MS lesions is a difficult sampling problem as atrophy, edema and density of axons can change and influence total number. In addition, finding age- and area-matched control samples is often complicated.

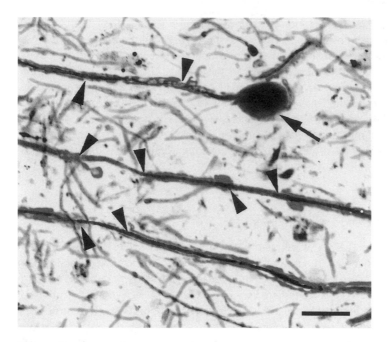

Figure 2 Axonal transection in MS lesion. Free floating sections were stained with neurofilament (*black*) and myelin (*gray*) antibodies. Three large, neurofilament-positive axons are undergoing demyelination (*arrowheads*) at the edge of an active lesion. One axon ends in a large terminal ovoid (*arrow*). Three-dimensional analysis using confocal microscopy established that most ovoids were terminal ends of axons, indicating axonal transection during demyelination. Scale bar = 45 μm. (From Ref. 7.)

Using an axonal sampling protocol that accounts for both atrophy and axonal loss, total axon numbers in chronic spinal cord MS lesions were determined; 6 lesions from 3 patients with SP-MS and 2 lesions from a patient with PP-MS. These patients were all severely disabled expanded disability status scale (EDSS > 7.5) and represented disease duration ranging from 12 to 46 years. The analyzed spinal cord lesions exhibited a 45 to 81% (mean 65%) loss of axons compared to similar areas in controls (33) (Fig. 3). To varying extent, lost axons appeared to be replaced by astrogliosis, as revealed by double labeling for the astrocyte-specific intermediate filament glial fibrillary acidic protein (GFAP). In the spinal cord of an ambulatory RR-MS patient with 8 months disease duration analyzed for comparison, a 20% axonal loss was detected in an area containing descending tracts distal to a brain stem lesion. Three other spinal cord areas in the RR-MS patient had normal axon numbers. The extensive loss of axons observed in lesions from these chronic MS patients provides additional evidence that axonal degeneration constitutes an important component of the pathogenesis in the disease. The severe functional impairment of the patients support the hypothesis that axonal degeneration may be a major determinant of the irreversible neurological disability seen during progressive stages of MS (see below).

Neuronal Pathology in Cortical MS Lesions

In addition to the more commonly described white matter locations, MS lesions can also involve gray matter (34–36). However, the histopathological features as well as the clinical

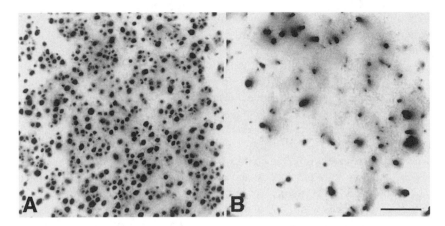

Figure 3 Axonal loss in the spinal cord of a paralyzed SP-MS patient. Neurofilament staining demonstrates axonal density in control (A) and in a demyelinated area in the gracile fasciculus of MS cervical spinal cord (B). This chronic MS lesion exhibits severe axonal loss. Scale bar = 25 µm. (From Ref. 24.)

significance of such lesions are not completely understood. MS lesions in the cerebral cortex are less obvious than white matter lesions on conventional T2-weighted images (36). Gray matter lesions are also difficult to detect macroscopically and histologically. Histologically, the frequency of cortical lesions has often been underestimated. Recently, Kidd *et al.* demonstrated that the use of gadolinium-enhancement resulted in an increased detection of cortical lesions on MRI scans by 140%. Twenty six percent of these enhancing lesions arose within or adjacent to the cerebral cortex (36). This study also suggested that conventional MRI underreports the presence of cortical lesions compared to neuropathological analysis.

In a recent portmortem study on MS brains using immunohistochemistry and confocal microscopy, the characteristics of gray matter lesions were described (37). In addition to inflammatory differences between gray and white matter lesions, injury to neurons was observed within the cortical lesions. Gray matter lesions contained fewer inflammatory cells, no perivascular cuffs, consisted mainly of reactive microglia, in contrast to white matter lesions that contained numerous lymphocytes, macrophages and perivascular cells. The cortical lesions also contained neuritic swellings, as well as dendritic and axonal transection. It has been hypothesized that injury to neurons in cortical or subcortical lesion may provide the biological correlate to the cognitive dysfunction many MS patients experience (36,38). In fact, executive and cognitive functional deficits arise in 40 to 70% of these patients (39–42). Increased knowledge regarding mechanisms of neuronal damage in cortical MS lesions will contribute to the understanding of the functional significance of such lesions.

III. AXONAL DEGENERATION AND TISSUE ATROPHY

A number of reports indicate that disease progression in MS is reflected by volume loss of central nervous system (CNS) tissue (3,14,15,23). This is important, as atrophy might be a useful surrogate marker for monitoring disease progression and the efficiency of MS therapeutics. The most commonly used surrogate marker for disease progression is total brain lesion volume as measured on T2 weighted MRI scans. This measurement has relatively low pathological specificity and its correlation to clinical performance is poor (23,43). In addition, measures of clinical disability such as EDSS are not sensitive to underlying pathological processes during RR-MS (44,45). Recent MRI studies, however, have demonstrated a correlation between clinical disability and atrophy of cerebellum (3), spinal cord (14) and cerebral tissue (15). Reliable methods of measuring the rate of tissue atrophy in MS from early stages of the disease could therefore be useful for the monitoring of MS patients.

The spinal cord, frequently affected in MS patients (46), is considered a suitable model to study the relation between atrophy and clinical progression due to the impact of motor disability on EDSS (23). Spinal cord atrophy as determined by MRI, but not total brain lesion load, correlates with clinical disability in MS (14,47,48). In spinal cords from chronic MS patients with severe disability (EDSS > 7.5) and significant axonal loss in spinal cord lesions (see above), average cervical spinal cord cross section area was reduced by 25% (33). The amount of cervical cord atrophy in a comparable patient subgroup investigated by MRI was 28% (14). Considering the correlation between atrophy and disability as well as the substantial loss of axons in chronic spinal cord lesions, these data suggest that axonal loss contribute to spinal cord atrophy in MS.

In the brain, the periventricular white matter is frequently affected by MS lesions, which might contribute to the progressive enlargement of the lateral ventricles often observed in MS patients (9,34,49) (Fig. 4). In a serial MRI study, progressive cerebral atrophy as determined by the volume calculated from four central brain slices was significantly more pronounced in patients with worsening disability indicating axonal damage or degeneration (15). Interestingly, progressive brain atrophy as seen by MRI has also been reported in RR-MS patients with short disease duration. During the 2 years of observation, brain atrophy in RR-MS patients with mild to moderate disability increased yearly, in many cases without clinical manifestations (45,49). As indicated by the presence of gadolinium-enhanced lesions in these brains, the course of atrophy seems to be influenced by general

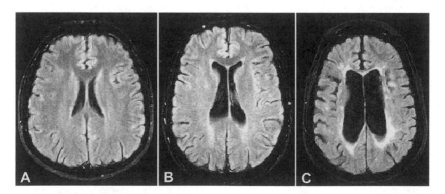

Figure 4 Progressive brain atrophy during the course of MS. Magnetic resonance images from a control subject without disease (male, age 31) (A); a patient with relapsing-remitting MS (female, age 36) with disease duration of 2 years (B); and a secondary-progressive MS patient (female, age 43) with disease duration of 19 years (C). As shown in B and C, brain tissue volume decreases and ventricular volume increases with disease severity. Demyelination and axonal loss contributes to tissue loss. (From Ref. 9.)

inflammatory disease activity. On the same population of relapsing patients, a new sensitive measure of whole-brain atrophy was applied (45). The brain parenchymal fraction (BPF), defined as the ratio of brain parenchyma to the total volume within the brain surface contour, was highly reproducible, thus allowing precise comparison of individual brain volumes from year to year. The BPF declined at a highly significant rate during each of 2 years of follow-up in these patients and was significantly reduced compared with age- and sex-matched control individuals.

Although demyelination and reduced axon diameter may decrease CNS tissue volume, axonal loss from the onset of disease is a plausible contributor to atrophy in MS for the reasons discussed above (9,23,45,49). However, the lack of correlation between axonal loss and atrophy in some spinal cord lesions of chronic MS patients (33), and the prominent upregulation of GFAP observed in many chronic MS lesions suggest that other factors such as the extent and nature of compensatory astrogliosis can influence tissue volume in MS. Astrogliosis may also, in theory, lead to tissue contraction. It is therefore likely that atrophy in MS is the net result of several contributing factors, of which axonal loss is one.

IV. NAA AS A MARKER FOR AXONAL LOSS IN MS

Considering the role of axonal injury in the pathogenesis of MS, noninvasive axonal monitoring could become usable for the study of disease progression in MS patients as well as for evaluation of ongoing therapy. MRI generally lacks pathological specificity as many factors influence image contrast (50,51). However, measurements of the neuron specific marker N-acetyl aspartic acid (NAA) might allow monitoring of axonal loss in MS. NAA is the second most abundant amino acid in the adult CNS after glutamate, and is localized primarily in neurons and neuronal processes (52–54). NAA can be measured by magnetic resonance spectroscopy (MRS), a noninvasive technique (51). Decreased levels of NAA, as measured by MRS, have been demonstrated in a number of neurodegenerative disorders including MS (51,55,56). Hence, measurements of NAA levels by MRS might be useful for non invasive axonal monitoring in vivo.

A. Magnetic Resonance Spectroscopy Studies

Axonal damage in MS is supported by in vivo MRS data describing decreased levels of NAA in MS brains (2,5,12,13,16,17,51,57). In acute stages of the disease, reduced NAA is partly reversible, restricted to lesion area, and correlates with reversible functional impairment (2,12,16,57). In chronic stages of MS, reduced NAA is also detected in normal-appearing white matter, suggesting axonal damage or Wallerian degeneration outside MS lesions (5,17,51). In addition, NAA levels correlate with disability over time (2,17,22) and with executive function in MS (42).

Decreased NAA in MS was initially interpreted as a result of irreversible axonal loss. However, the observation that NAA in acute MS lesions is, to some extent, reversible indicated that NAA levels also reflect reversible axonal dysfunction. The function of NAA is unknown, although participation in protein synthesis, osmotic regulation, and metabolism of neurotransmitters such as aspartate and N-acetyl-glutamate has been suggested (52,58–60). After synthesis in mitochondria from L-aspartate and acetyl-CoA, NAA is transported to the neuronal cytoplasm where it is present in high concentrations (61,62). It has recently been suggested that neuronal NAA is released into the extracellular space and subsequently taken up and degraded by astrocytes (63). Myelin or myelin forming cells can dynamically influence various axonal properties such as the distribution of axolemmal ion channels (64–66), phosphorylation or dephosphorylation of neurofilaments (67) and axon caliber (68,69). Analogously, it is possible that inflammatory demyelination and remyelination may dynamically influence the activity of axonal enzymes involved in NAA metabolism, thereby transiently affecting NAA levels. In addition, it is possible that NAA metabolism is related to neuronal activity in a tract. For example, acute deafferentation in the CNS causes trans synaptic decreases of NAA levels without ultrastructural abnormalities, indicating that impaired function reduces neuronal NAA (70). Reduced levels of NAA might therefore reflect a number of mechanisms, such as reversible neuronal/axonal damage due to inflammatory demyelination, altered neuronal/axonal metabolism, changes in neuronal activity, or axonal loss (2,51,57,70).

B. High-Performance Liquid Chromatography Measurements

In addition to MRS, NAA can also be measured by high-performance liquid chromatography (HPLC). In HPLC experiments performed on postmortem spinal cord tissue from disabled chronic MS patients, average NAA levels were reduced, supporting a correlation between reduced NAA levels and disability in MS (33). The reduced tissue concentrations of NAA (expressed as nanomoles per milligram of tissue) in these chronic MS cords, suggests that the decreased NAA levels are not exclusively due to spinal cord atrophy (see above). In order to address NAA levels in relation to white matter axons, lesions from MS spinal cords, MS nonlesion and control white matter areas were sampled and analyzed with HPLC and immunohistochemistry. In chronic lesions, average NAA levels were significantly reduced (60 to 65% decrease) compared to normal-appearing MS white matter areas and controls, and this reduction correlated with loss of total axonal volume. The decrease in axonal density by 50 to 80% in these lesions indicates that reduced axon volume reflects axonal loss (33). Therefore, measurements of NAA levels by proton MRS should be useful for noninvasive axonal monitoring of axonal loss in chronic MS in vivo (see below).

V. MECHANISMS OF AXONAL PATHOLOGY IN MS

The pathophysiology of axonal injury in MS is poorly understood. It is possible that several, principally different mechanisms of axonal degeneration occur at different stages of the disease. Elucidating the cellular and molecular mechanisms of axonal loss in MS will influence the development of future neuroprotective therapies.

The correlation between inflammatory activity and number of transected axons in cerebral MS lesions support the hypothesis that inflammatory demyelinating environments injure axons (4,7). At later stages of MS, axonal transection and Wallerian degeneration may occur as a direct consequence of the chronic demyelination (9,24). In addition, multiple lesions along a tract could result in accumulation of axonal loss distally due to Wallerian degeneration, especially in long white matter tracts of the spinal cord. It is also possible that individual axons with multiple hits of demyelination become more vulnerable to transection and degeneration, compared to axons with a single demyelinated segment. A direct immunologic attack on the axon has been discussed as a possible cause of nerve fiber degeneration in MS. A primary immune-mediated attack on axons has been reported in the acute motor axonal neuropathy (AMAN) form of Guillain-Barré syndrome (GBS), an autoimmune disease of the PNS (71,72). However, data supporting a similar pathogenesis in MS is currently lacking. Since most axons survive the acute demyelinating process, a generalized immunologic attack on axons seems unlikely. It is still possible, however, that immune-mediated mechanisms might target axonal subpopulations (9).

A. Axonal Injury and Inflammation

All current knowledge suggests that MS is a primary inflammatory demyelinating disease of the CNS. Moreover, several lines of evidence indicate that disease activity reflect CNS inflammation even when the disease is subclinical (73). For example, most RR-MS patients exhibit progressive brain atrophy and persistent inflammation, as identified by gadolinium-enhanced lesions on MRI scans, regardless of the presence of clinical symptoms, and will also exhibit progressive disease on subsequent MRI examinations (45,49,74). Since axon pathology and frequency of transected axons in cerebral MS lesions correlate with the degree of inflammation (4,7), early axonal transection might occur due to vulnerability of demyelinated axons to inflammation (Fig. 5). Indeed, the inflammatory microenvironment contains a variety of substances that potentially could injure axons, such as proteolytic enzymes, cytokines, oxidative products and free radicals produced by activated immune and glial cells (75). In addition, the inflammatory edema might cause ischemic or mechanical damage to axons due to increased extracellular pressure. The spinal cord might be particularly vulnerable in this aspect, as the space for tissue expansion is more limited in the cord compared to the brain. Increased endoneurial fluid pressure due to edema, supposedly interfering with axonal blood supply, has been suggested as an ischemic mechanism of axon degeneration in GBS (76). Most likely, inflammation causing irreversible tissue damage is a major factor behind accumulating axonal pathology at early stages of MS. Therefore, aggressive anti-inflammatory treatment during RR-MS might also have, in addition to effects on the inflammation, indirect effects in preventing axonal injury.

B. Axonal Degeneration and Chronic Demyelination

Although myelin-forming cells influence axonal morphology and long-term viability, little is known about the molecular mechanisms involved. However, valuable insights are

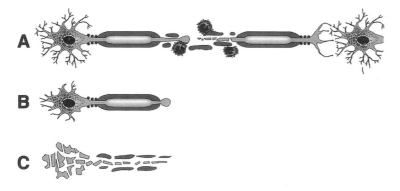

Figure 5   Axonal transection during inflammatory demyelination (A) causes irreversible loss of neuronal function and induces formation of terminal axonal ovoids. The distal axonal segment undergoes Wallerian degeneration (B), and retrograde neuronal degeneration (C) may occur. During relapsing-remitting MS, the CNS compensates for loss of axons.

emerging from studies on inherited human demyelinating diseases and relevant mutant animal models. A number of genes coding for myelin-related proteins—such as MAG, PLP, PMP22, P_0 and connexin 32, or for GM2/GD2 synthase, an enzyme involved in ganglioside biosynthesis—have been identified as essential for maintaining axonal structure, function and viability (77–82). Consequently, chronic demyelination may lead to axonal degeneration due to the lack of such support from myelin forming cells (Fig. 6). In this sense, remyelination can be considered a neuroprotective event for demyelinated axons.

Late-Onset Axonal Degeneration in Mice Lacking MAG and PLP

Myelin-associated glycoprotein (MAG), a member of the immunoglobulin gene superfamily with receptor- or ligand-like properties (83–85), is enriched in the adaxonal membrane of myelin internodes (79,86,87). MAG inhibits neurite outgrowth [88,89] and causes growth cone collapse in vitro (90), suggesting that it can modulate the axonal cytoskeleton. In MAG-deficient mice, myelination progresses as in wild type animals with normal amounts of myelin. However, from the age of 5 weeks, progressive axonal—atrophy including reduced axonal caliber, reduced neurofilament spacing, reduced neurofilament phosphorylation, and Wallerian degeneration—was observed. The findings indicate that MAG has direct or indirect long term modulating effects on the cytoskeleton via axonal kinases or phosphatases (79).

Recently, mice with disrupted gene for a key enzyme in the biosynthesis of complex gangliosides, GM2/GD2 synthase, were generated. These animals develop decreased central myelination, axonal degeneration in both CNS and PNS, and demyelination in peripheral nerves (82). The neurodegenerative features were similar to those observed in sciatic nerves of MAG-deficient mice described above (79). Interestingly, the ganglioside-deficient animals also have reduced MAG expression in the CNS. These studies raise the possibility that complex gangliosides are endogeneous binding partners for MAG, playing a role in maintenance of axons and myelin sheaths (82).

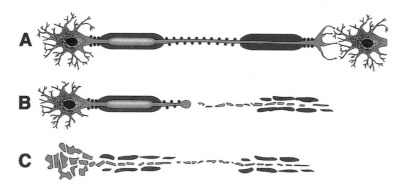

Figure 6 Degeneration of chronically demyelinated axon (A). Oligodendrocyte-derived factors have a trophic effect on axons. The lack of trophic support may cause axonal transection and Wallerian degeneration distally (B) or retrograde neuronal death (C). This mechanism of axonal loss may cause atrophy and progression of neurological disability during secondary-progressive MS when inflammatory activity is reduced.

Proteolipid protein (PLP), a major structural protein of compact CNS myelin, has been proposed to stabilize the intraperiod line of central myelin sheaths (91). Mutations, deletions, or duplications involving the PLP gene cause Pelizaeus Merzbacher disease (PMD) and spastic paraplegia of varying severity in humans (92–94). In the *jimpy* mouse, PLP mutations result in premature oligodendrocyte death and dysmyelination (95). Many of these phenotypes, however, are considered "gain of function" effects due to toxicity of misfolded proteins encoded by the mutated genes. In contrast, the PLP null-mutant mice form normal amounts of compact myelin with slightly altered periodicity. From the age of 6 weeks, PLP-deficient mice exhibit focal axonal swellings containing dense bodies and mitochondria in CNS regions containing mainly small diameter axons (80). The accumulation and distribution of organelles and neurofilaments in axonal swellings indicate impairment of retrograde axonal transport. After 12 months of age, slow progressive axonal degeneration in the absence of primary demyelination was observed. Subsequent motor impairment at 16 months of age suggests that a threshold of axonal loss manifests in neurological disability. Late onset axonal degeneration and progressive neurological disability is also seen in transgenic mice that moderately overexpress the PLP gene (96). Taken together, these studies indicate that long-term survival of CNS axons depends on correct expression of the PLP gene.

Late-onset axonal pathology in mice lacking MAG and PLP suggest that long-term survival of myelinated axons is dependent upon trophic support from myelin or myelin-forming cells after myelination has been completed and that MAG and PLP are essential for mediating these effects. Since MAG-deficient and PLP-deficient mice myelinate normally and do not contain dysmyelination or "gain of function" mutations, these animals are particularly informative and support, in principal, the hypothesis of axonal degeneration as a consequence of chronic demyelination (Fig. 6).

Axonal Pathology as a Result of Alterations in Myelin-related Genes

Additional knowledge regarding mechanisms underlying axonal pathology as a consequence of myelin pathology or loss has been provided from peripheral nerves of mice and humans with inherited alterations in genes coding for myelin-related molecules. Peripheral nerves may be useful in this respect, as they are relatively accessible technically, and also allow transplantation approaches that cannot be performed in CNS models. Studies on the inherited peripheral neuropathy Charcot-Marie-Tooth disease (CMT) have been particularly informative. The most common demyelinating form of CMT, CMT1A is usually caused by duplication of the peripheral myelin protein 22 (PMP22) gene (97). The other two demyelinating forms, CMT1B and CMTX, are caused by point mutations in the genes of protein P_0 and connexin 32 respectively (98,99). In patients with CMT1, progressive reduction in number of motor axons correlates with functional disability (100). Mutant mouse models of CMT1B and CMTX, show peripheral neuropathy with axonal involvement (77,78,101). Hence, in addition to the demyelination itself, axonal degeneration secondary to demyelination seem to contribute to the clinical manifestation of these neuropathies (97,102). Trembler (*Tr*) mice have a demyelinating peripheral neuropathy characterized by abnormally thin myelin, reduced axonal caliber, and cytoskeleton changes due to a PMP22 mutation (67,103). Wild-type axons regenerating through *Tr* mice grafts display *Tr* phenotype, indicating that *Tr* Schwann cells locally modulate axonal pathology (67,104). Normal mouse axons regenerating through xenografts from CMTX or CMT1A patients become ensheathed by CMTX or CMT1A Schwann cells and exhibit abnormal cytoskeletal organization, axonal degeneration and fiber loss locally (81,105). Together, these results indicate that myelin-forming glia influence axons at a local level, and that the axonal cytoskeleton might play a central role in the pathogenesis of axonal degeneration secondary to demyelination.

C. Animal Models of Axonal Injury During Inflammatory Demyelination

Axonal Loss and Neurological Disability in Experimental Allergic Encephalomyelitis (EAE)

Insights regarding pathophysiological mechanisms and functional consequences of axonal injury in inflammatory demyelinating disease has been obtained from animals with experimental allergic encephalomyelitis (EAE), the most common animal model of MS. EAE is produced by the injection of myelin antigens or by the transfer of antigen-specific T cells into susceptible animals (106–108). Axonal dystrophy and swellings indicating axonal transection has been described in mouse (19) and guinea pig (20) models of EAE. Mice of the SWR/SJL strain immunized with proteolipid protein peptides develop inflammatory demyelination of the spinal cord and consistent progression from relapsing disease to chronic disability (109). Immunohistochemical examination revealed axonal pathology and a progressive axonal loss in spinal cord white matter, which started relatively early in the disease course (110). At the initial exacerbation, there was a poor correlation between clinical disability and the extent of axonal loss. At a chronic stable endstage of the disease, however, mice exhibited irreversible functional impairment of varying severity, and a striking correlation between axonal loss in spinal cord and neurological disability. Mice that lacked clinical signs at the chronic EAE stage had relatively modest (20 to 30%) loss of white matter axons, while severely disabled animals showed extensive (50 to 60%) axonal loss. In the most disabled end-stage mice, some lesions appeared almost devoid of normal axonal profiles (110).

These data indicate that acute reversible disability in EAE results from mechanisms other than axonal transection. At chronic stages, on the other hand, axonal degeneration most likely constitutes a major cause of the neurological disability in these EAE mice. The development of new neuroprotective drugs for MS requires suitable animals models. This relapsing EAE model resembles many aspects of MS. First, similar to most cases of MS, the disease course is initially relapsing but subsequently progresses to chronic disability. Second, these mice respond to interferon beta treatment with milder symptoms and less frequent relapses (109). Third, the magnitude of axonal loss in the spinal cord of chronic paralyzed mice is comparable to that observed in spinal cord lesions of severely disabled chronic MS patients (33). This relapsing EAE model may be suitable for testing efficiency of novel neuroprotective drugs aimed for MS patients.

Genetic Background and Susceptibility to Axonal Injury

The disease course of MS is highly variable between patients. Both environmental factors and genetic predisposition contribute to susceptibility and clinical heterogeneity of the disease (111,112). Current evidence indicates that interactions between multiple genes influence the outcome of MS in individual patients (113). For example, genetically determined response of various tissue components to inflammation could influence the development of tissue damage in MS. Data suggesting a genetic component in the axonal response to inflammatory demyelination is provided from Theiler's murine encephalomyelitis virus

(TMEV) disease, a virus induced model of inflammatory CNS demyelination. Infected animals with susceptible genetic background develop neurological impairment and pathological changes comparable to those in MS (114,115). Infected SJL/J mice develop chronic demyelination, neurological deficits, and extensive loss of axons in the spinal cord (116). Mice lacking the major histocompatibility complex (MHC) class I, in a strain usually resistant to TMEV induced disease (C57BL/6 x 129 mice), develop a similar distribution and extent of demyelinated lesions as SJL/J mice after infection but no functional disability. Reduced neurological symptoms in these mice were attributed to increased axolemmal sodium channel densities and relative preservation of demyelinated axons (116). In contrast, C57BL/6 x 129 mice lacking MHC class II developed various neurological signs such as stiffness and paralysis and exhibited axonal pathology and axonal degeneration in spinal cord white matter 4 months after infection (21). The neurological symptoms in these class II–deficient mice were suggested to result from axonal injury. Together, these results highlight the possible role of genetic influence on the development of axonal degeneration and neurological symptoms during inflammatory demyelination. In addition, they indicate that MHC class I is involved in this process. Considering the genetic component in MS, the variation in individual susceptibility, and the differences in clinical course between patients (111–113), it is possible that genes involved in axonal responses to inflammatory demyelination influence the outcome of MS in individual patients.

VI. FUNCTIONAL CONSEQUENCES

What are the functional consequences, short and long term, of cumulative axonal degeneration during the course of MS? The evolving concept of an inflammatory neurodegenerative component to MS provides a hypothetical framework that explains disease progression and development of permanent neurological disability in affected patients (Fig. 7). As discussed above, inflammatory demyelination itself may cause episodes of disability during RR-MS. However, as it is well established that demyelinated axons, after axolemmal remodeling, can regain their ability to conduct impulses (26–28), it is unlikely that demye-

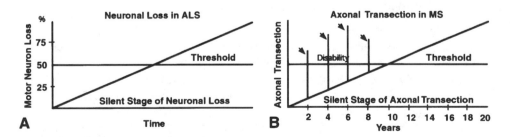

Figure 7 Neuronal loss is clinically silent during initial stages of neurodegenerative diseases. A. In amytrophic lateral sclerosis (ALS), patients may lose 50% of their lower motor neurons (*solid oblique line*) before neurological symptoms appear (disability threshold; *horizontal line*). B. In MS, axonal loss begins at disease onset but is clinically silent until reaching the disability threshold, where the CNS cannot compensate for the accumulative axonal loss. During this initial stage (relapsing-remitting MS), neurological deficits are associated with new inflammatory lesions or relapses (*arrows*). After reaching the disability threshold, functional impairment and axonal loss increase concomitantly (secondary-progressive MS). Relapses at onset of disease allow early identification and treatment of MS patients.

lination is the only cause of chronic disability in MS (9,24,51). The histopathology of MS, including the irreversible destructive process affecting white matter axons, therefore provides a pathological substrate for the progressive disability many chronic MS patients experience.

Although axonal loss begins at disease onset, it is subclinical during RR-MS, because the CNS has a remarkable ability to compensate for neuronal loss (4,7,9,73). An initial silent stage of neuronal cell loss is characteristic for all neurodegenerative diseases (Fig. 7A). For example, in amyotrophic lateral sclerosis (ALS) and in Parkinson's disease it has been estimated that 50 to 80% of target neurons respectively may be lost before these patients present with neurological symptoms (117,118). In RR-MS, lesions outnumber clinical relapses by as much as 10:1 (119). Moreover, correlations between clinical status and T2 lesion load on MRI scans are usually poor (74,120). However, the correlation between progressive disability and increasing brain atrophy in individual patients is strong, and likely reflects accumulating axonal loss (15). Mews *et al.* reported an average axonal loss of 64% in MS lesions from individuals without reported neurological symptoms (121). The lack of clinical signs was attributed to lesion site, neuronal redundancy, low levels of total axon loss, and remyelination. Also, clinical features during RR-MS are often poor predictors of subsequent disability progression (73). Hence, episodes of reversible functional disability during RR-MS might primarily be associated with acute inflammatory lesions in articulate parts of the CNS.

Most RR-MS patients develop chronic neurological disability (SP-MS) 8 to 15 years after the diagnosis. However, the time point when a patient reaches this progressive stage varies between individuals and most likely depends on a number of factors such as location of lesions, disease activity, medication and various aspects of genetic susceptibility. Approximately 10% of all patients diagnosed with MS develop benign MS, which is characterized by full functional ability in all neurological systems 15 years after onset of disease (122). We have proposed that the transition from RR-MS to SP-MS, and the subsequent development of progressive permanent disability, occurs when a threshold of neuronal or axonal loss is reached (9,25) (Fig. 7B).

VII. CLINICAL IMPLICATIONS

In addition to being a primary inflammatory demyelinating disease, MS can also be considered an inflammatory neurodegenerative disease. In contrast to most neurodegenerative diseases, however, MS patients can usually be identified at initial stages of the disease because of symptomatic episodes caused by inflammatory demyelination–relapses (Fig. 7). The axonal and neuronal destruction begins early in the disease course, and has important clinical implications regarding disease progression and treatment strategies.

During RR-MS, periods of deterioration respond relatively well to anti-inflammatory and immunomodulatory drugs. In contrast, SP-MS is characterized by decreasing response to anti-inflammatory treatment, and satisfactory therapies for progressive MS are currently lacking. The goal of treatment in all neurological diseases must be to prevent permanent functional disability. Cumulative irreversible axonal damage during RR-MS, as a cause of subsequent permanent neurological disability during SP-MS, highlights the importance of a proactive treatment approach (73). At present, there are a number of drugs with documented effect during RR-MS—for example, interferon beta and glatiramer acetate (113,123). Given the role of persistent inflammation as a cause of axonal injury, even during clinically silent stages of RR-MS, early, aggressive anti-inflammatory treatment might therefore also have indirect neuroprotective effects. In other words, intervention with disease-modifying therapy at relapsing stages of MS should be used continuously in order to prevent and delay accumulating axonal degeneration and thereby prevent and delay development of neurological impairment. In addition, neuroprotective therapies should be added to the anti-inflammatory and immunomodulatory treatments presently used for MS patients. For this reason, the development of neuroprotective drugs that apply to MS is an urgent goal for the MS research field.

The role of cumulative axonal degeneration in the development of permanent disability in MS suggests that neuronal or axonal markers could be used as a general monitor of these patients. Conventional MRI is generally believed to lack pathological specificity in MS (50,51), although association between decreased axonal density and hypointensity in T1-weighted images has been suggested (8,18). On the other hand, MRS measurements of the neuronal marker NAA demonstrate correlations between decreased brain NAA levels and changes in disability (see above). Moreover, axonal loss correlate with decreased levels of NAA in chronic MS lesions (33). Together, these data support axonal loss as the major cause of reduced NAA levels in chronic stages of MS. Since this axonal loss is a major contributor to neurological disability, whole brain NAA measured by MRS combined with the brain parenchymal fraction may be useful for monitoring disease progression and to determine response to therapy in MS patients (45,51).

VIII. CONCLUSIONS

This chapter summarizes data indicating that axonal injury is an integral part of MS and that loss of axons contributes to the irreversible functional impairment observed in affected individuals. Axonal involvement in the disease has been discussed by different investigators for more than a century. Recent reports however, describing various aspects of axonal injury in MS using a number of different methods, have increased our understanding of the role of axonal pathology in the development of permanent symptoms during the disease course. Several lines of evidence indicate that primary inflammatory demyelination is a major factor underlying axon loss during RR-MS. This axonal loss, however, is clinically silent. We and other have suggested that the transition from RR-MS to SP-MS, and the subsequent development of permanent neurological symptoms, occurs when a threshold of axonal loss is reached and the CNS compensatory resources are exhausted. The rate of inflammatory neurodegeneration during RR-MS determines the time point when a patient enters the secondary progressive stage of the disease.

The concept of MS as an inflammatory neurodegenerative disease has several clinical implications: First, surrogate markers of axonal loss are needed to monitor these patients. Second, considering the loss of axons from onset of disease and the role of inflammation causing axonal injury during RR-MS, early aggressive anti-inflammatory and immunomodulatory treatment should be provided in order to prevent or delay disability. Third, neuroprotection should be considered as a future therapeutic option in MS. Finally, studies of the molecular mechanisms behind axonal injury in MS are essential for the development of novel therapeutic strategies.

ACKNOWLEDGMENTS

This work was supported by NIH grants NS35058, NS38667 and by a pilot study grant (B.D.T.) and a postdoctoral fellowship (C.B.) from the National Multiple Sclerosis Society. The authors thank Dr. Angela Chang for assistance with the illustrations.

REFERENCES

1. Barnes D, Munro PMG, Youl BD, Prineas JW, McDonald WI. The longstanding MS lesion. Brain 1991; 114:1271–1280.

2. Arnold DL, Reiss GT, Matthews PM, Francis GS, Collins DL, Wolfson C, Antel JP. Use of proton magnetic resonance spectroscopy for monitoring disease progression in multiple sclerosis. Ann Neurol 1994; 36:76–82.

3. Davie CA, Barker GJ, Webb S, Tofts PS, Thompson AJ, Harding AE, McDonald WI, Miller DH. Persistent functional deficit in multiple sclerosis and autosomal dominant cerebellar ataxia is associated with axon loss. Brain 1995; 118:1583–1592.

4. Ferguson B, Matyszak MK, Esiri MM, Perry VH. Axonal damage in acute multiple sclerosis lesions. Brain 1997; 120:393–399.

5. Narayanan S, Fu L, Pioro E, De Stefano N, Collins DL, Francis GS, Antel JP, Matthews PM, Arnold DL. Imaging of axonal damage in multiple sclerosis: Spatial distribution of magnetic resonance imaging lesions. Ann Neurol 1997; 41:385–391.

6. Lassmann H. Neuropathology in multiple sclerosis: New concepts. Mult Scler 1998; 4:93–98.

7. Trapp BD, Peterson J, Ransohoff RM, Rudick R, Mörk S, Bö L. Axonal transection in the lesions of multiple sclerosis. N Engl J Med 1998; 338:278–285.

8. van Waesberghe JHTM, Kamphorst W, De Groot CJA, van Walderveen MAA, Castelijns JA, Ravid R, Lycklama a Nijeholt GJ, van der Valk P, Polman CH, Thompson AJ, Barkhof F. Axonal loss in multiple sclerosis lesions: Magnetic resonance imaging insights into substrates of disability. Ann Neurol 1999; 46:747–754.

9. Trapp BD, Ransohoff RM, Fisher E, Rudick RA. Neurodegeneration in multiple sclerosis: Relationship to neurological disability. Neuroscientist 1999; 5:48–57.

10. Kornek B, Lassman H. Axonal pathology in multiple sclerosis. A historical note. Brain Pathol 1999; 9:651–656.

11. Charcot, M. Histologie de le sclerose en plaques. Gazette Hopitaux 1868; 141:554–558.

12. Davie CA, Hawkins CP, Barker GJ, Brennan A, Tofts PS, Miller DH, McDonald WI. Serial proton magnetic resonance spectroscopy in acute multiple sclerosis lesions. Brain 1994; 117:49–58.

13. De Stefano N, Matthews PM, Antel JP, Preul M, Francis G, Arnold DL. Chemical pathology of acute demyelinating lesions and its correlation with disability. Ann Neurol 1995; 38:901–909.

14. Losseff NA, Webb SL, O'Riordan JI, Page R, Wang L, Barker GJ, Tofts PS, McDonald WI, Miller DH, Thompson AJ. Spinal cord atrophy and disability in multiple sclerosis: A new reproducible and sensitive MRI method with potential to monitor disease progression. Brain 1996; 119:701–708.

15. Losseff NA, Wang L, Lai HM, Yoo DS, Gawne-Cain ML, McDonald WI, Miller DH, Thompson AJ. Progressive cerebral atrophy in multiple sclerosis: A serial MRI study. Brain 1996; 119:2009–2019.

16. Matthews PM, Pioro E, Narayanan S, De Stefano N, Fu L, Francis G, Antel J, Wolfson C, Arnold DL. Assessment of lesion pathology in multiple sclerosis using quantitative MRI morphometry and magnetic resonance spectroscopy. Brain 1996; 119:715–722.

17. Fu L, Matthews PM, De Stefano N, Worsley KJ, Narayanan S, Francis GS, Antel JP, Wolfson C, Arnold DL. Imaging axonal damage of normal-appearing white matter in multiple sclerosis. Brain 1998; 121:103–113.

18. van Walderveen MAA, Kamphorst W, Scheltens P, van Waesberghe JHTM, Ravid R, Valk J, Polman CH, Barkhof F. Histopathologic correlate of hypointense lesions on T1-weighted spin-echo MRI in multiple sclerosis. Neurology 1998; 50:1282–1288.

19. Brown A, McFarlin DE, Raine CS. Chronologic neuropathology of relapsing experimental allergic encephalomyelitis in the mouse. Lab Invest 1982; 46:171–185.

20. Raine CS, Cross AH. Axonal dystrophy as a consequence of long-term demyelination. Lab Invest 1989; 60:714–725.

21. Njenga MK, Murray PD, McGavern D, Lin X, Drescher KM, Rodriguez M. Absence of spontaneous central nervous system remyelination in class II-deficient mice infected with Theiler's virus. J Neuropathol Exp Neurol 1999; 58:78–91.

22. De Stefano N, Matthews PM, Fu L, Narayanan S, Stanley J, Francis GS, Antel JP, Arnold DL. Axonal damage correlates with disability in patients with relapsing-remitting multiple sclerosis: Results of a longitudinal magnetic resonance spectroscopy study. Brain 1998; 121:1469–1477.

23. Losseff NA, Miller DH. Measures of brain and spinal cord atrophy in multiple sclerosis. J Neurol Neurosurg Psychiatry 1998; 64:S102–S105.

24. Bjartmar C, Yin X, Trapp BD. Axonal pathology in myelin disorders. J Neurocytol 1999; 28:383–395.

25. Waxman SG. Demyelinating diseases—New pathological insights, new therapeutic targets. N Engl J Med 1998; 338:223–225.

26. Bostock H, Sears TA, The internodal axon membrane: Electrical excitability and continuous conduction in segmental demyelination. J Physiol (Lond) 1978; 280:273–301.

27. Foster RE, Whalen CC, Waxman SG. Reorganization of the axon membrane in demyelinated peripheral nerve fibers: Morphological evidence. Science 1980; 210:661–663.

28. Felts PA, Baker TA, Smith KJ. Conduction in segmentally demyelinated mammalian central axons. J Neurosci 1997; 17:7267–7277.

29. Marburg O. Die sogenannte "akute multiple Sklerose" (Encephalomyelitis peraxialis scleroticans). Jahrb Neurol Psychiatry 1906; 27:211–312.

30. Putnam TJ. Studies in multiple sclerosis. Arch Neurol Psychiatry 1936; 35:1289–1308.

31. Greenfield JG, King LS. Observations on the histopathology of the cerebral lesions in disseminated sclerosis. Brain 1936; 59:445–458.

32. Koo EH, Sisodia SS, Archer DR, Martin LJ, Weidemann A, Beyreuther K, Fischer P, Masters CL, Price DL. Precursor of amyloid protein in Alzheimer disease undergoes fast anterograde axonal transport. Proc Nat Acad Sci USA 1990; 87:1561–1565.

33. Bjartmar C, Kidd G, Mörk S, Rudick R, Trapp BD. Axonal loss correlates with reduced N-acetyl-aspartate levels in chronic multiple sclerosis lesions of the spinal cord (abstr). J Neurochem 2000; 74:S13. (Suppl for American Society for Neurochemistry.)

34. Brownell B, Hughes JT. The distribution of plaques in the cerebrum in multiple sclerosis. J Neurol Neurosurg Psychiatry 1962; 25:315–320.

35. Lumsden CE. The neuropathology of multiple sclerosis. In: Vinken PJ, Bruyn GW, eds. Handbook of Clinical Neurology, vol 9. Amsterdam: North-Holland, 1970, pp 217–309.

36. Kidd D, Barkhof F, McConnell R, Algra PR, Allen IV, Revesz T. Cortical lesions in multiple sclerosis. Brain 1999; 122:17–26.

37. Peterson JW, Bö L, Chang A, Mörk S, Trapp BD. Neuropathology of cortical lesions in multiple sclerosis (abstr). J Neurochem 2000; 74:S13. (Suppl for American Society for Neurochemistry.)

38. Damian MS, Schilling G, Bachmann G, Simon C, Stoppler S, Dorndorf W. White matter lesions and cognitive deficits: Relevance of lesion pattern? Acta Neurol Scand 1994; 90:430–436.

39. Rao SM, Leo GJ, Bernardin L, Unverzagt F. Cognitive dysfunction in multiple sclerosis: I. Frequency, patterns, and prediction. Neurology 1991; 41:685–691.

40. Ron MA, Callanan MM, Warrington EK. Cognitive abnormalities in multiple sclerosis: A psychometric and MRI study. Psychol Med 1991; 21:59–68.

41. Beatty WW, Paul RH, Wilbanks SL, Hames KA, Blanco CR, Goodkin DE. Identifying multiple sclerosis patients with mild or global cognitive impairment using the Screening Examination for Cognitive Impairment (SEFCI). Neurology 1995; 45:718–723.

42. Foong J, Rozewics L, Davie CA, Thompson AJ, Miller DH, Ron MA. Correlates of executive

function in multiple sclerosis: The use of magnetic resonance spectroscopy as an index of focal pathology. J Neuropsychiatr Clin Neurosci 1999; 11:45–50.

43. Stevenson VL, Miller DH. Magnetic resonance imaging in the monitoring of disease progression in multiple sclerosis. Mult Scler 1999; 5:268–272.

44. Isaac C, Li DK, Genton M, Jardine C, Grochowski E, Palmer M, Kastrukoff LF, Oger J, Paty DW. Multiple sclerosis: A serial study using MRI in relapsing patients. Neurology 1988; 38:1511–1515.

45. Rudick RA, Fisher E, Lee JC, Simon J, Jacobs L. Use of the brain parenchymal fraction to measure whole brain atrophy in relapsing-remitting MS. Multiple Sclerosis Collaborative Research Group. Neurology 1999; 53:1698–1704.

46. Oppenheimer DR. The cervical cord in multiple sclerosis. Neuropathol Appl Neurobiol 1978; 4:151–162.

47. Kidd D, Thorpe JW, Thompson AJ, Kendall BE, Mosley IF, MacManus DG, McDonald WI, Miller DH. Spinal cord MRI using multi-array coils and fast spin echo: II. Findings in multiple sclerosis. Neurology 1993; 43:2632–2637.

48. Filippi M, Colombo B, Rovaris M, Pereira C, Martinelli V, Comi G. A longitudinal magnetic resonance imaging study of the cervical cord in multiple sclerosis. J Neuroimaging 1997; 7: 78–80.

49. Simon JH, Jacobs LD, Campion MK, Rudick MA, Cookfair DL, Herndon RM, Richert JR, Salazar AM, Fisher JS, Goodkin DE, Simonian N, Lajaunie M, Miller DE, Wende K, Martens-Davidson A, Kinkel RP, Munschauer FE, Brownscheidle CM, The Multiple Sclerosis Collaborative Research Group (MSCRG). A longitudinal study of brain atrophy in relapsing multiple sclerosis. Neurology 1999; 53:139–148.

50. Brück W, Bitsch A, Kolenda H, Brück Y, Stiefel M, Lassman H. Inflammatory central nervous system demyelination: Correlation of magnetic resonance imaging findings with lesion pathology. Ann Neurol 1997; 42:783–793.

51. Matthews PM, De Stefano N, Narayanan S, Francis GS, Wolinsky JS, Antel JP, Arnold DL. Putting magnetic resonance spectroscopy studies in context: Axonal damage and disability in multiple sclerosis. Semin Neurol 1998; 18:327–336.

52. Birken DL, Oldendorf WH. N-acetyl-L-aspartic acid: A literature review of a compound prominent in ^{1}H-NMR spectroscopic studies of brain. Neurosci Biobehav Rev 1989; 13:23–31.

53. Moffett JR, Namboodiri MAA, Cangro CB, Neale JH. Immunohistochemical localization of N-acetylaspartate in rat brain. Neuroreport 1991; 2:131–134.

54. Simmons ML, Frondoza CG, Coyle JT. Immunocytochemical localization of N-acetyl-aspartate with monoclonal antibodies. Neuroscience 1991; 45:37–45.

55. Graham GD, Blamire AM, Howseman AM, Rothman DL, Fayad PB, Brass LM, Petroff OA, Shulman RG, Prichard JW. Proton magnetic resonance spectroscopy of cerebral lactate and other metabolites in stroke patients. Stroke 1992; 23:333–340.

56. Pioro E, Antel JP, Cashman NR, Arnold DL. Detection of cortical neuron loss in motor neuron disease by proton magnetic resonance spectroscopic imaging in vivo. Neurology 1994; 44:1933–1938.

57. Narayana PA, Doyle TJ, Dejian L, Wolinsky JS. Serial proton magnetic resonance spectroscopic imaging, contrast-enhanced magnetic resonance imaging, and quantitative lesion volumetry in multiple sclerosis. Ann Neurol 1998; 43:56–71.

58. Clarke DD, Greenfield S, Dicker E, Tirri LJ, Ronan EJ. A relationship of N-acetylaspartate biosynthesis to neuronal protein synthesis. J Neurochem 1975; 24:479–485.

59. Cangro CB, Namboodiri MA, Sklar LA, Corigliano-Murphy A, Neale JH. Immunohistochemistry and biosynthesis of N-acetylaspartylglutamate in spinal sensory ganglia. J Neurochem 1987; 49:1579–1588.

60. Lee JH, Arcinue E, Ross BD. Brief report: Organic osmolytes in the brain of an infant with hypernatremia. N Engl J Med 1994; 331:439–442.

61. Patel TB, Clark JB. Synthesis of N-acetyl-L-aspartate by rat brain mitochondria and involvement in mitochondrial/cytosolic carbon transport. Biochem J 1979; 184:539–546.

62. Truckenmiller ME, Namboodiri MAA, Brownstein MJ, Neale JH. N-acetylation of L-aspartate in the nervous system: Differential distribution of a specific enzyme. J Neurochem 1985; 45:1658–1662.

63. Sager TN, Thomsen C, Valsborg JS, Laursen H, Hansen AJ. Astroglia contain a specific transport mechanism for N-acetyl-L-aspartate. J Neurochem 1999; 73:807–811.

64. Rosenbluth J. Role of glial cells in the differentiation and function of myelinated axons. Int J Dev Neurosci 1988; 6:3–24.

65. Dugandzija-Novakovic S, Koszowski AG, Levinson SR, Shrager P. Clustering of Na+ channels and node of Ranvier formation in remyelinating axons. J Neurosci 1995; 15:492–503.

66. Kaplan MR, Meyer-Franke A, Lambert S, Bennett V, Duncan ID, Levison SR, Barres BA. Induction of sodium channel clustering by oligodendrocytes. Nature 1997; 386:724–728.

67. de Waegh SM, Lee VM-Y, Brady ST. Local modulation of neurofilament phosphorylation, axonal caliber, and slow axonal transport by myelinating Schwann cells. Cell 1992; 68:451–463.

68. Windenbank AJ, Wood P, Bunge RP, Dyck PJ. Myelination determines the caliber of dorsal root ganglion neurons in culture. J Neurosci 1985; 5:1563–1569.

69. Sanchez I, Hassinger L, Paskevich PA, Shine HD, Nixon RA. Oligodendroglia regulate the regional expansion of axon caliber and local accumulation of neurofilaments during development independently of myelin formation. J Neurosci 1996; 16:5095–5105.

70. Rango M, Spagnoli D, Tomei G, Bamonti F, Scarlato G, Zetta L. Central nervous system trans-synaptic effects of acute axonal injury: A ^{1}H magnetic resonance spectroscopy study. Magn Reson Med 1995; 33:595–600.

71. Hafer-Macko C, Hsieh S-T, Li CY, Ho TW, Sheikh K, Cornblath DR, McKhann GM, Asbury AK, Griffin JW. Acute motor axonal neuropathy: An antibody-mediated attack on axolemma. Ann Neurol 1996; 40:635–644.

72. Ho TW, McKhann GM, Griffin JW. Human autoimmune neuropathies. Ann Rev Neurosci 1998; 21:187–226.

73. Rudick RA, Goodman A, Herndon RM, Panitch HS. Selecting relapsing remitting multiple sclerosis patients for treatment: the case for early treatment. J Neuroimmunol 1999; 98:22–28.

74. Simon JH, Jacobs LD, Campion M. Magnetic resonance studies of intramuscular interferon β-1a for relapsing multiple sclerosis. Ann Neurol 1998; 43:79–87.

75. Hohlfeld R. Biotechnological agents for the immunotherapy of multiple sclerosis. Principles, problems and perspectives. Brain 1997; 120:865–916.

76. Powell HC, Myers RR. The axon in Guillain-Barré syndrome: Immune target or innocent bystander? Ann Neurol 1996; 39:4–5.

77. Giese KP, Martini R, Lemke G, Soriano P, Schachner M. Mouse P_0 gene disruption leads to hypomyelination, abnormal expression of recognition molecules, and degeneration of myelin and axons. Cell 1992; 71:565–576.

78. Anzini P, Neuberg DH, Schachner M, Nelles E, Willecke K, Zielasek J, Toyka KV, Suter U, Martini R. Structural abnormalities and deficient maintenance of peripheral nerve myelin in mice lacking the gap junction protein connexin 32. J Neurosci 1997; 17:4545–4551.

79. Yin X, Crawford TO, Griffin JW, Tu P, Lee VM-Y, Li C, Roder J, Trapp BD. Myelin-associated glycoprotein is a myelin signal that modulates the caliber of myelinated axons. J Neurosci 1998; 18:1953–1962.

80. Griffiths I, Klugmann M, Anderson T, Yool D, Thomson C, Schwab MH, Schneider A, Zimmermann F, McCulloch M, Nadon N, Nave K-A. Axonal swellings and degeneration in mice lacking the major proteolipid of myelin. Science 1998; 280:1610–1613.

81. Sahenk Z, Chen L, Mendell JR. Effects of PMP22 duplication and deletions on the axonal cytoskeleton. Ann Neurol 1999; 45:16–24.

82. Sheikh KA, Sun J, Liu Y, Kawai H, Crawford TO, Proia RL, Griffin JW, Schnaar RL. Mice lacking complex gangliosides develop Wallerian degeneration and myelination defects. Proc Nat Acad Sci USA 1999; 96:7532–7537.

83. Salzer JL, Holmes WP, Colman DR. The amino acid sequences of the myelin-associated glycoproteins: Homology to the immunoglobulin gene superfamily. J Cell Biol 1987; 104: 957–965.

84. Arquint M, Roder J, Chia L-S, Down J, Wilkinson O, Bayley H, Braun P, Dunn R. Molecular cloning and primary structure of myelin-associated glycoproteins. Proc Nat Acad Sci USA 1987; 84:600–604.

85. Lai C, Brow MA, Nave K-A, Noronha AB, Quarles RH, Bloom FE, Milner RJ, Sutcliffe JG. Two forms of 1B236/myelin-associated glycoprotein (MAG), a cell adhesion molecule for postnatal neural development, are produced by alternative splicing. Proc Nat Acad Sci USA 1987; 84:4337–4341.

86. Sternberger NH, Quarles RH, Itoyama Y, Webster HD. Myelin-associated glycoprotein demonstrated immunocytochemically in myelin and myelin forming cells of developing rats. Proc Nat Acad Sci USA 1979; 76:1510–1514.

87. Trapp BD, Andrews SB, Cootauco C, Quarles RH. The myelin-associated glycoprotein is enriched in multivesicular bodies and periaxonal membranes of actively myelinating oligodendrocytes. J Cell Biol 1989; 109:2417–2426.

88. McKerracher L, David S, Jackson DL, Kottis V, Dunn RJ, Braun PE. Identification of myelin-associated glycoprotein as a major myelin-derived inhibitor of neurite growth. Neuron 1994; 13:805–811.

89. Mukhopadhya G, Doherty P, Walsh FS, Crocker P, Filbin MT. A novel role for myelin-associated glycoprotein as an inhibitor of axonal regeneration. Neuron 1994; 13:757–767.

90. Li M, Shibata A, Li C, Braun PE, McKerracher L, Roder J, Kater SB, David S. Myelin-associated glycoprotein inhibits neurite/axon growth and causes growth cone collapse. J Neurosci Res 1996; 46:404–414.

91. Duncan ID, Hammang JP, Trapp BD. Abnormal compact myelin in the myelin-deficient rat: Absence of proteolipid protein correlates with a defect in the intraperiod line. Proc Nat Acad Sci USA 1988; 84:6287–6291.

92. Hodes ME, Pratt VM, Dlouhy SR. Genetics of Pelizaeus-Merzbacher disease. Dev Neurosci 1993; 15:383–394.

93. Seitelberger F. Neuropathology and genetics of Pelizaeus-Merzbacher disease. Brain Pathol 1995; 5:267–273.

94. Inoue K, Osaka H, Imaizumi K, Nezu A, Takanashi J, Arii J, Murayama K, Ono J, Kikawa Y, Mito T, Shaffer LG, Lupski JR. Proteolipid protein gene duplications causing Pelizaeus-Merzbacher disease: Molecular mechanism and phenotypic manifestations. Ann Neurol 1999; 45:624–632.

95. Griffiths IR, Schneider A, Anderson J, Nave K-A. Transgenic and natural mouse models of proteolipid protein (PLP) related dysmyelination and demyelination. Brain Pathol 1995; 5: 275–281.

96. Anderson TJ, Schneider A, Barrie JA, Klugmann M, McCulloch MC, Kirkham D, Kyriakides E, Nave K-A, Griffiths IR. Late-onset neurodegeneration in mice with increased dosage of the proteolipid protein gene. J Comp Neurol 1998; 394:506–519.

97. Hanemann CO, Müller HW. Pathogenesis of Charcot-Marie-Tooth IA (CMTIA) neuropathy. Trends Neurosci 1998; 21:282–286.

98. Hayasaka K, Himoro M, Sato W, Takada G, Uyemura K, Shimizu N, Bird TD, Coneally PM, Chance PF. Charcot-Marie-Tooth neuropathy type 1B is associated with mutations of the myelin P0 gene. Nature Genet 1993; 5:31–34.

99. Bergoffen J, Scherer SS, Wang S, Oronzi Scott M, Bone LJ, Paul DL, Chen K, Lensch MW, Chance PF, Fischbeck KH. Connexin mutations in X-linked Charcot-Marie-Tooth disease. Science 1993; 262:2039–2042.

100. Dyck PJ, Karnes JL, Lambert EH. Longitudinal study of neuropathic deficits and nerve conduction abnormalities in hereditary motor and sensory neuropathy type 1. Neurology 1989; 39:1302–1308.

101. Scherer SS, Xu YT, Nelles E, Fischbeck K, Bone LJ. Connexin32-null mice develop demyelinating peripheral neuropathy. Glia 1998; 24:8–20.

102. Scherer S. Axonal pathology in demyelinating diseases. Ann Neurol 1999; 45:6–7.

103. Low PA, McLeod JG. Hereditary demyelination neuropathy in the Trembler mouse. J Neurol Sci 1975; 26:565–574.

104. Aguayo A, Attiwell M, Trecarten J, Perkins S, Bray G. Abnormal myelination in transplanted Trembler mouse Schwann cells. Nature 1977; 265:73–75.

105. Sahenk Z, Chen L. Abnormalities in the axonal cytoskeleton induced by a Connexin32 mutation in nerve xenografts. J Neurosci Res 1998; 51:174–184.

106. Raine CS. Biology of disease. Analysis of autoimmune demyelination: Its impact upon multiple sclerosis. Lab Invest 1984; 50:608–635.

107. Owens T, Sriram S. The immunology of multiple sclerosis and its animal model, experimental allergic encephalomyelitis. Neurol Clin 1995; 13:51–73.

108. Linington C. Experimental animal models. In: Zhang J, Hafler D, Hohlfeld R, Miller A, eds. Immunotherapy in Neuroimmunologic Diseases. London: Martin Dunitz, 1998, pp 11–28.

109. Yu M, Nishiyama A, Trapp BD, Tuohy V. Interferon-β inhibits progression of relapsing-remitting experimental autoimmune encephalomyelitis. J Neuroimmunol 1996; 64:91–100.

110. Wujek JR, Bjartmar C, Richer E, Yu M, Tuohy V, Trapp BD. Loss of spinal cord axons in the experimental allergic encephalomyelitis animal model of multiple sclerosis (abstr). J Neurochem 2000; 74:S46. (Suppl for American Society for Neurochemistry; 74:546).

111. Bell JI, Lathrop GM. Multiple loci for multiple sclerosis. Nature Genet 1996; 13:377–378.

112. Ebers GC, Dyment DA. Genetics of multiple sclerosis. Semin Neurol 1998; 18:295–299.

113. Noseworthy JH. Progress in determining the causes and treatment of multiple sclerosis. Nature 1999; 399(suppl):A40–A47.

114. Rodriguez M, Oleszak E, Leibowitz J. Theiler's murine encephalomyelitis: A model of demyelination and persistence of virus. Crit Rev Immunol 1987; 7:325–365.

115. Drescher KM, Pease LR, Rodriques M. Antiviral immune responses modulate the nature of central nervous system (CNS) disease in a murine model of multiple sclerosis. Immunol Rev 1997; 159:177–193.

116. Rivera-Quinones C, McGavern D, Schmelzer JD, Hunter SF, Low PA, Rodriguez M. Absence of neurological deficits following extensive demyelination in a class I-deficient murine model of multiple sclerosis. Nature Med 1998; 4:187–193.

117. Lloyd KG. CNS compensation to dopamine neuron loss in Parkinson's disease. Adv Exp Med Biol 1977; 90:255–266.

118. Bradley WG. Recent views on amyotrophic lateral sclerosis with emphasis on electrophysiological studies. Muscle Nerve 1987; 10:490–502.

119. McFarland HF, Frank JA, Albert PS, Smith ME, Martin R, Harris JO, Patronas N, Maloni H, McFarlin DE. Using gadolinium-enhanced magnetic resonance imaging lesions to monitor disease activity in multiple sclerosis. Ann Neurol 1992; 32:758–766.

120. Filippi M, Paty DW, Kappos L, Barkhof F, Compston DA, Thompson AJ, Zhao GJ, Wiles CM, McDonald WI, Miller DH. Correlations between changes in disability and T2-weighted brain MRI activity in multiple sclerosis: a follow-up study. Neurology 1995; 45:255–260.

121. Mews I, Bergmann M, Bunkowski S, Gullotta F, Brück W. Oligodendrocyte and axon pathology in clinically silent multiple sclerosis lesions. Mult Scler 1998; 4:55–62.

122. Lublin FD, Reingold SC. Defining the clinical course of multiple sclerosis: Results of an international survey. Neurology 1996; 46:907–911.

123. Rudick RA, Cohen JA, Weinstock-Guttman B, Kinkel RP, Ransohoff RM. Management of multiple sclerosis. N Engl J Med 1997; 337:1604–1611.

14

Cerebrospinal Fluid

JOHN N. WHITAKER

University of Alabama at Birmingham and the Neurology and Research Services of the Birmingham Veterans Medical Center, Birmingham, Alabama

KHURRAM BASHIR and ETTY N. BENVENISTE

University of Alabama at Birmingham, Birmingham, Alabama

I. INTRODUCTION

The examination of cerebrospinal fluid (CSF) preceded neuroimaging and evoked potentials by decades as the first method to provide laboratory confirmation of a clinical diagnosis of multiple sclerosis (MS) (1). CSF continues to yield valuable clinical information for establishing the presence of MS and monitoring its activity (2,3). Because of its direct contact with the central nervous system (CNS), CSF has also been important for investigating the etiology and pathogenesis of MS.

The CSF in MS can be totally normal. However, the typical profile (Table 1) of stable or chronic progressive MS is 5 or fewer mononuclear cells per cubic millimeter, a normal total protein in 60% of patients and under 70 mg/dL in nearly all patients, normal glucose, a quantitative and relative (to albumin) increase of immunoglobulin G (IgG), and qualitative changes of immunoglobulin in the form of oligoclonal bands (OCBs). The immunoglobulin abnormalities reflect changes occurring inside the blood-brain barrier (BBB). During periods of acute demyelination, myelin basic protein (MBP)-like material appears in CSF (4) and, less consistently, a slight pleocytosis is evident (5). Measurements of soluble adhesion molecules, cytokines and related materials in CSF are of pathogenic interest and are beginning to have more clinical meaning.

II. CELLULAR COMPOSITION

In nearly every instance where CSF is sampled in a MS patient, it is done via a lumbar puncture. It is highly desirable to obtain CSF free of trauma, because the influx of blood

Table 1 Clinically Related Changes of CSF in MS

Total protein
  Normal value in 60% of MS patients
  >100 mg/dL very rare
Leukocytes
  Normal value in 66%
  Lymphocytes, >5/mm^3 in 33%
  Irregularly correlated with relapses
  Lymphocyte subsets
    >80% CD3+
    2:1 ratio of CD4+:CD8+
    16–18% B lymphocytes
    Plasma cells rarely found
Glucose values normal
Immunoglobulin
  Increased in amount
  Increaed IgG index (>0.7)
  Increased IgG synthetic rate (>3.3 mg/dL)
  Oligoclonal IgG bands present
  Increased κ/λ light chain ratio
Tissue markers
  Increased MBP-like material in active phases

---

components will obscure some of the abnormalities that should be detected. The number of cells in the CSF of MS patients is increased—that is, >5 lymphocytes per cubic millimeter, in one-third of cases—with the pleocytosis in the range of 10 to 20 mononuclear cells per cubic millimeter (6). CSF leukocyte counts of >50 mm^3 are rare in MS, and >100 mm^3 should lead to the likely diagnosis of another condition. Although some differences of opinion exist (5), there seems to be no consistent correlation between CSF pleocytosis and clinical disease activity (2). In addition, although the number of cells in CSF correlates positively with gadolinium (Gd)-enhancing lesion volume, it has no correlation with T2-weighted (T2W) lesion volume on cranial magnetic resonance imaging (MRI) (7). The literature on the analysis of leukocytes in CSF of MS patients is extensive. The CSF profile need not bear a close relationship to the cellular composition of CNS lesions, but it does show differences compared to blood.

The cells in the brain (8) and CSF (9–12) are the source for the intra-BBB synthesis of immunoglobulins. Under normal conditions, a very small number of T lymphocytes are present in the brain, making them almost undetectable by immunohistochemical methods (13–16). In MS, these cells increase in number and are readily detectable within the brain parenchyma (17–19). A proportionate increase in the CSF is usually not apparent where, as noted above, the cell count is within or relatively close to the normal range (6). The increased plasma cell content of the brain is also not paralleled in the CSF, where plasma cells are rarely found (6). All CSF lymphocytes are ultimately derived from the blood pool via transmigration across the BBB or blood-CSF barrier (20,21). There is evidence of rapid movement of cells from blood into CSF (22), and the cell-mediated immunity induced by systemic stimulation against tetanus toxoid can be detected in cells of the CSF (23). However, even with this rapid movement of cells from blood to CSF and, presumably, vice versa, the distribution of lymphocyte subsets in CSF is different from that of peripheral blood (24). In the CSF, the percentage of T lymphocytes, which express the CD3 marker, accounts for 80% or more of the lymphocytes present compared to 65% of those in peripheral blood (5). The percentage of CD4+ (T-helper/inducer) and CD8+ (T-suppressor/cytotoxic) cells remains at approximately the same 2:1 ratio as exists in blood (5,25,26). This may be due to a "lymphocyte subset-selective barrier" that regulates the passage of T cells between the blood and CSF (27). However, CNS inflammatory disorders, such as MS, may disrupt this barrier in ways that the ratio of lymphocyte subsets in CSF in these conditions is a result of selective as well as nonselective transfer. Compared to blood lymphocytes, CSF-derived lymphocytes demonstrate enhanced adhesion to vascular endothelial cells (28). CSF lymphocytes also express a greater number of interleukin-2 (IL-2) cell surface receptors and have increased mRNA and DNA synthesis, suggesting cellular activation (29–31). These observations suggest that CSF-derived lymphocytes represent a selected subpopulation of T cells in blood. The percentage of B cells in CSF is also approximately the same, 16 to 18%, as that in blood (26). There has been no characteristic change or consistent difference noted in the relative percentages of T or B lymphocytes or in the distribution of T lymphocyte subsets in MS patients who are in relapse versus chronic progressive phases of disease activity (5,32). In addition, lymphocyte subsets and their relative proportions do not help in distinguishing MS from other neurologic diseases (33).

During any immune reaction, two patterns of immunologic response can be recognized based on different T-lymphocyte functions and cytokine profiles (34,35). T helper type 1 (Th1) cells secrete proinflammatory cytokines such as IL-2, interferon gamma (IFN-γ), and tumor necrosis factor-alpha (TNF-α) which leads to stimulation of macrophages, induction of inflammation and inhibition of CD8+ suppressor T cells. On the other hand, Th2 cells produce anti-inflammatory cytokines, such as interleukin-4 (IL-4), interleukin-5 (IL-5), and interleukin-10 (IL-10), which inhibit production of cytokines from Th1 cells, suppress cell mediated immune responses, and enhance fibrosis (36,37). This immune response dichotomy appears to be active in a number of autoimmune diseases including MS. The T cells present in active lesions of experimental autoimmune encephalomyelitis (EAE) and MS have predominantly a Th1 phenotype, suggesting a role for these cells in the pathogenesis of the disease (38,39). Over 90% of lymphocytes derived from the CSF of progressive MS patients are T lymphocytes, and of these 70% are CD4+ T helper cells while 30% are CD8+ T suppressor cells (25,40). The proportion of T suppresser cells in CSF drops even further during acute MS relapses, implying an interaction between these two lymphocyte subtypes in the immunopathogenesis of MS (41). B cells secreting antibodies against myelin, MBP, and various MBP peptides, proteolipid protein (PLP), and myelin-associated glycoprotein (MAG) are present in the CSF of MS and optic neuritis patients (42–45). The significance and pathogenetic relevance of these antibody-secreting CSF cells in MS is not clear. They may represent an antibody response against myelin antigens that is either an integral part of the underlying pathogenic process or a result of myelin breakdown.

A major limitation in the analysis of CSF cells is the low number that can be recovered. This quantitative limitation has been addressed in several ways. One has been through a modification of techniques to permit microcultures (46). With this method, a compartmentalized response to MBP of CSF cells in MS could be detected when it could not be demonstrated in blood lymphocytes (47). Evidence derived from the same method also suggested polyclonal B-cell activation in CSF of MS patients (48). There is no apparent correlation between the presence of MBP in the CSF (discussed later) and the existence of CSF cells sensitized to MBP (49). Other modifications of techniques have dealt with examination of more sensitive cellular functions. For example, it has been shown that an increased percentage of lymphocytes in the CSF of MS patients are in the Gl phase of the proliferative cycle during all phases of disease activity, but especially during active phases (50), and that the population of cells in the CSF appears to be selected for a higher frequency of response to autologous and allogeneic cell antigens (51). This later finding is suggestive of a lymphocyte response to altered self-antigens. However, evidence is lacking for autonomously proliferating lymphocytes in CSF, as might be expected with transformed T cells (52). Newer techniques utilizing the polymerase chain reaction (53) should permit a delineation of the features of CSF cells in MS.

In summary, the low level of CSF pleocytosis in MS should be acknowledged, and there is evidence that CSF cells in MS are abnormal. However, the CSF cell profile in MS appears to be of little clinical value at present (33). The possibility that changes in the CSF cellular composition and function may be the result of soluble factors released from infiltrating or activated cells in the brain rather than cell migration from brain into CSF requires further assessment (54). This subject is approached more completely by analyzing CSF for cytokines, their receptors and soluble adhesion molecules (see Sec. V).

III. IMMUNOGLOBULIN

A. Characteristics of the Immunoglobulin Molecule

Although all five isotypes, IgG, IgA, IgM, IgD, and IgE, may be detected in CSF with appropriate assays, IgG is by far the dominant isotype present. The typical immunoglobulin molecule, and IgG in particular, is a glycoprotein consisting of four polypeptide chains, two identical heavy chains of approximately 50,000 molecular weight, and two identical light chains of approximately 22,000 molecular weight (55) (Fig. 1). The light and heavy chains each have variable ends which react with antigen and constant ends which, especially for the heavy chain, account for an array of biological effects triggered by the reaction of IgG with antigen. The IgG molecule also has antigenic features based on amino acid sequences, which can be recognized by other antibodies. These take the form of isotypes, allotypes, and idiotypes.

B. Historical Aspects

Quantitative abnormalities of total protein in CSF are sometimes noted in MS, but values of over 70 mg/dL are unusual (6). Higher elevations may be attributable to previous myelographic procedures and arachnoiditis or coexistent demyelinating polyneuropathy (56,57) but should always prompt a careful reexamination of the diagnosis.

Observations made in recent years have dealt mostly with quantitative changes of selected components, particularly IgG, of CSF proteins and their qualitative features. Abnormalities of protein components of CSF in MS were initially sought with a number of chemical reagents with procedures previously applied in cases of neurosyphilis (1,2). Two of the most commonly used methods were those of the Pandy and colloidal gold tests. The Pandy test was abnormal if a precipitate of globulins formed after phenol was added to CSF. The turbidity of the treated CSF was rated on a semiquantitative scale with little or no turbidity being normal and turbidity increasing with either an increase in total protein or an increase in the relative amount of globulin. The colloidal gold test consisted of 10

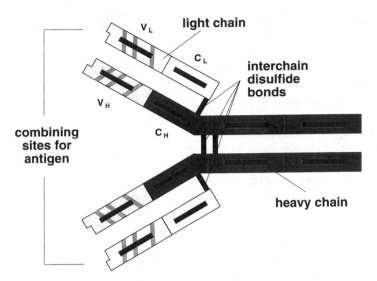

Figure 1 Immunoglobulin G molecule consisting of two identical heavy and two identical light chains covalently linked by interchain disulfide bonds. The heavy and light chains have constant regions in which the sites determining isotypes and allotypes are located. The variable regions of the light and heavy chains create the antigen-binding site. Idiotypes are present in the variable regions (VH and VL), especially in the hypervariable portions (represented by the slanted lines).

tubes prepared by adding serial dilutions of CSF to a rust-colored colloidal gold solution and examining the change in appearance of the mixture (1). A positive first-zone colloidal gold test was found in neurosyphilis, especially general paresis, and MS, and was subsequently shown to be associated with elevated levels of gamma globulin or, as it is now known, immunoglobulin. This complex reaction most likely arose from a precipitation by gamma or beta globulin and the prevention of this by albumin (58). The ratios of the facilitating and inhibitory proteins gave rise to different results and different zones of precipitation.

A major advance in the technology of examining and quantitating immunoglobulins in any body fluid occurred in the late 1930s in the Svedberg Laboratory in Uppsala, with the description of free-moving electrophoresis by Tiselius and the application of this methodology by Tiselius and Kabat (59–61). With this method, Kabat and coworkers were able to show the similarities of serum and CSF proteins (58–62) and that 65 to 85% of patients with MS had an elevation of CSF immunoglobulins that could occur when the total protein was normal (63). Over the ensuing 60 years a number of studies have been conducted to delineate the features of CSF immunoglobulins in health and disease and to provide guidelines for the examination and interpretation of changes in CSF immunoglobulins in MS.

C. Quantitation of CSF Immunoglobulins

Given the knowledge that the ratio of protein in the serum and CSF is approximately 200 to 300:1 and that the BBB is altered in MS, particularly during acute phases of disease (64), studies have been performed to determine the source of the increased immunoglobulin in CSF and to devise ways of maximizing the information obtained on CSF immunoglobulin removed for clinical purposes. Although the isotypes IgG, IgM, and IgA may each be increased in the CSF of MS patients (65), most of the studies have been of IgG only. The IgG content of CSF may be quantitatively increased when there is a change in the BBB permeability, when an increased serum IgG equilibrates to also raise CSF IgG, and by the production of IgG inside the BBB by plasma cells in the CNS. A number of studies have revealed both the cellular basis for such immunoglobulin synthesis in the CNS (8) and the increase in immunoglobulin in the brains of patients with MS (66). In the instances of permeability changes in the BBB or the normal transfer of increased serum protein levels, the CSF IgG and albumin ratio should correspond to that in the serum, but when IgG is synthesized in the CNS, the CSF IgG should be disproportionately raised compared to albumin. Thus, the combination of plasma cells secreting immunoglobulin as well as some change in BBB permeability are the two main factors that must be considered in the interpretation of the level of CSF IgG.

To interpret the ratio of IgG and albumin in CSF, it is necessary also to quantitate IgG and albumin in serum. Once this has been accomplished, a dimensionless index, standardized by Link and colleagues (67,68) can then be expressed in which the ratio of CSF IgG and CSF albumin is related to the ratio of serum IgG and serum albumin:

$$\text{CSF IgG index} = \frac{\text{CSF IgG/CSF albumin}}{\text{serum IgG/serum albumin}}$$

On the basis of extensive studies, a ratio of 0.7 or higher indicates that IgG is being synthesized within the CNS.

A number of formulas have also been proposed whereby a more quantitative statement of the amount of IgG produced in the CNS per hour or per day is derived. One of the goals of such calculations is to state more precisely the amount of IgG produced that can be subsequently monitored for a relationship to changes in the natural history of disease or its modification with therapy. The most widely used formula is the one developed by Tourtellotte (3,6,69). The amount of IgG produced is based on the same four measurements of CSF and serum IgG and albumin concentrations used for calculating the Link index but is expressed in milligrams per 24 h and determined by the following formula:

$$\left[\left(\text{CSF IgG} - \frac{\text{serum IgG}}{369} \right) - \left(\text{CSF albumin} - \frac{\text{serum albumin}}{230} \right) \times \left(\frac{\text{serum IgG}}{\text{serum albumin}} \right) (0.43) \right] \times 5$$

The concentrations are in milligrams per deciliter, the number 369 is the average normal serum/CSF ratio of IgG, the number 230 is the average normal serum/CSF ratio of albumin, and 0.43 is the molecular weight ratio of albumin to IgG. The multiplier of 5 is included because of the presumed production of 5 dL of CSF per 24 h. The in vivo validation of this formula has been demonstrated by isotopic dilution in a small number of patients (70).

This formula and others are helpful, but all have limitations in the degree of accuracy that can be attained (68,71,72). The major reservation about the formulas is the assumed constancy of the transfer of albumin and IgG from serum to CSF in areas of increased BBB permeability (68). The formula also does not take into account the catabolism of IgG or albumin in CSF, which will influence their values (72). Nevertheless, an index of

0.7 or higher and a synthetic rate of >3.3 mg/24 h indicate that the amount of IgG being synthesized inside the BBB is increased. An abnormal index or synthetic rate can be found in approximately 90% of patients with MS, but it is not disease-specific and may also occur in over 50% of patients with inflammatory and infectious disease of the CSF (73).

D. Qualitative Features

The in situ immune response in the CNS, expressed in the elevated IgG index and synthetic rate, is also associated with the presence of OCBs in CSF (Table 2). IgG molecules are the products of plasma cells that arise from clones of B lymphocytes. Each B-cell clone and the population of plasma cells produced through proliferation of the clone synthesize immunoglobulin molecules that are identical in amino acid sequence of heavy and light chains and electrical charge. By subjecting CSF proteins to electrophoretic separation, in which the immunoglobulin molecules migrate toward the cathode, the heterogeneity of charges and, by inference, the array of clones expressed in the production of IgG can be recognized by the banding pattern. In normal serum and CSF the IgG molecules are polyclonal, i.e., they are the products of many clones, and appear as a diffuse band. If a single clone has proliferated, as occurs in multiple myeloma, a single molecular species of immunoglobulin is produced and a single monoclonal band or spike is noted. Patients with MS have CSF IgG that shows two or more bands, designated by Lowenthal et al. as oligoclonal (74); this is presumed to be the product of a few B-cell clones which reached the CNS, proliferated, and ultimately transformed to plasma cells. Unless highly sensitive methods are used, serum from the same patient should not have OCBs. Should serum also contain OCBs, the number of OCBs in the CSF should outnumber those in the serum. The CSF OCBs appear as distinct bands through protein staining and can be characterized further by binding to antibodies specific for IgG and kappa or lambda light chains by a technique referred to as *immunofixation*.

Table 2 CSF Oligoclonal Immunoglobulin Bands in MS

Incidence
90% of MS
30% of inflammatory or infectious neurological disease controls
5–10% of noninflammatory neurological disease controls
Demonstration
CSF
Two or more discrete bands of immunoglobulin
By immunofixation stains for immunoglobulin heavy chain and a light chain, may be free light chains
Serum
No oligoclonal banding
Other features
Persistent in MS
Most have no known antibody activity
No clear relationship to disease activity or progression

Plasma cells are abundant in most (8) but not all (75) MS CNS, and extracts of CNS tissue from MS cases reveal OCBs (76). Whether different clones reside in different sites in the CNS of a single MS patient (76) or are spread throughout the CNS (77) is unresolved. The demonstration of distinct histopathological subtypes in MS (78) with their different profiles and possibly differences in roles of T and B cells (79) makes this an important distinction to resolve. The detection of OCBs in sera of MS patients implies that a more systemic and restricted immune stimulation may occur in MS (80). Cultured and stimulated blood mononuclear cells from MS patients secrete oligoclonal IgG (81). Serum OCBs are best detected with very sensitive tests, such as isoelectric focusing with immunofixation (82). Oligoclonal IgM (83) and IgA (84) may also be noted in CSF of MS patients, but they are less common and have no recognized clinical significance beyond that seen with IgG.

OCBs are not unique to MS patients (73). They are found in other conditions, such as neurosyphilis and subacute sclerosis panencephalitis, in which an *in situ* hyperimmune humoral response occurs. The frequency of OCBs found in MS CSF is dependent on the tests used (62). Two or more OCBs must be seen. A single band has no diagnostic significance because it may occur in a variety of conditions (85). In general, CSF OCBs are found in over 90% of MS patients, 30% of CNS inflammatory and infectious disease controls, and 5 to 10% of other, noninflammatory neurological disease controls (86,87). With increasing sensitivity, specificity may be sacrificed. In MS, once OCBs appear, they may increase in number but do not disappear. The CSF OCBs in controls are less likely to persist (77). CSF OCBs may also be detected in the monosymptomatic forms of MS (88) and, when present in optic neuritis, are predictive of a greater chance that MS will ultimately develop (89).

The CSF OCBs in MS may be superimposed on a background of polyclonal IgG (90). The latter is presumed to arise from either a variety of B-cell clones in the CNS or from an altered BBB. The polyclonal and oligoclonal IgG contribute to the increased concentration of CSF IgG and the higher index and synthetic rate for IgG. A number of anti-inflammatory and immunosuppressive regimens lower the index and rate but do not alter the OCB pattern or intensity (see Sec. VI). Oligoclonal IgG patterns may change over time (91) but do not correlate with severity, duration, or disease activity of MS (92). However, because OCBs cannot be quantitated, small changes might go unnoted. Two-dimensional electrophoresis offers even greater resolution (77) and may be potentially quantifiable through scanning and densitometric analysis. Two-dimensional gels also show stability of the clones of IgG, IgA, and IgM in MS CSF (77).

Allotypes

The heightened synthesis or oligoclonality of IgG and other immunoglobulins *in situ* within the CNS is of practical importance in studies of CSF. A more detailed analysis has been made of the molecular features of the IgG in MS patients. Gamma chain marker (Gm) allotypes are genetically determined regions of the sequences in the constant portions of heavy and light chains (Fig. 1) of the IgG molecule. An increase in certain Gm allotypes, though inconsistently (93), in the CSF of MS patients has been reported (94). While clones producing IgG of a selected allotype might be more likely to respond or proliferate, their significance is unclear.

Idiotypes

Idiotypes (Id) are genetically determined markers in the variable regions of the heavy or light chains of the immunoglobulin molecule (Fig. 1). The portion of the immunoglobulin molecule that binds with the epitope of an antigen is called the *paratope*. The Id of an immunoglobulin is found in the hypervariable portions of the variable regions of the immunoglobulin molecule—the heavy chain, the light chain, or both—and serves as an antigen for an antibody, referred to as an *anti-Id*. Anti-Ids have been studied because they may reveal abnormalities in the germline for immunoglobulin production and afford insight into the humoral immune basis for autoimmune diseases. If there is a genetic abnormality for production of the variable portion of the immunoglobulin molecule, the Id of these immunoglobulins may be similar and show cross-reactivity with anti-Id. Using whole immunoglobulin as the Id-bearing antibody and not based on any antigenic specificity, cross-reactive Ids have been detected in only a small number of MS patients studied (95–97). More recently, evidence for cross-reactive Ids in the CSF of MS has been obtained with the Id-bearing antibody directed to MBP peptide 80-89. Using the technique of reverse transcriptase polymerase chain reaction and Southern blot, the CSF of 45% (14 of 31) of MS patients had B-cell gene product related to this Id compared to 10% (2 of 19) of controls ($p = 0.0134$) (98). With a different technique, immunoblotting, an anti-Id also directed to the Id-bearing antibody recognizing MBP 80–89 detected a cross-reactive Id in the CSF of 79% (45 of 57) of MS patients compared to 16% (7 of 45) of other neurological disease controls ($p = <0.0001$) (99). These findings imply that immunoglobulin V–region gene restriction exists among MS patients and may relate to a shared genetic influence or a common antigen inducing the response.

Kappa/Lambda Ratios

Another qualitative abnormality reflecting an intra-BBB synthesis of CSF immunoglobulins in MS is an increased ratio of kappa/lambda light chains compared to the serum (100). The normal ratio of kappa to lambda light chains in humans is $70:30$, but in the CSF of MS patients, this ratio is higher. Furthermore, free kappa light chains, not covalently bound to functional immunoglobulin molecules, are present in MS CSF (101,102), implying a discordance in the synthesis of heavy and light chains.

E. Mechanism for In Situ CNS Synthesis of Immunoglobulins

The origin of *in situ* synthesis of immunoglobulins in the CNS and the formation of OCBs are imprecisely understood. Based on studies in animals, it is evident that the normal brain supports the development of humoral immunity and that B cells can cross an intact BBB (103). Following intrathecal injection of antigen, CSF specific antibody are detected by day 14 subsequent to antigen processing in draining cervical lymph nodes. Since plasma cells do not circulate, B cells can enter the CNS and differentiate into plasma cells in the CNS where the antigen is located.

F. Antibody Activity and Specificity

The presence of quantitatively increased immunoglobulin and OCBs in CSF of MS patients has prompted numerous studies (104) to attempt to identify the specificity of the antibody present in CSF and to determine whether the OCBs contain antibody activity. The antigens tested have typically been viruses or their components, CNS tissue, myelin extracts, or specific myelin components. In neurosyphilis (105), mumps meningitis (106), and subacute sclerosing panencephalitis (107), there is CSF antibody to the etiological agent, and the presence of specific antibody has been detected in the OCBs of CSF. There is evidence that some antiviral antibody, especially to the measles virus, is produced in the CNS, implied by the relatively higher antiviral titer in CSF of MS patients compared to serum (104). Although some MS patients may synthesize 100 mg of IgG in their CNS per 24 h (6), the specific reactivity of the bulk of the increased IgG and the immunoglobulin in OCBs (108) remains uncertain.

Several explanations have been offered for failure to detect specific antibody in MS CSF IgG. First, an increase in CSF IgG may arise from a poorly suppressed clonal stimulation from such an assortment of immunogens that no specific reactivity dominates. This explanation is especially favored by the immunoregulatory defect of diminished suppressor cell function in MS discussed earlier and in Chap. 7. Second, the appropriate antigen or antigenic fragment may not have been examined in a sufficiently sensitive assay. There are, for example, antigen-specific responses to fragments of MBP that are not detected with the intact MBP molecule (109). Third, the antibody present may be aggregated or complexed with antigen(s) preventing detection of its presence. Immune complexes occur in the CSF of MS patients (110), and CSF antibody to MBP appears to be present in both free (111–113) and bound (112,113) forms. A report of the correlation of free antibody to MBP with relapses of MS and bound antibody to MBP with chronic progressive phases in MS (113) is of considerable interest because it could be of diagnostic and prognostic significance. The portion of the MBP molecule against which the CSF antibody is directed appears to be in the region of residues 85-96 of the MBP molecule of 170 residues (114). This MBP epitope in peptide 85-96 is very similar to an epitope recognized by T cells cultured from the blood of MS patients (115). This similarity of T and B cell epitopes has implications about the pathogenic role for antibodies to MBP in the pathogenesis of MS (116). Furthermore, the specificity of CSF antibody may influence the immune-mediated changes in MS. Thus, CSF antibody to PLP is less common and less associated with inflammation than is CSF antibody to MBP (117).

IV. OTHER NONCELLULAR COMPONENTS

In addition to the cellular content and the immunoglobulin components of CSF, CSF also has a variety of substances which have been examined in patients with MS for clues to etiology and other aspects of the disease (1,2,6). Most of these analyses have centered on the changes either for diagnostic import or for disease activity relationships in MS. As previously reviewed (4), the materials sought have included (1) components of myelin that might enter CSF, (2) glial components that might represent responses to injury, and (3) proteinases and other materials that might be derived from the inflammatory cells or induced in resident glial cells of the CNS. Of the myelin components, only with MBP has sufficient information been acquired to characterize its role as a marker of disease activity. Studies of other myelin components, such as PLP (118), MAG (119), 2′, 3′-cyclic nucleotide 3′ phosphodiesterase (120), and a number of lipids and lipid-related enzymes (6,121–124) have revealed absent, minimal, or inconsistent abnormalities and have not been further pursued. The glial-derived components, such as the S-100 protein (125) and glial fibrillary acidic protein, have also revealed no information of dependable clinical value (126). Because of the increased level of proteinases in CNS lesions in MS (127), the levels of proteinases in the CSF have been examined in a number of laboratories. The specificity of the enzyme assays and the identity of the proteinases were often uncertain, making interpretation difficult. Except for occasional reports of abnormalities (128), these studies of proteinases have yet to reveal changes that would strongly encourage further study (127). Other substances that have been found to be elevated in CSF, such as neopterin, a cofactor in the synthesis of neurotransmitters and produced by macrophages

(129,130), and somatostatin (131), await further confirmation and analysis. Changes in the level of complement components in CSF (54,132) show no clear relationship to disease activity of MS.

Matrix metalloproteinases (MMPs) are enzymes, secreted by activated T-cells, macrophages, and multiple other cell types: they act on and degrade collagen present in the extracellular matrix and vascular endothelial basement membrane (133–137), convert procytokines—such as that for TNF-α (138–141)—to active molecules, degrade myelin proteins such as MBP (142,143), and possibly assist in remyelination (136). Through their action on basement membrane, MMPs enhance the ability of cells to transmigrate from the vascular lumen to the CNS parenchyma. Two members of this group, MMP-9 and MMP-2, have been demonstrated in the CNS of MS patients in and around MS lesions (144). CSF MMP-9 levels are higher in both RR and PP MS, and, in the case of former, there is a further increase during relapses (145–147). MMP-2, on the other hand, is present in the CSF of both inflammatory and noninflammatory CNS disorders, suggesting that it may be a constitutive enzyme (145). High serum MMP-9 levels correlate with Gd enhancement on cranial MRI, and this increase may precede the development of active lesions (148,149). Several lines of evidence suggest that an increase in serum MMP-9, either absolute or relative to the tissue inhibitors of metalloproteinases, is involved in the pathogenesis of MS, and these findings may have implications for future therapeutic development.

Initial proof that myelin-related materials could enter CSF as a result of myelin damage was provided by the observation that CNS myelin structures were present in the CSF sediment of individuals who had recent acute myelin damage (150). Beginning with this observation and supported by more sensitive radioimmunoassays reported since the mid-1970s (151,152), it has become evident that MBP or a fragment thereof may enter CSF and provide information about the status of CNS myelin damage as well as the potential response of the myelin damage to treatment. As with many radioimmunoassays, the analysis of CSF for content of MBP-like material is subject to many variables, among which are the antisera and the form of the assay utilized. Many antisera to MBP do not detect any material in the CSF and, depending on the radioligand used in the assay, different numbers and results may be obtained (153,154). Thus some of the information obtained from individual commercial or research laboratories or with MBP assay kits may differ because of different assays and reagents. The variation in assays and maintenance of quality of results has limited the utility of results obtained (2).

MBP has been studied extensively because of its ability to induce experimental allergic encephalomyelitis (EAE), a model of inflammatory demyelinating disease (155). It is synthesized by the oligodendrocyte or Schwann cell (156), in which it is encoded by a single gene of seven exons on chromosome 18 (157). MBP accounts for 30% of CNS myelin protein. The dominant form of MBP in the human has a molecular weight of 18,500 and is composed of 170 residues (156). Several investigators have demonstrated that MBP, immunochemically detected in CSF and referred to as MBP-like, is a marker for recent CNS myelin damage (4,151,152). Normally, CSF has no detected MBP-like materials within the valid sensitivity limits of the assay. Following an acute relapse of MS, MBP-like material rises quickly to the range of nanograms per milliliter and rapidly declines and disappears. The presence of MBP-like material in CSF in chronic and slowly progressive phases of the disease is unusual but may sometimes be detected in low levels, depending on the assay used for detection (154). The level of CSF MBP-like material is related to both the mass and time of myelin damage. Large lesions, especially those in the cervical spinal cord, and within 5 days of onset are correlated with high values. The appearance of CSF MBP-like material is not disease specific and may occur in other diseases, such as cerebral infarctions, in which CNS myelin is damaged. When the features of the MBP-like material in CSF have been carefully examined as to size, it has been demonstrated that the MBP-like material in MS tends to be smaller and to follow a closer time course with disease activity than is the case with cerebral infarcts (112) and head injury (158). The level of CSF MBP-like material is unrelated to CSF protein level, level of IgG, presence of OCBs, or pleocytosis (152,159). In more detailed studies of the specific portion of MBP-like material in CSF, one of the dominant epitopes present is in the decapeptide of 80-89 and can be readily detected with radioimmunoassays using radioligands of MBP peptides 45-89 (152) and 69-89 (154). It is likely that other fragments of MBP also appear in CSF during acute myelin damage or at other phases of disease, but that has yet to be defined with certainty.

The clinical utility of the assay for MBP-like material in CSF is largely to document the presence continuation or resolution of CNS myelin damage. An elevated level of CSF MBP-like material may serve as an adjunct in the diagnosis of disease even though it is not specific for disease type. In individuals who have a disabling form of MS and in whom the degree of deficit is already marked, the presence of CSF MBP-like material may also provide documentation for another exacerbation when this is clinically uncertain. The studies in which MBP-like material, immunoglobulin changes in CSF, and blood lymphocyte subsets have been examined in the same patients, only the CSF MBP-like material was shown to correlate with disease activity (152). Although it has been suggested that the level of MBP-like material in CSF may have implications about the future course of MS (160), the clinical period for follow-up is still too brief for conclusions to be reached. Reductions in MBP-like material in CSF of patients with MS who have been treated with either immunosuppressant drugs (161) or glucocorticoids (162) correlate well with clinical improvement. Because of the known rapid changes in the MBP-like material in the CSF of untreated MS patients, proof of therapeutic efficacy with controlled studies of adequate duration is not yet available. However, an increase in CSF MBP-like material has predictive value for a better response to glucocorticoids given for worsening of disease in MS (163).

The studies of MBP-like material in CSF have provided more firm documentation for the release of myelin markers into CSF, which presumably might enter CSF, blood, or urine through the mechanisms of normal turnover, demyelination, or synthesis of MBP in excess of that incorporated into myelin. The detection of MBP-like material in body fluids other than CSF would be of great value because of the resulting improved feasibility for objectively monitoring the natural history of MS and response to therapy. Studies on blood have yet to produce a valid assay of MBP-like material. Studies on urine (164) provide evidence that MBP-like material, though different in its features from that in CSF, may provide a correlate not with acute demyelination (165) but with progression of disease in MS (166).

V. CYTOKINES, CYTOKINE RECEPTORS, AND ADHESION MOLECULES IN THE CSF

The MS lesion contains cytokines, chemokines, adhesion molecules, and other soluble mediators required for the entry of inflammatory cells into the CNS parenchyma. As such, the CSF has been intensely studied for markers that might reflect inflammatory changes and disease activity in the CNS of MS patients. Technical aspects of measuring these substances have improved over the past few years, making the data more reliable. Possibly reflecting different MS patient populations studied, data on soluble materials in the CSF of MS patients is neither consistent nor conclusive and remain controversial. However, the potential importance of these molecules in the pathogenesis of MS warrants close attention to the information available.

A. TNF-α

TNF-α is a proinflammatory cytokine recognized to be an important mediator of immunologic and inflammatory responses in a variety of tissues, including the CNS (for review see (167–169). It has multiple effects on various cell populations in the CNS—including the ability to mediate myelin and oligodendrocyte damage *in vitro* (170,171), and to induce astrocyte proliferation—leading to the reactive gliosis associated with MS lesions (172) and affecting the expression of adhesion molecules on brain endothelial cells and astrocytes (for review, see Ref. 173). Studies to examine TNF-α expression in the CSF of MS patients have yielded conflicting data. Two groups did not detect TNF-α in the CSF of MS patients (174,175). Hauser et al. (176) detected higher levels of TNF-α in the CSF from patients with active MS than in MS patients in remission or patients with other neurologic diseases. Since there was no correlation between the degree of CSF pleocytosis and cytokine expression, they suggested that the TNF-α in CSF originated from cellular elements within the CNS rather than from immune cells in the CSF. Maimone et al. (177) detected TNF-α in the CSF of ~20% of MS patients and ~30% of patients with other inflammatory neurological diseases, which agrees with another study in which TNF-α was detected in the CSF of ~15% of patients with chronic progressive MS (178). The most compelling evidence for an association of TNF-α with MS comes from Sharief, et al. (179), who reported that increased TNF-α expression in the CSF of MS patients correlated with disease progression. Another study demonstrated that patients with relapsing-remitting (RR) MS in relapse showed significantly higher CSF levels of TNF-α compared with MS patients in remission (180). Sharief et al. (181,182) then went on to demonstrate that a strong correlation exists between increased CSF levels of TNF-α, disruption of the BBB, CSF pleocytosis, and increased levels of soluble intercellular adhesion molecule-1 (sICAM-1) in both the serum and CSF of patients with active MS.

Several recent studies have also supported a role for TNF-α in MS disease activity. First, even though statistical significance was not achieved, a prospective analysis revealed that TNF-α concentrations in the CNS of MS patients with RR-MS is associated with bursts of Gd-DTPA enhancement on MRI (183). Second, additional evidence supported the finding that CSF concentrations of TNF-α correlated with the degree of disability in MS patients (184). Third, highly elevated levels of MBP-reactive TNF-α mRNA-expressing cells were detected in MS patients' CSF, particularly during clinical exacerbations (185).

There are a number of factors which can account for the differences in the ability to detect TNF-α in the CSF of MS patients and correlate levels with disease progression. These include differences in the patients examined, timing of CSF collection, and the short half-life of TNF-α *in vivo*. TNF-α secreted within the CNS is likely to interact with TNF-α receptors on a variety of cells (T cells, macrophages, microglia, astrocytes, oligodendrocytes, and neurons), leaving little to reach lumbar CSF. Furthermore, many cell types express TNF-α in a functional membrane bound form (186), making it unavailable for detection in the CSF.

B. Interleukin-6 (IL-6)

IL-6, like TNF-α, is a pleiotropic cytokine involved in the regulation of inflammatory and immunologic responses (for review, see Ref. 187). IL-6 serves as the principal cytokine for inducing terminal differentiation of activated B cells into immunoglobulin-secreting plasma cells. Given its ability to promote astrogliosis, immunoglobulin production, and T-cell activation, IL-6 has been implicated in contributing to CNS inflammation and immune responsiveness. However, IL-6 also has some immunosuppressive effects, such as inhibition of TNF-α expression by macrophages and astrocytes (188,189), inhibition of ICAM-1, and vascular cellular adhesion molecule-1 (VCAM-1) expression by astrocytes and microglia (190,191), and induction of expression of soluble TNF-α receptors and the IL-1 receptor antagonist (192). Studies have also documented a protective effect of IL-6 in Theiler's virus induced demyelination and EAE (193,194).

    As already noted (see Secs. III. C and D), one of the hallmarks of MS is intrathecal B-cell activation as evidenced by elevation of the CSF IgG index and the presence of OCBs in the CSF. Since IL-6 is involved in differentiation of B cells into immunoglobulin secreting plasma cells, there has been interest in determining whether elevated IL-6 levels could be responsible for local B-cell responses within the CNS. Results have been conflicting; three groups report that IL-6 is not detected in MS CSF (54,176,195), while two other studies suggest that IL-6 is elevated in MS CSF (177) and MS plasma (196). More recent studies have not resolved this conflict; Navikas et al. (197) demonstrated that numbers of IL-6 mRNA expressing cells were highly enriched in the CSF of MS patients, while Padberg et al. (198) detected no difference in IL-6 CSF levels between controls and MS patients. Interestingly, in the latter study, CSF levels of soluble gp130, the signaling component of the IL-6 receptor (187), were significantly lower in MS versus patients with other neurological diseases (198). The relevance of this finding is not clear at present. Thus, in MS patients, no relationship between the incidence or the amount of intrathecal IgG synthesis or OCBs and IL-6 expression in the CSF has been observed.

C. Soluble Cytokine Receptors

Other studies have been conducted to determine if levels of circulating soluble cytokine receptors provide a better correlate with disease progression. The results are conflicting with respect to soluble TNF-R (sTNF-R). One study found that MS patients with RR-MS during a relapse and those with chronic progressive MS had significantly increased CSF levels of sTNF-R (199). A longitudinal study of MS patients undergoing monthly MRI did not show significant fluctuations in sTNF-R levels, and no correlations were noted with enhancing lesions on MRI (183). Currently, the data on soluble cytokine receptors in the CSF are sparse and the utility of measuring them is unclear.

D. Soluble Adhesion Molecules

MS is characterized by the migration of lymphocytes and monocytes from blood into the CNS, and subsequent invasion of the CNS parenchyma. A variety of adhesion molecules have been implicated in this process, and measurement of these proteins may serve as an indicator for inflammatory activity in MS. A circulating soluble form of ICAM-1 (sICAM-1) can be detected in the serum of normal individuals, and increased levels are found during various pathological conditions including inflammatory, immune, and malignant diseases (200). At present, the function of sICAM-1 is unknown. Increased expression of sICAM-1 is detected in both the serum and CSF of MS patients, and its presence correlates with relapses and with enhancing lesions on cranial MRI (181,201–210). Activated brain endothelial cells and astrocytes can serve as a CNS source for sICAM-1 (211,212). In this regard, astrocytes, upon stimulation with TNF-α, are capable of expressing membrane-bound ICAM-1, and then, in time, soluble forms of ICAM-1 appear (212). The proteolytic cleavage process for the conversion of membrane-associated ICAM-1 to sICAM-1 is sensitive to two inhibitors of metalloproteinases, implicating this family of enzymes in the generation of sICAM-1 (212). The increased intrathecal release of sICAM-1 likely reflects a strong immune response within the CNS and may serve as a valuable immunologic marker of the disease activity in MS.

Increased CSF sVCAM-1 levels have been found in MS patients during relapses (201,206,208). The level of sVCAM-1 and MRI markers of MS disease activity have been reported to correlate directly (213), and a significant relationship between the CSF/serum ratio for sVCAM-1 and the area of Gd-enhancing lesions has been observed (208). However, in MS patients treated with IFNβ-1b, a cytokine reducing the number and severity of relapses in MS, increased serum levels of sVCAM-1 were detected and correlated with a decrease in MRI lesion (214). Recent studies demonstrated that on *in vitro* treatment with sVCAM-1 the expression of VLA-4 is downregulated in blood lymphocytes (215). This could be a mechanism for the IFNβ-1b-mediated downregulation of VLA-4 in MS. It is possible that sVCAM-1 may play a role in quenching autoimmune responses either by inhibiting leukocyte extravasation through the BBB or affecting T-cell activation.

VI. CHANGES IN CSF RELATED TO TREATMENT OF RELAPSES AND DISEASE COURSE

Besides their role in the diagnosis and investigation of the pathogenesis of MS, cellular and soluble components of CSF have also been examined for possible changes related to treatment and therapeutic efficacy. The number of studies is small and the results are somewhat mixed. Given the presumed autoimmune nature of MS, it was postulated that CSF IgG—especially intrathecal IgG synthesis, which can be quantitated—may provide objective evidence of immunosuppression and benefit of a reagent. Intrathecal IgG synthesis rates correlate well with burden of disease on T2W cranial MRI (216,217), however, the CSF IgG synthesis rate has only a weak association with disease duration and disability status (88,218–221). Moreover, T2W changes on cranial MRI have only a weak correlation with clinical disability (222,223).

Different doses and treatment schedules of intramuscular adrenocorticotrophic hormone (ACTH), intravenous methylprednisolone (MP), and oral prednisone have been consistently shown to reduce *de novo* intrathecal IgG synthesis (224–226). This decrease in CSF IgG synthesis is primarily due to a decrease in IgG1 and IgG3 subclasses (227), the predominant IgG subclasses in OCBs. This effect usually does not result in normal values, and the magnitude and duration of this effect is variable depending on the nature of ACTH or glucocorticoid preparation, route of administration, pharmacological level achieved in the CSF, and possibly, the dose (224,226). Following treatment with ACTH or glucocorticoids, most studies demonstrate no change in the number or pattern of CSF OCBs determined by the most sensitive techniques (224–226, 228–231). An occasional patient may have a reduction in number or even disappearance of the banding pattern of CSF OCBs following intrathecal or intravenous MP therapy, which typically reverts to the baseline number and pattern of OCBs after discontinuation of treatment (225,226,232). There is usually no change in the number or differential of CSF leukocytes following treatment with ACTH or glucocorticoids (226). A reduction in the CSF levels of anti-MBP antibodies and anti-MAG antibodies and circulating immune complexes following treatment with high-dose oral prednisone has been reported (162,233). In contrast to these observations, a more recent study demonstrated that treatment with 1000 mg/day of intravenous MP for 10 days resulted in a persistent decrease in CSF MBP, mononuclear cells, IgG synthesis rate, and the number of OCBs for up to 1.6 years (234). These CSF changes were associated with a decrease in relapse rate but not with progression to disability or the rate of progression of disability in RR and progressive MS patients.

There is no change in the CSF OCB number or pattern in patients who are administered natural interferon alpha (235,236). Similarly, patients treated with weekly intrathecal natural beta interferon over a 2-month period did not have a change in their CSF IgG, IgG/total protein ratio or OCB pattern (237). Intramuscular interferon beta1a (IFNβ-1a; Avonex) treatment resulted in a significant decrease in CSF cell count but had no effect on IgG index, kappa light chains or OCBs (7). Data on the effects of IFNβ-1b (Betaseron), IFNβ-1a (Rebif) and glatiramer acetate (Copaxone), on these CSF variables have not been published. Although the effects of pharmacologic intervention on CSF MMP-9 have not been studied to date, treatment with IFNβ-1b or glucocorticoids results in a reduction in serum MMP-9 levels (147,238–240).

CNS irradiation results in a transient reduction in CSF IgG in MS patients (241, 242). This effect was greater and persisted longer if CNS radiation was combined with intramuscular ACTH and oral prednisone. These experimental therapies, however, had no effect on CSF IgG OCB number and pattern or on CSF kappa/lambda ratio. A decrease in CSF lymphocyte count, typically <2 cells per cubic millimeter by the third or fourth week and a modest concurrent transient increase in the number of CSF monocytes was noted in all patients given CNS irradiation. At the same time, an increase in CSF albumin was also seen, presumably due to BBB damage, because it disappeared when glucocorticoids were co-administered with CNS radiation.

High dose oral cyclophosphamide shifts the ratio of T-helper cells and T-suppressor cells present in the CSF in favor of the latter (25). Intravenous treatment with cytarabine (cytosine arabinoside, ara-C) did not change CSF IgG synthesis, OCB pattern, or leukocyte count in MS patients (243). Combination therapy with antilymphocytic globulin, azathioprine, and prednisone also had no effect on CSF OCB (91). The BBB and blood-CSF barrier prevent entry of systemically administered intravenous immunoglobulin (IVIg) into the brain parenchyma and CSF under normal physiological conditions (244). However, when the BBB is damaged, as is especially the case in MS with acute lesions, there may be transudation of IgG into the brain. A small increase in CSF IgG has been detected following administration of intravenous IVIg for various conditions (245).

In summary, the major effect of immunosuppressive and immunomodulatory therapy employed in MS is alteration, commonly reduction, in the de novo IgG synthesis. Other CSF changes, if occurring at all, are less frequent and of lesser degree. A summary of changes in CSF of MS patients related to pharmacological intervention is given in Table 3.

Table 3 Changes in CSF as a Result of Pharmacological Intervention in MS

Agent	IgG synthesis	Total IgG	IgG/Alb ratio	Alb	MBP	OCB	Cell count	Anti-MBP Ab	CIC
Systemic ACTH/Glucocorticoid	↓				↓	NC	NC	↓	↓
Intrathecal Glucocorticoid	↓	↓	↓	NC		NC			
CNS-RT	↓			↑		NC	↓		
Natural IFN-α						NC			
Natural IFN-β		NC	NC			NC			
Recombinant IFNβ-1a	NC					NC	↓		
Ara-C	NC		NC			NC	NC		
ALG + Aza + Pred						NC			

Key: ACTH, adrenocorticotrophic hormone; Alb, albumin; ALG, antilymphocytic globulin; Anti-MBP Ab, anti-myelin basic protein antibody; Ara-C, Cytarabine; Aza, azathioprine; CIC, circulating immune complexes; CNS-RT, central nervous system radiation therapy; IFN, interferon; IgG, immunoglobulin G; MBP, myelin basic protein; NC, no change; Pred, prednisone; OCB, oligoclonal bands; ↓, decreased; ↑, increased.

ACKNOWLEDGMENTS

The authors thank Mrs. Denise Ball and Ms. Linda Brent for assistance in the preparation of the manuscript.

REFERENCES

1. Merritt HH, Fremont-Smith F. The Cerebrospinal Fluid. Philadelphia, Saunders, 1937, pp 63–67, 270–272.
2. Fishman RA. Cerebrospinal Fluid in Diseases of the Nervous System. Philadelphia, Saunders, 1992, pp 213–214.
3. Walsh MJ, Tourtellotte WW. The cerebrospinal fluid in multiple sclerosis. In: Hallpike JF, Adams CMW, Tourtellotte WW, eds. Multiple Sclerosis. Baltimore, Williams & Wilkins, 1983, pp 275–358.
4. Whitaker JN, Snyder DS. Myelin components in the cerebrospinal fluid in diseases affecting central nervous system myelin. Clin Immunol Allergy 2:469–482, 1982.
5. Hauser SL, Reinherz EL, Hoban CJ, Schlossman SF, Weiner HL. CSF cells in multiple sclerosis: Monoclonal antibody analysis and relationship to peripheral blood T-cell subsets. Neurology 33:575–579, 1983.
6. Tourtellotte WW. The cerebrospinal fluid in multiple sclerosis. In: Vinken PJ, Bruyn GW, Klawans HL, Koetsier JC, eds. Handbook of Clinical Neurology, vol 47. Amsterdam: Elsevier, 1985, pp 79–130.
7. Rudick RA, Cookfair DL, Simonian NA, Ransohoff RM, Richert JR, Jacobs LD, Herndon RM, Salazar AM, Fischer JS, Granger CV, Goodkin DE, Simon JH, Bartoszak DM, Bourdette DN, Braiman J, Brownscheidle CM, Coats ME, Cohan SL, Dougherty DS, Kinkel RP, Mass MK, Munchsauer FE, OReilly K, Priore RL, Pullicino PM, Scherokman BJ, Wende K, Weinstock-Guttman B, Whitham RH. Cerebrospinal fluid abnormalities in a phase III trial of Avonex (IFN beta-1a) for relapsing multiple sclerosis. J Neuroimmunol 93(1–2):8–14, 1999.
8. Prineas JW. The Neuropathology of Multiple Sclerosis. In: Vinken PJ, Bruyn GW, Klawans HL, Koetsier JC, eds. Handbook of Clinical Neurology, vol 47. Amsterdam: Elsevier, 1985, pp 213–257.
9. Cohen S, Bannister R. Immunoglobulin synthesis within the central nervous system in disseminated sclerosis. Lancet 1:366–367, 1967.
10. Sandberg-Wollheim M, Zetterwall L, Muller R. In vitro synthesis of IgG by cells from the cerebrospinal fluid in a patient with multiple sclerosis. Clin Exp Immunol 4:401–405, 1969.

11. Henriksson A, Kam-Hansen S, Link H. IgM, IgA and IgG producing cells in cerebrospinal fluid in a patient with multiple sclerosis. Clin Exp Immunol 62:176–184, 1985.

12. Weber T, Rieckmann P, Jurgens S, Prange HW, Felgenhauer K. Immunocytochemical analysis of immunoglobulin-containing cells in CSF and blood in inflammatory disorders of the central nervous system. J Neurol Sci 86:61–72, 1988.

13. Hickey WF, Cohen JA, Burns JB. A quantitative immunohistochemical comparison of actively versus adoptively induced experimental allergic encephalomyelitis in the Lewis rat. Cell Immunol 109:272–281, 1987.

14. Barker CF, Billingham RE. Immunologically privileged sites. Adv Immunol 25:1–6, 1977.

15. Cruzner ML, Hayes GM, Newcombe J, Woodroofe MN. The nature of inflammatory components during demyelination in multiple sclerosis. J Neuroimmunol 20:203–209, 1988.

16. Hauser SL, Bhan AK, Gilles FH, Hoban CJ, Reinherz EL, Weiner HL. Immunohistochemical staining of human brain with monoclonal antibodies that identify lymphocytes, nomocytes and the Ia antigen. J Neuroimmunol 5:197–205, 1983.

17. Paterson PY, Day ED, Whitacre CC. Neuroimmunologic diseases: Effector cell responses and immunoregulatory mechanisms. Immunol Rev 55:89–120, 1981.

18. Paterson PY, Day ED. Current perspectives of neuroimmunologic disease: Multiple sclerosis and experimental allergic encephalomyelitis (1, 2). Clin Immunol Rev 1:581–697, 1982.

19. Traugott U, Scheinberg LC, Raine CS. On the presence of Ia positive endothelial cells and astrocytes in multiple sclerosis and its relevance to antigen presentation. J Neuroimmunol 8:1–9, 1985.

20. Wood JH. Neurobiology of cerebrospinal fluid. In: Wood JH, ed. Physiology, Pharmacology, and Dynamics of Cerebrospinal fluid, vol 1. New York: Plenum Press, 1980, pp 1–16.

21. Betz LA, Goldstein GM, Katzman R. Basic neurochemistry: molecular, cellular, and medical aspects. In: Siegal GJ, ed. Blood-Brain-Cerebrospinal Fluid Barriers. New York: Raven Press, 1989, pp 591–606.

22. Hafler DA, Weiner HL. In vivo labeling of blood T cells: Rapid traffic into cerebrospinal fluid in multiple sclerosis. Ann Neurol 22:89–93, 1987.

23. Burns J, Zweiman B, Lisak R. Tetanus toxoid reactive T lymphocytes in the cerebrospinal fluid of multiple sclerosis patients. Immunol Commun 13:361–369, 1984.

24. Svenningsson A, Andersen O, Edsbagge M, Stemme S. Lymphocyte phenotype and subset distribution in normal cerebrospinal fluid. J Neuroimmunol 63:39–46, 1995.

25. Brinkman CJJ, Nillesen WM, Hommes OR. T-cell subpopulations in blood and cerebrospinal fluid of multiple sclerosis patients: Effect of cyclophosphamide. Clin Immunol Immunopathol 29:341–348, 1983.

26. Bamborschke S, Heiss WD. Cerebrospinal fluid and peripheral blood leukocyte subsets in acute inflammation of the CNS. J Neurol Sci 79:1–2, 1987.

27. Kleine TO, Albrecht J, Zofel P. Flow cytometry of cerebrospinal fluid (CSF) lymphocytes: Alterations of blood CSF ratios of lymphocyte subsets in inflammation disorders of human central nervous system (CNS). Clin Chem Lab Med 37(3):231–241, 1999.

28. Elfont RM, Griffin DE, Goldstein GW. Enhanced endothelial cell adhesion of human cerebrospinal fluid lymphocytes. Ann Neurol 38(3):405–413, 1995.

29. DeFreitas EC, Sandberg-Wollheim M, Schonely K, et al. Regulation of interleukin-2 receptors on T cells from multiple sclerosis patients. Proc Natl Acad Sci USA 83:2637–2641, 1986.

30. Tournier-Lasserve E, Lyon-Caen O, Roullet E, et al. IL-2 receptor and HLA class II antigens on cerebrospinal fluid cells of patients with multiple sclerosis and other neurological diseases. Clin Exp Immunol 67:581–586, 1987.

31. Noronha A, Richman D, Arnason B. Multiple sclerosis: Activated cells in cerebrospinal fluid in acute exacerbations. Ann Neurol 18:722–725, 1985.

32. Reder AT, Arnason BGW. Immunology of multiple sclerosis. In: Vinken PJ, Bruyn GW,

Klawans HC, eds. Handbook of Clinical Neurology, vol 47. Amsterdam: Elsevier, 1985, pp 337–395.

33. Polman CH, deGroot CJA, Koetsier JC, Sminia T, Veerman AJP. Cerebrospinal fluid cells in multiple sclerosis and other neurological disease: An immunocytochemical study. J Neurol 234:19–22, 1987.

34. Cher DJ, Mosmann TR. Two types of murine helper T cell clone. II. Delayed-type hypersensitivity is mediated by TH1 clones. J Immunol 138(11):3688–3694, 1987.

35. Seder RA, Paul EW. Acquisition of lymphokine-producing phenotype by CD4+ T cells. Annu Rev Immunol 12:635–673, 1994.

36. Powrie F, Coffman RL. Cytokine regulation of T-cell function: Potential for therapeutic intervention. Immunol Today 14(6):270–274, 1993.

37. Mosmann TR, Coffman RL. TH1 and TH2 cells: Different patterns of lymphokine secretion lead to different functional properties. Annu Rev Immunol 7:145–173, 1989.

38. Kuchroo VK, Martin CA, Greer JM, Shyre-Te J, Sobel RA, Dorf ME. Cytokines and adhesion molecules contribute to the ability of myelin proteolipid protein-specific T cell clones to mediate experimental allergic encephalomyelitis. J Immunol 151:4371–4382, 1993.

39. Baron JL, Madri JA, Ruddle NH, Hashim G, Janeway CA. Surface expression of α4 integrin by CD4 T cells is required for their entry into brain parenchyma. J Exp Med 177(1):57–68, 1993.

40. Rotteveel FTM, Lucan CJ. T lymphocytes in the cerebrospinal fluid of patients with multiple sclerosis. Immunol Res 9:287–297, 1990.

41. Antonen J, Syrjala P, Oikarinen R, Frey H, Krohn K. Acute multiple sclerosis exacerbations are characterized by low cerebrospinal fluid suppressor/cytotoxic T-cells. Acta Neurol Scand 75:156–160, 1987.

42. Martino G, Olsson T, Fredrikson S, Hojeberg B, Kostulas V, Grimaldi LME, Link H. Cells producing antibodies specific for myelin basic protein region 70–89 are predominant in cerebrospinal fluid from patients with multiple sclerosis. Eur J Immunol 21:2971–2976, 1991.

43. Baig S, Olsson T, Yu-Ping J, B Höjeberg, Cruz M, Link H. Multiple sclerosis: Cells secreting antibodies against myelin-associated glycoprotein are present in cerebrospinal fluid. Scand J Immunol 33:73–79, 1991.

44. Soderstrom M, Link H, Xu Z, Fredriksson S. Optic neuritis and multiple sclerosis: Anti-MBP and anti-MBP peptide antibody-secreting cells are accumulated in CSF. Neurology 43: 1215–1222, 1993.

45. Sellebjerg FT, Frederiksen JL, Olsson T. Anti-myelin basic protein and anti-proteolipid protein antibody-secreting cells in the cerebrospinal fluid of patients with acute optic neuritis. Arch Neurol 51:1032–1036, 1994.

46. Levinson AI, Lisak RP, Zweiman B. A microtechnique for PHA transformation of 5000 separated lymphocytes. Cell Immunol 14:321–326, 1974.

47. Lisak RP, Zweiman B. In vitro cell-mediated immunity of cerebrospinal-fluid lymphocytes to myelin basic protein in primary demyelinating disease. N Engl J Med 297:850–853, 1977.

48. Levinson AI, Sandberg-Wollheim M, Lisak RP. Analysis of B-cell activation of cerebrospinal fluid lymphocytes in multiple sclerosis. Neurology 33:1305–1310, 1983.

49. Lisak RP, Zweiman B, Whitaker JN. Spinal fluid basic protein immunoreactive material and spinal fluid lymphocyte reactivity to basic protein. Neurology 31:180–182, 1981.

50. Noronha ABC, Richman DP, Arnason BGW. Detection of in vivo stimulated cerebrospinal-fluid lymphocytes by flow cytometry in patients with multiple sclerosis. N Engl J Med 303: 713–717, 1980.

51. Birnbaum G, Kotilinek L, Schwartz M, Sternad M. Spinal fluid lymphocytes responsive to autologous and allogeneic cells in multiple sclerosis and control individuals. J Clin Invest 74:1307–1317, 1984.

52. Birnbaum G, Aubitz S, Kotilinek L. Search for autonomously proliferating spinal fluid lymphocytes in patients with multiple sclerosis. Neurology 38:28–30, 1988.

53. Maier CC, Blalock JE. Cloning and sequencing immunoglobulin and T-cell receptor variable regions involved in neuroimmune disorders. Methods Neurosci 24:321–334, 1995.

54. Frei K, Leist TP, Meager A. Production of B-cell stimulatory factor-2 and interferon-γ in the central nervous system during viral meningitis and encephalitis: Evaluation in a murine model infection and in patients. J Exp Med 168:449–453, 1988.

55. Harlow E, Lane D. Antibodies: A Laboratory Manual. NY, Cold Spring Harbor Laboratory, 1988, pp 7–22.

56. Mendell JR, Kolkin S, Kissel JT, Weiss KL, Chakeres DW, Rammohan KW. Evidence for central nervous system demyelination in chronic inflammatory demyelinating polyradiculoneuropathy. Neurology 37:1291–1294, 1987.

57. Thomas PK, Walker RWH, Rudge P, et al. Chronic demyelinating peripheral neuropathy associated with multifocal central nervous system demyelination. Brain 110:53–76, 1987.

58. Kabat EA, Moore DH, Landow H. An electrophoretic study of the protein components in cerebrospinal fluid and their relationship to serum proteins. J Clin Invest 21:571–577, 1942.

59. Tiselius A, Kabat EA. An electrophoretic study of immune sera and purified antibody preparations. J Exp Med 69:119–131, 1939.

60. Kabat EA. Getting started 50 years ago-experiences, perspective, and problems of the first 21 years. Annu Rev Immunol 1:1–32, 1983.

61. Bibel DJ. Milestones in immunology. Berlin, Springer-Verlag, 1988, pp 94–98.

62. Kabat EA, Landow H, Moore DH. Electrophoretic patterns of concentrated cerebrospinal fluid. Proc Soc Exp Biol Med 49:260–263, 1942.

63. Kabat EA, Freedman DA, Murray JP, Knaub V. A study of the crystalline albumin, gamma globulin and total protein in the cerebrospinal fluid of one hundred cases of multiple sclerosis and in other diseases. Am J Med Sci 219:55–64, 1950.

64. Grossman RI, Gonzalez-Scarano F, Atlas SW, Galetta S, Silberberg DH. Multiple sclerosis: Gadolinium enhancement in MR imaging. Radiology 161:721–725, 1986.

65. Mingioli ES, Strober W, Tourtellotte WW, Whitaker JN, McFarlin DE. Quantitation of IgG, IgA and IgM in the CSF by radioimmunoassay. Neurology 28:991–995, 1978.

66. Tourtellotte WW, Parker PA. Multiple sclerosis: Correlation between immunoglobulin-G in cerebrospinal fluid and brain. Science 154:1044–1046, 1966.

67. Link H, Tibbling G. Principles of albumin and IgG analyses in neurological disorders: III. Evaluation of IgG synthesis within the central nervous system in multiple sclerosis. Scand J Clin Lab Invest 37:397–401, 1977.

68. Lefvert AK, Link H. IgG production within the central nervous system: A critical review of proposed formulae. Ann Neurol 17:13–20, 1985.

69. Tourtellotte W. On cerebrospinal fluid immunoglobulin G (IgG) quotients in multiple sclerosis and other diseases: A review and a new formula to estimate the amount of IgG synthesized per day by the central nervous system. J Neurol Sci 10:279–304, 1970.

70. Tourtellotte WW, Potvin AR, Fleming JO, et al. Multiple sclerosis: Measurement and validation of central nervous system IgG synthesis rate. Neurology 30:240–244, 1980.

71. Tourtellotte WW, Staugaitis SM, Walsh MJ, et al. The basis of intra-blood-brain-barrier IgG synthesis. Ann Neurol 17:21–27, 1985.

72. Whitaker JN. Quantitation of the synthesis of immunoglobulin G within the central nervous system. Ann Neurol 17:11–12, 1985.

73. Rudick RA, Whitaker JN. Cerebrospinal fluid tests for multiple sclerosis. In: Scheinberg P, ed. Neurology/Neurosurgery Update Series, vol. 7 (lesson 21). Princeton, NJ, CPEC, 1987, pp 1–8.

74. Lowenthal A, van Sande M, Karcher D. The differential diagnosis of neurological diseases by fractionating electrophoretically the CSF gamma-globulins. J Neurochem 6:51–56, 1960.

75. Farrell MA, Kaufmann JCE, Gilbert JJ, Noseworthy JH, Armstrong HA, Ebers GC. Oligoclonal bands in multiple sclerosis: clinical-pathological correlation. Neurology 35:212–218, 1985.

76. Mattson DH, Roos RP, Arnason BGW. Isoelectric focusing of IgG eluted from multiple sclerosis and subacute sclerosing panencephalitis brains. Nature 287:335–337, 1980.

77. Walsh MJ, Tourtellotte WW. Temporal invariance and clonal uniformity of brain and cerebrospinal IgG, IgA, and IgM in multiple sclerosis. J Exp Med 163:41–53, 1986.

78. Lucchinetti CF, Bruck W, Rodriguez M, Lassmann H. Distinct patterns of multiple sclerosis pathology indicates heterogeneity in pathogenesis. Brain Pathol 6(3):259–274, 1996.

79. Raine CS, Cannella B, Hauser SL, Genain CP. Demyelination in primate autoimmune encephalomyelitis and acute multiple sclerosis lesions: A case for antigen-specific antibody mediation. Ann Neurol 46(2):144–160, 1999.

80. Zeman AZJ, Keir G, Luxton R, Thompson EJ. Serum oligoclonal IgG is a common and persistent finding in multiple sclerosis, and has a systemic source. QJM 89(3):187–193, 1996.

81. Nagelkerken LM, Out TA. In vitro stimulated peripheral blood lymphocytes from multiple sclerosis patients produce idiotypes of oligoclonal CSF IgG. J Immunol 131:2328–2331, 1983.

82. Laurenzi MA, Mavra M, Kam-Hansen S, Link H. Oligoclonal IgG and free light chains in multiple sclerosis demonstrated by thin-layer polyacrylamide gel isoelectric focusing and immunofixation. Ann Neurol 8:241–247, 1980.

83. Keir G, Walker RWH, Thompson EJ. Oligoclonal immunoglobulin M in cerebrospinal fluid from multiple sclerosis patients. J Neurol Sci 57:281–285, 1982.

84. Grimaldi LME, Roos RP, Nalefski EA, Arnason BGW. Oligoclonal IgA bands in multiple sclerosis and subacute sclerosing panencephalitis. Neurology 35:813–817, 1985.

85. Bass BH, Armstrong H, Weinshenker B, Ebers GC, Noseworthy JH, Rice GPA. Interpretation of single band patterns in CSF protein electrophoresis. Can J Neurol Sci 15:20–22, 1988.

86. Kostulas VK, Link H, Lefvert AK. Oligoclonal IgG bands in cerebrospinal fluid: Principles for demonstration and interpretation based on findings in 1114 neurological patients. Arch Neurol 44:1041–1044, 1987.

87. Miller JR, Burke A, Bever CT. Occurrence of oligoclonal bands in multiple sclerosis and other CNS diseases. Ann Neurol 13:53–58, 1983.

88. Moulin D, Paty DW, Ebers GC. The predictive value of cerebrospinal fluid electrophoresis in "possible" multiple sclerosis. Brain 106:809–816, 1983.

89. Stendahl-Brodin L, Link H. Optic neuritis: Oligoclonal bands increase the risk of multiple sclerosis. Acta Neurol Scand 67:301–304, 1983.

90. Mattson DH, Roos RP, Arnason BW. Comparison of agar gel electrophoresis and isoelectric focusing in multiple sclerosis and subacute sclerosing panencephalitis. Ann Neurol 9:34–41, 1981.

91. Thompson EJ, Kaufmann P, Rudge P. Sequential changes in oligoclonal patterns during the course of multiple sclerosis. J Neurol Neurosurg Psychiatry 46:115–118, 1983.

92. Thompson AJ, Hutchinson M, Martin EA, Mansfield M, Whelan A, Feighery C. Suspected and clinically definite multiple sclerosis: The relationship between CSF immunoglobulins and clinical course. J Neurol Neurosurg Psychiatry 48:989–994, 1985.

93. Bulman DE, Pandey JP, Ebers GC. Gm allotypes in multiple sclerosis. In: Lowenthal A, Raus J, eds. Cellular and Humoral Immunological Components of Cerebrospinal Fluid in Multiple Sclerosis. New York: Plenum, 1987, pp 81–86.

94. Salier JP, Goust JM, Pandey JP, Fudenberg HH. Preferential synthesis of the G1m(1) allotype of IgG in the central nervous system of multiple sclerosis patients. Science 213:1400–1402, 1981.

95. Ebers GC. A study of CSF idiotypes in multiple sclerosis. Scand J Immunol 16:151–161, 1982.

96. Gerhard W, Taylor A, Sandberg-Wollheim M, Koprowski H. Longitudinal analysis of three intrathecally produced immunoglobulin subpopulations in MS patients. J Immunol 134:1555–1560, 1985.

97. Tachovsky TG, Sandberg-Wollheim M, Baird LG. Rabbit antihuman CSF IgG: I. Characterization of anti-idiotype antibodies produced against MS CSF and detection of cross-reactive idiotypes in several MS CSF. J Immunol 129:764–770, 1982.

98. Zhou SR, Maier CC, Mitchell GW, LaGanke CC, Blalock JE, Whitaker JN. A cross-reactive anti-myelin basic protein idiotope in cerebrospinal fluid cells in multiple sclerosis. Neurology 50(2):411–417, 1998.

99. LaGanke C, Freeman DW, Whitaker JN. Cross-reactive idiotypy in cerebrospinal fluid immunoglobulins in multiple sclerosis. Ann Neurol 47:87–92, 2000.

100. Link H, Muller H. Immunoglobulins in multiple sclerosis and infections of the nervous system. Arch Neurol 25:326–344, 1971.

101. Rudick RA, Pallant A, Bidlack JM, Herndon RM. Free kappa light chains in multiple sclerosis spinal fluid. Ann Neurol 20:63–69, 1986.

102. Rudick RA. Free light chain of immunoglobulins in multiple sclerosis: A Putative index of the intrathecal humoral immune response. In: Lowenthal A, Raus J, eds. Cellular and Humoral Immunological Components of Cerebrospinal Fluid in Multiple Sclerosis. New York: Plenum Press, 1987, pp 187–200.

103. Knopf PM, Harling-Berg CJ, Cserr HF, Basu D, Sirulnick EJ, Nolan SC, Park JT, Keir G, Thompson EJ, Hickey WF. Antigen-dependent intrathecal antibody synthesis in the normal rat brain: Tissue entry and local retention of antigen-specific B cells. J Immunol 161:692–701, 1998.

104. Ivanainen MV. The significance of abnormal immune responses in patients with multiple sclerosis. J Neuroimmunol 1:141–172, 1981.

105. Vartdal F, Vandvik B, Michaelsen TE, Loe K, Norrby E. Neurosyphilis: Intrathecal synthesis of oligoclonal antibodies to Treponema pallidum. Ann Neurol 11:35–40, 1982.

106. Vandvik B, Norrby E, Steen-Johnson J, Stensvold K. Mumps meningitis: Procerebrospinal fluid. Eur Neurol 17:13–22, 1978.

107. Vandvik B, Norrby E. Oligoclonal IgG antibody response in the central nervous system to different measles virus antigens in subacute sclerosing panencephalitis. Proc Natl Acad Sci USA 70:1060–1063, 1973.

108. Vartdal F, Norrby E. Viral and bacterial antibody responses in multiple sclerosis. Ann Neurol 8:248–255, 1980.

109. Whitaker JN, Chou CHJ, Chou FCH, Kibler RF. Molecular internalization of a region of myelin basic protein. J Exp Med 146:317–331, 1977.

110. Coyle PK, Brooks BR, Hirsh RL, et al. Cerebrospinal-fluid lymphocyte populations and immune complexes in active multiple sclerosis. Lancet 2:229–232, 1980.

111. Panitch HS, Hooper CJ, Johnson KP. CSF antibody to myelin basic proteins: Measurement in patients with multiple sclerosis and subacute sclerosing panencephalitis. Arch Neurol 37:206–209, 1980.

112. Bashir RM, Whitaker JN. Molecular features of immunoreactive myelin basic protein in cerebrospinal fluid of persons with multiple sclerosis. Ann Neurol 7:50–57, 1980.

113. Warren KG, Catz I. Diagnostic value of cerebrospinal fluid anti-myelin basic protein in patients with multiple sclerosis. Ann Neurol 20:20–25, 1986.

114. Warren KG, Catz I, Steinman L. Fine specificity of the antibody response to myelin basic protein in the central nervous system in multiple sclerosis: The minimal B-cell epitope and a model of its features. Proc Natl Acad Sci USA 92(24):11061–11065, 1995.

115. Wucherpfennig KW, Catz I, Hausmann S, Strominger JL, Steinman L, Warren KG. Recognition of the immunodominant myelin basic protein peptide by autoantibodies and HLA-DR2-restricted T cell clones from multiple sclerosis patients—Identity of key contact residues in the B-cell and T-cell epitopes. J Clin Invest 100(5):1114–1122, 1997.

116. Genain CP, Cannella B, Hauser SL, Raine CS. Identification of autoantibodies associated with myelin damage in multiple sclerosis. Nature Med 5(2):170–175, 1999.

117. Warren KG, Catz I, Johnson E, Mielke B. Anti-myelin basic protein and anti-proteolipid protein specific forms of multiple sclerosis. Ann Neurol 35:280–289, 1994.

118. Trotter JL, Wegerscheide CL, Garvey WF. Immunoreactive myelin proteolipid protein-like activity in cerebrospinal fluid and serum of neurologically impaired patients. Ann Neurol 14:464–469, 1983.

119. Yanagisawa K, Quarles RH, Johnson D, Brady RO, Whitaker JN. A derivative of myelin-associated glycoprotein (dMAG) in cerebrospinal fluid of normal subjects and patients with neurological disease. Ann Neurol 18:464–469, 1985.

120. Clapshaw PA, HW Müller, H Wiethölter, Seifert W. Simultaneous measurement of $2':3'$ cyclic-nucleotide $3'$ phosphodiesterase and RNase activities in sera and spinal fluids of multiple sclerosis patients. J Neurochem 42:12–15, 1984.

121. Neu IS. Essential fatty acids in the serum and cerebrospinal fluid of multiple sclerosis patients. Acta Neurol Scand 67:151–163, 1984.

122. Reiber H, Voss W. Cholesterol ester hydrolase activity in human cerebrospinal fluid. J Neurochem 34:1324–1326, 1980.

123. Ginns E, French J. A radioassay for G_{MI} ganglioside concentration in cerebrospinal fluid. J Neurochem 35:977–982, 1980.

124. Pitkänen ASL, Halonen TO, HO Kilpeläinen, Riekkinen PJ, et al. Cholesterol esterase activity in cerebrospinal fluid of multiple sclerosis patients. J Neurol Sci 74:45–53, 1986.

125. Massaro AR, Michetti F, Laudisio A, Bergonzi P. Myelin basic protein and S-100 antigen in cerebrospinal fluid of patients with multiple sclerosis in the acute phase. Ital J Neurol Sci 6:53–56, 1985.

126. Massaro AR, Carbone G. Cerebrospinal fluid markers in multiple sclerosis. In: Crescenzi GS, ed. A Multidisciplinary Approach to Myelin Disease. New York: Plenum, 1988, pp 267–274.

127. Bever CT, Whitaker JN. Proteinases in inflammatory demyelinating disease. Springer Semin Immunopath 8:235–250, 1985.

128. Inuzuka T, Sato S, Daba H, Mujatake T. Neutral protease in cerebrospinal fluid from patients with multiple sclerosis and other neurological diseases. Acta Neurol Scand 76:18–23, 1987.

129. Fredrikson S, Link H, Eneroth P. CSF neopterin as marker of disease activity in multiple sclerosis. Acta Neurol Scand 75:352–355, 1987.

130. Frederickson S, Eneroth P, Link H. Intrathecal production of neopterin in aseptic meningoencephalitis and multiple sclerosis. Clin Exp Immunol 67:76–81, 1987.

131. Sorensen KV. Somatostatin in multiple sclerosis. Acta Neurol Scand 75:161–167, 1987.

132. Gallo P, Piccinno M, Pagni S, Tavolato B. Interleukin-2 levels in serum and cerebrospinal fluid of multiple sclerosis patients. Ann Neurol 24:795–797, 1988.

133. Welgus HG, Campbell EJ, Cury JD, Eisen AZ, Senior RM, Wilhelm SM, Goldberg GI. Neutral metalloproteinases produced by human mononuclear phagocytes: Enzyme profile, regulation and expression during cellular development. J Clin Invest 86:1496–1502, 1990.

134. Conca W, Willmroth F. Human T lymphocytes express a member of the matrix metalloproteinase gene family. Arthritis Rheum 37:951–956, 1994.

135. Leppert D, Waubant E, Galardy R, Bunnett NW, Hauser SL. T cell gelatinases mediate basement membrane transmigration in vitro. J Immunol 154:4379–4389, 1995.

136. Uhm JH, Dooley NP, Oh LYS, Yong VW. Oligodendrocytes utilize a matrix metalloproteinase, MMP-9, to extend processes along an astrocyte extracellular matrix. Glia 22(1):53–63, 1998.

137. Birkedal-Hansen H, Moore WGI, Bodden MK, Windsor LJ, Birkedal-Hansen B, DeCarlo A, Engler JA. Metalloproteinases: A review. Crit Rev Oral Biol Med 4:197–250, 1993.

138. Gearing AJ, Beckett P, Christodoulou M, Churchill M, Clements J, Davidson AH, Drummond AH, Galloway WA, Gilbert R, Gordon JL, et al. Processing of tumour necrosis factor-alpha precursor by metalloproteinases. Nature 370(6490):555–557, 1994.

139. Crowe PD, Walter BN, Mohler KM, Otten-Evans C, Black RA, Ware CF. A metalloprotease inhibitor blocks shedding of the 80-kD TNF receptor and TNF processing in T lymphocytes. J Exp Med 181(3):1205–1210, 1995.

140. Arribas J, Coodly L, Vollmer P, Kishimoto TK, Rose-John S, Massague J. Diverse cell surface protein ectodomains are shed by a system sensitive to metalloprotease inhibitors. J Biol Chem 271(19):11376–11382, 1996.

141. Chandler S, Miller KM, Clements JM, Lury J, Corkill D, Anthony DCC, Adams SE, Gearing AJH. Matrix metalloproteinases, tumor necrosis factor and multiple sclerosis: An overview. J Neuroimmunol 72:155–161, 1997.

142. Proost P, Van Damme J, Opdenakker G. Leukocyte gelatinase-B cleavage releases encephalitogens from human myelin basic protein. Biochem Biophys Res Commun 192(3):1175–1181, 1993.

143. Chandler S, Coates R, Gearing A, Lury J, Wells G, Bone E. Matrix metalloproteinases degrade myelin basic protein. Neurosci Lett 201(3):223–226, 1995.

144. Cuzner ML, Gveric D, Strand C, Loughlin AJ, Paemen L, Opdenakker G, Newcombe J. The expression of tissue-type plasminogen-activator, matrix metalloproteinases and endogenous inhibitors in the central nervous system in multiple sclerosis: Comparison of stages in lesion evolution. J Neuropathol Exp Neurol 55:1194–1204, 1996.

145. Gijbels K, Masure S, Carton H, Opdenakker G. Gelatinase in the cerebrospinal fluid of patients with multiple sclerosis and other inflammatory neurological disorders. J Neuroimmunol 41:29–34, 1992.

146. Leppert D, Ford J, Stabler G, Grygar C, Lienert C, Huber S, Miller KM, Hauser SL, Kappos L. Matrix metalloproteinase-9 (gelatinase B) is selectively elevated in CSF during relapses and stable phases of multiple sclerosis. Brain 121:2327–2334, 1998.

147. Trojano M, Avolio C, Liuzzi GM, Ruggeiri M, Defazio G, Liguori M, Santacroce MP, Paolicelli D, Giuliani F, Riccio P, Livrea P. Changes of serum sICAM-1 and MMP-9 induced by rIFNβ-1b treatment in relapsing-remitting MS. Neurology 53:1402–1408, 1999.

148. Lee MA, Palace J, Stabler G, Ford J, Gearing A, Miller K. Serum gelatinase B, TIMP-1 and TIMP-2 levels in multiple sclerosis–A longitudinal clinical and MRI study. Brain 122:191–197, 1999.

149. Waubant E, Goodkin DE, Gee L, Bacchetti P, Sloan R, Stewart T, Andersson P-B, Stabler G, Miller K. Serum MMP-9 and TIMP-1 levels are related to MRI activity in relapsing multiple sclerosis. Neurology 53:1397–1401, 1999.

150. Herndon RM, Johnson M. A method for the electron microscopic study of cerebrospinal fluid sediment. J Neuropathol Exp Neurol 29:320–330, 1970.

151. Cohen SR, Herndon RM, McKhann GM. Radioimmunoassay of myelin basic protein in spinal fluid: An index of active demyelination. N Engl J Med 295:1455–1457, 1976.

152. Whitaker JN. Myelin encephalitogenic protein fragments in cerebrospinal fluid of persons with multiple sclerosis. Neurology 27:911–920, 1977.

153. Gupta MK, Whitaker JN, Johnson C, Goren H. Measurement of immunoreactive myelin basic protein peptide (45-89) in cerebrospinal fluid. Ann Neurol 23:273–280, 1988.

154. Whitaker JN, Herman PK. Human myelin basic protein peptide 69-89: Immunochemical features and use in immunoassays of cerebrospinal fluid. J Neuroimmunol 19:47–57, 1988.

155. Whitaker JN. Indicators of disease activity in multiple sclerosis: Studies of myelin basic protein-like materials. Ann NY Acad Sci 436:140–150, 1984.

156. Morell P, Quarles RH, Norton WT. Formation, structure and biochemistry of myelin. In: Siegel G, Agranoff B, Albers RW, Molinoff P, eds. Basic Neurochemistry. New York: Raven Press, 1989, pp 109–136.

157. Kamholz J, deFerra F, Puckett C, Lazzarini RA. Identification of three forms of human myelin basic protein by cDNA cloning. Proc Natl Acad Sci USA 83:4962–4966, 1986.

158. Karlsson B, Alling C. Molecular size of myelin basic protein immunoactivity in spinal fluid. J Neuroimmunol 6:141–150, 1984.

159. Warren KG, Catz I. The relationship between levels of cerebrospinal fluid myelin basic protein and IgG measurements in patients with multiple sclerosis. Ann Neurol 17:475–480, 1985.

160. Thompson AJ, Hutchinson M, Brazil J, Feighery C, Martin EA. A clinical and laboratory study of benign multiple sclerosis. QJ Med 58:69–80, 1986.

161. Lamers KJB, Uitdehaag BMJ, R HO., Doesburg W, Wevers RA, Geel WJA. The short-term effect of an immunosuppressive treatment on CSF myelin basic protein in chronic progressive multiple sclerosis. J Neurol Neurosurg Psychiatry 51:1334–1337, 1988.

162. Warren KG, Catz I, Carroll DJ. Effects of high-to-mega-dose synthetic corticosteroids on multiple sclerosis patients with special reference to cerebrospinal fluid antibodies to myelin basic protein. Clin Neuropharm 10:397–411, 1987.

163. Whitaker JN, Layton BA, Herman PK, Kachelhofer RD, Burgard S, Bartolucci AA. Correlation of myelin basic protein–like material in cerebrospinal fluid of multiple sclerosis patients with their response to glucocorticoid treatment. Ann Neurol 33:10–17, 1993.

164. Whitaker JN. The presence of immunoreactive myelin basic protein peptide in urine of persons with multiple sclerosis. Ann Neurol 22:648–655, 1987.

165. Whitaker JN, Williams PH, Layton BA, McFarland HF, Stone LA, Smith ME, Kachelhofer RD, Bradley EL, Burgard S, Zhao GJ, Paty DW. Correlation of clinical features and findings on cranial magnetic resonance imaging with urinary myelin basic protein-like material in patients with multiple sclerosis. Ann Neurol 35:577–585, 1994.

166. Whitaker JN, Kachelhofer RD, Bradley EL, Burgard S, Layton BA, Reder AT, Morrison W, Zhao GJ, Paty DW. Urinary myelin basic protein-like material as a correlate of the progression of multiple sclerosis. Ann Neurol 38:625–632, 1995.

167. Benveniste EN. The role of cytokines in multiple sclerosis/autoimmune encephalitis and other neurological disorders. In: Aggrawal B, Puri R, eds. Human Cytokines: Their Role in Research and Therapy. Boston: Blackwell, 1995, pp 195–216.

168. Merrill JE, Benveniste EN. Cytokines in inflammatory brain lesions: Helpful and harmful. Trends Neurosci 19(8):331–338, 1996.

169. Probert L, Selmaj K. TNF and related molecules: Trends in neuroscience and clinical applications. J Neuroimmunol 72(2):113–117, 1997.

170. Selmaj KW, Raine CS. Tumor necrosis factor mediates myelin and oligodendrocyte damage in vitro. Ann Neurol 23:339–346, 1988.

171. Robbins DS, Shirazi Y, Drysdale BE, Lieberman A, Shin HS, Shin ML. Production of cytotoxic factor for oligodendrocytes by stimulated astrocytes. J Immunol 139:2593–2597, 1987.

172. Selmaj KW, Farooq M, Norton WT, Raine CS, Brosnan CF. Proliferation of astrocytes in vitro in response to cytokines: A primary role for tumor necrosis factor. J Immunol 144:129–135, 1990.

173. Lee SJ, Benveniste EN. Adhesion molecule expression and regulation on cells of the central nervous system. J Neuroimmunol 98(2):77–88, 1999.

174. Gallo P, Piccinno MG, Krzalic L, Tavolato B. Tumor necrosis factor alpha (TNFα) and neurological diseases: Failure in detecting TNFα in the cerebrospinal fluid from patients with multiple sclerosis, AIDS dementia complex, and brain tumours. J Neuroimmunol 23:41–44, 1989.

175. Merrill JE, Strom SR, Elison GW, Myers LW. In vitro study of mediators of inflammation in multiple sclerosis. J Clin Immunol 9:84–96, 1989.

176. Hauser SL, Doolittle TH, Lincoln R, Brown RH, Dinarello CA. Cytokine accumulations in CSF of multiple sclerosis patients: Frequent detection of interleukin-1 and tumor necrosis factor but not interleukin-6. Neurology 40:1735–1739, 1990.

177. Maimone D, Gregory S, Arnason BGW, Reder AT. Cytokine levels in the cerebrospinal fluid and serum of patients with multiple sclerosis. J Neuroimmunol 32:67–74, 1991.

178. Franciotta DM, Grimaldi LME, Martino GV, Piccolo G, Bergamaschi R, Citterio A, Melzi

d'Eril GV. Tumor necrosis factor in serum and cerebrospinal fluid of patients with multiple sclerosis. Ann Neurol 26:787–789, 1989.

179. Sharief MK, Hentges R. Association between tumor necrosis factor-α and disease progression in patients with multiple sclerosis. N Engl J Med 325:467–472, 1991.

180. Tsukada N, Miyagi K, Matsuda M, Yanagisawa N, Yone K. Tumor necrosis factor and interleukin-1 in the CSF and sera of patients with multiple sclerosis. J Neurol Sci 102:230–234, 1991.

181. Sharief MK, Noori MA, Ciardi M, Cirelli A, Thompson EJ. Increased levels of circulating ICAM-1 in serum and cerebrospinal fluid of patients with active multiple sclerosis: Correlation with TNF-α and blood-brain barrier damage. J Neuroimmunol 43:15–22, 1993.

182. Sharief MK, Thompson EJ. In vivo relationship of tumor necrosis factor-α to blood-brain barrier damage in patients with active multiple sclerosis. J Neuroimmunol 38:27–34, 1992.

183. Spuler S, Yousry T, Scheller A, Voltz R, Holler E, Hartmann M, Wick M, Hohlfeld R. Multiple sclerosis: Prospective analysis of TNF-α and 55 kDa TNF receptor in CSF and serum in correlation with clinical and MRI activity. J Neuroimmunol 66(1–2):57–64, 1996.

184. Drulovic J, MostaricaStojkovic M, Levic Z, Stojsavljevic N, Pravica V, Mesaros S. Interleukin-12 and tumor necrosis factor-alpha levels in cerebrospinal fluid of multiple sclerosis patients. J Neurol Sci 147(2):145–150, 1997.

185. Matusevicius D, Navikas V, Soderstrom M, Xiao B-G, Haglund M, Fredrikson S, Link H. Multiple sclerosis: The proinflammatory cytokines lymphotoxin-α and tumour necrosis factor-α are upregulated in cerebrospinal fluid mononuclear cells. J Neuroimmunol 66:115–123, 1996.

186. Kriegler M, Perez C, DeFay K, Albert I, Lu SD. A novel form of TNF/cachectin is a cell surface cytotoxic transmembrane protein: ramifications for the complex physiology of TNF. Cell 53:45–53, 1988.

187. Taga T, Kishimoto T. gp130 and the interleukin-6 family of cytokines. Annu Rev Immunol 15:797–819, 1997.

188. Aderka D, Le J, Vilcek J. IL-6 inhibits lipopolysaccharide-induced tumor necrosis factor production in cultured human monocytes, U937 cells, and in mice. J Immunol 143:3517–3523, 1989.

189. Benveniste EN, Tang LP, Law RM. Differential regulation of astrocyte TNF-alpha expression by the cytokines TGF-beta, IL-6 and IL-10. Int J Dev Neurosci 13:341–349, 1995.

190. Shrikant P, Weber E, Jilling T, Benveniste EN. ICAM-1 gene expression by glial cells: Differential mechanisms of inhibition by interleukin-10 and interleukin-6. J Immunol 155:1489–1501, 1995.

191. Oh JW, VanWagoner NJ, RoseJohn S, Benveniste EN. Role of IL-6 and the soluble IL-6 receptor in inhibition of VCAM-1 gene expression. J Immunol 161(9):4992–4999, 1998.

192. Tilg H, Trehu E, Atkins MB, Dinarello CA, Mier JW. Interleukin-6 (IL-6) as an anti-inflammatory cytokine: induction of circulating IL-1 receptor antagonist and soluble tumor necrosis factor receptor p55. Blood 83:113–118, 1994.

193. Rodriguez M, Pavelko KD, McKinney CW, Leibowitz JL. Recombinant human IL-6 suppresses demyelination in a viral model of multiple sclerosis. J Immunol 153(8):3811–3821, 1994.

194. Willenborg DO, Fordham SA, Cowden WB, Ramshaw IA. Cytokines and murine autoimmune encephalomyelitis: inhibition or enhancement of disease with antibodies to select cytokine, or by delivery of exogenous cytokines using a recombinant vaccinia virus system. Scand J Immunol 41:31–41, 1995.

195. Houssiau FA, Bukasa K, Sindic CJM. Elevated levels of the 26K human hybridoma growth factor (interleukin 6) in cerebrospinal fluid of patients with acute infection of the central nervous system. Clin Exp Immunol 71:320–323, 1991.

196. Frei K, Fredrikson S, Fontona A, Link H. Interleukin-6 is elevated in plasma in multiple sclerosis. J Neuroimmunol 31:147–153, 1991.

197. Navikas V, Matusevicius D, Soderstrom M, Fredrikson S, Kivisakk P, Ljungdahl A, Hojeberg B, Link H. Increased interleukin-6 mRNA expression in blood and cerebrospinal fluid mononuclear cells in multiple sclerosis. J Neuroimmunol 64(1):63–69, 1996.

198. Padberg F, Feneberg W, Schmidt S, Schwarz MJ, Korschenhausen D, Greenberg BD, Nolde T, Muller N, Trapmann H, Konig N, Moller HJ, Hampel H. CSF and serum levels of soluble interleukin-6 receptors (sIL-6R and sgp130), but not of interleukin-6 are altered in multiple sclerosis. J Neuroimmunol 99:218–223, 1999.

199. Tsukada N, Matsuda M, Miyagi K, Yanagisawa N. Increased levels of intercellular adhesion molecule-1 (ICAM-1) and tumor necrosis factor receptor in the cerebrospinal fluid of patients with multiple sclerosis. Neurology 43(12):2679–2682, 1993.

200. Rothlein R, Mainolfi EA, Czajkowski M, Marlin SD. A form of circulating ICAM-1 in human serum. J Immunol 147:3788–3793, 1991.

201. Dore-Duffy P, Newman W, Balabanov R, Lisak RP, Mainolfi E, Rothlein R, Peterson M. Circulating, soluble adhesion proteins in cerebrospinal fluid and serum of patients with multiple sclerosis: Correlation with clinical activity. Ann Neurol 37:55–62, 1995.

202. Rieckmann P, Martin S, Weichselbraun I, Albrecht M, Kitze B, Weber T, Tumani H, Broocks A, Luer W, Helwig A, Poser S. Serial analysis of circulating adhesion molecules and TNF receptor in serum from patients with multiple sclerosis: cICAM-1 is an indicator for relapse. Neurology 44(12):2367–2372, 1994.

203. Rieckmann P, Nunke K, Burchhardt M, Albrecht M, Wiltfang J, Ulrich M, Felgenhauer K. Soluble intercellular adhesion molecule-1 in cerebrospinal fluid: An indicator for the inflammatory impairment of the blood-cerebrospinal fluid barrier. J Neuroimmunol 47(2):133–140, 1993.

204. Tsukada N, Miyagi K, Matsuda M, Yanagisawa N. Increased levels of circulating intercellular adhesion molecule-1 in multiple sclerosis and human T-lymphotropic virus type I-associated myelopathy. Ann Neurol 33:646–649, 1993.

205. H-P Hartung. Immune-mediated demyelination. Ann Neurol 33(6):563–567, 1993.

206. Droogan AG, Mcmillan SA, Douglas JP, Hawkins SA. Serum and cerebrospinal fluid levels of soluble adhesion molecules in multiple sclerosis: Predominant intrathecal release of vascular cell adhesion molecule-1. J Neuroimmunol 64(2):185–191, 1996.

207. Trojano M, Avolio C, Simone LL, Defazio G, Manzari C, De Robertis F, Calo A, Livrea P. Soluble intercellular adhesion molecule-1 in serum and cerebrospinal fluid of clinically active relapsing-remitting multiple sclerosis: Correlation with Gd-DTPA magnetic resonance imaging-enhancement and cerebrospinal fluid findings. Neurology 47:1535–1541, 1996.

208. Rieckmann P, Altenhofen B, Riegel A, Baudewig J, Felgenhauer K. Soluble adhesion molecules (sVCAM-1 and sICAM-1) in cerebrospinal fluid and serum correlate with MRI activity in multiple sclerosis. Ann Neurol 41(3):326–333, 1997.

209. Kraus J, Oschmann P, Engelhardt B, Schiel C, Hornig C, Bauer R, Kern A, Traupe H, Dorndorf W. Soluble and cell surface ICAM-1 as markers for disease activity in multiple sclerosis. Acta Neurol Scand 98(2):102–109, 1998.

210. Petersen AA, Sellebjerg F, Frederiksen J, Olesen J, Vejlsgaard GL. Soluble ICAM-1, demyelination, and inflammation in multiple sclerosis and acute optic neuritis. J Neuroimmunol 88(1–2):120–127, 1998.

211. Rieckmann P, Michel U, Albrecht M, Bruck W, Wockel L, Felgenhauer K. Cerebral endothelial cells are a major source for soluble intercellular adhesion molecule-1 in the human central nervous system. Neurosci Lett 186:61–64, 1995.

212. Lyons PD, Benveniste EN. Cleavage of membrane-associated ICAM-1 from astrocytes: Involvement of a metalloprotease. GLIA 22(2):103–112, 1998.

213. Giovannoni G, Lai M, Thorpe J, Kidd D, Chamoun V, Thompson AJ, Miller DH, Feldmann M, Thompson EJ. Longitudinal study of soluble adhesion molecules in multiple sclerosis: Correlation with gadolinium enhanced magnetic resonance imaging. Neurology 48(6):1557–1565, 1997.

214. Calabresi PA, Tranquill LR, Dambrosia JM, Stone LA, Maloni H, Bash CN, Frank JA, McFarland HF. Increases in soluble VCAM-1 correlate with a decrease in MRI lesions in multiple sclerosis treated with interferon β-1b. Ann Neurol 41:669–674, 1997.

215. Calabresi PA, Pelfrey CM, Tranquill LR, Maloni H, McFarland HF. VLA-4 expression on peripheral blood lymphocytes is downregulated after treatment of multiple sclerosis with interferon beta. Neurology 49(4):1111–1116, 1997.

216. Baumhefner RW, Tourtellote WW, Syndulko K, Ellison G, Myers L, Cohen SN, Shapshak P, Osborne M, Waluch V. Multiple sclerosis (MS): Correlations of quantified magnetic resonance imaged plaque area with clinical disability, instrumented neurologic function measurement (QENF), evoked potentials, and intra-BBB IgG synthesis. Neurology 37(suppl 1):231, 1987.

217. Baumhefner RW, Tourtellote WW, Syndulko K, Ellison G, Myers L, Cohen SN, Shapshak P, Osborne M, Waluch V. Quantitative multiple sclerosis plaque assessment with magnetic resonance imaging: Its correlation with clinical parameters, evoked potentials and intra-blood-brain-barrier IgG seynthesis. Arch Neurol 47(8):841–843, 1989.

218. Sand T, Sulg IA. Evoked potentials and CSF-immunoglobulins in MS: Relationship to disease duration, disability, and functional status. Acta Neurol Scand 82:217–221, 1990.

219. Ganes T, Brautaset NJ, Nyberg-Hansen R, Vandvik B. Multimodal evoked responses and cerebrospinal fluid oligoclonal immunoglobulins in patients with multiple sclerosis. Acta Neurol Scand 73:472–476, 1986.

220. Christensen O, Clausen J, Fog T. Relationships between abnormal IgG index, oligoclonal bands, acute phase reactants and some clinical data in multiple sclerosis. J Neurol 218:237–244, 1978.

221. Hutchinson M, Martin EA, Maguire P, Glynn D, Mansfield M, Feighery C. Visual evoked responses and immunoglobulin abnormalities in the diagnosis of multiple sclerosis. Acta Neurol Scand 68:90–95, 1983.

222. Thorpe JW, Kidd D, Moseley IF, Thompson AJ, Macmanus DG, Compston DAS, McDonald WI, Miller DH. Spinal MRI in patients with suspected multiple sclerosis and negative brain MRI. Brain 119(part 3):709–714, 1996.

223. Kidd D, Thorpe JW, Thompson AJ, Kendall BE, Moseley IF, MacManus DG, McDonald WI, Miller DH. Spinal cord MRI using multi-array coils and fast spin echo. II. Findings in multiple sclerosis. Neurology 43:2632–2637, 1993.

224. Durelli L, Cocito D, Riccio A, B C., Bergamasco B, Baggio GF, Perla F, Delsedime M, Gusmaroli G, Bergamini L. High-dose intravenous methylprednisolone in the treatment of multiple sclerosis: Clinical-immunologic correlations. Neurology 36:238–243, 1986.

225. Tourtellotte WW, Baumhefner RW, Potvin AR, Ma BI, Potvin JH, Mendez M, Syndulko K. Multiple sclerosis de novo CNS IgG synthesis: Effect of ACTH and corticosteroids. Neurology 30:1155–1162, 1980.

226. Baumhefner RW, Tourtellotte WW, Syndulko K, Staugaitis A, Shapshak P. Multiple sclerosis intra-blood-brain-barrier IgG synthesis: Effect of pulse intravenous and intrathecal corticosteroids. Ital J Neurol Sci 10:19–32, 1989.

227. Losy J, Michalowska-Wender G. The effect of large-dose Prednisone therapy on IgG subclasses in multiple sclerosis. Acta Neurol Scand 89:69–71, 1994.

228. Brooks BR, Jubelt B, Cohen S, P O'Donnell, Johnson TR, McKhann GM. Cerebrospinal fluid (CSF) myelin basic protein (MBP) in multiple sclerosis (MS): Effect of prolonged high single-dose alternate-day prednisone therapy. Neurology 29:548, 1979.

229. Olsson JE, Nilsson K. Gammaglobulins of CSF and serum in multiple sclerosis: Isoelectric focusing on polyacrylamide gel and agar gel electrophoresis. Neurology 29:1383–1391, 1979.

230. Hershey LA, Trotter JL. The use and abuse of the cerebrospinal fluid IgG profile in the adult: A practical evaluation. Ann Neurol 8:426–434, 1980.

231. Baumhefner RW, Mendex M, Ma BI, Tourtellotte WW. Modulation of de novo central ner-

vous system (CNS) IgG synthesis with preservation of oligoclonal IgG in multiple sclerosis (MS). Neurology 29:549, 1979.

232. Trotter JL, Garvey WF. Prolonged effects of large-dose methylprednisolone infusion in multiple sclerosis. Neurology 30:702–708, 1980.

233. Wajgt A, Gorny MK, Jenek R. The influence of high-dose prednisone medication on autoantibody specific activity and on circulating immune complex level in cerebrospinal fluid of multiple sclerosis patients. Acta Neurol Scand 68:378–385, 1983.

234. Frequin STFM, Lamers KJB, Barkhof F, Borm GF, Hommes OR. Follow-up study of MS patients treated with high-dose intravenous methylprednisolone. Acta Neurol Scand 90:105–110, 1994.

235. Panitch HS, Francis GS, Hooper CJ, Merigan TC, Johnson KP. Serial immunological studies in multiple sclerosis patients treated systemically with human alpha interferon. Ann Neurol 18:434–438, 1985.

236. Rice GPA, Talbot P, Woelfel EM, et al. Immunological observations in patients with multiple sclerosis treated with human alpha Interferon (abstr). Neurology 34(suppl 1):112, 1984.

237. Confavreux C, Chapuis-Cellier C, Arnaud P, Robert O, Aimard G, Devic M. Oligoclonal "fingerprint" of CSF IgG in multiple sclerosis patients is not modified following intrathecal administration of natural beta-interferon. J Neurol Neurosurg Psychiatry 49:1308–1312, 1986.

238. Leppert D, Waubant E, Burk MR, Oksenberg JR, Hauser SL. Interferon beta-1b inhibits gelatinase secretion and in vitro migration of human T cells: A possible mechanism for treatment efficacy in multiple sclerosis. Ann Neurol 40:846–852, 1996.

239. Stuve O, Dooley NP, Uhm JH, Antel JP, Francis GS, Williams G, Yong VW. Interferon β-1b decreases the migration of T lymphocytes in vitro: Effects on matrix metalloproteinase-9. Ann Neurol 40:853–863, 1996.

240. Rosenberg GA, Dencoff JE, Correa N, Reiners M, Ford CC. Effect of steroids on CSF matrix metalloproteinases in multiple sclerosis: Relation to blood-brain barrier injury. Neurology 46:1626–1632, 1996.

241. Tourtellotte WW, Murthy K, Brandes D, Sajben N, Ma B, Comiso P, Potvin A, Costanza A, Korelitz J. Schemes to eradicate the multiple sclerosis central nervous system immune reaction (abstr). Neurology 26(6):59–61, 1976.

242. Tourtellotte WW, Potvin AR, Baumhefner RW, Potvin JH, Ma BI, Syndulko K, Petrovich Z. Multiple sclerosis de novo CNS IgG synthesis. Effect of CNS Irradiation. Arch Neurol 37:620–624, 1980.

243. Tourtellotte WW, Potvin AR, Mendez M, Baumhefner RW, Potvin JH, Ma BI, Syndulko K. Failure of intravenous and intrathecal cytarabine to modify central nervous system IgG snythesis in multiple sclerosis. Ann Neurol 8:402–408, 1980.

244. Fazekas F, Deisenhammer F, StrasserFuchs S, Nahler G, Mamoli B. Treatment effects of monthly intravenous immunoglobulin on patients with relapsing–remitting multiple sclerosis: Further analyses of the Austrian immunoglobulin in MS study. Mult Scler 3(2):137–141, 1997.

245. Wurster U, Haas J. Passage of intravenous immunoglobulin interaction with the CNS. J Neurol Neurosurg Psychiatry 57:21–25, 1994.

15

Laboratory Tests: Evoked Potentials

MARC R. NUWER

UCLA School of Medicine and UCLA Medical Center, Los Angeles, California

I. INTRODUCTION

Evoked potentials (EPs) are electrical potentials generated by the nervous system that are evoked by certain sensory stimuli. These tests have been used for the past 25 years by clinicians seeking to diagnose multiple sclerosis (MS). They have also been applied in research into the pathophysiology of demyelination and as an adjunct in MS therapeutic trials. EPs have found a permanent role in these several diagnostic and research areas.

EPs are sensitive, objective, and reproducible; they can be quantified easily to two or three significant figures. They can detect "silent lesions," i.e. physiological changes not accompanied by physical signs or localizing symptoms. The finding of silent lesions can help diagnose MS by providing evidence of a second or third lesion. The tests are objective because they require no patient participation beyond lying quietly or watching a video screen. A patient cannot alter the results. The reader scores the tests in a standard manner, which leaves little room for subjective error. EPs are reproducible, yielding identical values as long as the conditions of the testing are well controlled. The fact that these tests can be readily quantified makes it easy to compare their results with normal values. Quantified parametric measurements and statistics are also substantially more powerful tools than discontinuous categorical variables (e.g., mild/moderate/severe or better/worse/unchanged scoring) for evaluating scientific hypotheses.

EPs represent electrical potentials (voltages) that are evoked by brief sensory stimuli. Nerve volleys associated with EPs are conducted along the peripheral and central nervous system pathways associated with the stimulated sensory modality. These nervous system signals become delayed or blocked when they cross through a demyelinated region. EP electrophysiology has been well studied, including the effects of demyelination (1–5). In classic demyelination, a delay in conduction occurs through the region of impairment, up to complete conduction blocks across a demyelinated region. The EPs generated from beyond the demyelination are abnormal because they are delayed, attenuated, or absent. Substantial knowledge exists about which EPs come from various locations around the nervous system. With this knowledge, the EP reader can determine the approximate level of the nervous system at which a delay or a block probably has occurred. In turn this allows a clinician to assess which parts of the nervous system have been impaired in an individual patient. However, EPs can test only a few selected portions of the nervous system: the central visual pathways, the brainstem auditory pathways, and the posterior column/medial lemniscus/internal capsule sensory pathways. There is not yet any EP that can test spinothalamic or cerebellar pathways. EP testing of the pyramidal tract central motor pathways is becoming clinically available as a diagnostic test (6–8).

EPs have also been used in many other areas of neurological practice beyond MS. Brainstem auditory EPs are used to screen for hearing impairment (9). All three EP sensory modalities (visual, auditory, and somatosensory) are used for evaluation of comatose patients, allowing quantified assessment of degree of impairment (10,11) and help in assessing locations of lesions. Hereditary-degenerative neurologic conditions are associated with specific patterns of changes in various EP peaks, which is sometimes useful in the diagnostic evaluation of these conditions (12). EPs can be monitored in the operating room, allowing for identification of nervous system impairment early enough to allow intervention to correct the impairment before it becomes permanent (13). The presence of normal EPs despite severe symptoms can help confirm conversion hysteria or malingering. EPs can also help separate peripheral from central or separate spinal from intracranial localization for a variety of sensory disorders, analogous to the use of the tendon reflexes for separating central from peripheral motor pathway disorders.

II. VISUAL EVOKED POTENTIALS

Visual EPs (VEPs) can be elicited with either a strobe flash or a checkerboard-patterned reversal device. Use of the flash technique for MS was described first (14), but the pattern reversal VEP technique subsequently was found to be clearly more sensitive for detecting demyelinating lesions (15). Pattern reversal is typically a checkerboard of black and white squares, in which each white square becomes black and each black square becomes white twice each second. This can be accomplished on a television screen controlled by a small computer or with a mirror and galvinometer. The subject is usually tested one eye at a time in a darkened room. Recordings are made over the occipital scalp. Measurements are made to the large positive electrical polarity peak seen about 100 ms after each checkerboard reversal. About 100 separate stimulus presentations are performed, and their results averaged together to help eliminate random background ''noise'' such as EEG and ECG. The positive polarity peak seen at 100 ms is usually called P100. This peak represents the culmination of a series of neurological events. These events begins with potentials conducted out of the eye along the optic nerve, across the chiasm, and down the optic tract to the lateral geniculate body. From there the signal travels up the optic radiations, passing directly through the periventricular white matter for rather long distances until it reaches occipital cortex. Substantial processing occurs at the occipital region for up to 50 ms after the initial impulse arrival there. Finally, a large electrical surface positive peak is generated from striate cortex and detectable at the occipital scalp as the P100 peak.

In MS, impairment may occur at several points along this pathway, not just at the optic nerve but also along the optic tract and especially in the periventricular white matter.

Prechiasmatic lesions at the optic nerve can be separated from the postchiasmatic lesions by testing the two eyes separately. Interocular discrepancies in P100 latencies are usually attributed to lesions at the optic nerve, for obvious anatomical reasons.

VEPs are more sensitive to demyelination than even a careful clinical examination of visual function (16–18). When VEPs were compared with to careful neuroophthalmologic examination in 198 MS patients, there was never an abnormality in the clinical examination when the VEP was normal (17). When the VEP was abnormal, various clinical examinations were often normal. For example, when the VEP was abnormal, 96% of patients had normal visual fields by confrontation, 55% had normal visual fields by formal testing, 74% had normal pupillary responses, 39% had normal appearance of the optic fundus, and there was no red color desaturation in 27% of patients carefully tested.

The checkerboard-reversal pattern VEP technique is abnormal in almost all patients who have a clear history of optic neuritis. In a summary of various reports in the medical literature (19–43), Chiappa (18) noted that about 90% of patients with optic neuritis showed abnormal pattern VEPs, with the percentage closer to 100% in many of the individual research reports. When there was no clinical evidence for optic neuritis, the VEPs still were abnormal in 51% of 715 MS patients. See Table 1.

VEPs tend to worsen monotonically. Once a lesion has occurred and the VEP has become delayed, only modest improvement occurs even after many years (44). In this way, VEPs can help to establish whether an episode of suspicious visual changes many years ago was indeed due to an episode of optic neuritis. This is, of course, of great value in diagnosis of MS. Patients presenting with single spinal cord or brainstem lesions are often referred for VEP studies to determine whether optic neuritis has occurred at any time in past years. The finding of such a second visual system lesion has helped substantially in establishing many a diagnosis of MS.

Other disorders can also affect VEP latencies. Some hereditary-degenerative neurologic conditions—e.g., Friedreich's ataxia (12) and adrenoleukodystrophy (45) as well as B12 deficiency (46), neurosyphillis (47) and other disorders (48)—can slow P100 latencies. Occasionally, these latter conditions may produce some interocular differences in P100 latencies. But a substantial difference in interocular latency is usually due to MS, and finding a large interocular latency difference does substantially help establish that a plaque of demyelination is the cause of a VEP abnormality. MS can sometimes cause symmetrical

Table 1 Rates of Abnormalities for Evoked Potentials in MS: Aggregate Results of 26–31 Separate Research Series

	Pattern visual	Brainstem auditory	Somatosensory
Number of patients	1950	1006	1006
Number of research series	26	26	31
Rates of EP abnormality:			
Definite MS	85%	67%	77%
Probable MS	58%	41%	67%
Possible MS	37%	30%	49%
Asymptomatic patients	51%	38%	42%
All patients	63%	46%	58% (upper extremity) 76% (lower extremity)

Source: From Ref. 18.

P100 delays by bilateral symmetrical demyelination. As such, the finding of bilaterally symmetrical P100 delays is considered confirmatory for an abnormality but nonspecific for the particular type of pathology. Overall, a VEP abnormality cannot be considered absolutely pathognomonic of MS. Clinical correlation is useful in each of these circumstances.

The VEP is about twice as sensitive as MRI for detecting demyelinating lesions in the optic nerves, chasm and optic tracts (49–52). In searching for a second lesion in patients with known optic neuritis, brain MRI is more sensitive than VEP of the unaffected eye (49,53). In patients with early MS, MRI has been compared to VEPs in several studies. Brain MRI was abnormal in 46 to 62% of these patients (52,54–55).

For patients with acute or chronic spinal cord lesions being evaluated for a diagnosis of MS, multimodality EPs had a higher yield of abnormalities (69% sensitivity) and a lower false-positive rate (5% false-positives for EPs compared to 9% for MRI). VEPs alone, however, had only a modest diagnostic yield (7 to 28%) in patients initially presenting with spinal lesions (57). VEPs are also helpful in clarifying the nature of signal enhancing MRI lesions by helping to separate MS from the dozen or so other causes of such lesions mimicking those of MS (58). The time course of resolution of gadolinium enhancement in optic neuritis parallels the time course of improvement in the VEP latency (59).

VEPs have been used to study the physiology of demyelination. The latencies and amplitudes can be affected by heat and by medications that alter conduction across a demyelinated plaque. Heat alters VEPs (60–62) in a way similar to the clinical Uhthoff's phenomenon or the hot bath test. For the VEP, these effects can be quantified more precisely. Hyperventilation can improve the VEP, causing some improved amplitudes and even shorter latencies (63). This is in keeping with previous observations that hyperventilation, alkalosis, and hypocalcemia can bring about transient improvements in clinical deficits. The calcium channel blocker verapamil (64) and the potassium channel blocker 4-aminopyridine (65) can also substantially improve VEPs transiently in some patients.

The genetics of MS have been studied using VEPs (66). A few symptomatic first-degree relatives of MS patients were found to have mildly abnormal P100 VEP interocular latency asymmetries. This may be related to a genetic predisposition toward subclinical pathology, such as plaques of edema without demyelination or with only subtle demyelination. For epidemiological reasons, most of these abnormalities are unlikely to go on to develop into frank clinical MS. Some additional factor is needed to change silent lesions like these into lesions associated with clinical MS. This may give some hints as to the underlying multifactorial nature of MS.

Overall, checkerboard-reversal-pattern VEPs have proven themselves to be a substantial help in clinical evaluation of individual patients when MS is under consideration. The finding of abnormalities in these visual pathways is common, even in patients with no other clinical indications of central visual pathway impairment. VEPs are more sensitive than MRI in detecting optic neuritis. In typical clinical circumstances, these tests are useful in clarifying whether a previous visual event was or was not optic neuritis, and in looking for visual pathway impairment in patients with single brainstem or spinal cord lesions.

II. BRAINSTEM AUDITORY EVOKED POTENTIALS

Signals from brainstem auditory pathway generators can be detected at the scalp. These signals represent activation of brainstem pathways after presentation of a 100-μs click through earphones. Pathways involved are probably those associated with the ability to localize an auditory stimulus in space rather than those used for speech or tone discrimination. These pathways lie exclusively in the pons and midbrain. These auditory EP tests are unable to detect lesions except for those located in the specific brainstem pathways tested here. They fail to detect lesions at or below the medulla or at the thalamus and above. But these tests are so sensitive that they can pick up a delay of just a fraction of a millisecond when it does lie in the specific brainstem pathways tested.

The eighth nerve is the generator of wave I. The presence of this wave I peripheral potential is valuable in assessing that the click stimulus had been adequately processed by the cochlea and other peripheral portions of the auditory pathway. Of course, this wave I is almost universally normal in MS patients who have no additional specific ear-related problems. The brainstem auditory EP (BAEP) has four succeeding waves, labeled II to V. They are shown in Fig. 1. These arise from within the brainstem itself. Wave II is generated around the cochlear nucleus, at the caudal pons. Wave III arises around the superior olive and trapezoid body in the central pons. Waves IV and V probably arise from regions around the lateral lemniscus bilaterally, as each of these pathways travels rostrally toward inferior colliculus. Central nervous system lesions can be localized by observing which of these waves has been disrupted or delayed. The left-right laterality of lesions is more difficult to assess for lower midbrain or upper pontine lesions. The laterality is fairly straightforward for lower pontine lesions. Impairment of the BAEP usually corresponds clinically to disruption of nuclei and pathways in the deep pons. Internuclear ophthalmoplegia is the most common clinical sign correlating with BAEP abnormalities. Other brainstem signs have a lesser degree of correlation. Vertigo, dysarthria, and dysphagia correlate poorly with BAEP abnormalities (see Table 2).

The typical abnormalities found in MS patients include a prolongation of waves II to V as determined by the I to V interpeak latencies and a loss of amplitude of wave V, determined by V/I amplitude ratio, and disappearance of V. Each of these types of

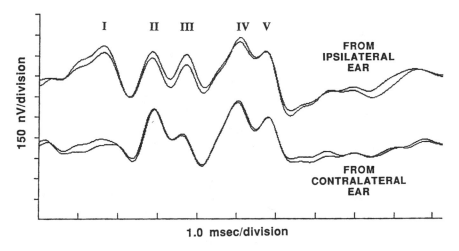

Figure 1 Brainstem auditory evoked potentials, identifying the five main peaks. (From Ref. 157.)

Table 2 Correlation Between Degree of Brainstem
Auditory EP Abnormality and MS Patient Signs and
Symptoms

Correlation with change in BAEPs	
	History
0.41	Diplopia
0.23	Dysphagia
0.16	Vertigo
0.12	Hearing impairment
0.10	Dysarthria
0.03	Facial sensory impairment
	Physical signs
0.39	Ocular dysmetria or gaze paresis
0.32	Nystagmus
0.29	Facial weakness
0.25	Dysarthria
0.23	Facial sensory loss
0.21	Slow tongue movements
0.09	Other brainstem signs
0.04	Subjective hearing threshold

Source: From Ref. 156.

abnormalities is about equally as common. Figure 2 shows examples of various degrees of BAEP abnormalities in MS patients.

Other types of neurological disorders can also affect the BAEPs. These include damage from tumors (67,68) and ischemia (68) as well as changes associated with some hereditary degenerative neurological disorders (12). As such, BAEP abnormalities cannot be considered pathognomonic of MS. Rather, these abnormalities just indicate the presence of impairment at a pontine or lower midbrain level.

Chiappa (18) has summarized aggregate results from research reports (32,70–92), which included approximately 1000 MS patients (see Table 1). Among these patients, 46% had abnormal BAEPs. Among patients having no history or physical signs of brainstem abnormalities, 38% had EP abnormalities, with abnormality rates in individual studies varying between 21 and 55%. The latter represent clinically silent lesions detected by these EP techniques.

BAEPs have repeatedly been found to be more sensitive to detecting pontine lesions than are MRI tests (93–96). Brain MRI is more sensitive than BAEP to inpatients undergoing an evaluation to diagnose MS. Among three studies directly comparing the two tests, brain MRI was abnormal among 68 to 83% of patients, whereas BAEP was abnormal among 41 to 50% of patients (55,95,97).

Overall, BAEP seems an appropriate clinical tool to confirm that cranial nerve or other signs or symptoms are due to central, brainstem impairment as opposed to impairment along the peripheral pathways. The test is sensitive to impairment at pons and lower midbrain. For that specific purpose, it is probably more sensitive than brain MRI. For

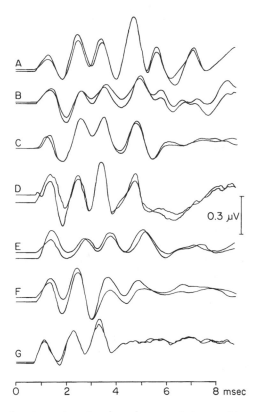

Figure 2 Examples of various degrees of abnormality in the brainstem auditory EP test in MS. The upper EP traces are less affected and the lower traces are more affected. Demyelination causes some prolongation of latencies, with loss of amplitude and eventual absence of peaks II to V. (From Ref. 156.)

the general setting of evaluating possible MS patients, brain MRI has a higher yield of abnormality.

IV. SOMATOSENSORY EVOKED POTENTIALS

Somatosensory modality testing usually begins with the delivery of a brief electrical stimulus to the median nerve at the wrist, or to the posterior tibial nerve at the ankle. Peripheral recordings are taken from electrodes located over the brachial plexus or the lumbar spinal cord. More rostral recording electrodes are placed over the cervical spinal cord and the scalp. Electrodes at these latter locations can detect electrical potentials signaling passage through progressively more rostral central nervous system tracts and nuclei. The pathways underlying somatosensory EPs (SEPs) are the posterior columns, medial lemniscus, and internal capsule. At present there are no satisfactory EPs for testing the spinothalamic pathways.

For median nerve EPs, the principle peaks detected are generated at the brachial plexus, midcervical cord, cervicomedullary junction, or nearby the thalamus, and finally at the rolandic fissure (see Fig. 3). For posterior tibial nerve EPs, reliable potentials are usually only found for the lumbar cord and rolandic fissure generator sites. Occasionally additional posterior tibial nerve SEP peaks can be detected over the rostral spinal cord or at brainstem levels, but these additional peaks are difficult to record in many normal subjects.

Comparison of the latencies and amplitudes of these various peaks can help the clinical reader determine the anatomic level of disruption along these sensory pathways. In many circumstances, EPs can locate specific levels of disruption along these pathways. This is useful in possible MS, where diagnosis requires finding lesions in separate locations. It is also useful in other neurological evaluations in which approximate anatomic localization is valuable.

Chiappa (18) has summarized the aggregate results from clinical studies on abnormality rates for median nerve SEPs in MS (29–35,44,77–80,98–119). Median nerve SEP abnormalities were seen in 42% of MS patients who had *no* signs of symptoms of sensory systems impairment and in 75% of patients who *did* have signs or symptoms of appropriate sensory abnormalities. Posterior tibial nerve SEPs have revealed a slightly greater rate of finding clinically silent abnormalities. See Table 1.

A variety of neurologic disorders can affect this SEPs. Peripheral neuropathy and other peripheral disorders can affect the peripheral conduction velocities. Fortunately, these peripheral effects can be removed from the analysis of central nervous system conduction by subtracting away the latencies of the peripheral peaks seen over the brachial plexus or lumbar spinal cord. A variety of hereditary-degenerative neurological conditions (12) can slow central conduction latencies in sensory pathways, as can some acquired metabolic disorders such as B_{12} deficiency (120). Focal lesions due to ischemia, tumors, myelopathy associated with spondylosis, and other focal disorders can disrupt conduction along the central portions of the somatosensory pathways. As such, information from SEPs must be integrated with other clinical information in order to assess whether EP changes are due to MS or due to other neurological disorders.

Brain magnetic resonance imaging (MRI) is more sensitive than either median nerve SEP or posterior tibial nerve SEP alone in MS. In one direct comparison in 46 suspected or confirmed MS 25 (54%) had abnormal median nerve SEPs, 33 (72%) had abnormal posterior tibial nerve SEPs, whereas 34 (74%) had an abnormal brain MRIs (97). In another study of 60 patients with definite, probable, or possible MS, 29 (48%) had abnormal median nerve SEPs, 37 (61%) had abnormal posterior tibial nerve SEPs, whereas 50 (83%) had an abnormal brain MRI (95). Similar results were seen for cervical MRI in 46 patients with spinal cord syndromes being evaluated for MS (57). In that study, 31 of 46 (67%) patients had an abnormal cervical MRI, whereas 26 of 46 (57%) had abnormal SEPs.

Figure 3 Examples of the peaks seen in normal short latency (A) median nerve and, (B) posterior tibial nerve, somatosensory EP testing. Negative potentials are upward deflections here. Recording sites EPi and EPc are at the shoulders; C5Sp and T12 over the spine; PF, K, and IC at the popliteal fossa, knee, and iliac crest; Ci, Cc, C'z and Fz on scalp. The several standard peaks are identified here. (From Ref. 158.)

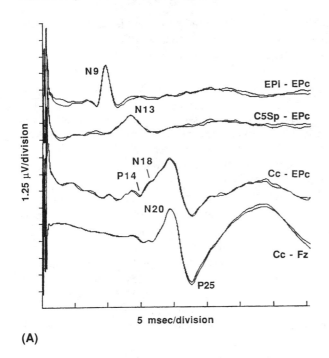

(A)

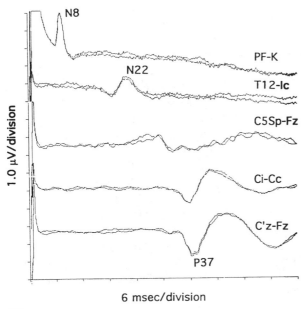

(B)

Overall, SEPs provide a useful tool for detecting clinically silent lesions that contribute to the diagnosis of MS. They provide a sensitive way to assess the spinal cord pathways, which can complement other testing such as brain MRI.

V. MOTOR EVOKED POTENTIALS

Brief electrical stimulation can discharge cortical pyramidal neurons. Such electrical stimulation can be delivered to exposed cortex at surgery. This stimulation also can be achieved through an intact skull. Considerable voltage is needed to drive electrical currents from the scalp through the skull to the cortex, e.g., 300 to 400 V. When patients are awake, such electrical stimulation is painful.

An ingenious solution to this painful situation has been devised. A powerful magnetic device held above the scalp can create a brief but extremely intense magnetic field. The skull is a resistor for electrical currents but offers no impedance to a magnetic field. According to the standard principles of electromagnetism, a fluctuating magnetic field invariably creates an electrical potential. The same principle is used in standard electric generators. The brief, intense magnetic field above the scalp creates an electric current within the cerebral cortex strong enough to discharge the neurons. The technique can be focused at the cells in a particular one square centimeter or so under the magnetic stimulator. Specific cortical regions can be stimulated by positioning the magnetic stimulator coil precisely over each such location.

This magnetic technique was popularized a decade ago by Barker and colleagues (121,122). Previously, investigators in MS and other neurological disorders had used transcrancial electrical stimulation to study motor pathways (123,124). In either technique, recordings can be made at muscles or large peripheral nerves. Using the transcranial electrical technique, studies demonstrated marked prolongation of central motor conduction times in most MS patients tested (6–8). With the advent of magnetic cortical stimulation, the clinical feasibility of the technique improved greatly. Clinicians studying motor pathway stimulation now generally use the magnetic techniques.

Several studies have demonstrated a high rate of central motor conduction time delays in MS (7,125–129). The techniques seem suited to identifying silent lesions in MS patients. They do correlate well with overall motor function and may prove an objective measure useful in MS therapeutic trials (130–132). The rate of abnormality is even higher for lower extremity recording than for the upper extremity.

Magnetically evoked motor potentials (MEPs) were compared to multimodality sensory evoked potentials (VEP, BAEP, SEP) and also to MRI testing by Ravnborg and colleagues (129). In that study, 68 patients clinically suspected of having MS were tested. Among the 40 of 68 (59%) eventually diagnosed as having MS, the MRI was positive in 88%, MEP 83%, VEP 67%, SEP 63%, and BAEP 42%. The MEP was abnormal also among one-third of the patients who eventually received other CNS diagnoses or no clear diagnosis. Among 10% of the MS patients, the MRI was normal but the neurophysiological tests were abnormal, confirming a CNS disorder. The paraclinical indicators as a whole were important for finding silent second lesions in 17 of 40 (43%) of the patients eventually diagnosed with MS. On overall diagnostic sensitive for finding silent lesions, the multimodality SEPs were best, followed by MRI and then MEP. If SEP were broken out by each individual modality, MRI and MEP had better sensitivities.

In another comparison of MEPs and sensory EPs in MS, Filippi and colleagues (133) found lower extremity SEPs to be abnormal most often (75% of patients), followed by lower extremity MEPs (65%) VEPs (64%) in upper extremity MEPs and SEPs (56% and 52%), and finally BAEPs (39%). They also noted that patients with chronic progressive MS had a high rate and greater degrees of EP abnormalities compared to patients with a more benign MS course. This paralleled similar findings with MRI plaque load among those same patients.

Central motor conduction tests can also demonstrate abnormalities in other neurological disorders. Slowed central motor conduction was found in motor neuron disease among 13 of 15 patients in one study (134) and 8 of 11 patients in another (135), whereas somatosensory evoked potentials were normal. Patients with hereditary motor and sensory neuropathy (HMSN) had delayed central conduction when they had clinical signs of pyramidal disease, with degrees of delay differed in different specific subtypes of HMSN disorders presumably corresponding to different specific pathophysiology (136).

Magnetically evoked central motor conduction tests should be considered a test available to search for clues in diagnosing MS and in the differential diagnosis of other possible central motor disorders.

VI. MULTIMODALITY EVOKED POTENTIAL TESTING

It is worthwhile to compare the three evoked potential modalities against each other, and also to compare multimodality EPs against MRI and cerebral spinal fluid findings in MS. This is useful for determining which modality is most sensitive for clinical diagnostic purposes in MS overall. Such comparisons can also be helpful in planning strategies for research studies such as therapeutic trials.

Chiappa (1990) has summarized the aggregate results of 26 to 31 original research reports of the rate of abnormality of the three EP modalities (19–44,70–92,98–119). A summary is provided in Table 1. Overall, this set of data encompasses several thousand patients in several dozen research series. Several specific features should be pointed out. The overall rates of abnormality are highest for pattern VEPs and lowest for BAEPs. SEPs have abnormality rates nearly as good as VEPs, even exceeding the latter's rate in the possible and probable MS category. Lower extremity somatosensory SEPs from peroneal and posterior tibial nerves are abnormal more often than median nerve SEPs. Silent lesions, i.e., EP abnormalities despite no signs or symptoms in that sensory modality, are seen in one-third to a half of the patients tested overall here.

Among patients with a more severe degree of MS, SEPs are even more likely to be abnormal. In one study (137) of all three EP modalities simultaneously in 101 patients with chronic progressive MS, pattern VEPs were abnormal in 75%; BAEPs in 48%; and median nerve SEPs in 93%. In most of these cases the EPs were abnormal but still present. This latter fact is important if one wishes to follow changes in EPs over time, since there is room in such cases for either improvement or deterioration. A more detailed comparison of the three sensory EPs modalities recorded in this study is presented in Table 3.

How useful are EPs in providing diagnostic information in patients being evaluated to rule out MS? Hume and Waxman (138) recently reported their findings on 2 1/2 year follow-up in 222 patients suspected of having MS. During follow-up, 48 of 222 patients initially suspected of having MS developed clinically definite MS. Among these 48 patients, 90% had had abnormal EPs during their initial clinical workup. In 65% of these 48 patients, the EPs had provided positive diagnostic evidence of a silent lesion previously unsuspected by the clinician or the patient. In the remaining 25% of these 48 patients, the EPs provided confirmatory information only. Among these same 48 patients, the VEPs

Table 3 Evoked Potentials Found Among 101 Patients with Chronic Progressive MS (Left and Right Sides Scored Separately)[a]

Pattern visual EPs	
Median P100 latency	119 ms (normal <105)
Number normal	50/202 (25%)
Present but abnormal	132/202 (65%)
Absent	20/202 (10%)
Median P100 amplitude	4.0 µV
Brainstem auditory EPs	
Median I–V interpeak latency	4.4 ms (normal <4.6)
Median V/I amplitude ratio	64% (normal >50%)
Number normal	105/202 (52%)
V present but abnormal	24/202 (12%)
V absent	63/202 (32%)
All peaks	2/202 (1%)
Median nerve somatosensory EPs	
Number normal	15/202 (7%)
Number N9 absent	0/202
N13 absent	70/202 (35%)
N20 absent	115/202 (57%)
Median N20 latency	26 ms
N20 amplitude	0.8 µV

[a] Small adjustments to normal limits for individual patients were made for age, gender, and height (details not shown here). Absent peaks were excluded from median latency determination here. Somatosensory normal limits were N20–N9 < 10.5 ms, N20–N13 < 7.0 ms plus N13–N9 < 4.3 ms; absolute latencies of N20 were not used in assessing normality.
Source: From Ref. 137.

were positive in 53%, SEPs in 26% and BAEPs in 13%. The VEP was the only positive EP in 14 patients (30% of the patients who developed definite MS); the SEP, in 5 (11%); and the BAEP in none. In that same study, 18 of the original 222 patients eventually received a diagnosis other than MS. Among these patients, EPs were usually all normal. Abnormal EPs were occasionally seen in these other disorders—e.g., an abnormal VEP in a patient with vasculitis. Overall, the false-positive rate for EPs appeared to be about 13% in this rule-out MS diagnostic paradigm.

In that same study, Hume and Waxman looked at the likelihood of disease progression in patients initially evaluated for possible MS. They found a 71% chance of clinical deterioration over 2 1/2 years if the patient had abnormal EPs, whereas there was only a 16% chance of clinical deterioration over the same time span if the patient had normal EPs. Several of cerebrospinal fluid (CSF) measures were not so accurate in predicting deterioration.

MRI has been compared to EP testing in several studies. Overall, mutltimodality EP testing is abnormal about as often as MRI among patients with definite or probable MS (51,55–56,93–97,138-139). Either type of test finds abnormalities in approximately 70% of patients evaluated across these various studies. Indeed, multimodality EP testing found slightly more abnormalities than MRI in several reported series (51,55–56,95,97). BAEPs appear to be better than MRI for detecting lesions in the pons (93,96). VEPs also appear to be better than MRI at detecting optic nerve lesions in MS. Some research reports have evaluated how well each type of test finds *multiple* abnormalities, helping thereby to confirm the multifocal nature of the disorder under evaluation. By this criterion, MRI can show multiplicity of lesions more effectively than multimodal EPs (51,96). In the Hume and Waxman (138) study following 222 rule-out MS patients for 2 1/2 years, MRI and multimodal EPs were equally effective in predicting that a patient would eventually be diagnosed as MS or have a deteriorating clinical course. Similar results were found by Lee et al. (54) among 200 patients.

The likelihood of an MS diagnosis enhanced by use of EPs alone in 7 of 25 (28%) patients studied by Gilmore et al (97). In the same study, brain MRI results along made the diagnosis more likely in 4 of 25 (16%). Among the remaining 14 of 25 (56%) patients, the EPs and MRI both made the diagnosis more likely by providing evidence of additional lesions and abnormalities typical of demyelinating disease. In a larger patient group studied by the same authors, EPs found a second, silent lesion in 21 of 58 (36%) of patients and brain MRI in 18 of 58 (31%).

In comparison to oligoclonal banding and similar CSF changes, multimodal EPs were slightly more likely to be abnormal in early or possible MS (54,117,138,140–143), although specific results did vary among reports.

When they are abnormal they predict with a higher degree of uncertainty that the patient will deteriorate after a several-year period. Patients with normal results on both EP and CSF studies are most likely to remain stable during follow-up. There does not appear to be any further relationship between CSF changes and any particular type of EP abnormality.

In a formal technology assessment, the American Academy of Neurology (AAN) Quality Standards Subcommittee looked at EPs in MS (144). They used a structured literature review to assess the usefulness of evoked potentials in identifying clinically silent lesions in patients with suspected multiple sclerosis. Based on this review and analysis, the AAN formally recommends using VEPs and SEPs to search for clinically silent lesions. For BAEPs, there is a trend in the direction of usefulness to search for silent lesions, but the magnitude of an effect is much less than for VEPs and SEPs. The report notes that there are other reasons for using EPs in MS beyond just searching for silent lesions. For example, EPs may help to localize lesions, confirm clinically ambiguous lesions or the organic basis of symptoms, and suggest demyelination as the cause of a suspicious lesion.

Finally, it is appropriate to look at the comparative resource utilization of EPs and MRI. In the United States, the Medicare fee schedule allows 29.12 relative value units (RVUs) for brain MRI, and 29.42 each for cervical and thoracic MRI. In contrast, all four evoked potential tests together are valued at 8.66 RVUs. This includes 1.24 RVUs for VEP, 3.31 RVUs for four extremity SEP, and 4.11 RVUs for BAEP. In this relative value assessment of resource utilization, all four EP tests cost 30% as much as one brain MRI; or, 10% the cost of combined brain, cervical, and thoracic MRI.

Overall, most investigators have concluded that the two types of tests are complementary, one assessing anatomy and the other assessing physiology. Each has its own niche in the diagnostic evaluation paradigm.

VII. USE OF EPs IN MS THERAPEUTIC TRIALS

EPs are clearly a useful measurement for MS therapeutic trials. Testing can be repeated annually or semiannually. The costs associated with such testing are reasonable, and can be integrated into most therapeutic trial budgets. Visual testing seems to be the best for use of therapeutic trials. This is because of the ease of measurement in this modality. Grouped data provide a reliable way to track accumulating disease burden (35,137,145).

In one large trial of azathioprine and steroids, visual and median nerve middle-latency SEPs both proved to have approximately equal statistical significance. Those two modalities were superior to BAEPs in predicting the overall outcome of that study (37). VEPs have the advantage that they do not require the annoying somatosensory electrical shocks on the wrist. The SEPs take more than twice as long to perform compared to VEPs. The somatosensory short-latency EPs, using peaks between 13 and 22 ms, are often unsatisfactory for therapeutic trials because those peaks tend to be absent in a large portion of patients who would be entered in such a trial. The middle-latency somatosensory peaks are preserved in essentially all patients (137), but most laboratories have much less familiarity with these than with short-latency SEPs.

The use of EPs in therapeutic trials is commensurate with the recommendations of the Ad Hoc Working Group on the Design of Clinical Studies to Assess Therapeutic Efficacy in Multiple Sclerosis (146). In that report it was stated, ''the unpredictability of the clinical course of MS makes it necessary for the investigator to be particularly critical in choosing methods for assessing the changes in patients relative to any putative therapy . . . the frequent occurrence of lesions in clinically silent areas provides part of the impetus for seeking to include laboratory parameters in modern therapeutic trials . . . made determinations that seem to be potentially most useful at the time of writing include visual evoked response (and several immunological tests).'' That belief has been substantiated in at least one well-designed, thorough study of EPs in a therapeutic trial. The use of MRI scans now also appears to be a highly recommended testing modality for following patients through therapeutic trials. The quantifiable aspects of MRI testing include the amount of plaque load, measure in cubic millimeters, and the number of plaques seen. Quantifying these require considerable sophistication, cost, time and effort. The sensitivity of MRI seems superior to EPs for this purpose, because the MRIs cover a much greater volume of deep white matter. The biggest disadvantages to the MRI study lie in the much greater amount of money, effort, and expertise needed to use the technique correctly in MS therapeutic trials. In many trials the VEPs may end up yielding the same general outcome data in a sensitive, objective, reproducible way. In the design of a therapeutic study, it is therefore important to weigh the advantages and disadvantages and the cost-effectiveness of the testing approach to be taken. In this author's opinion, VEPs will be found to be the more cost-effective alternative of the two approaches in many individual trials.

Some skepticism has been voiced about the usefulness of EPs in monitoring the course of MS disease activity. This is in part because the EPs often remain quite abnormal even when the MS becomes relatively inactive (44). This is actually, however, an advantage of EPs, since they tend to worsen in a monotonic fashion. EPs can detect the physiological remnants of a new plaque that appeared long before and may gradually have become relatively inapparent on MRIs.

The EP data do not appear to be redundant with any signs or symptoms that can easily be determined by physical examination or detailed history. This is because the EPs tend to pick up many silent lesions that are not reflected in any particular way in the physical examination or history.

The design of EPs for therapeutic trial also is important. There are appropriate ways in which to carry out the study, and other ways in which the testing may be of little or no benefit. This is particularly important when it comes to the scoring of the tests. The

VEPs ought to be scored in terms of the actual latency values of the EPs. Test-retest differences ought to be reassessed by direct, careful comparison of the actual EP traces themselves rather than by completely separate scoring of the individual traces. In this way, the reader can make sure that the scoring is based on exactly the same portion of the EP peaks when separate repetitions are scored. This substantially reduced the trial to trial variability. The statistics done with EPs also ought to be done using the actual latency values themselves. Year-to-year comparisons in the therapeutic trial can then be carried out using parametric statistics. This is far superior to the "better/worse/unchanged" or "changed/unchanged" or "normal/abnormal" scoring that has been used an unfortunately large number of reports of EPs in therapeutic MS trials. The latter techniques are not statistically powerful and defeat the goals of using a quantified tool in this type of scientific study.

EPs have shown themselves to be of value in two therapeutic trials we are discussing in their details. One is the case of azathioprine, antilymphocite globulin and steroid trial reported by Mertin et al. (147). In that study, VEPs, BAEPs, and short-latency median nerve SEPs were performed at the beginning and end of the 15-month treatment course. EP changes were scored as better, worse, or unchanged. The authors found that the BAEP and short latency SEP tests were difficult to interpret because of the complexity of the multiple peaks and absent peaks. The simpler visual-pattern-reversal EPs deteriorated in their control group, whereas the VEPs were more stable ($p = 0.06$) in their immunosuppressed group. These authors also found a small clinical improvement in the treatment group compared to the controlled group, although this was not statistically significant. One can learn from this study that the VEPs were better at detecting changes than the other modalities and that the VEPs were able to show a therapeutic effect even when the clinical data otherwise showed a trend that did not reach a statistical significance.

In the UCLA study of azathioprine with or without steroids in a three-year, double blind, placebo controlled therapeutic trial in chronic progressive MS (137), EPs substantially outperformed routine physical examination and disability scales in predicting the study outcome. VEPs, BAEPs, and median nerve middle-latency SEPs were performed annually during this 3-year study. Treatment-related VEP and SEP changes became statistically significantly different one year before corresponding differences were seen in the Standard Neurological Examination scores. Data regarding gradual changes is shown in Fig. 4. Note that at the bottom of each of these graphs the statistical significance of the results is shown. For the VEPs, the probability of a treatment-related difference was $p = 0.13$ even at year 1 in this 3-year study. By year 2, the difference had grown to $p = 0.02$, considered statistically significant, since it is $p < 0.05$. By year 3, the statistical significance of the difference had grown to $p = 0.002$, with the double-drug-treated group seeming to be stable over the course of this therapeutic trial. The statistical significance of this VEP difference was substantially greater in degree that was true for the Standard Neurological Examination score, which only reached a $p = 0.04$ level of statistical significance by the third year of this study. Overall, the authors of that study concluded that the statistical significance of EP changes was substantially greater than that seen for other clinical scales. The degree of significance was increased by using EP latency values rather than simple criteria for EP change. EPs were considered to be a sensitive, objective measurement useful in MS therapeutic trials.

By comparison, in that same study, EPs were evaluated using the much more common "better/worse/unchanged" criteria. When the VEPs were analyzed using 10-, 7-, and 5-ms criteria for "change," the group differences using a chi-square analysis did not

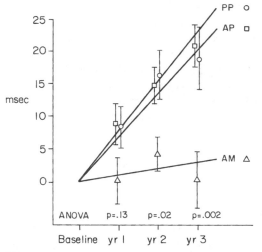

(A)

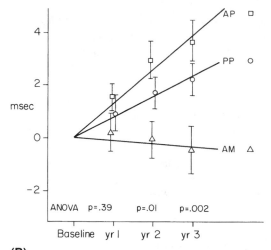

(B)

Figure 4 Effects of azathioprine and steroids on VEP (A), SEP (B), and Standard Neurological Examination Score (C) during a 3-year study in 57 patients. The three drug treatment groups are shown (AP, azathioprine; AM, azathioprine plus steroids; PP, placebo only). In each case increasing scores represent worsening. Statistical significance is shown above each horizontal axis. These data show that the double-drug-treated (AM) group remained stable or improved for each measurement. Error bars represent the standard error of the mean. Overall, the statistical significance of the group differences can be seen earlier and more strongly in the EP data. (From Ref. 137.)

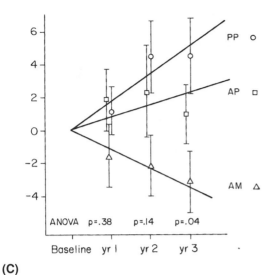

(C)

quite reach statistical significance. This should help drive home the very important lesson that EPs in a therapeutic trial must be applied by taking advantage of the quantified nature of actual latency values. Trial design should avoid the statistically less powerful, less effective better/worse/unchanged, or normal/abnormal, or changed/unchanged qualitative EP scoring schemes.

Other studies have also looked at EPs during MS therapeutic trials. Most of those investigators have not found EPs to be helpful. Some of these studies failed to use EPs in the quantified manner described above. In some other studies the treatment used probably was not effective, and the EPs were therefore quite correct in saying that there was no effect. For example, hyperbaric oxygen tests in MS did not change EPs (148,149). High-dose methylprednisolone was found to cause no change in any three EP modalities when retested at 1 week or at 1 month despite some clinical improvement in some patients (150). Among the several steroid regimens compared by LaMantia and colleagues (151), EP changes paralleled clinical changes at 6 months. In natural alpha interferon trials, EPs have confirmed the clinical findings using the Disability Status Scale and to the Scripps Neurological Rating Scale (152). In that study, EP changes were said to parallel exacerbations with some fluctuations independent of the clinical course, although details of EP testing was not actually not described. Studies of plasmapheresis found that EPs tended to corroborate clinical changes found in five reports (101,118,153–155).

Overall, EPs seem to be a reasonable, cost-effective tool that can be used to great advantage in clarifying and adding statistical significance to the results of an MS therapeutic trial. They are especially useful when used in a quantified manner.

REFERENCES

1. Waxman SG. Clinicopathological correlations in multiple sclerosis and related diseases. In: Waxman SG, Ritchie JM, eds. Demyelinating Disease: Basic and Clinical Electrophysiology. New York: Raven Press, 1981, pp 169–182.

2. Waxman SG, Ritchie JM. Electrophysiology of demyelinating disease: Future directions and questions. In: Waxman SG, Ritchie JM, eds. Demyelinating Disease: Basic and Clinical Electrophysiology. New York: Raven Press, 1981, pp 511–514.

3. Raminsky M. Hyperexcitability of pathologically myelinated axons and positive symptoms in multiple sclerosis. In: Waxman SG, Ritchie JM, eds. Demyelinating Disease: Basic and Clinical Electrophysiology. New York: Raven Press, 1981, pp 289–298.

4. Sears TA, Bostock H. Conduction failure in demyelination: Is it inevitable? In: Waxman SG, Ritchie JM, eds. Demyelinating Disease: Basic and Clinical Electrophysiology. New York: Raven Press, 1981, pp. 357–376.

5. Sedgwick EM. Pathophysiology and evoked potentials in multiple sclerosis. In: Hallpike JF et al, eds. Multiple Sclerosis: Pathology, Diagnosis and Management. Baltimore: Williams & Wilkins, 1983, pp 177–201.

6. Mills KR, Murray NMF. Corticospinal tract conduction time in multiple sclerosis. Ann Neurol, 1985; 18:601–605.

7. Hess CW, Mills KR, Murray NMF, Schriefer TN. Magnetic brain stimulation: Central motor conduction studies in multiple sclerosis. Ann Neurol 1987; 22:744–752.

8. Cowan JMA, Rothwell JC, Dick JPR, Thompson PD, Day BL, Marsden CD. Abnormalities in central motor pathway conduction in multiple sclerosis. Lancet 1984; 2:304–307.

9. Starr A, Amlie RN, Martin WH, Sanders S. Development of auditory function in newborn infants revealed by auditory brainstem potentials. Pediatrics 1977; 60:831–839.

10. Cant BR, Hume AL, Judson JA, Shaw NA. The assessment of severe head injury by short-latency somatosensory and brainstem auditory evoked potentials. Electroencephalogr Clin Neurophysiol 1986; 65:188–195.

11. Karnaze DS, Marshall LF, McCarthy CS, Klauber MR, Bickford RG. Localizing and prognostic value of auditory evoked responses in coma after closed head injury. Neurology 1982; 32:299–302.

12. Nuwer MR, Perlman SL, Packwood JW, Kark RAP. Evoked potential abnormalities in the various inherited ataxias. Ann Neurol 1983; 13:20–27.

13. Nuwer MR. Evoked Potential Monitoring in the Operating room. New York: Raven Press, 1986.

14. Richey ET, Kooi KA, Tourtellotte WW. Visually evoked responses in multiple sclerosis. J Neurol Neurosurg Psychiatry 1971; 34:275–280.

15. Halliday AM, McDonald WI, Mushin J. Delayed visual evoked response in optic neuritis. Lancet 1972; 1:982–985.

16. Kupersmith MJ, Nelson JI, Seiple WH, Carr RE, Weiss PA. The 20/20 eye in multiple sclerosis. Neurology 1983; 33:1015–1020.

17. Brooks EB, Chiappa KH. A comparison of clinical neuro-ophthalmological findings and pattern shift visual evoked potentials in multiple sclerosis. In: Courjan JJ, Mauguiere F, Revol M, eds. Clinical Applications of Evoked Potentials in Neurology. New York: Raven Press, 1982, 453–457.

18. Chiappa KH. Evoked Potentials in Clinical Medicine, 2nd ed., New York: Raven Press, 1990.

19. Halliday AM, McDonald WI, Mushin J. Delayed pattern evoked responses in optic neuritis in relation to visual acuity. Trans Ophthalmol Soc UK 1973; 93:314–324.

20. Halliday AM, McDonald WI, Mushin J. Visual evoked response in the diagnosis of multiple sclerosis. BMJ 1973; 4:661–664.

21. Asselman P, Chadwick DW, Marsden CD. Visual evoked responses in the diagnosis and management of patients suspected of multiple sclerosis. Brain 1975; 98:261–282.

22. Hume AL, Cant BR. Pattern visual evoked potentials in the diagnosis of multiple sclerosis and other disorders. Proc Austr Assoc Neurol 1976; 13:7–13.

23. Celesia GG, Daly RF. Visual electroencephalographic computer analysis (VECA). Neurology 1977; 27:637–641.

24. Matthews WB, Small DG, Small M, Pountney E. Pattern reversal evoked visual potential in the diagnosis of multiple sclerosis. J Neurol Neurosurg Psychiatry 1977; 40:1009–1014.

25. Cant BR, Hume AL, Shaw NA. Effects of luminance on the pattern visual evoked potential in multiple sclerosis. Electroencephalogr Clin Neurophysiol 1978; 45:496–504.

26. Duwaer AL, Spekreijse H. Latency of luminance and contrast evoked potentials in multiple sclerosis patients. Electroencephalogr Clin Neurophysiol 1978; 45:244–258.

27. Shahrokhi F, Chiappa KH, Young RR. Pattern shift visual evoked responses: Two hundred patients with optic neuritis and/or multiple sclerosis. Arch Neurol 1978; 35:65–71.

28. Tackmann W, Strenge H, Barth R, Sojka-Raytscheff A. Diagnostic validity for different components of pattern shift visual evoked potentials in multiple sclerosis. Eur Neurol 1979; 18:243–248.

29. Trojaborg W, Petersen E. Visual and somatosensory evoked cortical potentials in multiple sclerosis. J Neurol Neurosurg Psychiatry 1979; 42:323–330.

30. Chiappa KH. Pattern shift visual, brainstem auditory, and short-latency somatosensory evoked potentials in multiple sclerosis. Neurology 1980; 30(7 pt 2): 110–123.

31. Diener HC, Scheibler H. Follow-up studies of visual potentials in multiple sclerosis evoked by checkerboard and foveal stimulation. Electroencephalogr Clin Neurophysiol 1980; 49: 490–496.

32. Purves SJ, Low MD, Galloway J, Reeves B. A comparison of visual brainstem auditory, and somatosensory evoked potentials in multiple sclerosis. Can J Neurol Sci 1981; 8:15–19.

33. Kjaer M. Visual evoked potentials in normal subjects and patients with multiple sclerosis. Acta Neurol Scand 1980; 62:1–13.

34. van Buggenhout E, Ketelaer P, Carton H. Success and failure of evoked potentials in detecting clinical and subclinical lesions in multiple sclerosis patients. Clin Neurol Neurosurg 1982; 84:3–14.

35. Walsh JC, Garrick R., Cameron J, McLeod JG. Evoked potential changes in clinically definite multiple sclerosis: A two year follow up study. J Neurol Neurosurg Psychiatry 1982; 45: 494–500.

36. Wilson WB, Keyser RB. Comparison of the pattern and diffuse-light visual evoked responses in definite multiple sclerosis. Arch Neurol 1980; 37:30–34.

37. Lowitzsch K, Kuhnt U, Sakmann Ch, Maurer K. Hopf HC, Schott D, Thater K. Visual pattern evoked reponses and blink reflexes in assessment of MS diagnosis. J Neurol 1976; 213:17–32.

38. Mastaglia FL, Black JL, Collins DWK. Visula and spinal evoked potentials in the diagnosis of multiple sclerosis. BMJ 1976; 2:732.

39. Hennerici M, Wenzel D. Freund H-J. The comparison of small-size rectangle and checkerboard stimulation for the evaluation of delayed visual evoked response in patients suspected of multiple sclerosis. Brain 1977; 100:119–136.

40. Collins DWK, Black JL, Mastaglia FL. Pattern reversal visual evoked potential. J Neurol Sci 1978; 36:83–95.

41. Nilsson BY. Visual evoked responses in multiple sclerosis: Comparison of two methods for pattern reversal. J Neurol Neurosurg Psychiatry 1978; 41:499–504.

42. Wist ER, Hennerici M, Dichgans J. The Pulfrich spatial frequency phenomenon: A psychophysical method competitive to visual evoked potentials in the diagnosis of multiple sclerosis. J Neurol Neurosurg Psychiatry 1978; 41:1069–1077.

43. Rigolet MH, Mallecourt J, LeBlanc M, Chain F. Etude de la vision des couleurs et des potentiels evoqués dans diagnostic de la sclérose en plaques. J Fr Ophthalmol 1979; 2:553–560.

44. Matthews WB, Small DG. Serial recording of visual and somatosensory evoked potentials in multiple sclerosis. J Neurol Sci 1979; 40:11–21.

45. Mamoli B, Graf M, Toifl K. EEG, pattern-evoked potentials and nerve conduction velocity

in a family with adrenoleukodystrophy. Electroencephalogr Clin Neurophysiol 1979; 47: 411–419.

46. Krumholz A, Weiss HD, Goldstein PJ, Harris KC. Evoked responses in vitamin B-12 deficiency. Ann Neurol 1981; 9:407–409.

47. Lowitzsch K, Westhoff M. Optic nerve involvement in neurosyphillis: Diagnostic evaluation by pattern-reversal visual evoked potentials (VEP). EEG EMG 1980; 11:77–80.

48. Streletz LJ, Chambers RA, Bae SH, Israel HL. Visual evoked potentials in sarcoidosis. Neurology 1981; 31:1545–1549.

49. Frederiksen JL, Petrera J, Larsson HBW, Stigsby B, Olesen J. Serial MRI, VEP, SEP and biotesiometry in acute optic neuritis: Value of baseline results to predict the development of new lesions at one year follow up. Acta Neurol Scand 1996; 93:246–252.

50. Martinelli V, Comi G, Filippi M. Poggi A, Colombo B. Rodegher M, Scotti G, Triulzi F. Canal N. Paraclinical tests in acute-onset optic neuritis: Basal data and results of a short follow-up. Acta Neurol Scand 1991; 84:231–236.

51. Farlow MR, Markand ON, Edwards MK, Stevens JC, Kolar OJ. Multiple sclerosis: Magnetic resonance imaging, evoked responses, and spinal fluid electrophoresis. Neurology 1986; 36: 828–831.

52. Paty DW, Oger JJF, Kastrukoff LF, Hashimoto SA, Hooge JP, Eisen AA, Eisen KA, Purves SJ, Low MD, Brandejs V, Robertson WD, Li DKB. MRI in the diagnosis of MS: A prospective study with comparison of clinical evaluation, evoked potentials, oligoclonal banding and CT. Neurology 1988; 38:180–185.

53. Frederiksen JL, Larsson HBW, Olesen J. Stigsby G. MRI, VEP, SEP, and biothesiometry suggest monosymptomatic acute optic neuritis to be a first manifestation of multiple sclerosis. Acta Neurol Scand 1990; 83:343–350.

54. Lee KH, Hashimoto SA, Hooge JP, Kastrukoff LF, Oger JJF, Li DKB, Paty DW. Magnetic resonance imaging of the head in the diagnosis of multiple sclerosis: a prospective 2-year follow-up with comparison of clinical evaluation, evoked potentials, oligoclonal banding, and CT. Neurology 1991; 41:657–660.

55. Giesser BS, Kurtzberg D, Vaughan HG, Arezzo JC, Aisen ML, Smith CR, LaRocca NG, Scheinberg LC. Trimodal evoked potentials compared with magnetic resonance imaging in the diagnosis of multiple sclerosis. Arch Neurol 1987; 44:281–284.

56. O'Connor PW, Tansey CM, Detsky AS Mushlin, Kucharczyk W. The effect of spectrum bias on the utility of magnetic resonance imaging and evoked potentials in the diagnosis of suspected multiple sclerosis. Neurology 1996; 47:140–144.

57. Miller DH, McDonald WI, Blumhardt LD, du Boulay GH, Halliday AM, Johnson G, Kendall BE, Kingsley DPE, MacManus DG, Moseley IF, Rudge P, Sandercock AG. Magnetic resonance imaging in isolated noncompressive spinal cord syndromes. Ann Neurol 1987; 22: 714–723.

58. McDonald WI. The role of NMR imaging in the assessment of multiple sclerosis. Clin Neurol Neurosurg 1988; 90:3–9.

59. Youl BD, Turano G, et al. The pathophysiology of acute optic neuritis. Brain 1991; 114: 2437–2450.

60. Persson HE, Sachs C. VEPs during provoked visual impairment in multiple sclerosis. In: Barber C, ed. Evoked Potentials. Baltimore: University Park Press, 1980, pp. 575–579.

61. Regan D, Murray TJ, Silver R. Effect of body temperature on visual evoked potential delay and visual perception in multiple sclerosis. J Neurol Neurosurg Psychiatry 1977; 40:1083–1091.

62. Bajada S, Mastaglia FL, Black JL, Collins DWK. Effects of induced hyperthermia on visual evoked potentials and saccade parameters in normal subjects and multiple sclerosis patients. J Neurol Neurosurg Psychiatry 1980; 43:849–852.

63. Davies HD, Carroll WM, Mastaglia FL. Effects of hyperventilation on pattern-reversal visual

evoked potentials in patients with demyelination. J Neurol Neurosurg Psychiatry 1986; 49: 1392–1396.

64. Gilmore RL, Kasarskis EJ, McAllister RG. Verapamil-induced changes in central conduction in patients with multiple sclerosis. J Neurol Neurosurg Psychiatry 1985; 48:1140–1146.

65. Jones RE, Heron JR, Foster DH, Snelgar RS, Mason RJ. Effects of 4-aminopyridine in patients with multiple sclerosis. *J Neurol Sci* 1983; 60:353–362.

66. Nuwer MR, Visscher BR, Packwood JW, Namerow NS. Evoked potential testing in relatives of multiple sclerosis patients. Ann Neurol, 1985; 18:30–34.

67. House JW, Brackmann DE. Brainstem audiometry in neurotologic diagnosis. Arch Otolaryngol 1979; 105:305–309.

68. Brown RH, Chiappa KH, Brooks EG. Brainstem auditory evoked responses in 22 patients with intrinsic brainstem lesions: Implications for clinical interpretations. Electroencephalogr Clin Neurophysiol 1981; 51:38P.

69. Robinson K, Rudge P. Auditory evoked responses in multiple sclerosis. Lancet 1975; 1: 1164–1166.

70. Robinson K, Rudge P. Abnormalities of the auditory evoked potentials in patients with multiple sclerosis. Brain 1977; 100:19–40.

71. Robinson K, Rudge P. The early components of the auditory evoked potential in multiple sclerosis. Prog Clin Neurophysiol 1977; 2:58–67.

72. Robinson K, Rudge P. The use of the auditory evoked potential in the diagnosis of multiple sclerosis. J Neurol Sci 1980; 45:235–244.

73. Stockard JJ, Rossiter VS. (1977) Clinical and pathologic correlates of brain stem auditory response abnormalities. Neurology 1977; 27:316–325.

74. Lacquanti F, Benna P, Gilli M, Troni W, Bergamasco B. (1979) Brain stem auditory evoked potentials and blink reflex in quiescent multiple sclerosis. Electroencephalogr Clin Neurophysiol 1979; 47:607–610.

75. Mogensen F, Kristensen O. Auditory double click evoked potentials in multiple sclerosis. Acta Neurol Scand 1979; 59:96–107.

76. Chiappa KH, Harrison JL, Brooks EB, Young RR. Brainstem auditory evoked responses in 200 patients with multiple sclerosis. Ann Neurol 1980; 7:135–143.

77. Green JB, Price R. Woodbury SG. (1980) Short-latency somatosensory evoked potentials in multiple sclerosis. Comparison with auditory and visual evoked potentials. Arch Neurol 1980; 37:630–633.

78. Hausler R, Levine RA. Brain stem auditory evoked potentials are related to interaural time discrimination in patients with multiple sclerosis. Brain Res 1980; 191:589–594.

79. Stockard JJ, Sharbrough FW. Unique contributions of short-latency somatosensory evoked potentials in patients with neurological lesions. Prog Clin Neurophysiol 1980; 7:231–263.

80. Tackmann W, Strenge H, Barth R, Sojka-Raytscheff A. Evaluation of various brain structures in multiple sclerosis with multimodality evoked potentials, blink reflex and nystagmography. J Neurol 1980; 224:33–46.

81. Fischer C, Blanc A, Mauguiere F, Courjon J. Apport des potentiels evoqués auditifs précoces au diagnostic neurologique. Rev Neurol (Paris) 1981; 137:229–240.

82. Khoshbin S, Hallett M. Multimodality evoked potentials and blink reflex in multiple sclerosis. Neurology 1981; 31:138–144.

83. Parving A, Elbering C, Smith T. Auditory electrophysiology: Findings in multiple sclerosis. Audiology 1981; 20:123–142.

84. Shanon E, Himmelfarb MZ, Gold S. Pontomedullary vs pontomesencephalic transmission time: A diagnostic aid in multiple sclerosis. Arch Otolaryngol 1981; 107:474–475.

85. Barajas JJ. (1982) Evaluation of ipsilateral and contralateral brainstem auditory evoked potentials in multiple sclerosis patients. J Neurol Sci 1982; 54:69–78.

86. Elidan J, Sohmer H, Gafni M, Kahana E. Contribution of changes in click rate and intensity

on diagnosis of multiple sclerosis by brainstem auditory evoked potentials. Acta Naurol Scand 1982; 65:570–585.

87. Green JB, Walcoff M, Lucke JF. Phenytoin prolongs far-field somatosensory and auditory evoked potentials interpeak latencies. Neurology 1982; 32:85–88.

88. Prasher DK, Sainz M, Gibson WPR, Findley LJ. Binaural voltage summation of brain stem auditory evoked potentials: An adjunct to the diagnostic criteria for multiple sclerosis. Ann Neurol 1982; 11:86–91.

89. Tackmann W, Ettlin T. Blink reflexes elicited by electrical, acoustic and visual stimuli. II. Their relation to visual-evoked potentials and auditory brain stem evoked potentials in the diagnosis of multiple sclerosis. Eur Neurol 1982; 21:264–269.

90. Hutchinson M, Blandford S, Glynn D, Martin EA. Clinical correlates of abnormal brainstem auditory evoked responses in multiple sclerosis. Acta Neurol Scand 1984; 69:90–95.

91. Kayamori R, Dickins S, Yamada T, Kimura J. Brainstem auditory evoked potential and blink reflex in multiple sclerosis. Neurology 1984; 34:1318–1323.

92. Koffler B, Oberascher G, Pommer B. Brain-stem involvement in multiple sclerosis: A comparison between brain-stem auditory evoked potentials and the acoustic stapedius reflex. Neurology 1984; 231:145–147.

93. Baum K, Scheuler W, Hegerl U, Girke W, Schörner W. Detection of brainstem lesions in multiple sclerosis: Comparison of brainstem auditory evoked potentials with nuclear magnetic resonance imaging. Acta Neurol Scand 1988; 77:283–288.

94. Comi G, Canal N, Martinelli V, Medaglini S, Locatelli T, Triulzi F, Del Maschio A, Banfi G. Comparison between magnetic resonance imaging and other techniques in 39 multiple sclerosis patients. Riv Neurologia 1987; 57:44–47.

95. Comi G, Martinelli V, Medaglini S, Locatelli T, Filippi M, Canal N, Triulzi F, DelMaschio A. Correlation between multimodal evoked potentials and magnetic resonance imaging in multiple sclerosis. Neurology 1989; 236:4–8.

96. Culter JR, Aminoff MJ, Brant-Zawadzki M. Evaluation of patients with multiple sclerosis by evoked potentials and magnetic resonance imaging: A comparative study. Ann Neurol 1986; 20:645–648.

97. Gilmore RL, Kasarskis EJ, Carr WA, Norvell E. Comparative impact of paraclinical studies in establishing the diagnosis of multiple sclerosis. Electroencephalogr Clin Neurophysiol 1989; 73:433–442.

98. Abbruzzese G, Abbruzzese M, Favale E, Ivaldi M, Leandri M, Ratto S. The effect of hand muscle vibration on the somatosensory evoked potential in man: An interaction between lemoniscal and spinocerebellar inputs? J Neurol Neurosurg Psychiatry 1980; 43:433–437.

99. Anziska B, Cracco RQ, Cook AW, Feld EW. Somatosensory far field potentials: Studies in normal subjects and patients with multiple sclerosis. Electroencephalogr Clin Neurophysiol 1978; 45:602–610.

100. Chiappa KH, Choi S, Young RR. Short latency somatosensory evoked potentials following median nerve stimulation in patients with neurological lesions. Prog Clin Neurophysiol 1980; 7:264–281.

101. Dau PC, Petajan JH, Johnson KP, Panitch HS, Borenstein MB. Plasmapheresis in multiple sclerosis: Preliminary findings. Neurology 1980; 30:1023–1028.

102. Dorfman LJ, Bosley TM, Cummins KL. Electrophysiological localization of central somatosensory lesions in patients with multiple sclerosis. Electroencephalogr Clin Neurophysiol 1978; 44:742–753.

103. Eisen A, Nudleman K. Cord to cortex conduction in multiple sclerosis. Neurology 1979; 29:189–193.

104. Eisen A, Odusote K. Central and peripheral conduction times in multiple sclerosis. Electroencephalogr Clin Neurophysiol 1980; 48:253–265.

105. Eisen A, Stewart J, Nudleman K, Cosgrove JBR. Short-latency somatosensory repsonses in multiple sclerosis. Neurology 1979; 827–834.

106. Eisen A, Paty D, Purves S, Hoirch M. Occult fifth nerve dysfunction in multiple sclerosis. Can J. Neurol Sci 1981; 8:221–225.

107. Eisen A, Purves S, Hoirch M. Central nervous system amplification: Its potential in the diagnosis of early multiple sclerosis. Neurology 1982; 32:359–364.

108. Ganes T. Somatosensory evoked response and central afferent conduction times in patients with multiple sclerosis. J Neurol Neurosurg Psychiatry 1980; 43:948–953.

109. Kazis A, Vlaikidis N, Xafenias D, Papanastasiou J, Pappa P. Fever and evoked potentials in multiple sclerosis. J Neurol 1982; 227:1–10.

110. Kjaer M. The value of brainstem auditory, visual and somatosensory evoked potentials and blink reflexes in the diagnosis of multiple sclerosis. Acta Neurol Scand 1980; 62:220–236.

111. Mastaglia FL, Black JL, Edis R, Collins DWK. The contribution of evoked potentials in the functional assessment of the somatosensory pathway. Clin Exp Neurol 1978; 15:279–298.

112. Matthews WB, Esiri M. Multiple sclerosis plaque related to abnormal somatosensory evoked potentials. J Neurol Neurosurg Psychiatry 1979; 42:940–942.

113. Namerow NS. Somatosensory evoked response in multiple sclerosis patients with varying sensory loss. Neurology 1968; 18:1197–1204.

114. Namerow NS. Somatosensory recovery functions in multiple sclerosis patients. Neurology 1970; 20:813–817.

115. Noel P, Desmedt JE. Cerebral and far-field somatosensory evoked potentials in neurological disorders involving the cerevical spinal cord, brainstem, thalamus and cortex. Prog Clin Neurophysiol 1980; 7:205–230.

116. Small DG, Matthews WB, Small M. The cervical somatosensory evoked potential (SEP) in the diagnosis of multiple sclerosis. J Neurol Sci 1978; 35:211–224.

117. Trojaborg W, Bottcher J. Saxtrup O. Evoked potentials and immunoglobulin abnormalities in multiple sclerosis. Neurology 1981; 31:866–871.

118. Weiner HL, Dawson DM. Plasmapheresis in multiple sclerosis: preliminary study. Neurology 1980; 30:1029–1033.

119. Larrea LG, Mauguicre F. Latency and amplitude abnormalities of the scale far-field P14 to median nerve stimulation in multiple sclerosis: A SEP study of 122 patients recorded with a non-cephalic reference montage. Electroencephalogr Clin Neurophysiol 1988; 71:180–186.

120. Fine EJ, Hallet M. Neurophysiological study of subacute combined degeneration. J Neurol Sci 1980; 45:331–336.

121. Barker AT, Jalinous R, Freeston IL. Non-invasive magnetic stimulation of human motor cortex. Lancet 1985; 2:1106–1107.

122. Barker AT, Freeston IL, Jalinous R, Jarratt JA. Clinical evaluation of conduction time measurements in central motor pathways using magnetic stimulation of the human brain. Lancet 1986; 1:1325–1326.

123. Merton PA, Morton HB. Stimulation of the cerebral cortex in the intact human subjects. Nature 1980; 285:227.

124. Merton PA, Morton HB, Hill DK, Marsden CD. Scope of a technique for electrical stimulation of human brain, spinal cord and muscle. Lancet 1982; 2:596–600.

125. Hess CW, Mills KR, Murray NMF. Measurement of central motor conduction in multiple sclerosis by magnetic brain stimulation. Lancet 1986; 2:596–600.

126. Ingram, DA, Thompson AJ, Swash M. Central motor conduction in multiple sclerosis: evaluation of abnormalities revealed by transcutaneous magnetic stimulation of the brain. J. Neurol Neurosurg Psychiatry 1988; 51:487–494.

127. Jones SMJ, Streletz LJ, Raab VE, et al. Lower extremity motor evoked potentials in multiple sclerosis. Arch Neurol 1991; 48:944–948.

128. Mayr N, Baumgartner C, Zeitlhofer J, Deecke L. The sensitivity of transcranial cortical magnetic stimulation in detecting pyramidal tract lesions in clinically definite multiple sclerosis. Neurology 1991; 41:566–569.

129. Ravnborg M, Liguori R, Christiansen P, Larsson H, Sørenson PS. The diagnostic reliability

of magnetically evoked motor potentials in multiple sclerosis. Neurology 1992; 42:1296–1301.

130. Kandler RH, Jarratt JA, et al. Magnetic stimulation as a quantifier of motor disability. J Neurol Neurosurg Psychiatry 1989; 52:1205.

131. Kandler RH, Jarratt JA, et al. The role of magnetic stimulation as a quantifier of motor disability in patients with multiple sclerosis. J Neurol Sci 1991; 106:31–34.

132. Andersson T, Siden A, et al. A comparison of motor evoked potentials and somatosensory evoked potentials in patients with multiple sclerosis and potentially related conditions. Electromyogr Clin Neurophysiol 1995; 35:17–24.

133. Filippi M, Campi A, Mammi S, Martinelli V, Locatelli T, Scotti G, Amadio S, Canal N, Comi G. Brain magnetic resonance imaging and multimodal evoked potentials in benign and secondary progressive multiple sclerosis. J Neurol Neurosurg Psychiatry 1995; 58:(1)31–37.

134. Hugon J, Lubeau M, Tabaraud F, Chazot F, Vallat JM, Dumas M. Central motor conduction in motor neuron disease. Ann Neurol 1987; 22:544–546.

135. Berardelli A, Inghilleri M, Formisano R, Accornero N, Manfredi M. Stimulation of motor tracts in motor neuron disease. J Neurol Neurosurg Psychiatry 1987; 50:732–737.

136. Claus D, Waddy HM, Harding AE, Murray NMF, Thomas PK. Hereditary motor and sensory neuropathies and hereditary spastic paraplegia: A magnetic stimulation study. Ann Neurol 1990; 28:43–49.

137. Nuwer MR, Packwood JW, Myers LW, Ellison GW. Evoked potentials predict the clinical changes in multiple sclerosis drug study. Neurology 1987; 37:1754–1761.

138. Hume AL, Waxman SG. Evoked potentials in suspected multiple sclerosis: Diagnostic value and prediction of clinical course. J Neurol Sci 1988; 83:191–210.

139. Guerit JM, Argile AM. The sensitivity of multimodal evoked potentials in multiple sclerosis: A comparison with magnetic resonance imaging and cerebrospinal fluid analysis. Electroencephalogr Clin Neurophysiol 1988; 70:230–238.

140. Bartel DR, Markand ON, Kolar OJ. The diagnosis and classification of multiple sclerosis: Evoked responses and spinal fluid electrophoresis. Neurology 1983; 33:611–617.

141. Miller JR, Burke AM, Bever CT. Occurrence of oligoclonal bands in multiple sclerosis and other CNS diseases. Ann Neurol 1983; 13:53–58.

142. Cosi V, Citterio A, Battelli G, Bergamaschi R, Grampa G, Callieco R. Multimodal evoked potentials in multiple sclerosis: A contribution to diagnosis and classification. Ital J Neurol Sci 1987; 8:(suppl 6):109–112.

143. Ganes T, Brautaset NJ, Nyberg-Hansen, Vandvik B. Multimodal evoked response and cerebrospinal fluid oligoclonal immunoglobulins in patients with multiple sclerosis. Acta Neurol Scand 1986; 73:472–476.

144. Gronseth GS, Ashman EJ. The usefulness of evoked potentials in identifying clinically silent lesions in patients with suspected multiple sclerosis (an evidence-based review): Report of the Quality Standards Subcommittee of the American Academy of Neurology. Neurology 2000; 54:1720–1725.

145. Brigell M, Kaufman DI, et al. The pattern visual evoked potential: A multicenter study using standardized techniques. Documenta Ophthalmologica 1994; 86:65–79.

146. Brown JR, Beebe GW, Kurtzke JF, et al. (1979) The design of clinical studies to assess the therapeutic efficacy in multiple sclerosis. Neurology 1979; 29(9, pt 2):1–23.

147. Mertin J, Rudge P, Kremer M, et al. Double-blind controlled trial of immunosuppression in the treatment of multiple sclerosis: Final report. Lancet 1982; 2:351–354.

148. Neiman J, Nilsson BY, Barr PO, Perkins DJD. Hyperbaric oxygen in chronic progressive multiple sclerosis: visual evoked potentials and clinical effects. J Neurol Neurosurg Psychiatry 1985; 48:497–500.

149. Harpur GD, Suke R, Bass BH, et al. Hyperbaric oxygen therapy in chronic stable multiple sclerosis: double-blind study. Neurology 1986; 36:988–991.

150. Smith T, Zeeberg I, Sjo O. Evoked potentials in multiple sclerosis before and after high-dose methylprednisolone infusion. Eur Neurol 1986; 25:67–73.

151. La Mantia L, Riti F, Milanese C, Salmaggi A, Eoli M, Ciano C, Avanzini G. Serial evoked potentials in multiple sclerosis bouts: Relation to steroid treatment. J Neurol Sci 1994; 15: 333–340.

152. Sipe JC, Knobler RL, Braheny SL, Rice GPA, Panitch HS, Oldstone MBA. A neurologic rating scale (NRS) for use in multiple sclerosis. Neurology 1984; 34:1368–1372.

153. Sorenson PS, Wanscher, et al. Plasma exchange combined with azathioprine in multiple sclerosis using serial gadolium-enhanced MRI to monitor disease activity. Neurology 1996; 46:1620–1625.

154. Khatri BO, McQuillen MP, Harrington GJ, Schmoll D, Hoffmann RG. Chronic progressive multiple sclerosis: Double-blind controlled study of plasmapheresis in patients taking immunosuppressive drugs. Neurology 1985; 35:312–319.

155. Gordon PA, Carroll DJ, Etches WS, et al. A double-blind controlled pilot study of plasma exchange versus sham apheresis in chronic progressive multiple sclerosis. Can J Neurol Sci 1985; 12:39–44.

156. Nuwer MR, Packwood JW, Ellison GW and Meyers LW. A parametric scale for BAEP latencies in multiple sclerosis. Electroencephalogr Clinical Neurophysiol 1988; 71:33–39.

157. Nuwer MR, Aminoff M, Goodin D, Matsuoka S, Mauguière F, Starr A, Vibert JF. IFCN recommended standards for brain-stem auditory evoked potentials. Electroencephalogr Clin Neurophysiol 1984; 91:12–17.

158. Nuwer MR, Aminoff M, Desmedt J, Eisen AA, Goodin D, Matsuoka S, Mauguière F, Shibasaki H, Sutherling W, Vibert JF. IFCN recommended standards for short latency somatosensory evoked potentials. Electroencephalogr Clin Neurophysiol 1994; 91:6–11.

16

Neuroimaging and the Use of Magnetic Resonance in Multiple Sclerosis

LAEL A. STONE

Cleveland Clinic Foundation, Cleveland, Ohio

NANCY RICHERT

Clinical Center, National Institutes of Health, Bethesda, Maryland

HENRY F. MCFARLAND

National Institute of Neurological Disorders and Stroke, National Institutes of Health, Bethesda, Maryland

I. INTRODUCTION

The past decade has seen remarkable progress in multiple sclerosis. Advances include an improved understanding of the natural history of the disease, three new approved therapies in the United States, and a better understanding of the pathogenesis of the disease. Magnetic Resonance Imaging (MRI) in MS has contributed to all of these advances. MRI studies from the 1980s forward have shown that the illness is often active even during the early relapsing remitting phase of disease and during periods when the disease appears inactive clinically. This finding points toward a need to consider therapy early in the course of the illness. Studies of the relationship between progression of clinical disease and MRI measures of disease activity indicate that progression of disability may be more closely related to the destructive elements of the MS lesion than to the early acute inflammatory stage. These preliminary findings indicate that progression of disease may be related to a complicated series of steps in lesion development. The findings also suggest that MRI may be an effective tool to monitor this stage of the illness and to determine if treatments can alter the natural history of the destructive phase of MS. Finally, all of the currently approved therapies have been studied by MRI scans to further understanding of the therapeutic effect. The effect of treatment on MRI measures of disease activity played an important role in the approval of the first drug approved for use in MS, interferon beta 1b. Thus, overall, MRI has played a central role in almost all aspects of MS research over the past decade. This chapter examines the MRI techniques currently being used to study the disease, discusses the relationship between MRI measures of disease activity and clinical disease, and examines the role of MRI as a tool for monitoring new therapies. The previous edition of this chapter, written in 1995, relegated the non-imaging applications of MR technology in MS to the final few paragraphs of the discussion. At this writing, quantitative MR techniques are gaining more prominence in MS, but remain of limited use in clinical practice. Thus, although the quantitative MR techniques involving magnetization transfer, MR spectroscopy, apparent diffusion coefficient, and T1 and T2 relaxation time have more space devoted to them in this chapter, it will probably be 5 years before they are used commonly in clinical practice or trials in MS. Overall, there remain many unresolved questions with regard to the use of MRI to monitor MS. Further technical advances in the use of MRI are progressing very rapidly and the use of the newer techniques present new problems in interpretation. In these discussions we will attempt to identify both the strengths and weaknesses of the use of MRI in MS research and practice.

A. MRI Principles

Although the principles of nuclear magnetic resonance (NMR) were elucidated in the 1940s, imaging of humans required large-bore magnets that were constructed in the late 1970s. In 1981, the first inversion recovery scans were made of the brains of eight clinically definite MS patients, and these scans showed focal areas of abnormality around the ventricles. The power of MRI in MS was quickly realized both by the research and clinical community, and the diagnostic criteria published only 2 years later included MRI as a paraclinical test that could contribute to the diagnosis of MS.

A full discussion of the basic principles of MRI is beyond the scope of this chapter, although a brief overview is provided and the reader is referred to several excellent texts on the subject. MRI is based on the principle that protons (positively charged hydrogen nuclei) emit signals that can be processed into images. MRI takes advantage of the abundance of hydrogen atoms (protons) in intra- and extracellular water, lipids, and other more complex molecules, all of which are readily found in MS plaques.

When a person lies in the magnetic field of an MR unit, the protons align with the longitudinal (z axis) of the magnet in an equilibrium state. The protons wobble around the z axis in a process known as *precession*. The precession frequency, which is proportional to the strength of the magnetic field, can be calculated using the Larmor equation, which defines the precessional frequency as the magnetic field strength of the magnet multiplied by the constant of proportionality of the precessional frequency of a specific nucleus at 1.0 (T) tesla (the gyromagnetic ratio, or lambda).

To perturb the protons from their equilibrium position, a radiofrequency (RF) pulse, which is equal to the precession frequency, is transmitted through the head coil. The RF pulse rotates the protons from the longitudinal z axis toward the transverse (XY) axis. A 90-degree RF pulse rotates the protons into the XY plane, whereas a 180-degree pulse produces twice the degree of rotation. When the 90-degree RF pulse is turned off, there is regrowth of the longitudinal magnetization along the z axis (T1 relaxation) and loss of transverse magnetization (T2) with time. The T1 and T2 relaxation times are usually mono-exponential and reflect the environment in which the protons reside. For example, free water and cerebrospinal fluid (CSF) have long T1 and T2 relaxation times, compared with fat (short T1, long T2), gray matter, and white matter, which have intermediate T1 and T2 relaxation times. MS lesions have T1 and T2 relaxation properties like CSF because of the increased free water associated with edema and inflammation and because of tissue destruction.

By varying the pattern and timing of the RF pulse, in combination with changes in the main magnetic field with the additional magnetic field gradients, one can impart spatial information to the NMR signals to create an MR image. The combination of specifically orchestrated RF and magnetic field gradient pulses used to create an MR image are known as *pulse sequences*. Pulse sequences used for MRI are known as *spin-echo* (SE), *gradient-recalled echo* (GRE), and *inversion recovery* (IR) pulse sequences. Spin-echo pulse sequences are the most versatile and commonly used sequences to image MS patients today. The SE pulse sequences produce images that favor or are "weighted" toward one or the other relaxation time [i.e., T1 weighted (T1W) or T2 weighted (T2W)]. The weighting is produced by changes in the scanning variables, known as *repetition time* (TR) and *echo time* (TE). In general, T1W images have a short TR (<700 ms) and a short TE (<20 ms), whereas T2W images have a long TR (>2000 ms) and long TE (>60 ms). Proton density-weighted images are produced with a mixture of T1 weighting and T2 weighting, using a long TR and a short TE.

B. Recent Technical Advances in MRI and General Scanning Issues

Several variables including slice thickness and magnetic field strength have changed in the last few years; these affect the quality of images. Signal-to-noise ratio increases with magnets of higher field strength, and 1.5-tesla magnets have become the norm. The "open" magnets are lower in field strength and may not offer optimal resolution for MS lesions, particularly those in the spine. In addition, the available contrast agent for T1W scans, gadopentetate, is less visible when used in the lower-field-strength magnets without very careful adjustment of scanning parameters, thus limiting the use of these magnets for measuring disease activity. Most researchers prefer interleaved or contiguous slices (no gap between slices), but a small interslice gap may not be detrimental to scans done solely for diagnosis. Scans should include the entire brain, although MS lesions are most frequent in the periventricular region. Slices of 3 to 5 mm are most commonly obtained in the straight transverse or oblique transverse planes in the cerebrum. As scanner hardware continues to be developed, it may be feasible to use three-dimensional (3D) techniques to improve the resolution and decrease the partial volume effects of small plaques. Sagittal images may be particularly useful in distinguishing nonspecific white matter hyperintensities from MS plaques, although axial transverse images are the most commonly obtained images in MS.

C. Pulse Sequences Commonly Used in MS Imaging

T2W Imaging

Conventional T2W sequences (conventional spin-echo, or CSE), with long TR (2000 to 3000 ms) and long TE (60 to 100 ms) produce images where CSF is bright, and MS plaques appear as hyperintense foci that may be confluent with the ventricles and each other (Fig. 1) Both active and chronic inactive lesions are visualized as hyperintense T2W lesions, but they cannot be reliably distinguished from one another. The advantages of T2W images are that a large number of MS plaques are well seen, particularly in the centrum semiovale or adjacent to the ventricles. Ovoid lesions may also be seen in the cerebellar peduncles, cerebellar hemisphere, and midbrain. The disadvantages of the T2W images are that the distinction between the border of the lateral ventricles and plaques may

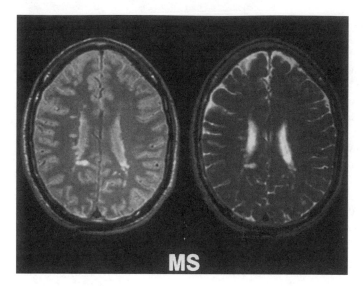

Figure 1 Examples of T2-weighted white matter hyperintensities of MS and proton density images in the same patient.

be difficult to ascertain and that lesions in the posterior fossa may be partially obscured by flow artifacts.

Proton-Density Images

Proton-density images provide much of the same information as the T2W images in MS, with certain advantages in terms of contrast with CSF and scan time (Fig. 1). Proton-density (PD) images are often obtained with a long TR (>2000 ms and a short TE (<30 ms). The PD images are usually obtained as the first echo of a conventional T2W spin-echo sequence. MS lesions are hyperintense on proton-density images, but the CSF is more hypointense (darker) than on T2W images. Thus, the border between ventricle and periventricular lesion is more apparent.

Fast Spin-Echo (FSE)

Fast spin-echo (FSE) imaging is a simple modification of CSE whereby a single 90-RF pulse is followed by multiple refocusing pulses to produce a large train (4 to 64) echoes. The reduction in image acquisition time is proportional to the length of the echo train; thus scanning time is reduced. Comparison of CSE with FSE has demonstrated comparable sensitivity in lesion detection (1), but others maintain that FSE is less sensitive than CSE due to blurring around the edges of the plaques and thus does not justify the time saving.

Fluid-Attenuated Inversion Recovery (FLAIR)

Fluid-attenuated inversion recovery (FLAIR) imaging has come into wider use over the last few years as MR scanners have been upgraded to be able to perform this sequence (Fig. 2). It is perhaps, the most sensitive imaging sequence for white matter abnormalities but has several disadvantages that are worth noting. FLAIR overcomes the difficulty with conventional T2W images, where the signal intensity from the adjacent plaques can be indistinguishable. In FLAIR, a CSE or FSE (fast FLAIR) T2W pulse sequence is preceded by a 180-degree inversion pulse to null the signal from CSF. FLAIR produces striking

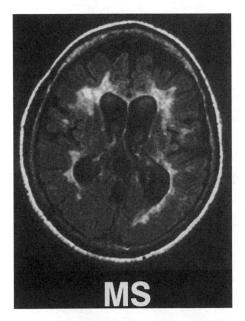

Figure 2   Example of fluid attenuated inversion recovery (FLAIR) scan in an MS patient.

images of periventricular hyperintense abnormalities in MS, but it is prone to artifacts, particularly from vascular structures, and is relatively insensitive to lesions in the posterior fossa. Studies have demonstrated that FLAIR imaging detects two to three times the number of lesions seen on T2W imaging.

Contrast-Enhanced Imaging

T1W images may be obtained with or without the addition of an intravenous contrast agent made up of a paramagnetic substance, gadolinium, in various chelates (Fig. 3) The addition of a paramagnetic contrast agent shortens the T1 and T2 relaxation times of the tissues. With disruption of the blood-brain barrier (BBB), the gadolinium chelate diffuses into the extracellular space of the abnormal brain parenchyma and alters the relaxation time of the tissue. This process results in an area of brightness, called *enhancement* (i.e., hyperintensity) on a T1W spin-echo image.

Postcontrast enhanced T1W images are most useful for distinguishing active lesions, with BBB breakdown. Contrast-enhanced lesions usually enhance for approximately 1-month in the cerebrum, although they may enhance for a longer time period in the spine and occur most commonly in relapsing remitting patients, as discussed below. The disruption of the BBB is believed to be an early if not the earliest event in the development of an MS lesion (2). Vascular structures are sometimes misclassified as enhancing lesions, and gliotic lesions may occasionally have an intermediately bright ring surrounding them, which does not change with contrast injection. Flow artifacts in the posterior fossa make the distinction of active lesions in that area very difficult.

Increased number and volume of contrast-enhancing lesions may be obtained by increasing the dose of contrast agent or delaying the time from contrast injection to image acquisition to allow for greater seepage of contrast agent though the open BBB. Both triple-dose contrast agent and delayed scanning increase the cost of scanning, though, and generally are not used in routine clinical work.

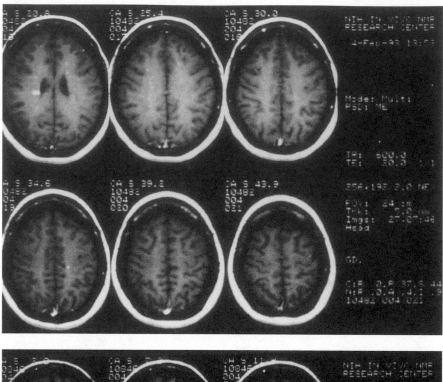

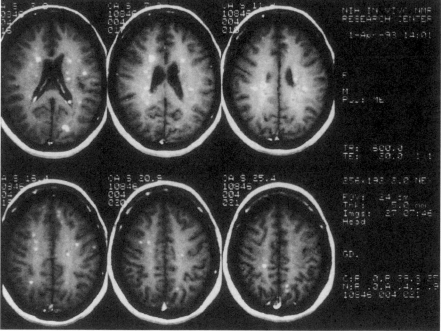

Figure 3 Examples of contrast-enhancing lesions coming and going over a several-month period in the same MS patient, showing T1W hypointensity as well.

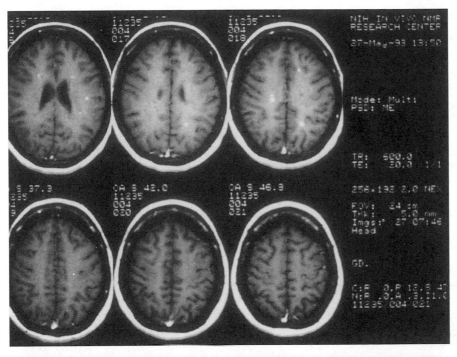

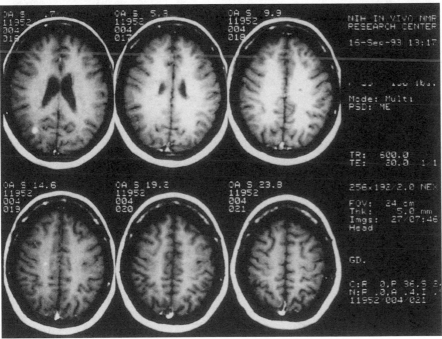

Magnetization Transfer Imaging

Magnetization transfer imaging is a relatively new quantitative MR technique. It is based on the principle that there is an equilibrium exchange between protons bound to macromolecules and freely mobile protons in solution. Only the mobile protons contribute to the signal intensity of the image. The technique employs a prolonged off-resonance broadbandwidth saturation pulse to selectively saturate the macromolecular protons prior to each excitation. The magnetization transfer exchange between saturated protons and free protons causes the signal intensity of the image to be reduced. By obtaining duplicate sets of images with and without a saturation pulse, the magnetization transfer ratio can be calculated, and this ratio indirectly reflects macromolecular structural integrity of the tissue. This technique is discussed in more detail in the section on quantitative techniques, below (Sec. III.E). This method promises to reveal knowledge about the biochemistry and physiology of MS, although much remains to be understood about the appropriate processing methods and standardization over scanners for magnetization transfer ratios and images.

II. IMAGING OF THE SPINAL CORD AND OPTIC NERVE

MRI of the spinal cord or optic nerve in MS constitutes a special case, and both may be of particular value in the diagnosis of MS. Patients may have prominent enhancing abnormalities of the spinal cord with little to no abnormalities seen in cranial MRI. Spinal MRI requires a few modifications, including the use of surface receiver coils. Motion artifacts from cardiac and respiratory motion and long scanning times degrade image quality in spinal cord imaging. Low-field strength (open) scanners may not be able to image the intramedullary lesions of MS well, and several of the techniques in use for studying of the cerebrum (FLAIR, MTC, diffusion weighting, and spectroscopy) are difficult to apply to the spinal cord. Several groups have begun to apply magnetization transfer (MT) histograms in particular to the cervical cord in MS, with abnormalities correlating with the degree of disability in ambulation (3). Lesions of the optic nerve, common during optic neuritis, may be best visualized by fat-suppressed SE images or STIR, which detect lesion in the optic nerves in up to 84% of symptomatic patients (4). Postcontrast enhanced T1W images with a fat saturation pulse visualize acute plaques in the optic nerves, and this enhancement correlates with visual dysfunction. Orbital surface coils may be used to provide high-resolution studies of the optic nerve.

A. The Use of MRI in the Diagnosis and Differential Diagnosis of MS

The diagnosis of MS remains a clinical decision, which requires the demonstration of characteristic symptoms and signs of central nervous system (CNS) lesions separated in space and time. A characteristic MRI is not a condition for diagnosis but is valuable in support of the diagnosis of MS. For a diagnosis of clinically definite MS, the Washington (Poser) (5) criteria require that a patient be 10 to 59 years of age and have had two attacks characteristic of MS at least 1 month apart, with a clinical examination showing evidence of two separate CNS lesions and the proviso that there is no better alternative diagnosis. Characteristic abnormalities of MRI or evoked potential recordings may be used as paraclinical evidence of one of the lesions. The sensitivity of MRI to abnormalities in MS is quite high, although a few patients may clearly have MS in the presence of a completely normal MRI at presentation. The exact sensitivity of MRI in MS is unknown but is undoubtedly increasing with the use of higher-strength magnets and FLAIR imaging. MRI is the most sensitive of paraclinical tests that are currently available. The majority of MS patients have the typical MRI scans findings of ovoid lesions with well-defined margins asymmetrically located perpendicularly (Dawson's fingers) to the corpus callosum, in the corpus callosum, or in the subcortical white matter, middle cerebellar peduncle, pons, or medulla.

The specificity of characteristic abnormalities on MRI in MS is more problematic. Several groups (6–8) have attempted to develop criteria for the characteristic abnormalities of MS on MRI, as discussed below. The major difficulty is the differentiation from normal changes seen in aging, in which multi-focal white matter lesions may be seen on T2W images, presumably caused by small vessel disease. Thus, MRI has a lower specificity in older patients and those with risk factors for unidentified bright objects (UBOs), such as hypertension, smoking, and migraine headaches. In some patients, another nonpathological condition may result in high signal intensities on T2W images: enlarged Virchow-Robin spaces (VRS). These dilated perivascular spaces filled with CSF may be asymmetrical and may be distinguished from MS because VRS have the same signal intensity as CSF on all pulse sequences (hence they disappear on proton density images), while MS lesions are hyperintense on PD. VRS are typically located in the anterior commissure, basal ganglia, centrum semiovale, midbrain, and pons.

The sensitivity of the criteria of any test indicates its ability to pick up abnormalities, including false-positive results, whereas the specificity of a test refers to its accuracy in selecting only the truly abnormal. Thus a highly specific test is subject to false-negative results. The Fazekas criteria (6,7) for T2W images consistent with MS require at least two of the following three findings to be present: a lesion next to the body of the lateral ventricles, an infratentorial lesion, and a lesion larger than 5 mm in diameter. When these criteria were applied to 1500 consecutive patients, a sensitivity of 81% and a specificity of 96% were obtained. Another set of criteria (8) requires at least four hyperintense lesions or three lesions larger than or equal to 3 mm, with at least one periventricular lesion for an MRI strongly suggestive of MS. The sensitivity and specificity are both quoted as 92% for these latter criteria, but the false-positive rate is 8%. A third set of criteria published in 1997 (9) uses a four-parameter dichotomized MRI model to predict conversion to clinically definite MS in patients with a single episode of demyelination. This model, which includes contrast enhancement, had an accuracy rate of 80% in visualizing juxtacortical, intratentorial, and periventricular lesions and may have greater applicability to MR scans in MS in general.

Although the list of disorders causing hyperintense abnormalities on T2W images is long (Table 1), most of these may be easily distinguished from MS on a combination of clinical and MRI grounds. A few disorders, such as neurosarcoidosis and the vasculitides can also cause problems diagnostically, as they can appear similar to MS both clinically and by MRI. Until recently, the therapies for these conditions were relatively similar. However, as we become more able to treat MS in a more specific manner, directed toward the underlying mechanisms, this differentiation will become increasingly important. The pattern of abnormalities on MRI in sarcoidosis may be differentiated on the basis of contrast enhancement, with meningeal enhancement around the base of the brain (hypothalamus and optic chiasm) (Fig. 4) or in a beaded pattern over the spinal cord found in sarcoid but not in MS. The MRI in systemic lupus erythematosus most commonly demonstrates predominantly subcortical white matter lesions rather than the periventricular lesions seen in MS.

Table 1 Conditions That Produce
Hyperintensities on T2W Images

Demyelinating diseases
  MS
  ADEM
  PML
  Osmotic (central pontine myelinolysis)
Dysmelinating diseases
  Leukodystrophies
  Storage diseases
Other diseases
  Systemic lupus
  Neurosarcoidosis
  CNS vasculitides
  Behcet's syndrome
  CNS lymphoma
  Lyme disease
  Migraine
  Irradiation
  HTLV-1
  Syphillis
  Cerebral infarction
Other nondisease conditions
  Normal aging
  Virchow-Robin spaces

Key: MS, multiple sclerosis; ADEM, acute disseminated encephalomyelitis; PML, progressive
multifocal encephalopathy; CNS, central nervous system; HTLV-1, human T-cell leukemia/
lymphoma virus type 1.

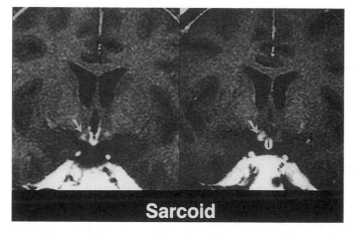

Figure 4 Example of neurosarcoidosis as seen on an MRI of the brain.

Other special cases of white matter demyelination causing hyperintensities that are worthy of brief mention here are acute demyelinating enchephalomyelitis (ADEM), progressive multifocal leukoencephalopathy (PML), and the leukodystrophies (Fig. 5). ADEM is a monophasic episode of inflammatory demyelination usually following a viral illness (e.g., measles) or vaccination (e.g., rabies or tetanus). Certain MRI characteristics of ADEM have been well delineated in the pediatric population where the condition is more common and almost always includes delirium (10). These characteristics, as listed in Table 2, appear relevant for the adult population as well. PML involves demyelination due to viral infection of oligodendrocytes in patients who are immunocompromised from a variety of causes. The MRI shows confluent white matter lesions, usually in the parietal occipital region and perhaps crossing the corpus callosum. U fibers are involved, but there is no contrast enhancement. Dysmyelinating diseases such as adrenal leukodystrophy,

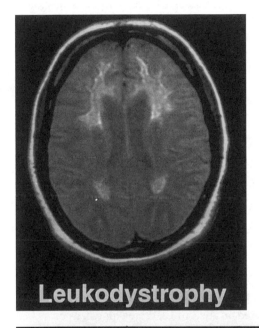

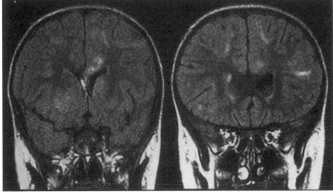

Figure 5 Examples of white matter hyperintensities seen in ADEM and leukodystrophy. Courtesy of Gilbert Vegina, Children's National Medical Center, Washington, DC.

Table 2 Multiple Sclerosis Versus Acute Disseminated Encephalomyelitis (ADEM) on MRI

MRI characteristic	Multiple Sclerosis	ADEM
Contour of lesion	Discrete	ill-defined
Location of lesion	Periventricular	Basal ganglia
	Dawson's fingers	Thalamus
	Corpus callosum	Cortical gray matter
Contrast enhancement	Discrete, may be ring-enhancing	No contrast enhancement

which shows bilateral symmetrical demyelination in occipital parietal areas, may show contrast enhancement at the leading edge. Metachromatic leukodystrophy shows diffuse white matter disease sparing the subcortical U fibers. Lyme disease may also show T2W abnormalities, simulating MS. In some cases, the characteristic enhancement of cranial nerve roots 3, 5, and 7 as well as leptomeningeal enhancement and the peripheral enhancement of lesions may be helpful in distinguishing Lyme disease from MS.

The sensitivity and specificity of MRI for the initial diagnosis of MS may be increased by the use of contrast agents, as mentioned above (11). Fifty-seven patients with neurological symptoms suggestive of MS were studied prospectively by a set of investigators who obtained T2W and T1W postcontrast images in all patients and also of CSF in 34 patients (12). Oligoclonal bands and typical findings in CSF had a sensitivity of 69% and a specificity of 38%, whereas T2W images had a sensitivity of 94% and specificity of 55% by liberal criteria. The use of contrast enhanced images increased the specificity to 80%, with a loss of sensitivity to 59%. In older individuals, MRIs of the spine are particularly useful diagnostically as the age-related changes seen in the cerebrum are not seen in the spinal cord, and additional paraclinical tests may be needed to supplement the diagnostic process in individuals with questionable MRI findings.

B. Histopathological Correlation with Magnetic Resonance Imaging

As stated in the previous edition of this chapter, despite some histological studies of MS lesions obtained by biopsy or autopsy following imaging, the complete nature of the complex relationship between signal changes on MRI and histopathology of MS plaques remains unclear. While previous work has focused on areas of BBB breakdown, as discussed further on, newer work has come back to older concepts of atrophy, tissue loss, and axonal transection studied in the pre-MRI era. Histological examination has been performed on the brain of a patient with severe secondary progressive MS who died within 10 days of an MRI. This examination that revealed several contrast-enhancing lesions (13) and, as expected evidence of both old and recent lesions was found. In an area that corresponded to an enhancing lesion, a dramatic perivascular inflammatory response was observed. Studies of biopsied lesions have also shown active demyelination and marked macrophage infiltration, but less inflammation was seen than that in the previously mentioned patient who died of secondary progressive disease (14). Maximal activity with numerous perivascular inflammatory cells, macrophages and primary demyelination was seen in lesions with inhomogeneous contrast enhancement, such as ring-enhancing lesions. Samples taken from outside the area of radiological abnormality appeared normal except for occasional perivascular inflammation and astrogliosis, although some of the normal-appearing white matter did contain thinly myelinated axons as well as many small round glial cells with the morphological features of oligodendrocytes.

Hypointensities on T1W, or "T1 holes," are a subset of chronic lesions seen on T2W that have extensive tissue destruction (15–17) (Fig. 3). In the evolutionary pathway of an MS plaque, T1W hypointensities may represent an end-stage lesion lacking reparative potential. T1W hypointense lesions were first described in MS patients by Uhlenbreck and Sehlen (18) and were subsequently termed "T1 black holes" by Truyen and colleagues (17). Histopathologically, T1W hypointensities represent areas of extensive demyelination, axonal loss, reactive astrocytosis, and matrix destruction (14,19). The term *hole* is somewhat misleading as these areas may not represent an area of actual tissue volume loss, as they exhibit varying degrees of hypointensity ranging from gray to black. *In vivo* studies have shown that the degree of hypointensity correlates with a progressive decrease in the magnetization transfer ratio (20,21) and with axonal loss as measured by a reduction in the *N*-acetylaspartate (NAA) peak on MR spectroscopy (22). Recent postmortem studies on unfixed tissues have confirmed that the hypointensity of a T1 hole is proportional to axonal loss ($r = -0.7, p < 0.001$) and matrix\destruction ($r = 0.45, p = 0.05$) but does not correlate with the extent of demyelination or to the number of reactive astrocytes (19,23).

C. Information Gained by the use of Various MRI Parameters in MS

T2W Studies

The first studies of serial unenhanced MRI in patients with relapsing remitting MS (RRMS) showed lesions developing and enlarging and a high percentage of clinically silent lesions. Lesions were observed to often increase in size over 1 to 2 months and then to become smaller over the next 1 to 2 months, resolving to small residual areas of hyperintensity on T2W images (24). The placebo arm of the multicenter cyclosporine trial as well as the placebo arm of the interferon beta-1b multicenter trial involved serial measures of abnormal white matter on MRI, showing an apparent increase in abnormal white matter over time. These studies found an increase in visualized abnormal white matter of approximately 10% per year (25). A small-scale study of seven RRMS patients, scanned monthly for up to 36 months, also showed accumulation of abnormal high signal intensity over time (26). This smaller study was able to look at the heterogeneity of rates of increase between patients; in addition, because scans were obtained at frequent intervals, month-to-month fluctuations in abnormal white matter signal were observed. These month-to-month fluctuations were thought to be partly due to the BBB breakdown seen on corresponding T1W contrast-enhanced scans and partly to some as yet not understood aspect of the pathophysiology of the MS lesions. T2W burden has been accepted as a quantitative measure of disease burden and has been used as an outcome measure in all recent phase III clinical trials, as discussed below.

Despite excellent spatial correlation between T2W hyperintense lesions and MS plaques on postmortem examination (14), there is only a weak correlation between T2W hyperintense lesion load and clinical disability as measured by the Expanded Disability Status Score (EDSS) (27,28). One explanation for the poor correlation is the lack of pathological specificity of T2W signal intensity. Hyperintense lesions on T2W images may represent focal areas of inflammation, edema, demyelination, axonal loss, or gliosis, but only axonal loss and/or demyelination would be expected to cause permanent neurological deficit. Another partial explanation is that the EDSS is a nonlinear scale that represents mainly spinal cord disease activity, as small lesions in the spinal cord may be more important in determining disability than large lesions in the brain (29). Future work incorporating cognitive testing may yield a higher correlation with T2W burdens. Last, T2W images may underrepresent the amount of diseased white matter, as microscopic pathology of otherwise normal-appearing white matter may contribute to disability. One recent study examined the presence of diffuse abnormalities or poorly demarcated high-signal areas as seen on both PD and T2W in the brain (30). These types of abnormalities may be most important in the primary progressive type of MS.

Bakshi and colleagues have recently presented work on T2W hypointensities, "black T2." This study attempts to describe and characterize this phenomenon which is noted in the thalamus, putamen, and caudate of many MS patients over time. This finding, which is believed to be due to abnormal iron deposition, may prove to be helpful in understanding neuronal degeneration in MS (31).

Contrast-Enhanced T1W Images

Several groups of investigators have now examined the natural history of early RRMS by frequent serial contrast-enhanced imaging. These studies have shown that considerable disease activity occurs during periods in which the patients are clinically stable. Contrast enhancement occurs in almost all the new lesions from patients with RRMS or secondary progressive MS (SPMS). Enhancement after a standard dose of contrast agent usually lasts from 4 to 8 weeks (32,33). A 15% increase in the number of lesions may be observed by scanning at weekly intervals instead of monthly (34). Enhancement depends on the dose of contrast, the time delay between contrast administration and scanning, and the magnitude of BBB disruption. The use of triple-dose contrast (0.3 mmol/kg) and a scanning delay of 20 to 40 min after contrast injection will increase the number of enhancing lesions by 80% (35,36).

The overall level of disease activity can be approximated by a study of 68 patients with RRMS images for 3 months (37). More than 75% of the patients had an enhancing lesion on a least one of the three monthly images and two-thirds of the patients had evidence of contrasting enhancing lesions on each of the three monthly examinations. This same study showed that contrast enhancement was more common in those patients with scores of greater than or equal to 3.5 on the Extended Disability Status Scale (EDSS) and early age of onset of disease. Gender and age did not appear as significant independent factors. Other studies have shown that primary progressive MS patients and so-called benign MS patients have the least contrast enhancement, whereas RRMS and secondary progressive patients who still have exacerbations have the most (38).

Several groups have attempted to correlate the level of MRI activity to various circulating compounds in the blood, CSF, or urine. A significant positive correlation has been reported between changes in the numbers of cells secreting interleukin 2 (IL-2) and contrast-enhancing lesions on MRI over a 6-month period (39). A weaker association was found between contrast-enhancing lesions and cells secreting interferon gamma or lymphotoxin alpha (40). Another study found a correlation between soluble intracellular adhesion molecule type 1(ICAM-1) and contrast-enhancing lesions (41).

Because contrast-enhancing lesions occur five to ten times more frequently than clinical relapses (11), this MRI measure has also been used in clinical trials to reduce the number of patients and the time period required to demonstrate a beneficial clinical effect (42–45). As with T2W hyperintense lesions, there is only weak correlation between contrast-enhancing lesion activity and future clinical disability (46). The number of contrast-enhancing lesions correlates with the onset and severity of clinical relapses (33,47) predicts future enhancing lesion activity as well as T2W lesion load 1 to 2 years later (48,49).

There is little information on whether contrast- enhancing lesions predict clinical status over the long term, although they are not strongly predictive over a 2-year horizon. Kappos and colleagues performed a metanalysis of five natural history and four placebo groups from clinical trials (44). Regression analysis confirmed that contrast-enhancing lesions were a risk for relapse but not for progression of disability at 2-years.

Thus evidence from evaluation of changes on T2W images, occurrence of contrasting-enhancing lesions, and—as shown further on—atrophy measures indicates that the disease is progressive and active from the initial stages in most patients. To improve the correlation between clinical measures and MRI measures of disease activity, researchers are investigating new imaging sequences that can identify the pathological substrate of MS lesions. These new methods include magnetization transfer imaging, MR spectroscopy, T1 holes, and cerebral and spinal atrophy.

T1W Hypointensities or "Black Holes"

T1W hypointensities or T1 holes, are subsets of chronic T2 lesions, which appear hypointense on T1W images and have extensive tissue destruction (15–17). T1W hypointensities occur more frequently in SPMS patients than in RRMS patients (17). They are rarely found infratentorially and represent 15 to 30% of the total lesion load (38). Compared to T2W lesions or contrast-enhancing lesions, T1 holes show the best correlation with baseline disability (EDSS) and disease progression in SPMS patients. In a longitudinal study of 17 SPMS patients followed for 3 years, the accumulation of T1 holes (T1 lesion load) strongly correlated with increasing disability (SRCC = 0.81 $p < 0.0001$) (17).

At the time of contrast enhancement, 80% of enhancing lesions show some degree of hypointensity on T1W scans and demonstrate a significant decrease in the magnetization transfer ratio (MTR) in the area of the lesion (50). Over the subsequent 6 months, the majority (60%) of these enhancing lesions become isointense to white matter, and the MTR returns toward that of normal-appearing white matter. A smaller fraction of enhancing lesions (40%) remains hypointense, with low MTR, and become T1 holes.

Predictive factors for the development of T1 holes in MS patients would be important to identify. A recent study (51) found that the T1-hole lesion load at baseline was the strongest predictor for subsequent T1 holes ($r = 0.68$, $p < 0.01$). Because T1 holes evolve from contrast-enhancing lesions, there is also a weaker correlation with the frequency of enhancing lesions ($r = 0.42$). Neither the pattern of enhancement nor the volume of the enhancing lesion is correlated with T1-hole formation, but persistent enhancement for >2 months may be a contributing factor (52).

D. Role of MRI as a Surrogate Outcome Measure

Considerable confusion surrounds the use of MRI measures of disease activity as a surrogate outcome measure in clinical studies. Much of the confusion relates to differences in the use of the term *surrogate*. Generally speaking terms a surrogate is an outcome other than disability or mortality that predicts the clinical outcome. However, in the field of experimental therapeutics, a well-defined criterion for a validated surrogate exists. The criterion stipulates that the surrogate must be shown to predict the clinical outcome and that, based on the examination of various classes of therapies that affect the clinical outcome, the treatments must be shown to modify the clinical disease through their effects on the surrogate (53). Thus, the surrogate must represent a step in causing the clinical outcome and not simply a marker associated with the outcome. This criterion distinguishes a validated surrogate from a biological marker that may reflect the disease process but does not entirely account for the progression of disease or for the clinical outcome. An example is the value of CD4 counts as a surrogate in HIV disease. It is now clear that that correlation between CD4 counts and survival in clinical trials is incomplete (54).

It is evident that no single MRI measure meets the criterion for a validated surrogate. Several studies demonstrate that the extent of disease seen on T2W images at the time of presentation predicts outcome in clinically isolated syndromes (CIS) with a reasonable degree of confidence (27,55). However, we lack clear evidence that therapies that modify T2W images also modify clinical outcome. Two clinical trials of interferon beta will soon be presented, but even in the case of a strongly positive effect on both MRI and clinical outcome, the need to demonstrate a similar effect of other classes of therapy will exist. In addition to CIS, the frequency of enhancing lesions shows a consistent relationship with exacerbation frequency and has some predictive value for relapse rate (33,46,48). Further, studies of treatment with the beta interferons show that a reduction in exacerbation rate is correlated with a reduction in the frequency of enhancing lesions (56). However, the recently conducted study of the effect of glatiramer acetate on MRI activity demonstrated a reduction in relapse rate similar to that seen in the large pivotal clinical trial, but with a reduction in enhancing-lesion frequency considerably less than that seen with beta interferon (57). This observation raises the possibility that glatiramer acetate reduces exacerbation frequency through mechanisms at least partially independent of events involved in the initiation of an enhancing lesion and reflects the care that must be used in the use of surrogate outcome measures. Although a trial of glatiramer acetate with MRI as a surrogate could have identified a treatment effect, the number of patients needed would have been considerably greater than what would have been expected based on results from interferon beta.

The use of MRI as a surrogate in SPMS is even more complicated than in RRMS or CIS. Conventional MRI measures—such as enhancing activity and lesion load seen on T2W images—exhibit a poor correlation with or prediction for clinical disease (58). However, recent studies suggest that measurements of brain atrophy or measures of more pathological specific changes that may contribute to disability such as axonal loss or irreversible demyelination, may correlate with disability, as discussed below. A combination of MRI measures may provide the best outcome measure both in RRMS and SPMS. Unfortunately, only short duration clinical trials are currently available, which limits assessment of the predictive value of these types of measurements. Further, the effect of various therapies on these MRI measures is largely unknown. Consequently, we lack sufficient evidence at present that MRI can represent a validated surrogate in any stage of MS.

Currently regulatory authorities in the United States allow the conditional use of un-validated surrogates. The surrogate must be determined to be reasonably likely to predict clinical outcome. In the case of MRI, it is reasonably likely that changes seen on MRI reflect the pathological process in the illness; on this basis, efforts have been begun to explore the potential strengths and weaknesses of studies that use MRI measures of disease activity as a primary outcome measure. There is now considerable agreement that MRI merits use as a primary outcome measure in preliminary trials of new therapies. However, the choice of MRI measures must be carefully considered in relation to the proposed mechanism of action of the new therapy and with regard to the phase of disease to be studied. Clinical trials with MRI outcomes that could be done with smaller sample sizes and over a shorter duration than current placebo-controlled studies with clinical outcomes are attractive at a time in which three approved therapies exist. The approval of a treatment shown to be effective in a clinical study of insufficient size or duration to provide confirmatory clinical outcome data would be problematic. Such studies could fail to identify the full safety profile of the treatment. These issues represent an important challenge for the MS research community. In distinction to its use as a surrogate outcome measure, MRI used in the measurement of disease has substantial value in providing biological markers of disease activity that can offer important insights into the cause of the disease and the effect of new therapies. In this regard MRI remains in invaluable tool in clinical trials.

E. Quantitative Magnetic Resonance Techniques

Magnetization Transfer Imaging

Magnetization transfer (MT) imaging measures the exchange of magnetization between bound (macromolecular) protons and free (mobile) protons in tissues (59,60). If an off-resonance RF pulse selectively saturates the bound proton fraction, the signal intensity of the images is reduced because of the transfer reaction between the two proton pools. The percent reduction in signal intensity on images obtained with the saturation pulse compared to images obtained without the pulse is expressed as the *magnetization transfer ratio* (MTR).

Factors, that affect the equilibrium of the two proton pools, will reduce MTR. Edema and inflammation, which increase the free proton pool, cause a 3 to 5% reduction in MTR. Demyelination, axonal loss, and disruption of the structural integrity of tissues produce a more profound reduction in MTR (61–64). MS lesions on T2W scans have a wide range of MTR values, (20,61,65–67), which is consistent with the known pathological heterogeneity. Lesions with extensive tissue destruction (e.g., T1 holes) have extremely low MTR values (<0.1), which is comparable to the MTR of CSF. Lesions with a 10 to 30% reduction in MTR are probably in various stages of demyelination or remyelination (16). There is an inverse correlation between lesion MTR and clinical disability in cross-sectional studies (68). Serial studies show that MTR decreases dramatically at the time of lesion enhancement and gradually recovers toward normal MTR over the following 1 to 6 months. (50,67–69). Several longitudinal studies have also demonstrated a small but statistically significant decrease in MTR prior to lesion enhancement (70,71), but others have not confirmed this (72). The decrease in MTR prior to contrast enhancement suggests that there may be earlier in lesion formation that is below the threshold of detection by conventional MRI.

Abnormal MTR values have also been detected in the normal-appearing white matter (NAWM) in MS patients (30,73), which confirms previous reports from pathological specimens. (74) To quantitate global white matter disease burden in MS patients, van Buchem and colleagues (75,76) have calculated MTR values for each voxel and plotted the distribution of whole-brain MTR values as a histogram. Their results showed that the height of the histogram peak in MS patients was lower than that of normal controls due to a shift of voxels to lower, abnormal MTR values. Others have also noted a shift of the histogram peak in MS patients, and there is good correlation between the MTR histogram metrics and cognitive or physical disability (77,78).

Two of the current authors have evaluated MTR histogram analysis as an outcome measure in clinical trials. In a small study, 8 RRMS patients were followed by serial monthly MTR studies during a 6-month crossover treatment trial with interferon beta-1b

(IFNbeta-1b) (79). During the baseline period, the histogram peak (Hp) in the MS patients was below that of normal control subjects. The extent of shift in the Hp correlated with the total T2 lesion load. Treatment with IFNβ-1b had no effect on MTR histogram profile during the first 6 months of treatment. Moreover, there were persistent fluctuations in MTR histogram peak during IFNβ-1b treatment, which suggests that there is ongoing inflammation and edema in chronic lesions or in NAWM.

Magnetic Resonance Spectroscopy

In vivo proton magnetic resonance spectroscopy (^{1}H-MRS) measures tissue metabolites and thus biochemical changes in lesions and NAWM of MS patients. MRS with long echo times (TE = 136 ms or TE = 272 ms), identifies four major resonance peaks: *N*-acetylaspartate (NAA), choline, creatine, and lactate. NAA is found exclusively in neurons (80,81), and a decrease in NAA reflects axonal damage or dysfunction (82). The choline (Cho) peak measures membrane phospholipids, and an increase in choline indicates increased membrane turnover with release of lipids and breakdown products of myelin (83). The creatine peak (Cr) is relatively constant and is used to normalize the signal intensities of other metabolites. The lactate peak is generally not detectable but can be associated with acute lesions (84). MRS with short echo times (TE 10 to 30 ms) measures mobile lipids, myoinositol and neurotransmitters. An increase in the mobile lipid peaks has been observed in MS lesions (85,86) and in NAWM (87), suggesting that demyelination can occur in NAWM in the absence of focal inflammation and BBB disruption. MR spectroscopy can be performed using single-voxel, multivoxel, single-slice, or multislice techniques (MRSI), which can simultaneously acquire spectra from 4 × 15 slices (88).

Early single-voxel studies of MS patients demonstrated a reduction of NAA in acute and chronic MS lesions, reflecting neuronal/axonal loss. Subsequent studies, however, found that the 30 to 70% reduction in NAA in acute lesions was partially reversible and the recovery of NAA was associated with recovery of function (89). This suggests that a transient loss of the NAA signal can occur when there are metabolic or structural changes in the axon, caused by inflammation and edema (90). As mentioned above, T1 holes show extensive loss of NAA (23) and are probably the most relevant lesions for clinical disability in SPMS (17).

NAA is also reduced in NAWM of MS patients (30,85,90–96), and the reduction is greater in SPMS patients than in RRMS patients (97–100). To what extent these changes represent diffuse microscopic disease in NAWM (74) or Wallerian degeneration of damaged axons projecting from the lesions is unclear. In a recent study of three patients with a large isolated MS lesion, a transient mirror-image reduction of NAA occurred in the contralateral hemisphere and recovered over the following 6 months (101). The excellent correlation between NAA and clinical disability has generated the axonal hypothesis, which proposes that axonal loss (or dysfunction) rather than demyelination is responsible for functional impairment and disability in MS. Cross-sectional studies showed an inverse correlation of NAA with EDSS (102), and in MS patients with cerebellar ataxia NAA correlated with disability (103). A progressive loss of NAA can be demonstrated in RRMS patients over time. In a 30-month longitudinal study, the decrease in NAA but not T2W lesion load correlated with disease progression as measured by change in EDSS ($p <$ 0.001) (104). Reversible changes in NAA also show a strong correlation ($r = 0.7$, $p <$ 0.001) with relapses and remissions (105).

The results of MRS coupled with the recent findings of axonal transection in MS lesions (106,107) suggest that axonal loss occurs early in disease, is progressive with time, and can cause increasing disability. These findings have important implications for future therapeutic approaches in MS.

F. New Analysis Techniques: Measurement of Atrophy

Atrophy is a global measure of tissue loss in response to injury. In MS patients, axonal loss (106,107) and demyelination (108) contribute to atrophy, but the relative contributions of structural reorganization, loss of macromolecular water, and gliosis are not known. Cerebral atrophy has been recognized for many years in MS patients by radiological criteria: increased size of the lateral ventricles, prominent sulci, increased volume of CSF spaces, and decreased AP diameter of the cervical spinal cord. However, reproducible MRI measurements of atrophy have only recently been obtained.

Spinal cord atrophy was first quantitated by Kidd and the Queen's Square group (109), who manually traced the cross-sectional area of the cord at four vertebral levels (C5, T1, T7, and T11). The mean cord diameter in 80 MS patients was significantly reduced compared to normal controls and showed an inverse correlation with EDSS. Longitudinal studies to determine the rate of atrophy were complicated by technical difficulties (e.g., errors in patient re-positioning, low signal-to-noise ratio between the cord and CSF, flow artifacts) and led to conflicting results (110–113). Finally, Losseff, also of the Queen's Square group (114), developed a highly reproducible semiautomated method of measuring spinal cord diameter at C2 and showed a strong correlation between cord diameter and EDSS ($r = -0.7$, $p < 0.001$) and disease duration ($r = 0.52$, $p < 0.001$) in 60 MS patients. Longitudinal studies of this patient cohort showed progressive reduction in the cord area at C2 over the subsequent 12 months, but there was no definite correlation between cord atrophy and progression of disease as measured by EDSS (115). These studies also showed that the cord diameter was significantly smaller in SPMS patients than in RRMS patients at baseline, but the rate of atrophy over 12 months was greater in RRMS patients. Recent 3D volumetric measurements of the cervical cord at C1-C3 (116) show a modest correlation with EDSS ($p < 0.05$) but a stronger correlation with combined Functional Systems Scores ($r = -0.5$, $p < 0.01$).

Cerebellar atrophy correlates with the degree of ataxia in MS patients (103) and with the Scripps Neurological Rating score (114). Cerebral atrophy has been estimated by regional measurements, which are presumed to reflect a global loss of tissue. Measurements of the corpus callosum (117–123), the width or volume of the lateral ventricles and third ventricle (114,116), and CSF volume (122) have been used.

Recently, global measures of cerebral atrophy have been performed using a central slab of tissue (four contiguous slices 5 mm thick) in the periventricular region (124) and an automated 3D segmentation program that quantitates the brain parenchymal fraction (BPF), the ratio of the brain parenchymal tissue/total brain volume within the outer surface contour (125). Losseff and his group (124) first demonstrated that progressive cerebral atrophy occurred in 29 MS patients over a very short period of time (18 months). Atrophy was observed more frequently in SPMS patients than in RRMS patients, and those patients who had a significant progression of atrophy had greater change in EDSS ($p < 0.05$). Using BPF measurements and a larger group of 172 MS patients, Rudick and colleagues (125) recently demonstrated that atrophy also occurs in early RRMS patients (EDSS 1 to 3.5) over a 2-year period. While there was a correlation between BPF and EDSS at baseline ($r = -0.29$, $p < 0.001$), there was no correlation between the progression of atrophy and change in EDSS during the follow-up period. At baseline, brain volume (BPF) also correlated equally well with disease duration, volume of T1 holes and T2W lesion load ($r =$ -0.29 to 0.49, $p < 0.001$) but not with contrast enhancing lesions or relapse rate. The T2W lesion load was the only factor that predicted subsequent atrophy ($p = 0.01$), and the change in T2 lesion volume correlated with progression of atrophy ($p = 0.05$). However, these correlations are relatively weak.

It is possible that cerebral atrophy correlates better with neurocognitive function than with motor disability on EDSS. Several cross-sectional studies using regional measurements of atrophy (corpus callosum and ventricular size) have shown a positive correlation with cognitive dysfunction (122,126,127), but others show a only a trend (128). Perhaps future studies comparing global atrophy and cognitive function will clarify this issue.

The correlation between cerebral atrophy and other MRI parameters is also unclear. Simon and his collaborators (117) found that contrast-enhancing lesions on the baseline exam were the best predictor of cerebral atrophy measured by increased size of the lateral ($p = 0.046$) and third ventricles ($p = 0.02$). However in the same patient population Rudick and Fisher and colleagues (125) found that enhancing lesions had no predictive value for global cerebral atrophy (BPF). Similarly, T2W lesion load showed no correlation with atrophy in the study of Losseff (124) but did correlate with regional atrophy measures (117) and BPF (125) in early RRMS patients. It is possible that cerebral atrophy is measuring a pathological process that is independent of focal inflammation and T2W lesions but is rather a global disease process that is also quantitated by MTR histogram measurements (129). In this regard it is interesting that 1b (manuscript in preparation), and Interferon B-1a both of which significantly reduce contrast enhancing lesions and T2 burden of disease have no effect on atrophy during the first 12 months of treatment (125). Similarly, IFNβ-1b does not affect the MTR histogram profile during the first 6 months of treatment (79).

G. Future Directions—Functional Techniques and More Quantitative Methods

Several new techniques that will play a prominent role in future imaging studies of MS patients are diffusion-weighted imaging (DWI), functional MRI (fMRI), and measurement of T1 and T2 relaxation times. DWI measures the diffusion properties of water in brain white matter. It is thus the most sensitive MRI imaging method for the diagnosis of ischemic brain infarcts (130). An increase in the apparent diffusion coefficient (ADC) has been demonstrated in MS plaques and in NAWM of MS patients compared to normal white matter of healthy controls (131). Gadolinium-enhancing lesions, and T1W holes have the highest ADC (132), which suggests that this technique may be able to define lesion pathology.

In fMRI, cortical activation to motor or visual stimuli is measured by a change in signal intensity that results from changes in blood levels of deoxyhemoglobin. Several fMRI studies have been reported in MS patients (133,134). fMRI could be a sensitive method for identifying reversible vs. irreversible functional deficits in MS patients and could also be used for testing cognitive function. One major goal for MRI in evaluating of MS patients in future treatment trials would be a comprehensive imaging protocol that would evaluate both cerebral and spinal cord activity as well as cognitive function.

Another functional imaging technique, positron emission tomography (PET), may prove useful in the next 5 to 10 years as well, as the resolution improves to closer what is needed for MS lesions and as we come to understand the more diffuse areas of abnormality in the disease as well. Initial studies have shown both regional and global cerebral hypometabolism in MS (135).

Measurement of the T1 and T2 relaxation times of protons can provide information about the tissue water environment. The use of T1 relaxation time measurement has been limited until recently by the long acquisition time, which limited the clinical application of this technique. MS lesions exhibit a wide range of T1 and T2 relaxation times, which may reflect histopathological heterogeneity. Many plaques show biexponential or multiexponential T2 relaxation, perhaps due to increased extracellular space. These time constants may be of particular interest in studies involving NAWM in the future (136).

III. SUMMARY

The use of MRI in MS has provided valuable insights into the course of the illness and has helped to identify new therapies that have at least a partial effect on disease activity. Thus, MRI has played a pivotal role in the remarkable advances made in the study and treatment of MS over the past decade. Current advances in MRI technology along with increasing well defined studies of pathological correlations of disease seen on MRI and on clinical correlations with disease activity seen on MRI will produce further advances in our understating of the disease. Although there are valid concerns about the use of MRI as a surrogate outcome measure in clinical trials of new therapies, MRI as an outcome measure represents an important option, as it is clearly necessary to consider how we will test new therapies in the future. The MS research community will need to deal with this important issue.

Further, the rapidly evolving technology will present new challenges. Newer techniques are often less stable and less reproducible from center to center, and they present new challenges in analysis. The use of these techniques in an optimal manner requires cooperation between investigators and increased levels of support. Despite these limitations, the potential of MRI as a tool in the study and care of patients with MS seems almost unlimited. Evolving techniques are beginning to define in a precise manner the steps involved in evolution of the MS lesion. These findings, in turn, will lead to more logical design and application of therapies in the disease. Studies of the early RR phase of MS have already provided strong arguments for consideration of early therapy in the illness. It is likely that this single application of MRI to MS will have a significant effect on the natural history of the illness. Advances in the design of more specific therapies and careful application of MRI measures of disease activity to testing new therapies will allow progress to continue at a rapid rate over the next decade.

REFERENCES

1. Thorpe JW, Halpin SF, MacManus DG, Miller DH. A comparison between fast spin echo and conventional spin echo in the detection of multiple sclerosis lesions. Neuroradiology 1994; 35:388–392.
2. Kermode AG, Thompson AJ, Tofts P, MacManus DG, Kendall BE, Kingsley DP, Moseley IF, Rudge P, McDonald WI. Breakdown of the blood-brain barrier precedes symptoms and other MRI signs of new lesions in multiple sclerosis. Pathogenetic and clinical implications. Brain 1990; 113:1477–1489.
3. Filippi M, Bozzali M, Horsfield MA, Rocca MA, Sormani MP, Iannucci G, Colombo B, Comi G. A conventional and magnetization transfer MRI study of the cervical cord in patients with MS. Neurology 2000; 54:207–213.

4. Miller DH, Newton MR, Van der Poel JC, du Boulay EP, Halliday AM, Kendal BE, Johnson G, MacManus DG, Moseley IF, McDonald I. Magnetic resonance imaging of the optic nerve in optic neuritis. Neurology 1988; 38:175–179.

5. Poser CM, Paty DM, Scheinberg L, Mcdonald WI, Davis FA, Ebers GC, Johnson KP, Sibley WA, Silverberg DH, Tourtellotte WW. New diagnostic criteria for multiple sclerosis: Guidelines for research protocols. Ann Neurol 1983; 13:227–231.

6. Fazekas F, Offenbacher H, Fuchs S, Schmidt R, Niederkorn K, Horner S, Lechner H. Criteria for an increased specificity of MRI interpretation in elderly subjects with suspected multiple sclerosis. Neurology 1988; 38:1822–1825.

7. Offenbacker H, Fazekas F, Schmidt R, Freidl W, Flooh E, Payer F, Lechner H. Assessment of MRI criteria for a diagnosis of MS. Neurology 1993; 43:905–909.

8. Paty DW, Oger JJ, Kastrukoff LF, Hashimoto SA, Hooge JP, Eisen AA, Eisen KA, Purves SJ, Low MD, Brandejs V. MRI in the diagnosis of MS: A prospective study with comparison of clinical evaluation, evoked potentials, oligoclonal banding, and CT. Neurology 1988; 38: 180–185.

9. Barkhof, Filippi M, Miller DH, Scheltens P, Campi A, Polman CH, Comi G, Ader HJ, Losseff N, Valk J. Comparison of MRI criteria at first presentation to predict conversion to clinically definite multiple sclerosis. Eur Neurol 1998; 39:80–89.

10. O'Riordan JK, Gomez-Anson B, Moseley IF, Miller DH. Long term MRI follow-up of patients with post infectious encephalomyelitis: Evidence for a monophasic disease. J Neurol Sci 1999; 167:132–136.

11. Miller DH, Barkhof F, Nauta JJ. Gadolinium enhancement increases the sensitivity of MRI in detecting disease activity in multiple sclerosis. Brain 1993; 116:1077–1094.

12. Tas MW, Barkhof F, van Walderveen MAA, Polman CH, Homes OR, Valk J. The effect of gadolinium on the sensitivity and specificity of MR in the initial diagnosis of multiple sclerosis. AJNR 1995; 16:259–264.

13. Katz D, Taubenberger JK, Cannella B, McFarlin DE, Raine CS, McFarland HF. Correlation between magnetic resonance imaging findings and lesion development in chronic, active multiple sclerosis. Ann Neurol 1993; 34:661–669.

14. Bruck W, Bitsch A, Kolenda H, Bruck Y, Stiefel M, Lassmann H. Inflammatory central nervous system demyelination: Correlation of magnetic resonance imaging findings with lesion pathology. Ann Neurol 1997; 42:783–793.

15. van Walderveen MA, Barkhof F, Hommes OR, Polman CH, Tobi H, Frequin ST, Valk J. Correlating MRI and clinical disease activity in multiple sclerosis: Relevance of hypointense lesions on short-TR/short-TE (T1-weighted) spin-echo images. Neurology 1995; 45:1684–1690

16. Hiehle JF Jr. Grossman RI, Ramer KN, Gonzalez-Scarano F, Cohen JA. Magnetization transfer effects in MR-detected multiple sclerosis lesions: Comparison with gadolinium-enhanced spin-echo images and nonenhanced T1-weighted images. AJNR 1995; 16:69–77.

17. Truyen L, van Waesberghe JH, van Walderveen MA, van Oosten BW, Polman CH, Hommes OR, Ader HJ, Barkhof F. Accumulation of hypointense lesions (''black holes'') on T1 spin-echo MRI correlates with disease progression in multiple sclerosis. Neurology 1996; 47: 1469–1476.

18. Uhlenbrock D, Sehlen S. The value of T1-weighted images in the differentiation between MS, white matter lesions, and subcortical arteriosclerotic encephalopathy (SAE). Neuroradiology 1989; 31:203–212.

19. van Walderveen MA, Kamphorst W, Scheltens P, van Waesberghe JH, Ravid R, Valk J, Polman CH, Barkhof F. Histopathologic correlate of hypointense lesions on T1-weighted spin- echo MRI in multiple sclerosis. Neurology 1998; 50:1282–1288.

20. Loevner LA, Grossman RI, McGowan JC, Ramer KN, Cohen JA. Characterization of multiple sclerosis plaques with T1-weighted MR and quantitative magnetization transfer. AJNR 1995; 16:1473–1479.

21. Hiehle JF, Jr., Lenkinski RE, Grossman RI, Dousset V, Ramer KN, Schnall MD, Cohen JA, Gonzalez-Scarano F. Correlation of spectroscopy and magnetization transfer imaging in the evaluation of demyelinating lesions and normal appearing white matter in multiple sclerosis. Magn Reson Med 1994; 32:285–293.

22. van Walderveen MA, Barkhof F, Pouwels PJ, van Schijndel RA, Polman CH, Castelijns JA. Neuronal damage in T1-hypointense multiple sclerosis lesions demonstrated in vivo using proton magnetic resonance spectroscopy. Ann Neurol 1999; 46:79–87.

23. van Waesberghe JH, Kamphorst W, De Groot CJ, van Walderveen MA, Castelijns JA, Ravid R, Lycklama a Nijeholt GJ, van der Valk P, Polman CH, Thompson AJ, Barkhof F. Axonal loss in multiple sclerosis lesions: Magnetic resonance imaging insights into substrates of disability. Ann Neurol 1999; 46:747–54.

24. Issac C, Li DKB, Genton M, Jardine C, Grochowski E, Palmer M, Kastrukoff LF, Oger J, Paty DW. Multiple sclerosis: a serial study using MRI in relapsing patients. Neurology 1988; 38:1511–1515.

25. Paty DW, Li DK. Interferon beta-1b is effective in relapsing-remitting multiple sclerosis. II. MRI analysis results of a multicenter, randomized, double blind, placebo-controlled trial. UBC MS/MRI Study Group and the IFNB Multiple Sclerosis Study Group. Neurology 1993; 43:662–667.

26. Stone LA, Albert PS, Smith ME, DeCarli C, Armstrong MR, McFarlin DE, Frank JA, McFarland HF. Changes in the amount of diseased white matter over time in patients with relapsing remitting multiple sclerosis. Neurology 1995; 45:1808–1814.

27. Filippi M, Paty DW, Kappos L, Barkhof F, Compston DA, Thompson AJ, Zhao GJ, Wiles CM, McDonald WI, Miller DH. Correlations between changes in disability and T2-weighted brain MRI activity in multiple sclerosis: a follow-up study. Neurology 1995; 45:255–260.

28. Barkhof F. MRI in multiple sclerosis: Correlation with expanded disability status scale (EDSS). Mult Scler 1999; 5:283–286.

29. Kurtzke JF. Rating neurologic impairment in multiple sclerosis: An expanded disability status scale (EDSS). Neurology. 1983; 33:1444–1452.

30. Filippi M, Campi A, Dousset V, Baratti C, Martinelli V, Canal N, Scotti G, Comi G. A magnetization transfer imaging study of normal-appearing white matter in multiple sclerosis. Neurology 1995; 45:478–482.

31. Bakshi R, Shaikh ZA, Janardhan V. MRI T2 shortening ('black T2') in multiple sclerosis: Frequency, location, and clinical correlation. Neuroreport 2000; 11:15–21.

32. Grossman RI, Braffman BH, Brorson JR, Goldberg HI, Silberberg DH, Gonzalez-Scarano F. Multiple sclerosis: Serial study of gadolinium-enhanced MR imaging. Radiology 1988; 169:117–122.

33. Smith ME, Stone LA, Albert PS, Frank JA, Martin R, Armstrong M, Maloni H, McFarlin DE, McFarland HF. Clinical worsening in multiple sclerosis is associated with increased frequency and area of gadopentetate dimeglumine–enhancing magnetic resonance imaging lesions. Ann Neurol 1993; 33:480–489.

34. Lai M, Hodgson T, Gawne-Cain M, Webb S, MacManus D, McDonald WI, Thompson AJ, Miller DH. A preliminary study into the sensitivity of disease activity detection by serial weekly magnetic resonance imaging in multiple sclerosis. J Neurol Neurosurg Psychiatry 1996; 60:339–341.

35. Silver NC, Good CD, Barker GJ, MacManus DG, Thompson AJ, Moseley IF, McDonald WI, Miller DH. Sensitivity of contrast enhanced MRI in multiple sclerosis. Effects of gadolinium dose, magnetization transfer contrast and delayed imaging. Brain 1997; 120:1149–1161.

36. Filippi M, Capra R, Campi A, Colombo B, Prandini F, Marciano N, Gasparotti R, Comi G. Triple dose of gadolinium-DTPA and delayed MRI in patients with benign multiple sclerosis. J Neurol Neurosurg Psychiatry 60:526–530, 1996.

37. Stone LA, Smith ME, Albert PS, Bash CN, Maloni H, Frank JA, McFarland HF. Blood brain barrier disruption as measured by contrast enhanced MRI in patients with mild relapsing

remitting multiple sclerosis: Relationship to course gender and age. Neurology 1995; 45: 1122–1126.

38. Nijeholt GJ, van Walderveen MA, Castelijns JA, van Waesberghe JH, Polman C, Scheltens P, Rosier PF, Jongen PJ, Barkhof F. Brain and spinal cord abnormalities in multiple sclerosis. Correlation between MRI parameters, clinical subtypes and symptoms. Brain 1998; 121:687–697.

39. Calabresi PA, Fields NS, Farnon EC, Frank JA, Bash CN, Kawanshi T, Maloni H, Jacobson S, McFarland H. ELI-spot of Th-1 cytokine secreting PBMCs in multiple sclerosis: Correlation with MRI lesions. J Neuroimmunol 1998; 85:212–219.

40. Hartung H-P, Reiners K, Archelos JJ, Michels M Seeldrayers P, Heidenreich F Pflughaupt KW, Toyka KV. Circulating adhesion molecules and tumor necrosis factor receptor in multiple sclerosis: Correlation with magnetic resonance imaging. Ann Neurol 1995; 38:186–193.

41. Giovannoni G, Kieseier B, Hartung HP. Correlating immunological and magnetic resonance imaging markers of disease activity in multiple sclerosis. J Neurol Neurosurg Psychiatry 1998; 64 (suppl 1):S31–S36.

42. Frank JA, Stone LA, Smith ME, Albert PS, Maloni H, McFarland HF. Serial contrast-enhanced magnetic resonance imaging in patients with early relapsing-remitting multiple sclerosis: implications for treatment trials. Ann Neurol 1994; 36 (suppl):S86–S90.

43. Tubridy N, Ader HJ, Barkhof F, Thompson AJ, Miller DH. Exploratory treatment trials in multiple sclerosis using MRI: Sample size calculations for relapsing-remitting and secondary progressive subgroups using placebo controlled parallel groups. J Neurol Neurosurg Psychiatry 1998; 64:50–55.

44. Nauta JJ, Thompson AJ, Barkhof F, Miller DH. Magnetic resonance imaging in monitoring the treatment of multiple sclerosis patients: statistical power of parallel-groups and crossover designs. J Neurol Sci 1994; 122:6–14.

45. Truyen L, Barkhof F, Tas M, Van Walderveen MA, Frequin ST, Hommes OR, Nauta JJ, Polman CH, Valk J. Specific power calculations for magnetic resonance imaging (MRI) in monitoring active relapsing-remitting multiple sclerosis (MS): Implications for phase II therapeutic trials. Mult Scler 1997; 2:283–290.

46. Kappos L, Moeri D, Radue EW, Schoetzau A, Schweikert K, Barkhof F, Miller D, Guttmann CR, Weiner HL, Gasperini C, Filippi M. Predictive value of gadolinium-enhanced magnetic resonance imaging for relapse rate and changes in disability or impairment in multiple sclerosis: A meta-analysis. Gadolinium MRI Meta-analysis Group. Lancet 1999; 353:964–969.

47. Khoury SJ, Guttmann CR, Orav EJ, Hohol MJ, Ahn SS, Hsu L, Kikinis R, Mackin GA, Jolesz FA, Weiner HL. Longitudinal MRI in multiple sclerosis: Correlation between disability and lesion burden. Neurology 1994; 44:2120–2124.

48. Molyneux PD, Filippi M, Barkhof F, Gasperini C, Yousry TA, Truyen L, Lai HM, Rocca MA, Moseley IF, Miller DH. Correlations between monthly enhanced MRI lesion rate and changes in T2 lesion volume in multiple sclerosis. Ann Neurol 1998; 43:332–339.

49. Simon JH, Jacobs LD, Campion M, Wende K, Simonian N, Cookfair DL, Rudick RA, Herndon RM, Richert JR, Salazar AM, Alam JJ, Fischer JS, Goodkin DE, Granger CV, Lajaunie M, Martens-Davidson AL, Meyer M, Sheeder J, Choi K, Scherzinger AL, Bartoszak DM, Bourdette DN, Braiman J, Brownscheidle CM, Whitham RH. Magnetic resonance studies of intramuscular interferon beta-1a for relapsing multiple sclerosis: The Multiple Sclerosis Collaborative Research Group. Ann Neurol 1998; 43:79–87.

50. van Waesberghe JH, van Walderveen MA, Castelijns JA, Scheltens P, Lycklama a Nijeholt GJ, Polman CH, Barkhof F. Patterns of lesion development in multiple sclerosis: Longitudinal observations with T1-weighted spin-echo and magnetization transfer MR. AJNR 1998; 19:675–683.

51. van Walderveen MA, Truyen L, van Oosten BW, Castelijns JA, Lycklamaa Nijeholt GJ, van Waesberghe JH, Polman C, Barkhof F. Development of hypointense lesions on T1weighted

spin-echo magnetic resonance images in multiple sclerosis: Relation to inflammatory activity. Arch Neurol 1999; 56:345–351.

52. Ciccarelli O, Giugni E, Paolillo A, Mainero C, Gasperini C, Bastianello S, Pozzilli C. Magnetic resonance outcome of new enhancing lesions in patients with relapsing-remitting multiple sclerosis. Eur J Neurol 1999; 6:455–459.

53. Bucher HC, Guyatt GH, Cook DJ, Holbrook A, McAlister FA. The evidence-based medicine working group. JAMA 282:771–778, 1999.

54. Fleming, TR. Surrogate markers in AIDS and cancer trials. Statistics in Medicine 1994; 13: 1423–1440.

55. O'Riordan JI, Thompson AJ, Kingsley DP, MacManus DG, Kendal BE, Rudge P, McDonald WI, Miller DH. The prognostic value of brain MRI in clinically isolated syndromes of the CNS. A 10 year follow-up. Brain 1998; 121:495–503.

56. Comi G, Filippi M, Barkhof F, Durelli L, Edan G, Fernandez O. Hartung HP, Seeldrayers P, Soelberg-Sorensen P, Rovaris M, Martinelli F, Homes OR, and the ETOMS study group. Interferon beta 1a (Rebif) in patients with acute neurological syndromes suggestive of multiple sclerosis: A multi-center, randomized, double-blind, placebo-controlled study. Neurology 54 (suppl 3): A85, 2000.

57. Ge Y, Grossman RI, Udupa JK, Fulton J, Constantines CS, Gonzales-Scarano F, Babb JS, Mannon LJ, Kolson DL Cohen JA. Glatiramer acetate (Copaxone) treatment in relapsing–remitting MS: Quantitative MR assessment. Neurology 2000; 54 (suppl 3): A86, (Suppl 3).

58. Miller DH. Multiple sclerosis: Use of MRI in evaluating new therapies. Semin Neurol 1998; 18:317–325.

59. Wolff SD, Balaban RS. Magnetization transfer contrast (MTC) and tissue water proton relaxation in vivo. Magn Reson Med 1989; 10:135–144.

60. Wolff SD, Balaban RS. Magnetization transfer imaging: Practical aspects and clinical applications. Radiology 1994; 192:593–599.

61. Dousset V, Grossman RI, Ramer KN, Schnall MD, Young LH, Gonzalez-Scarano F, Lavi E, Cohen JA. Experimental allergic encephalomyelitis and multiple sclerosis: Lesion characterization with magnetization transfer imaging [published erratum appears in Radiology 1992 Jun;183(3):878]. Radiology 1992; 182:483–491.

62. Lexa FJ, Grossman RI, Rosenquist AC. Dyke Award paper. MR of wallerian degeneration in the feline visual system: characterization by magnetization transfer rate with histopathologic correlation. AJNR 1994; 15:201–212.

63. Dousset V, Armand JP, Huot P, Viaud B, Caille JM. Magnetization transfer imaging in AIDS-related brain diseases. Neuroimaging Clin North Am 1997; 7:447–460.

64. Dousset V, Armand JP, Lacoste D, Mieze S, Letenneur L, Dartigues JF, Caill JM. Magnetization transfer study of HIV encephalitis and progressive multifocal leukoencephalopathy. Groupe d'Epidemiologie Clinique du SIDA en Aquitaine. AJNR Am J Neuroradiol 1997; 18:895–901.

65. Brochet B, Dousset V. Pathological correlates of magnetization transfer imaging abnormalities in animal models and humans with multiple sclerosis. Neurology 53:S12–S7, 1999.

66. Campi A, Filippi M, Comi G, Scotti G, Gerevini S, Dousset V. Magnetisation transfer ratios of contrast-enhancing and nonenhancing lesions in multiple sclerosis. Neuroradiology 1996; 38:115–119.

67. Gass A, Barker GJ, Kidd D, Thorpe JW, MacManus D, Brennan A, Tofts PS, Thompson AJ, McDonald WI, Miller DH. Correlation of magnetization transfer ratio with clinical disability in multiple sclerosis. Ann Neurol 1994; 36:62–67.

68. Dousset V, Gayou A, Brochet B, Caille JM. Early structural changes in acute MS lesions assessed by serial magnetization transfer studies. Neurology 51:1150–51998.

69. Lai HM, Davie CA, Gass A, Barker GJ, Webb S, Tofts PS, Thompson AJ, McDonald WI, Miller DH. Serial magnetisation transfer ratios in gadolinium-enhancing lesions in multiple sclerosis. J Neurol 244:308–311, 1997.

70. Filippi M, Rocca MA, Martino G, Horsfield MA, Comi G. Magnetization transfer changes in the normal appearing white matter precede the appearance of enhancing lesions in patients with multiple sclerosis. Ann Neurol 1998; 43:809–814.

71. Goodkin DE, Rooney WD, Sloan R, Bacchetti P, Gee L, Vermathen M, Waubant E, Abundo M, Majumdar S, Nelson S, Weiner MW. A serial study of new MS lesions and the white matter from which they arise. Neurology 1998; 51:1689–97.

72. Silver NC, Lai M, Symms MR, Barker GJ, McDonald WI, Miller DH. Serial magnetization transfer imaging to characterize the early evolution of new MS lesions. Neurology 1998; 51: 758–764.

73. Loevner LA, Grossman RI, Cohen JA, Lexa FJ, Kessler D, Kolson DL. Microscopic disease in normal-appearing white matter on conventional MR images in patients with multiple sclerosis: Assessment with magnetization-transfer measurements. Radiology 1995; 196:511–515.

74. Allen IV, McKeown SR. A histological, histochemical and biochemical study of the macroscopically normal white matter in multiple sclerosis. J Neurol Sci 1979; 41:81–91.

75. van Buchem MA, McGowan JC, Kolson DL, Polansky M, Grossman RI. Quantitative volumetric magnetization transfer analysis in multiple sclerosis: estimation of macroscopic and microscopic disease burden. Magn Reson Med 1996; 36:632–636.

76. van Buchem MA, Udupa JK, McGowan JC, Miki Y, Heyning FH, Boncoeur-Martel MP, Kolson DL, Polansky M, Grossman RI. Global volumetric estimation of disease burden in multiple sclerosis based on magnetization transfer imaging. AJNR Am J Neuroradiol 1997; 18:1287–1290.

77. van Buchem MA, Grossman RI, Armstrong C, Polansky M, Miki Y, Heyning FH, Boncoeur-Martel MP, Wei L, Udupa JK, Grossman M, Kolson DL, McGowan JC. Correlation of volumetric magnetization transfer imaging with clinical data in MS. Neurology 1998; 50:1609–1617,

78. Rovaris M, Filippi M, Falautano M, Minicucci L, Rocca MA, Martinelli V, Comi G. Relation between MR abnormalities and patterns of cognitive impairment in multiple sclerosis. Neurology 1998; 50:1601–1608.

79. Richert ND, Ostuni JL, Bash CN, Duyn JH, McFarland HF, Frank JA. Serial whole-brain magnetization transfer imaging in patients with relapsing-remitting multiple sclerosis at baseline and during treatment with interferon beta-1b. AJNR 1998; 19:1705–1713.

80. Urenjak J, Williams SR, Gadian DG, Noble M. Proton nuclear magnetic resonance spectroscopy unambiguously identifies different neural cell types. J Neurosci 1993; 13:981–989.

81. Urenjak J, Williams SR, Gadian DG, Noble M. Specific expression of N-acetylaspartate in neurons, oligodendrocyte type 2 astrocyte progenitors, and immature oligodendrocytes in vitro. J Neurochem 59:55–61, 1992.

82. McDonald WI. Rachelle Fishman-Matthew Moore Lecture. The pathological and clinical dynamics of multiple sclerosis. J Neuropathol Exp Neurol 1994; 53:338–343.

83. Arnold DL, Wolinsky JS, Matthews PM, Falini A. The use of magnetic resonance spectroscopy in the evaluation of the natural history of multiple sclerosis. J Neurol Neurosurg Psychiatry 1998; 64 (suppl 1):S94–S101.

84. Clanet M, Berry I. Magnetic resonance imaging in multiple sclerosis. Curr Opin Neurol 1998; 11:299–303.

85. Davie CA, Hawkins CP, Barker GJ, Brennan A, Tofts PS, Miller DH, McDonald WI. Serial proton magnetic resonance spectroscopy in acute multiple sclerosis lesions. Brain 1994; 117: 49–58.

86. Wolinsky JS, Narayana PA, Fenstermacher MJ. Proton magnetic resonance spectroscopy in multiple sclerosis. Neurology 1990; 40:1764–1769.

87. Narayana PA, Doyle TJ, Lai D, Wolinsky JS. Serial proton magnetic resonance spectroscopic imaging, contrast-enhanced magnetic resonance imaging, and quantitative lesion volumetry in multiple sclerosis. Ann Neurol 1998; 43:56–71.

88. Duyn JH, Moonen CT. Fast proton spectroscopic imaging of human brain using multiple spin-echoes. Magn Reson Med 1993; 30:409–414.

89. Miller DH, Austin SJ, Connelly A, Youl BD, Gadian DG, McDonald WI. Proton magnetic resonance spectroscopy of an acute and chronic lesion in multiple sclerosis (letter) (see comments). Lancet 1991; 337:58–59.

90. Arnold DL, Matthews PM, Francis GS, O'Connor J, Antel JP. Proton magnetic resonance spectroscopic imaging for metabolic characterization of demyelinating plaques. Ann Neurol 1992; 31:235–241.

91. Bruhn H, Frahm J, Merboldt KD, Hanicke W, Hanefeld Γ, Christen HJ, Kruse B, Bauer HJ. Multiple sclerosis in children: cerebral metabolic alterations monitored by localized proton magnetic resonance spectroscopy in vivo. Ann Neurol 1992; 32:140–150.

92. Matthews PM, Francis G, Antel J, Arnold DL. Proton magnetic resonance spectroscopy for metabolic characterization of plaques in multiple sclerosis [published erratum appears in Neurology 1991 Nov;41(11):1828]. Neurology 1991; 41:1251–1256.

93. De Stefano N, Matthews PM, Narayanan S, Francis GS, Antel JP, Arnold DL. Axonal dysfunction and disability in a relapse of multiple sclerosis: longitudinal study of a patient. Neurology 1997; 49:1138–41.

94. Matthews PM, De Stefano N, Narayanan S, Francis GS, Wolinsky JS, Antel JP, Arnold DL. Putting magnetic resonance spectroscopy studies in context: Axonal damage and disability in multiple sclerosis. Semin Neurol 18:327–336, 1998.

95. Arnold DL, Matthews PM, Francis G, Antel J. Proton magnetic resonance spectroscopy of human brain in vivo in the evaluation of multiple sclerosis: Assessment of the load of disease. Magn Reson Med 1990; 14:154–159.

96. Arnold DL, Riess GT, Matthews PM, Francis GS, Collins DL, Wolfson C, Antel JP. Use of proton magnetic resonance spectroscopy for monitoring disease progression in multiple sclerosis. Ann Neurol 1994; 36:76–82.

97. Husted CA, Goodin DS, Hugg JW, Maudsley AA, Tsuruda JS, de Bie SH, Fein G, Matson GB, Weiner MW. Biochemical alterations in multiple sclerosis lesions and normal-appearing white matter detected by in vivo 31P and 1H spectroscopic imaging. Ann Neurol 1994; 36: 157–165.

98. Fu L, Matthews PM, De Stefano N, Worsley KJ, Narayanan S, Francis GS, Antel JP, Wolfson C, Arnold DL. Imaging axonal damage of normal-appearing white matter in multiple sclerosis. Brain 1998; 121:103–113.

99. Sarchielli P, Presciutti O, Pelliccioli GP, Tarducci R, Gobbi G, Chiarini P, Alberti A, Vicinanza F, Gallai V. Absolute quantification of brain metabolites by proton magnetic resonance spectroscopy in normal-appearing white matter of multiple sclerosis patients. Brain 1999; 122:513–521.

100. Tourbah A, Stievenart JL, Gout O, Fontaine B, Liblau R, Lubetzki C, Cabanis EA, Lyon-Caen O. Localized proton magnetic resonance spectroscopy in relapsing remitting versus secondary progressive multiple sclerosis. Neurology 1999; 53:1091–1097.

101. De Stefano N, Narayanan S, Matthews PM, Francis GS, Antel JP, Arnold DL. In vivo evidence for axonal dysfunction remote from focal cerebral demyelination of the type seen in multiple sclerosis. Brain 1999; 122:1933–1939.

102. Matthews PM, De Stefano N, Narayanan S, Francis GS, Wolinsky JS, Antel JP, Arnold DL. Putting magnetic resonance spectroscopy studies in context: Axonal damage and disability in multiple sclerosis. Semin Neurol 1998; 18:327-36.

103. Davie CA, Barker GJ, Webb S, Tofts PS, Thompson AJ, Harding AE, McDonald WI, Miller DH. Persistent functional deficit in multiple sclerosis and autosomal dominant cerebellar ataxia is associated with axon loss. Brain 1995; 118:1583–1592.

104. De Stefano N, Matthews PM, Fu L, Narayanan S, Stanley J, Francis GS, Antel JP, Arnold DL. Axonal damage correlates with disability in patients with relapsing-remitting multiple

sclerosis. Results of a longitudinal magnetic resonance spectroscopy study. Brain 1998; 121: 1469–1477.

105. Ferguson B, Matyszak MK, Esiri MM, Perry VH. Axonal damage in acute multiple sclerosis lesions. Brain 1997; 120:393–399.

106. Trapp BD, Peterson J, Ransohoff RM, Rudick R, Mork S, Bo L. Axonal transection in the lesions of multiple sclerosis (see comments). N Engl J Med 1998; 338:278–285.

107. Raine CS, Scheinberg LC. On the immunopathology of plaque development and repair in multiple sclerosis. J Neuroimmunol 1988; 20:189–201.

108. Prineas JW, Connell F. The fine structure of chronically active multiple sclerosis plaques. Neurology 1978; 28:68–75.

109. Kidd D, Thorpe JW, Thompson AJ, Kendall BE, Moseley IF, MacManus DG, McDonald WI, Miller DH. Spinal cord MRI using multi-array coils and fast spin echo: II. Findings in multiple sclerosis. Neurology 1993; 43:2632–2637.

110. Kidd D, Thorpe JW, Kendall BE, Barker GJ, Miller DH, McDonald WI, Thompson AJ. MRI dynamics of brain and spinal cord in progressive multiple sclerosis. J Neurol Neurosurg Psychiatry 1996; 60:15–19.

111. Thorpe JW, Kidd D, Moseley IF, Kenndall BE, Thompson AJ, MacManus DG, McDonald WI, Miller DH. Serial gadolinium-enhanced MRI of the brain and spinal cord in early relapsing-remitting multiple sclerosis. Neurology 1996; 46:373–378.

112. Filippi M, Campi A, Colombo B, Pereira C, Martinelli V, Baratti C, Comi G. A spinal cord MRI study of benign and secondary progressive multiple sclerosis. J Neurol 1996; 243:502–505.

113. Losseff NA, Webb SL, O'Riordan JI, Page R, Wang L, Barker GJ, Tofts PS, McDonald WI, Miller DH, Thompson AJ. Spinal cord atrophy and disability in multiple sclerosis. A new reproducible and sensitive MRI method with potential to monitor disease progression. Brain 1996; 119:701–708.

114. Stevenson VL, Leary SM, Losseff NA, Parker GJ, Barker GJ, Husmani Y, Miller DH, Thompson AJ. Spinal cord atrophy and disability in MS: A longitudinal study. Neurology 1998; 51:234–238.

115. Liu C, Edwards S, Gong Q, Roberts N, Blumhardt LD. Three dimensional MRI estimates of brain and spinal cord atrophy in multiple sclerosis. J Neurol Neurosurg Psychiatry 1999; 66:323–330.

116. Edwards SG, Gong QY, Liu C, Zvartau ME, Jaspan T, Roberts N, Blumhardt LD. Infratentorial atrophy on magnetic resonance imaging and disability in multiple sclerosis. Brain 1999; 122:291–301.

117. Simon JH, Jacobs LD, Campion MK, Rudick RA, Cookfair DL, Herndon RM, Richert JR, Salazar AM, Fischer JS, Goodkin DE, Simonian N, Lajaunie M, Miller DE, Wende K, Martens-Davidson A, Kinkel RP, Munschauer FE III, Brownscheidle CM. A longitudinal study of brain atrophy in relapsing multiple sclerosis. The Multiple Sclerosis Collaborative Research Group (MSCRG). Neurology 1999; 53:139–148.

118. Huber SJ, Paulson GW, Shuttleworth EC, Chakeres D, Clapp LE, Pakalnis A, Weiss K, Rammohan K. Magnetic resonance imaging correlates of dementia in multiple sclerosis. Arch Neurol 1987; 44:732–736.

119. Dietemann JL, Beigelman C, Rumbach L, Vouge M, Tajahmady T, Faubert C, Jeung MY, Wackenheim A. Multiple sclerosis and corpus callosum atrophy: Relationship of MRI findings to clinical data. Neuroradiology 1988; 30:478–480.

120. Pelletier J, Habib M, Lyon-Caen O, Salamon G, Poncet M, Khalil R. Functional and magnetic resonance imaging correlates of callosal involvement in multiple sclerosis. Arch Neurol 1993; 50:1077–1082.

121. Pozzilli C, Bastianello S, Padovani A, Passafiume D, Millefiorini E, Bozzao L, Fieschi C. Anterior corpus callosum atrophy and verbal fluency in multiple sclerosis. Cortex 1991; 27: 441–445.

122. Barkhof FJ, Elton M, Lindeboom J, Tas MW, Schmidt WF, Hommes OR, Polman CH, Kok A, Valk J. Functional correlates of callosal atrophy in relapsing-remitting multiple sclerosis patients. A preliminary MRI study. J Neurol 1998; 245:153–158.

123. Dastidar P, Heinonen T, Lehtimaki T, Ukkonen M, Peltola J, Erila T, Laasonen E, Elovaara I. Volumes of brain atrophy and plaques correlated with neurological disability in secondary progressive multiple sclerosis. J Neurol Sci 1999; 165:36–42.

124. Losseff NA, Wang L, Lai HM, Yoo DS, Gawne-Cain ML, McDonald WI, Miller DH, Thompson AJ. Progressive cerebral atrophy in multiple sclerosis: A serial MRI study. Brain 1996; 119:2009–2019.

125. Rudick RA, Fisher E, Lee JC, Simon J, Jacobs L. Use of the brain parenchymal fraction to measure whole brain atrophy in relapsing-remitting MS. Multiple Sclerosis Collaborative Research Group (in process citation). Neurology 1999; 53:1698–1704.

126. Comi G, Filippi M, Martinelli V, Sirabian G, Visciani A, Campi A, Mammi S, Rovaris M, Canal N. Brain magnetic resonance imaging correlates of cognitive impairment in multiple sclerosis. J Neurol Sci 1993; 115 (suppl):S66–S73.

127. Pozzilli C, Passafiume D, Anzini A, Borsellino G, Koudriavsteva T, Sarlo G, Fieschi C. Cognitive and brain imaging measures of multiple sclerosis. Ital J Neurol Sci 1992; 13:133–136.

128. Rao SM, Glatt S, Hammeke TA, McQuillen MP, Khatri BO, Rhodes AM, Pollard S. Chronic progressive multiple sclerosis. Relationship between cerebral ventricular size and neuropsychological impairment. Arch Neurol 1985; 42:678–682.

129. Phillips MD, Grossman RI, Miki Y, Wei L, Kolson DL, van Buchem MA, Polansky M, McGowan JC, Udupa JK. Comparison of T2 lesion volume and magnetization transfer ratio histogram analysis and of atrophy and measures of lesion burden in patients with multiple sclerosis. AJNR 1998; 19:1055–1060.

130. Schabitz WR, Fisher M. Diffusion weighted imaging for acute cerebral infarction. Neurol Res 1995; 17:270–274.

131. Horsfield MA, Lai M, Webb SL, Barker GJ, Tofts PS, Turner R, Rudge P, Miller DH. Apparent diffusion coefficients in benign and secondary progressive multiple sclerosis by nuclear magnetic resonance. Magn Reson Med 1996; 36:393–400.

132. Droogan AG, Clark CA, Werring DJ, Barker GJ, McDonald WI, Miller DH. Comparison of multiple sclerosis clinical subgroups using navigated spin echo diffusion-weighted imaging. Magn Reson Imaging 1999; 17:6536–6561.

133. Yousry TA, Berry I, Filippi M. Functional magnetic resonance imaging in multiple sclerosis. J Neurol Neurosurg Psychiatry 1998; 64 (suppl 1):S85–S87.

134. Gareau PJ, Gati JS, Menon RS, Lee D, Rice G, Mitchell JR, Mandelfino P, Karlik SJ. Reduced visual evoked responses in multiple sclerosis patients with optic neuritis: Comparison of functional magnetic resonance imaging and visual evoked potentials. Mult Scler 1999; 5:161–164.

135. Bakshi R, Kinkel PR, Miletich RS, Emmet ML, Kinkel WR. High-resolution flurodeoxyglucose positron emission tomography shows both global and regional hypometabolism in multiple sclerosis. J Neuroimaging 1998; 8:228–234.

136. Van Walderveen MA, Barkhof F. Measures of T1 and T2 relaxation. In: Rudick R, Goodkin D, eds. Multiple Sclerosis Therapeutics. London: Martin Dunitz, 1999, pp. 91–106.

17

The Natural History of Multiple Sclerosis

SANDRA VUKUSIC and CHRISTIAN CONFAVREUX

Hôpital Neurologique Lyon, France

I. INTRODUCTION

The natural history of multiple sclerosis has been the topic of numerous studies for decades. The analysis of large and disease-representative cohorts of patients with a sufficient follow-up at close enough intervals, and the use of appropriate modern statistical techniques such as survival analysis, have made it possible to clearly delineate the overall prognosis of multiple sclerosis, which is currently well known. In this respect, results are consistent between the major series of the literature. However, there is also a considerable diversity of outcomes among individuals. This being said, the accumulation of disability within a given individual follows a remarkably steady progression, as shown by serial quantitative neurological examination. At present, the prediction of outcome in a given patient is still quite impossible when using clinical putative predictors, notably at the very onset of the disease, when therapeutic interventions are to be decided on or refrained from. Hopefully, the emerging magnetic resonance techniques will be more helpful in this respect in the near future.

For decades, many authors have been tempted to describe the overall course and prognosis of this so-called unpredictable disease (1–27). One of the key issues in providing information about its natural history is to define an adequate cohort. Several authors have discussed the qualities of an ideal natural history cohort of multiple sclerosis patients (28). Such a cohort must be population-based so as to avoid the referral bias of hospital- and clinic-based series. The follow-up must be prospective and longitudinal, and should begin near the onset of the disease, which is not so easy, considering the delay in establishing the diagnosis and the difference between the biological and clinical onset. The follow-up should be long enough, in respect with the length of the disease course, without any bias

433

toward the most severe cases. Last, the ideal cohort must be "natural," and the patients should not have been treated with any disease-modifying agent. Steroids are the only tolerated therapy.

II. DEFINITIONS AND CLASSIFICATIONS

The clinical course of the disease is made up of two distinct types of neurological episodes, exacerbations and progression, which lead to two distinct phases of multiple sclerosis.

An exacerbation—for which relapse, attack, and bout are alternative designations—is defined as the appearance, the reappearance, or the worsening of symptoms of neurological dysfunction lasting more than 24 h. It has a subacute onset. The initial phase is followed by a plateau, and usually by an improvement (remission), which may be complete or not. Some authors distinguish between exacerbations with and those without sequelae. A transient worsening of symptoms associated with an increase in body temperature, infec-

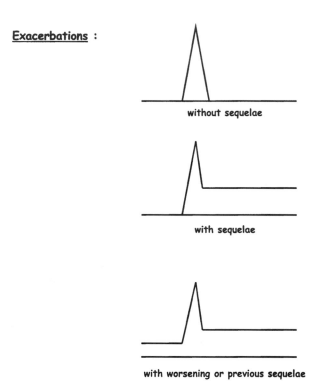

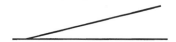

Figure 1   Two types of neurological episodes.

tion, or stress is not considered as an exacerbation. Fatigue alone is also not considered an exacerbation. By definition, exacerbations must be separated by at least 1 month, and symptoms occurring within a month are considered part of the same episode.

Progression is defined as a continuous neurological deterioration for a minimum of 6 months. Some authors prefer a minimum time window of 12 months. There is no universally accepted minimum amount of neurological worsening. Some authors leave it to the appreciation of the experienced neurologist, while others require a minimum of 0.5 worsening on the Kurtzke EDSS scale. Still others do require one full point at least. Assessment of the onset of progression and the progression per se is left to the judgment of the neurologist. Once started, the progression will go on indefinitely, sometimes with temporary plateaus. The date of onset of clinical progression is assessed in retrospect once the 6 (or 12) months of continuous neurological worsening have been confirmed. That always leaves some uncertainty regarding this parameter. Relapses can be superimposed on the progression, either at the onset of progression, during the progression, or both. An example of the different types of exacerbations and their connection to progression are shown in Fig. 1.

Exacerbations and progression allow one to consider two distinct phases of multiple sclerosis. The relapsing-remitting phase of the disease is characterized by the occurrence of exacerbations separated by periods of clinical inactivity. A period without sequelae and a period with sequelae may be considered according to the absence or the presence of sequelae between the relapses. The progressive phase is characterized by the clinical progression, as defined above. It may or may not be superimposed upon exacerbations.

III. ONSET OF MULTIPLE SCLEROSIS

A. Two Types of Clinical Onset

Two separate conditions can be observed for the clinical onset of multiple sclerosis: an initial exacerbation followed by a remission with or without sequelae defines the cases with an exacerbating-remitting onset; an initial progression with or without a superimposed relapse defines the cases with a progressive onset (Fig. 2).

From one series to another the proportion of patients with an exacerbating-remitting onset varies from 63% (8) to 89% (18). In the Lyon Multiple Sclerosis cohort (4), a progressive onset was found in 18% of the patients. In the London, Ontario, cohort (14), 18.7% of the patients were classified as chronic progressive, but 14.8% of the patients were also classified as being relapsing progressive. Differences in the definition of a progressive onset presumably explain the wide range of percentages among these studies. One should also notice that the proportion of progressive patients dramatically decreases when one takes into account only the patients seen at the very early stage of the disease—for instance, within the first year. A first explanation is that it takes a longer time for the patient to come to see the neurologist when the onset of symptoms is insidious. Another explanation is the possibility of a recall bias, the patients forgetting an initial relapse when data are collected retrospectively.

B. Age at Onset

Results are consistent from one series to another. Mean age at clinical onset of multiple sclerosis is 30 years on average (Table 1). In the Lyon MS cohort (4), 10% of the cases started before 20 years, 70% between 20 and 40 years, and 20% after 40 years.

<u>**Exacerbating-remitting onset**</u> :

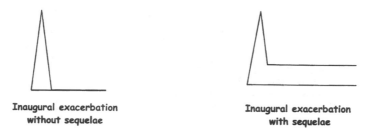

Inaugural exacerbation   Inaugural exacerbation
without sequelae   with sequelae

<u>**Progressive onset**</u> :

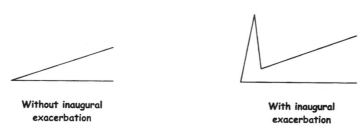

Without inaugural   With inaugural
exacerbation   exacerbation

Figure 2   Two types of clinical onset.

C.   Symptoms at Onset

It is difficult to compare the results of the different published series due to the lack
of consensus in classification and nomenclature of the symptoms and signs in multiple
sclerosis. In our opinion, a proper classification must be patient-driven, as clinical
onset of multiple sclerosis is often assessed in retrospect. For instance, it is not rare
for a patient to complain of disorders of balance, although examination will show a

Table 1   Age at Onset in Multiple Sclerosis

Authors	Mean age at onset (years)	Patients age at onset (years)		
		<20	20–40	≥40
Confavreux et al. (4)	31.3	11%	69%	20%
Weinshenker et al. (10)	30.5	12%	68%	20%
Trojano et al. (20)	26	NA	NA	NA
Kantarci et al. (24)	27.6	NA	NA	NA

Table 2 Symptoms at Clinical Onset
of Multiple Sclerosis[a]

Optic neuritis	17.2%
Diplopia/vertigo	12.9%
Ataxia	13.2%
Sensory symptoms	45.4%
Motor weakness	20.1%

[a] In percentages of 1096 patients.
Source: From Ref. 12.

pyramidal syndrome. Others may complain of fatigability for a cerebellar syndrome. Table 2 shows a list of symptoms of multiple sclerosis according to some series in the literature.

D. Influence of Clinical Variables on the Onset Phenotype of Multiple Sclerosis

There are interrelationships between the type of onset of multiple sclerosis and different clinical variables such as gender, age, and symptoms. For instance, the gender distribution in multiple sclerosis usually shows a female preponderance of about two-thirds, as observed in other autoimmune diseases. As a matter of fact, this figure is quite different in cases with a progressive onset, the distribution being either symmetrical or with a slight male preponderance (52 to 63% of males). A female preponderance in cases with a progressive onset has been found only by MacDonnel (68%) (23). The interplay between age at onset, type of onset, and symptoms at onset may be summarized as follows: the later the onset in life, the higher the proportion of cases with a progressive onset and with long tracts symptoms. By contrast, the earlier the onset in life, the higher the proportion of cases with an exacerbating-remitting onset and with optic neuritis (Table 3).

Table 3 Distribution (percentage) of Types and Symptoms at Onset Regarding Patient's Age at Presentation

	Age at onset (years)				
	<20 N = 131	20–29 N = 435	30–39 N = 310	40–49 N = 173	>50 N = 47
Type of onset of multiple sclerosis					
Exacerbating-remitting onset	82.4	80.9	62.3	37.0	25.5
Progressive onset	17.6	19.1	37.7	63.0	74.5
Symptoms					
Optic neuritis	22.9	22.8	13.2	9.2	6.3
Diplopia vertigo	17.6	12.4	11.0	16.8	12.8
Ataxia	13.7	11.3	14.8	12.7	10.6
Sensory symptoms	46.5	52.2	44.2	33.5	31.9
Motor weakness	9.9	13.5	21.3	33.5	51.0

Source: From Ref. 12.

IV. COURSE OF MULTIPLE SCLEROSIS

A. Course Classification

According to the scheme with two phases in the clinical expression of multiple sclerosis, there is a logical sequence in the possible combination of them. If the clinical onset is of the exacerbating-remitting type, the course may persist that way only. In some cases, it may convert to a progressive phase, secondary to the relapsing-remitting phase. By contrast, if the clinical onset of the disease is of the progressive type, the course will follow this pattern only. Concretely, three main categories can be considered: relapsing-remitting, secondary progressive, and primary progressive. It is important to note that for both progressive forms of multiple sclerosis, either secondary to a relapsing-remitting phase or primary, superimposed exacerbations may or may not be observed. For these two forms, a further distinction must be made according to two subtypes—"relapsing" versus "non-relapsing." This is shown in Fig. 3. In parallel, this figure shows the presently accepted classification established after an international survey in 1996 (29).

The relative proportions of these three main categories of disease course among a population of multiple sclerosis patients vary among series in the literature. With respect to the proportion of cases with a primary progressive course, the reader may refer to Sec. III.A above. What is less clear from the literature is the relative proportion of cases with superimposed relapses to those without among the population of cases with a primary progressive course of multiple sclerosis. For Weinshenker et al., of 267 patients with a progressive onset of the disease, 162 (61%) had superimposed relapses.

Concerning the proportion of relapsing-remitting forms and secondary progressive forms, the data available in the literature show also some variability (Table 4). An explanation could be that the fate of a majority of relapsing-remitting forms is to convert to a secondary progression. This change is time-dependent: the longer the duration of the follow-up, the higher the proportion of patients having switched from the relapsing-remitting phase to the secondary progressive phase. In other words, secondary progressive forms could be regarded as relapsing-remitting forms that have had time to progress (4).

B. Time Interval Between the First Two Neurological Episodes

In cases with an exacerbating-remitting onset, the second neurological episode may be either a relapse or the onset of the progressive phase. The median time to this second episode is about 2 years. It is important to raise here a methodological issue that is valid for the assessment of time intervals to entry into another state (e.g., a second relapse, a given level of nonreversible disability, the onset of progression), which may occur very late in the disease course, far beyond the mean follow-up of the population of patients under survey or which, in some cases, may never occur. The classic and presently out of date approach is to consider only the patients who have indeed reached the endpoint at the time of the closure of the survey. This leads to a systematic bias towards shorter estimates than the actual figure, as the patients who have not yet reached the endpoint at the time of the closure of the survey and who will likely reach this endpoint later on are not taken into account. The strength of survival analysis, like the Kaplan-Meier technique, is to weigh the estimate by taking into account the patients who have not reached the endpoint at the time of the closure of the survey, either because they have been followed up until the time of closure without reaching the endpoint or because they have been lost to follow-up before this time of closure, again without reaching the endpoint. For this

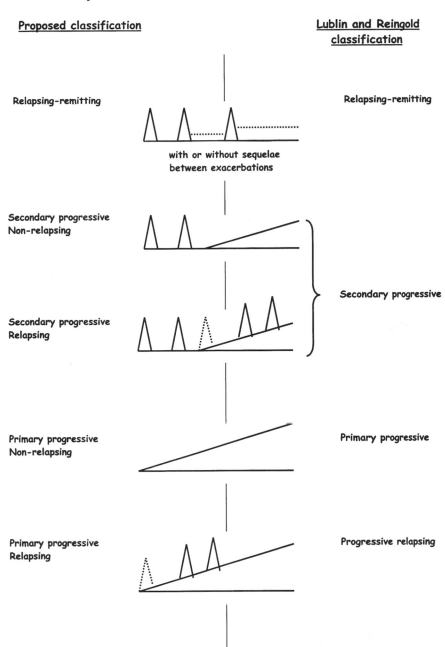

Figure 3   Course classification.

Table 4   Distribution of Patients in Two Published Series

	Confavreux *Brain*, 1980[4]	Weinshenker et al. *Brain*, 1989[12]
Disease duration (all patients), year		
Mean ± SD	9.0	12.0
Median (range)	NA	10
Course classification, % of patients		
Relapsing-remitting	58	66
Secondary-progressive course		
All	24	NA
Primary-progressive course		
All	18	34
With superimposed relapse	NA	15
Without superimposed relapse	NA	19

reason, it is important to mention whether the estimates are based upon crude observed data or are derived from survival analysis.

C.   Relapse Frequency in the Exacerbating-Remitting Phase

A number of contributions have dealt with this issue. The answer is not straightforward, as there are numerous possible biases. The source population must be representative of the disease. In this respect, figures derived from the placebo arms of therapeutic trials are presumably overestimated. In these trials, notably those for which the primary outcome criterion is the relapse frequency or the time to the first attack after enrollment, patients are usually selected upon a high disease activity in terms of relapse frequency. In natural history series, it is not always clear whether the relapse frequency is assessed on the relapsing-remitting phase only or by including also the secondary progressive phase of the disease or even the primary progressive phase. Ascertainment of relapses during the follow-up is also influenced by the frequency of the visits, with a positive correlation between the latter and the frequency of relapses (1). Presently available disease-modifying drugs, but also long-standing used drugs such as azathioprine (30), are able to reduce relapse frequency by about one-third. The degree of certainty of the relapses has also rarely been taken into account. Despite these numerous sources of variability and unreliability, the general consensus is that, in a representative population of multiple sclerosis patients, the average relapse frequency is about once every other year. It is higher, between 0.9 an 1.8, in the first year. It decreases thereafter as long as the disease evolves.

D.   Onset of the Progressive Phase in Cases with an Exacerbating-Remitting Onset

Though important, this issue has not been addressed very often in the literature, especially since the emergence of the new statistical techniques such as survival analysis. In the Lyon Database (4), for the 83 patients with a secondary progressive course, the mean time to progression was 6.8 (±5.4) years. This was an observed figure and, for the reasons stated above, a very likely underestimated figure. When taking into account all patients, exacerbating-remitting or progressive at onset, in an actuarial analysis, 30% entered the progressive phase by 5 years and 50% by 11 years. In 1993, using a survival analysis,

Runmarker found a median time to progression of about 9 years. But the analysis was done in all the patients of the series, including those with a progressive onset. Accordingly, this figure then is also an underestimate.

V. OVERALL PROGNOSIS

With the emergence of partially effective therapies, one of the most difficult issues for the clinician facing a patient with multiple sclerosis is the prediction of the forthcoming disability. The therapeutic decision derives from it. A series of available data provides some clues. When a given level of disability has been sustained for 6 months, the chance for it to be nonreversible approaches 100%. This is one of the requisites for the definition of progression according to Schumacher et al. (28). The overall prognosis of multiple sclerosis is presently well known, as well as a striking interindividual variability of the outcome and intraindividual fixedness of progression of disability.

A. Overall Outcome

Several studies on well-documented (1–25) cohorts and the use of appropriate statistical techniques such as life-table analysis provide a precise assessment of the time intervals from disease onset to reach defined key steps. It takes an average of 8 years to reach DSS4 (limited walking distance, but without aid, and over 500 without rest), 20 years to reach DSS6 (walking with unilateral support), and 30 years to reach DSS7 (walking limited to a few steps at home). Global survival is slightly reduced (31) (Table 5).

B. Interindividual Variability

These time intervals represent only the median, and confidence intervals may be quite large. Concretely, the overall severity of the disease varies considerably from one patient to another, with a full span ranging from benign forms compatible with a normal life to malignant forms that are rapidly disabling. There are also asymptomatic forms (32) as well as acute life-threatening forms.

It is difficult to assess the relative frequency of these forms with a different final outcome. In the series of the literature, the mean duration of multiple sclerosis at the time of the survey is 10 years at best, which is not a lot, considering that life expectancy is

Table 5 Transition from Clinical Onset (All Patients) to Nonreversible Entry into Kurtzke Disability Scores

	Median time (years) since MS onset		
	Confavreux *Brain* 1980[4] $N = 349$	Weinshenker *Brain* 1991[15] $N = 1099$	Confavreux *Rev Neurol* 1998[25] $N = 1191$
DSS3	—	8	—
DSS4	6	—	7
DSS6	—	15	—
DSS7	18	—	29
DSS8	—	47	—
Decease	>30	?	45

around 40 years after the clinical onset of multiple sclerosis. In other words, the patients who have not yet reached a significant level of nonreversible disability at the time of the survey and who could be classified as benign cases will reach this level later on and will have to be classified in another category of disease severity. There is no universally accepted consensus for the definition of these categories. However, an outstanding international effort has been conducted in 1996 (29), which has made it possible to suggest a definition for benign cases as a disease in which the patient remains fully functional in all neurological systems 15 years after disease onset. By contrast, malignant cases rapidly evolve to ''significant disability in multiple sclerosis systems, or death, in a relatively short time after disease onset.''

Some clues may be derived from the Lyon MS cohort (4) by updating the formulation of the key disability levels. In this work, the moderate disability is equivalent to the DSS4 level of disability on the Kurtzke scale and severe disability to DSS7. Therefore, by combining nonreversible disability scores and disease duration, the disease severity classification becomes the following:

> The benign forms were defined by a nonreversible DSS level of disability equal to 0 to 3 for a minimum disease duration of 10 years or equal 4 to 5 for a minimum of 15 years of disease duration. This definition is less conservative than the present one (29).
>
> ''Hyperacute,'' ''acute,'' ''subacute,'' and ''intermediate'' forms were defined by a time interval from the clinical onset of multiple sclerosis to nonreversible entry into the DSS7 level of disability, which was less than 5 years, 5 to 10 years, 10 to 15 years, and more than 15 years, respectively.
>
> ''Nonclassified'' forms were defined by a DSS0 level of 3 of nonreversible disability and a disease duration shorter than 10 years or a DSS4 to 5 and a duration shorter than 15 years.

According to this classification, benign cases represented 14% of the whole MS population, whereas hyperacute, acute, subacute, and intermediate cases represented 8, 8, 5, and 4% respectively.

C. Intraindividual Fixedness

In apparent contradiction with the preceding data, showing a very high variability of outcomes among multiple sclerosis patients, but also in apparent contradiction with the usually exacerbating and remitting symptomatic course of the disease, there is paradoxically a striking fixedness of the slope of the accumulation of neurological abnormalities and disability in a given individual. This was elegantly demonstrated by Fog and Linneman in the 1960s (1). These authors conducted a systematic prospective study of 73 patients with multiple sclerosis. They performed a standardized quantitated neurological examination of these patients, usually at quarterly intervals, over several years. For each patient, the successive scores were plotted on a diagram. Following a regression analysis, the mathematical curve (which can be derived from the observed curve) that fits the best is of a linear type in most cases. Its slope varies from one patient to another but remains stable for a given patient. It even allowed extrapolation of the outcome for the subsequent years (Fig. 4).

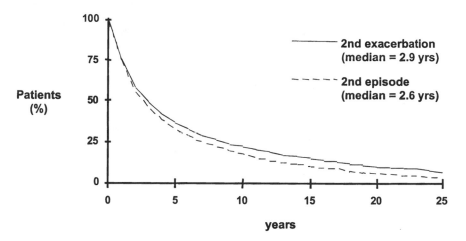

Figure 4 Transition from the first neurological exacerbation in relapsing-remitting cases to the second neurological episode. Survival analysis (Kaplan-Meier technique).

VI.   MULTIPLE SCLEROSIS AND DAILY LIFE

A.   Heat-Sensitivity

The Uhthoff phenomenon can easily be confounded with an exacerbation. As a matter of fact, it is a pseudoexacerbation, as it is not related to multiple sclerosis activity but only to a transient blockade of nerve conduction in the demyelinated fibers. Classically, it is illustrated by a transient and reversible decrease in visual acuity associated with physical exercise or increase in body temperature. In practice, the Uhthoff phenomenon may be observed in other areas, such as internuclear ophtalmoplegia. Its presence following a first episode of optic neuritis could have a pejorative predictive value: conversion to clinically definite multiple sclerosis could occur earlier (34).

B.   Pregnancy

Generally speaking, the relapse rate has been thought to decrease during pregnancy and to increase in the postpartum period. However, conclusions have long failed to be definitive, as studies have been small and some have reached different conclusions (35–40). Knowledge in this field has become more reliable following the publication of the results of the European multicentre Pregnancy In Multiple Sclerosis (PRIMS) study (41). A total of 269 pregnancies among 254 women with MS have been followed. A decrease in the relapse rate was observed during the 9-month pregnancy compared to the prepregnancy year, this decrease being most marked in the last 3 months of pregnancy. Conversely, the relapse rate increased dramatically in the first 3 months postpartum and came back to its rate prior to pregnancy during the next months postpartum. As a matter of fact, pregnancy seems to modify the relapse chronology, since the relapse rate during the pregnancy year (pregnancy plus 3 months postpartum) is comparable to that of the year prior to pregnancy (Table 6). It must be stressed that about one-third of the women will suffer from at least one exacerbation during pregnancy. Similarly, about one-third of the women will suffer from an exacerbation in the first 3 months postpartum. This means that the majority of

Table 6   Relapse Frequency During Pregnancy
Among the 227 Women in the PRIMS Study

Prepregnancy year	0.7 (±0.9)	*p* value[a]
Pregnancy		
First quarter	0.5 (±1.3)	*p* = 0.03
Second quarter	0.6 (±1.6)	*p* = 0.17
Third quarter	0.2 (±1.0)	*p* < 0.001
Postpartum		
First quarter	1.2 (±2.0)	*p* < 0.001
Second quarter	0.9	*p* = 0.17
Third quarter	0.9	*p* = 0.17
Fourth quarter	0.6	*p* = 0.59

[a] compared to the prepregnancy year.

the women will not suffer from an exacerbation during pregnancy and the postpartum period. Pregnancy does not seem to worsen disability. Peridural analgesia and breast-feeding have no impact on the relapse rate and the disability worsening. Obstetrical data and state of health of infants at birth are similar to those obtained with healthy patients.

These results confirm the influence of pregnancy on the course of multiple sclerosis. It is logical to establish a correlation between the variations of disease activity and the modifications of the sex hormones and immunity during pregnancy and after delivery with a shift in the cytokine balance towards Th2 responses during pregnancy and Th1 responses during delivery. These observations seem to open a new therapeutic era.

C. Vaccines

Controversy about the relationship between vaccination and multiple sclerosis has been revived after the campaign of vaccination against hepatitis B in France. A first question is related to the risk of triggering the clinical onset of multiple sclerosis in asymptomatic persons. The case-control epidemiological study requested by the French Medical Agency and aiming at determining whether the hepatitis B vaccine would trigger multiple sclerosis or a similar disease has revealed that there is no increased risk (odds ratio 1.4, confidence interval 0.4 to 4.5; results not yet published). A second issue concerns the risk of triggering a clinical exacerbation in patients with established multiple sclerosis. Influenza vaccine is the only one to show harmlessness in a placebo, double-blind, multicenter study (42). Attenuated live vaccines are often advised against (measles, rubella, varicella), notably the yellow fever and poliomyelitis vaccines. As a matter of fact, this policy is justified in dealing with patients who are given immunosuppressors. It may not be justified in dealing with other patients. As regards the other vaccines, it is reasonable to assess the risk of vaccination compared to the expected benefits considering patient's exposure to the disease. The results of a European multicenter study addressing this issue are being submitted for publication.

VII. CONCLUSION

Our knowledge of the natural history of multiple sclerosis has greatly improved with the establishment and appropriate follow-up of representative cohorts of patients and with the use of modern statistical techniques. The natural course and prognosis of multiple sclerosis are well known today from a statistical point of view. Similarly, the influence of pregnancy and delivery and, hopefully soon, the influence of vaccines on the clinical activity of multiple sclerosis are also better assessed from a statistical point of view. This being said, the early prediction of outcome in an individual remains an impossible bet. The only presently known technique is the prospective clinical follow-up of the patient with successive quantitated neurological examinations. The longer the follow-up, the more precise the assessment of the slope of the progression of disability. However, this determinist approach becomes informative too late and provides what could be called an ''a posteriori prognosis.'' It is likely that the clinical approach in this field has reached its cognitive limits. Hopefully, the emerging of magnetic resonance techniques applied to the analysis of the brain and spinal cord will provide earlier, more sensitive, and more reliable tools. This is becoming an emergency. Effective disease-modifying drugs are coming out. They must be restricted to patients who really need them and not given to those who will follow a naturally benign course.

REFERENCES

1. Fog T, Linneman F. The course of multiple sclerosis in 73 cases with computer designed curves. Acta Neurol Scand 1970; 46(suppl 47):1–175.
2. Percy AK, Nobrega FT, Okazaki H, Glattre E, Kurland LT. Multiple sclerosis in Rochester, Minn: A 60-year appraisal. Arch Neurol 1971; 25:105–111.
3. Kurtzke JF, Beebe GW, Nagler B, Kurland LT, Auth TL. Studies on the natural history of multiple sclerosis—Early prognostic features of the later course of the illness. J Chronic Dis 1977; 30:819–830.
4. Confavreux C, Aimard G, Devic M. Course and prognosis of multiple sclerosis assessed by the computerized data processing of 349 patients. Brain 1980; 103:281–300.
5. Clark VA, Detels R, Visscher BR, Valdiviezo NL, Malmgren RM, Dudley JP. Factors associated with a malignant or benign course of multiple sclerosis. JAMA 1982; 248:856–860.
6. Poser S, Poser W, Schlaf G, et al. Prognostic indicators in multiple sclerosis. Acta Neurol Scand 1986; 74:387–392.
7. Phadke JG. Survival pattern and cause of death in patients with multiple sclerosis: Results from an epidemiological survey in north-east Scotland. J Neurol Neurosurg Psychiatry 1987; 50:523–531.
8. Minderhoud JM, Van der Hoeven JH, Prange AJA. Course and prognosis of chronic progressive multiple sclerosis. Results of an epidemiological study. Acta Neurol Scand 1988; 78:10–15.
9. Riise T, Gronning M, Aarli JA, Nyland H, Larsen JP, Edland A. Prognostic factors for life expectancy in multiple sclerosis analised by Cox-models J Clin Epidemiol 1988; 41(10):1031–1036.
10. Weinshenker BG, Bass B, Rice GPA, et al. The natural history of multiple sclerosis: a geographical based study. I. Clinical course and disability. Brain 1989; 112:133–146.
11. Goodkin DE, Hertsgaard D, Rudick RA. Exacerbation rates and adherence to disease type in a prospective followed-up population with multiple sclerosis: Implications for clinical trials. Arch Neurol 1989; 46(10):1107–1112.
12. Weishenker BG, Bass B, Rice GPA, et al. The natural history of multiple sclerosis: A geographical based study—II. Predictive value of the early clinical course. Brain 1989; 112:1419–1428.
13. Phadke JG. Clinical aspects of multiple sclerosis in north-east Scotland with particular reference to its course and prognosis. Brain 1990; 113:1597–1628.

14. Weinshenker BG, Rice GPA, Noseworthy JH, Cariere W, Baskerville J, Ebers GC. The natural history of multiple sclerosis: A geographical based study—III. Multivariate analysis of predictive factors and models of outcome. Brain 1991; 114:1045–1056.

15. Weinshenker BG, Rice GPA, Noseworthy JH, Carniere W, Baskerville J, Ebers GC. The natural history of multiple sclerosis: A geographical based study—IV. Applications to planning and interpretation of clinical therapeutic trials. Brain 1991; 114:1057–1067.

16. Miller DH, Hornabrook RW, Purdie G. The natural history of multiple sclerosis: A regional study with some longitudinal data. J Neurol Neurosurg Psychiatry 1992; 55(5):341–346.

17. Riise T, Gronning M, Fernandez O, Lauer K, Midgard R, Minderhoud JM, et al. Early prognostic factors for disability in multiple sclerosis: A European multicenter study. Acta Neurol Scand 1992; 85:212–218.

18. Runmarker B, Andersen O. Prognostic factors in a multiple sclerosis incidence cohort with twenty five years of follow-up. Brain 1993; 116:117–134.

19. Runmarker B, Andersson C, Oden A, Andersen O. Prediction of outcome in multiple sclerosis based on multivariate models. J Neurol 1994; 241:597–604.

20. Trojano M, Avolio C, Manzari C, Calo A, De Robertis F, Serio G, et al. Multivariate analysis of predictive factors of multiple sclerosis with a validated method to assess clinical events. J Neurol Neurosurg Psychiatry 1995; 58:300–306.

21. Weinshenker BG, Issa M, Baskerville J. Long-term and short-term outcome of multiple sclerosis: A 3-year follow-up study. Arch Neurol 1996; 53:353–358.

22. Thompson AJ, Polman CH, Miller DH, McDonald WI, Brochet B, Filippi M, et al. Primary progressive multiple sclerosis. Brain 1997; 120:1085–1096.

23. McDonnel GV, Hawkins SA. Clinical study of primary progressive multiple sclerosis in Northern Ireland, UK. J Neurol Neurosurg Psychiatry 1998; 64:451–454.

24. Kantarci O, Siva A, Eraksoy M, Karabudak R, Sutlas N, Agaoglu J, et al. Survival and predictors of disability in Turkish MS patients. Turkish Multiple Sclerosis Study Group (TUMSSG). Neurology 1998; 51(3):765–772.

25. Confavreux C, Grimaud J, Vukusic S, Moreau T. Peut-on prédire l'évolution de la sclérose en plaques? Rev Neurol 1998; 154(8–9):624–628.

26. Kremenchutzky M, Cottrel D, Rice G, Hader W, Baskerville J, Koopman W, et al. The natural history of multiple sclerosis: A geographical based study—VII. Progressive-relapsing and relapsing-progressive multiple sclerosis: a reevaluation. Brain 1999; 122:1941–1949.

27. Amato MP, Ponziani G, Bartolozzi ML, Siracusa G. A prospective study on the natural history of multiple sclerosis: Clues to the conduct and interpretation of clinical trials. J Neurol Sci 1999; 168(2):96–106.

28. Ebers GC. Natural history of multiple sclerosis. In: Compston A, Ebers G, Lassmann H, McDonald I, Matthews B, Wekerle H, eds. McAlpine's Multiple Sclerosis, 3rd ed. London: Churchill Livingstone, 1998.

29. Lublin FD, Reingold SC, for the National Multiple Sclerosis Society (USA) Advisory Committe on Clinical Trials of New Agents in Multiple Sclerosis. Defining the clinical course: Results of an international survey. Neurology 1996; 46:907–911.

30. Yudkin PL, Ellison GW, Ghezzi A., et al. Overview of azathioprine treatment in multiple sclerosis. Lancet 1991; 338:1051–1055.

31. Bronnum-Hansen H, Koch-Henriksen N, Hyllested K. Survival of patients with multiple sclerosis in Denmark: A nationwide, long-term epidemiologic survey. Neurology 1994; 44(10): 1901–1907.

32. Gilbert JJ, Sadler M. Unsuspected multiple sclerosis. Arch Neurol 1983; 40:533–536.

33. Schumacher GA, Beebe G, Kibler RF, et al. Problems of experimental trials of therapy in MS: Report by the panel on the evaluation of experimental trials of therapy in MS. Ann NY Acad Sci 1965; 122:552–568.

34. School GB, Song HS, Wray SH. Uhthoff's symptom in optic neuritis: Relationship to magnetic resonance imaging and development of multiple sclerosis. Ann Neurol 1991; 30:180–184.

35. Douglass LH, Jorgensen CL. Pregnancy and multiple sclerosis. Am J Obstet Gynecol 1948; 55:332–336.

36. Tillman AJB. The effect of pregnancy on multiple sclerosis and its management. Res Publ Assoc Res Nerv Ment Dis 1950; 28:548–582.

37. Sweeney WJ. Pregnancy and multiple sclerosis. Am J Obstet Gynecol 1953; 66:124–130.

38. Birk K, Rudick R. Pregnancy and multiple sclerosis. Arch Neurol 1986; 43:719–726.

39. Hutchinson M. Pregnancy in multiple sclerosis. J Neurol Neurosurg Psychiatry 1993; 56: 1043–1045.

40. Abramsky O. Pregnancy and multiple sclerosis. Ann Neurol 1994; 36 (suppl):S39–S41.

41. Confavreux C, Hutchinson M, Hours MM, Cortinovis-Tourniaire P, Moreau T, and the Pregnancy in Multiple Sclerosis Group. Rate of pregnancy-related relapse in multiple sclerosis. N Engl J Med 1998; 339:285–291.

42. Miller AE, Morgante LA, Buchwald LY, Nutile SM, Coyle PK, Krupp LB, et al. A multicenter, randomised, double-blind, placebo-controlled trial of influenza immunization in multiple sclerosis. Neurology 1997; 48:312–314.

18

Prognostic Factors in Multiple Sclerosis

ORHUN H. KANTARCI and BRIAN G. WEINSHENKER

Mayo Clinic and Foundation, Rochester, Minnesota

I. INTRODUCTION

Since the introduction of long-term disease-modifying treatments such as interferon-β to clinical practice (1) there has been an increasing tendency to initiate treatment early in the course of disease of patients with MS. A need for treatments that act early and over the long term is evident from growing evidence that irreversible axonal damage begins early (2) and disability accumulates over time. However, to maximize the long-term benefit and minimize toxicity of a treatment, physicians should select the right patient at the right stage of disease. Given the short follow-up periods of clinical trials relative to time over which disability develops in MS, the need to demonstrate long-term benefit of these chronic treatments is evident. Especially in the setting of expensive and dedicated treatment strategies, physicians need reliable measures to predict the course and outcome of MS in order to initiate treatment early.

MS belongs to a heterogeneous spectrum of disorders that we have referred to as idiopathic inflammatory demyelinating diseases (IIDDs) with highly variable pathological phenotypes, disease course and outcome (3–5) (Fig. 1). Even patients with "prototypical" relapsing-remitting MS exhibit interindividual and intraindividual variation over time in disease course. They may or may not develop secondary progressive disease.

Disease severity can be conceived as a function of severity, extent of pathology, and time (Fig. 1). A self-limited syndrome may result in major, rapidly acquired disability (e.g., fulminant IIDDs, such as Marburg's variant), whereas other, more pathologically limited syndromes with relatively little inflammation (e.g., primary progressive MS) may result in disability because of their tendency to progress inexorably over time. An IIDD with limited distribution in the CNS may be associated with severe acute and permanent

449

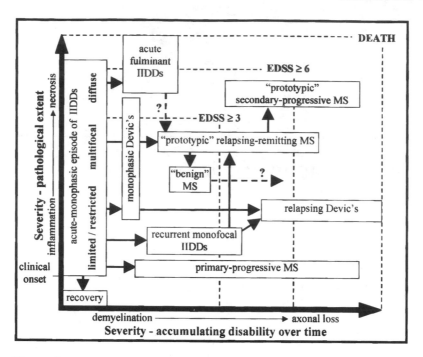

Figure 1   Schematic of the dynamic spectrum of idiopathic inflammatory demyelinating disorders of the CNS in relation to disease severity as defined by disability status (EDSS). Clinical severity is a function of pathological extent ranging from limited-restricted CNS involvement to multifocal or diffuse disease and pathological severity ranging from inflammation to necrosis (*y* axis); it is also a function of time-dependent conversion from predominant demyelination to axonal loss (x-axis). Patients may convert from one state to another, as illustrated.

disability when the lesions occur in critical locations and produce necrotizing inflammation (e.g., Devic's neuromyelitis optica with predilection for upper cervical cord involvement). Consequently, prognostic factors include those that determine whether and when a patient converts from a given self-limited syndrome (e.g., relapsing remitting MS) to a more extensive or chronic syndrome (e.g. secondary progressive MS) within the spectrum. Furthermore, prognostic factors can also be defined based on whether they predict early or long-term outcome (Fig. 2). Even during the preclinical period [asymptomatic MS (6)], where the disease is biologically active, prognostic factors can be defined that predict whether patients will remain asymptomatic or develop clinically manifest MS. At this stage the distinction between susceptibility factors and prognostic factors is blurred. Early (within the first 5 years of clinical disease) outcome measures include initial disease course, early attack frequency, recovery from attacks, early disability, and MRI lesion load. As discussed further on, these intermediate outcomes may be analyzed as predictors of long-term outcome. Long-term or definitive outcome measures include evolution of secondary progressive disease, disability levels attained by 25 years, or death. Our concept of prognostic factors is dynamic, with some factors being considered ''outcomes'' at one stage of disease and ''predictors'' at others.

Prognostic factors can be grouped into five major categories (Fig. 2). Genetic and environmental factors are expected to operate at every stage from susceptibility to long-

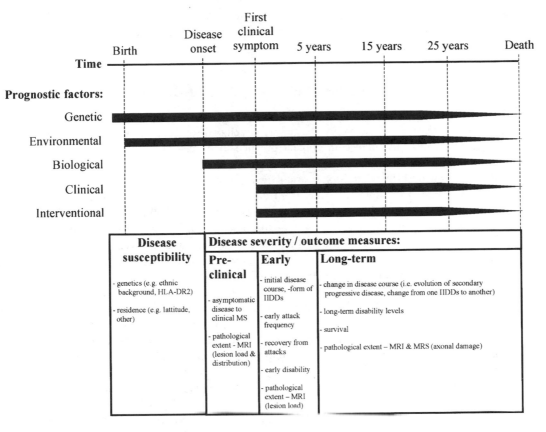

Figure 2 Prognostic factors as related to the time at which they are operative during the disease and severity measures that can be used at each stage.

term outcome, though different genes and environmental factors may predominate at different stages. Clinical and demographic predictors (e.g., nature of first symptoms, age at onset) are most probably helpful in early disease. Later clinical factors may have stronger predictive value [e.g. Expanded Disability Status Scale (EDSS) score at 5 years] but— as substantial disability may have already developed—these factors may be less useful. Biological measures such as magnetic resonance imaging (MRI) and immunological factors, on the other hand, reflect the disease process itself. However, they can be measured at the early stages of disease and may predict behavior of the disease. Current disease-modifying interventions (e.g., interferon β, glatiramer acetate) are probably most effective in changing the prognosis when instituted during the early disease course. Since the introduction of such treatments to clinical practice, it is harder to study untreated populations. Treatment modalities must be integrated into studies addressing predictors of outcome. For example, a favorable effect of socioeconomic status on disease outcome could be confounded by better access to expensive long-term therapies in those with higher incomes. Nevertheless, for the purpose of this chapter, treatment effects are not discussed.

Although many population studies have been conducted to study prognostic factors, the results have not been decisive. Predicting the long-term outcome in a given individual at or before the onset of clinical symptoms or during the early course of disease still remains a problem to be resolved. In this chapter, we review clinical and biological prognostic indicators in MS, emphasize established determinants of outcome, and highlight areas that require further study.

II. SPECTRUM OF IIDDs AND RELEVANCE TO PROGNOSIS

The first step is to distinguish MS from other treatable causes of a similar syndrome. Using Poser's criteria (7), which were mainly developed for the research setting but also gained widespread acceptance in clinical practice, one needs to confirm that no other neurological cause accounts for the disease, and lesions have to be disseminated in time and space. However, this definition restricts the early diagnosis of other IIDDs, necessitating further criteria to separate IIDDs from other mimics of demyelinating disease (8). During the initial clinical presentation, it is hard to predict whether the course will be monophasic, relapsing, or progressive. On the other hand, this is the period when the physician is often confronted with questions about outcome and whether to initiate treatment. Long-term prophylactic treatments (e.g., interferon β) are theoretically more effective at this stage than in patients with advanced disability.

IIDDs differ from one another by the extent and location of the lesions within the central nervous system (CNS) and also by the outcome of the illness (Fig. 1). Hence, the specific diagnosis of the subtype of the IIDD has prognostic as well as diagnostic implications. Isolated demyelinating syndromes (e.g., optic neuritis, partial transverse myelitis, isolated brainstem event) may later develop into ''prototypical'' MS (including relapsing-remitting and secondary-progressive disease) or other chronic forms of IIDDs (Fig. 1). Whether or not relapsing course ensues is often the predictor of the outcome in a given individual.

For example, a patient with an acute optic neuritis (ON) may recover and have no further problems (monophasic isolated syndrome), may develop successive attacks of ON of the same eye (recurrent isolated ON), attacks of myelitis without evidence of brain involvement (Devic's disease), attacks involving brain and/or spinal cord (prototypical relapsing-remitting MS), or a later progression after one or more attacks with gradual onset of impairment and disability (secondary progressive MS). Each of these diagnostic categories is associated with a different prognosis. The isolated syndrome and the recurrent ON attacks represent the most benign and Devic's syndrome and secondary progressive MS the most serious possibilities. Defining patients at risk for the more serious syndromes will help guide the decision about early institution of prophylactic therapy. Predictors of conversions from one syndrome to another are discussed below.

A. Prognostic Factors in Clinically Isolated Monophasic Syndromes of Demyelination

Several studies have examined predictors of conversion to MS in isolated IIDDs. The presence of MS-like lesions on MRI is the most important prognostic factor in predicting risk of conversion to MS. However, the presence of HLA-DR2 and oligoclonal bands in cerebrospinal fluid (CSF) also increases the risk (9,10).

Among a hospital-based cohort of 44 patients with isolated ON, 17 with isolated brainstem and 28 with isolated spinal cord syndromes, 72% of those with abnormal brain MRI at presentation and 6% with normal brain MRI developed MS within 5 years (9).

The frequencies increased to 82% and 12% by 10 years in a later updated study (11). Among those with abnormal scans at presentation, higher T2 lesion load on the initial MRI scan correlates with higher rates of conversion to MS, both at 5 and 10 years of follow-up (12). A lesion load of > 3 cm^3 in the initial scan invariably predicts conversion to clinically definite MS by 10 years, while a lesion load of ≤ 3 cm^3 is associated with conversion to MS in 78% of the cases.

For those who develop subsequent neurologic events leading to a diagnosis of definite MS, a high baseline lesion load at the time of first symptoms is also associated with a higher chance of developing secondary progression and greater disability. At 10 years of follow-up, 45% of patients with > 3 cm^3 lesions reach an EDSS score greater than 6 (requiring a cane to walk half a block), while only 18% of patients with ≤ 3 cm^3 lesions reach the same level. However, the absolute lesion volume at 5 years from onset is not associated with the change in EDSS in the next 5 years. Furthermore, the number of lesions do not increase as significantly beyond 5 years from onset as during the first 5 years, suggesting that the observed changes in lesion volume after this time are due to enlargement of the existing lesions rather than new lesion formation (12). Hence, the initial MRI studies are more valuable in predicting long-term disability than those performed beyond the first 5 years following the clinically isolated syndrome.

ON is the most common and benign form of isolated syndromes. Based on the Optic Neuritis Treatment Trial data (13), 5-year cumulative probability of developing MS following an event of optic neuritis in adults (range: 18 to 46 years at age of onset) is 30%. In this study, 16% of the patients with no involvement of the other eye and no lesions on initial MRI developed MS. Lack of pain, severe optic disk edema, and relatively mild loss of visual acuity were associated with reduced risk of developing MS in cases of monocular ON. The risk of conversion to MS is apparently lower in children: 13% in 10 years and 26% in 40 years (14). A history of infection preceding the onset of ON by 2 weeks decreases the risk, and bilateral sequential or recurrent ON episodes increases the risk of conversion to MS. Söderström et al (10) have followed 147 consecutive adults with acute monosymptomatic ON for an average of 25 months. They have shown that three or more MRI lesions and oligoclonal bands in CSF ($n = 38$) predicted development of clinically definite MS in 100% of patients, while less than three lesions and no oligoclonal bands ($n = 25$) consistently predicted no conversion to MS. The sensitivity of only three or more lesions on MRI or oligoclonal bands in CSF in predicting MS independently was 85 and 96%. Although less sensitive (57%), HLA-DR2 was also associated with increased risk for future conversion to definite MS in this study.

Predicting recovery from a demyelinating event is an issue separate from predicting conversion to MS. Miller et al. have found that long lesions on MRI that involve the intracanalicular portion of the nerve are associated with slow or incomplete recovery from an ON attack (15). ON is a discrete, relatively easy-to-study syndrome. Steroid treatment for the initial attack of ON has no effect on recovery (16).

Conversion to multiple sclerosis has also been studied for isolated acute transverse myelitis (ATM). ATM is usually a limited, steroid-responsive, monophasic disease of the spinal cord with rare relapses (17–19). Combined sensory and motor involvement and symmetry at presentation are the most important features distinguishing ATM from MS (20). Conversion to MS has been reported in 2 to 21 %, depending on the diagnostic criteria for ATM considered (19,21). Although the characteristic sausage-shaped, swollen, elongated MRI lesion of the spinal cord in ATM is different from the multifocal, relatively small spinal cord lesions in MS (19,22–24), the most important predictor of subsequent relapses is the presence of suspect demyelinating lesions on cerebral MRI and oligoclonal bands in the CSF (20,25).

B. Prognostic Factors in Devic's Syndrome (Neuromyelitis Optica)

Neuromyelitis optica (NMO) represents a special clinical situation, which according to the criteria of Poser, could be classified as clinically definite MS. However, there are features that distinguish this syndrome. In contrast to prototypical MS, there is a racial predilection for non-Caucasians (50% of IIDDs in Japan are NMO) (26,27); NMO is confined to the optic nerve and spinal cord clinically, and lesions are rarely observed on cerebral MRI; longitudinally extensive lesions in the spinal cord, which are more typical of ATM, are found; oligoclonal bands are uncommon; neutrophilic pleocytosis in CSF is common during attacks (28). The prognosis of NMO is worse than that of prototypical MS in terms of recovery from attacks, long-term cord-related disability, and mortality (Fig. 1). Hence distinguishing this disease from MS at its earliest stages is important for future management.

Wingerchuk et al have recently published a large series of NMO (28). The most important determinant of outcome was whether the course was monophasic (32.4%) or relapsing (67.6%). While the attack-related impairment was more severe in the monophasic group, the 5-year survival was 90% in the monophasic and 68% in the relapsing group. Long-term neurological impairment in relapsing cases is much greater. The main predictor of a monophasic rather than relapsing course is (near) simultaneous bilateral ON and myelitis (within 1 month). Conversely, isolated ON or myelitis at first presentation, relatively longer time interval between index events, female sex, older age at onset, and other systemic autoimmune disease are associated with a relapsing course.

C. Prognosis in Acute Fulminant IIDDs: Marburg's Variant of MS, Acute Disseminated Encephalomyelitis (ADEM), Balo's Concentric Sclerosis

Most patients with isolated IIDDs recover from their attacks spontaneously or after corticosteroid treatment. The acute fulminant syndromes, on the other hand, are characterized by severe attacks often with limited recovery despite corticosteroids. Cerebral involvement in these disorders ranges from innumerable perivenous lesions with extensive inflammation and relatively less demyelination in ADEM to large, tumor-like lesions with large, confluent demyelination in Marburg's variant and Balo's concentric sclerosis. These disorders are rare and large series with prognostic data are not available. However, even after putting aside the difficulties of publication bias, these syndromes apparently have a much worse prognosis than prototypical MS. In a recently completed double-blind, placebo-controlled, randomized study at the Mayo Clinic, plasmapheresis limited to patients with acute (duration less than 3 months) severe episodes of demyelination refractory to steroids has been shown to dramatically improve short-term outcome of the individual attack in 42% of cases (29). Significant recovery was uncommon in those failing to improve on active treatment (2 of 13 patients). In an earlier study, this effect was observed as a trend restricted to acute, severe attacks of MS but had not reached significance when all relapses were considered together (30). Recognizing these acute severe attacks as a separate subgroup of IIDDs might refine treatment approaches and influence outcome. Diagnostic features in MRI at presentation can help distinguish these syndromes early. Diffuse involvement with large, confluent lesions with enhancement of the cerebral hemispheres and lack of oligoclonal bands in CSF suggests Marburg's variant (31). However, one patient has been reported to improve following corticosteroid treatment and then to develop prototypical MS within 4 years (32). ADEM is more commonly a severe, postinfectious monophasic syndrome of children associated with diffuse enhancing white matter lesions. Some patients with ADEM may also have MS-like lesions and may be difficult to distinguish from patients with prototypical MS (33). Factors that predict degree of recovery from the acute event and whether subsequent conversion to MS occurs are unclear, but increased use of treatment modalities as alternatives to or following unsuccessful treatment with corticosteroids [e.g., intravenous immune globulin (IVIG) and plasmapheresis] may improve the outcome of the immediate attack and more of these patients may survive to develop ''prototypical'' MS later on.

A solitary mass lesion with a concentric whorled appearance on MRI suggests Balo's concentric sclerosis and has been generally reported to portend a grave prognosis, although some patients had lesions that regressed following corticosteroid treatment (34,35). Large tumor-like demyelinating lesions without concentric appearance, on the other hand, respond very well to corticosteroids and usually are monophasic syndromes with some chance of developing MS in the future (36). Biopsy is often required to differentiate the lesions from tumors.

D. Primary Progressive MS: A Distinct Prognostic Category

Primary progressive MS (PP-MS) is the most common of the chronic IIDDS other than ''prototypic'' MS. Consequently, it has been included in studies addressing prognostic factors in MS, emerging as the most important predictor of outcome in MS. It is usually possible to identify patients who will follow a primary progressive course at the beginning of their disease, as they typically develop symptoms insidiously rather than acutely. This may not be entirely clear at the early stages of the disease and the distinction from other patients with MS is further obscured for patients who later recall a single, often not well-documented remote ''attack'' that might or might not be related to MS. Other features may help to distinguish this entity from prototypical MS. Older age at onset (35 to 40), lack of female preponderance, slowly worsening paraparesis as dominant clinical feature, and relative paucity of intracranial lesions on MRI are the main distinguishing features (37). Other studies have examined the MRI appearances of abnormal and normal-appearing white matter to define distinctive characteristics of this disorder (see Sec. III.B). The differentiation is not absolute and ancillary tests to distinguish this distinct prognostic category of IIDDS from other forms of MS remain to be established. Immunogenetic differences [e.g., HLA-DR4 predominance (38,39)] may predict a primary progressive course.

III. PROGNOSTIC FACTORS IN PROTOTYPICAL MS

Prototypical MS is a relapsing remitting disease involving optic nerves, brain and spinal cord that is distinct from the aforementioned IIDDs. It commonly evolves into a secondary progressive course, which is believed to represent the crossing of a threshold of axonal damage resulting from previous or ongoing inflammatory episodes, which initially targeted myelin or oligodendrocytes. Most studies examined predictive factors in patients for whom a diagnosis of prototypical MS has been established (Table 1). This is a potential shortcoming, since application of disease-modifying treatments may be most effective at the time first symptoms (i.e. isolated demyelinating syndrome) develop.

Table 1 Clinical Prognostic Factor Studies in "Protoypic" MS That Have Used Comparable Outcome Measures[a]

	Phadke[47] 1990	Weinshenker[48] 1991	Riise[49] 1992	Runmarker[50] 1994	Kantarci[52] 1998
Male gender	±	−	±	−	−
Older age at onset	−	−	−	−	−
Initial symptoms					
Optic neuritis	+	+	±	+	+
Pyramidal		±(acute onset)	−	−	−
Sensory	+	±	±	+	+
Brainstem	+	±	±		±[b]
Cerebellar	−	−			
Spinal cord/sphincter	−				−
Higher early attack frequency		−		±	−
Shorter first interattack interval	−	−			
Moderate disability reached by 5 years		−			−

Key: −, unfavorable; +; favorable; ±; no effect.
[a] Progressive disease is uniformly associated with a worse prognosis and hance is not listed in the table.
[b] Brainstem and cerebellar symptoms analyzed together.

The outcome of MS can be assessed in several ways. A simple, robust outcome is survival. However, 50% of MS patients die from causes other than their primary disease (40). Nevertheless, some of the factors that influence disability—such as gender, age at onset, and the initial symptoms—also influence survival when large populations have been examined (41,42), presumably because the MS-specific causes are overrepresented and death from MS is largely associated with advanced disability. A more sensitive alternative is to consider disability rating scales, of which the EDSS (43) is the most commonly used. Measuring disability level reached at a specific time or application of survival methods stratified for prognostic factors have been the approaches most commonly taken. Another measurable endpoint often considered is the time to the onset of secondary progressive course. This discussion concentrates on predictors that have been identified consistently among different MS populations. Outcome measures are discussed in the next chapter.

A. Clinical and Demographic Factors that Determine Outcome in Prototypical MS

The demographic and clinical prognostic variables associated with poor outcome in MS have been reviewed previously (44). The factors that have been consistently established that cross ethnic barriers are male sex; older age at onset (>40); motor, cerebellar, or sphincter symptoms at initial presentation; polyregional onset; relatively frequent attacks, especially within the first 5 years; short interval between the first 2 attacks; relatively short time to reach an EDSS level of 4; and a progressive course (Table-1) (45–52). The disability status at 5 years correlates well with the long-term outcome, and the behavior of the disorder seems to be relatively established by this time. Therefore the course in the first 5 years usually predicts future outcome. However, this is not absolutely true in all cases, and some seemingly benign cases may later develop into progressive disease (53).

As pointed out by Confavreux (54), most of the early clinical predictors of outcome are interrelated. For example, in the study from Turkey (52), male sex, older age, and motor or sphincter symptoms at onset are strongly correlated with a primary progressive course, consistent with the clinical characteristics of primary progressive disease as recently discussed by Thompson (37). When primary progressive and prototypical MS cases are analyzed together, age of onset, sphincter symptoms and progressive disease emerge as strong independent predictors of outcome. When the primary progressive group is discarded and the group with prototypical MS is analyzed separately, male sex emerges as an independent predictor of outcome. Gender has an independent direct effect on the outcome of prototypical but not primary progressive MS. In primary progressive MS, the effect is indirect: i.e., it increases the probability of primary progressive disease. Similarly, motor symptoms at onset are strongly associated with the outcome but also with sphincter symptoms at onset, primary progressive course, and male sex. Since these factors are stronger determinants of outcome in this study, the effect of motor symptoms, which is evident in the univariate analysis, is lost in the multivariate analyses. The strongest independent predictors of long-term disability are a high number of attacks within the first 5 years of the disease and a progressive course.

Since some patients remain in remission with only mild or moderate disability levels throughout the course of disease (i.e., "benign" MS), it is important to predict which patients will develop secondary progression. How early and reliably is it possible to predict transition to progressive disease? Progressive MS is defined as "a gradual, nearly continuous, worsening baseline with minor fluctuations but no distinct relapses" (55). Although certain determinants that can be established early in the course of disease (e.g., male sex, older age at onset, high number of relapses within the first 5 years and shorter interval between the first two relapses) are associated with a later progressive course in large populations, their predictive value in a given patient is limited. Confavreux (56) reported that factors associated with the course of MS influence the time to reach EDSS 4.0 but not EDSS 7.0. This suggests that these established prognostic factors determine the onset of a progressive course (which generally begins when EDSS is approximately 4.0). The factors influencing behavior of the disease after that point may be different, perhaps because of a switch from inflammation to axonal injury as the major force in the disease course (57). More reliable measures of this change, such as immunological or MRI markers, would be more useful as predictors of the behavior of progressive MS.

B. Role of Early MRI Findings in Determining Long-Term Outcome in MS

Neuroimaging techniques are promising to be a good or better biological measure of disease activity than clinical scales, suggesting that inclusion of new MRI criteria together with clinical outcome scales may refine prediction of disease activity and severity (58–62).

MR spectroscopic findings may identify patients at risk of progressive disease. Loss of axonal markers such as N-acetylaspartate in the normal-appearing white matter in progressive MS patients (63–65) and progressive CNS atrophy (66,67) in serial conventional MRI can be indicators of axonal loss (68). Decreasing N-acetylaspartate levels in the normal appearing white matter is correlated with disability (changes in EDSS) in relapsing-remitting cases (69). Magnetization transfer imaging can detect white matter abnormalities when conventional MRI methods cannot (70). A recent MRI study conducted in patients with primary, secondary, and transitional progressive MS (i.e., patients that are in evolution from relapsing phase to a secondary progressive phase of the disease) demonstrates that the lesion load assessed in a cross-sectional manner after disease course is established does not correlate with EDSS, while measures of atrophy of the brain and the spinal cord does correlate with EDSS (71). In a longitudinal metanalysis of 307 prototypical MS patients examining monthly gadolinium-enhancing lesions for a period of 6 months after disease onset, Kappos et al. identified a weak predictive effect of enhancing lesion counts on early attack rate but not on EDSS change within the first 2 years (72). However, EDSS is insensitive to short-term changes in disability and may have underestimated the sensitivity of the MRI measure.

The studies discussed above correlate MRI findings with the clinical course and outcome in cross-sectional analysis or short follow-up times. Prospective studies in patients at the early stages of the disease with long-term follow-up will be necessary to establish MRI parameters as truly excellent predictors of outcome. Currently, most of the MRI techniques seem to be more useful for monitoring disease activity in clinical trials than in predicting long-term outcome early in the disease. Nevertheless, the role of MRI in predicting long-term disability in MS is promising.

C. Genetic Markers That Determine Long-Term Outcome in Prototypical MS

Genetic factors are established to influence susceptibility to MS, but recently there has been greater interest in their role in disease course and severity. Intrafamilial clustering of age at onset, disease course or severity has been demonstrated in MS (73). The concordance for course among siblings (74,75) is more evident for like-sex pairs with primary progressive disease. There is also concordance for disease severity in sib-pairs from France (76) and in like-sex pairs from Great Britain (75). A trend has also been demonstrated in a small Canadian study (74). Based on these data, there has recently been a growing interest in identifying genetic markers of disease severity in MS. HLA is the most extensively studied gene complex. No clear association with disease severity has been demonstrated (44,77). The HLA-DR2 genotype does not influence the prognosis after prototypical MS develops. However, it is associated with susceptibility to MS in case-control studies and predicts conversion to MS in clinically isolated syndromes. Susceptibility and outcome may be independently determined. Common genetic polymorphisms that in healthy individuals may have no phenotype may affect the biological behavior of a disease once established. The area of identifying disease "prognosis genes" is in its infancy and a comprehensive evaluation of non-HLA genes has not yet been undertaken. The only genes that have been studied and shown to influence disease severity in MS are polymorphisms of IL-1β, IL1-receptor antagonist, APOE, and immunoglobulin-G Fc-receptor (FcγR) genes (78–84). Given the potential confounders in case-control studies such as population stratification (variations in genotype related to ethnic differences), these findings need to be confirmed in other data sets before they can be considered as predictors of outcome that can be identified at the time of diagnosis. Variants in other genes have been studied but not associated with disease severity (85,86).

IV. CONCLUSION

Clinical predictors of outcome have been extensively studied. None of the single identified factors is sufficiently robust to predict the course and severity of MS in a given individual with a high degree of confidence, especially early in the disease. Prognostic factors are "dynamic." Intermediate outcomes (e.g., evolution of a secondary progressive course, disability reached by 5 years) serve as stronger prognostic factors than those ascertained at diagnosis. However, these measures are not helpful, especially for the decision of initiating long-term treatments, since disease behavior is established by the time they can be determined. Hence, the predictive value of clinical measures becomes more definitive during follow-up but the usefulness declines. Separate prognostic factors for conversion to clinically definite MS (e.g., HLA-DR2), for development of early disability or for onset of secondary progressive MS and rate of axonal loss once the patient is in the progressive phase need to be studied. Genetic factors are potential predictors that can be determined earliest during the disease if they can be established reliably across different, ethnically diverse populations. Similarly, improvements in conventional MRI and MR spectroscopic techniques will enable clinicians to predict the early biological nature of the disease.

REFERENCES

1. TheIFNβ Multiple Sclerosis Study Group. Interferon beta-1b is effective in relapsing-remitting multiple sclerosis: I. Clinical results of a multicenter, randomized, double-blind, placebo-controlled trial. Neurology 1993; 43:6655–661.
2. Storch M, Lassmann H. Pathology and pathogenesis of demyelinating diseases. Curr Opin in Neurol 1997; 10:186–192.
3. Lucchinetti CF, Brück W, Rodriguez M, Lassmann H. Distinct patterns of multiple sclerosis pathology indicates heterogeneity in pathogenesis. Brain Pathol 1996; 6:259–274.
4. Weinshenker BG. The natural history of multiple sclerosis: Update 1998. Semin Neurol 1998; 18(3):301–307.
5. Siva A, Kantarci O. An introduction to the clinical spectrum of inflammatory demyelinating disorders of the central nervous system. In: Siva A, Kesselring J, Thompson A, eds, Frontiers in Multiple Sclerosis, vol II. London: Martin Dunitz, 1999, pp 1–9.
6. Allen IV. Asymptomatic multiple sclerosis: what does it mean? In: Siva A, Kesselring J, Thompson A, eds. Frontiers in Multiple Sclerosis, vol II. London: Martin Dunitz, 1999, pp 11–15
7. Poser CM, Paty DW, Scheinberg L, et al. New diagnostic criteria for multiple sclerosis: Guidelines for research protocols. In: Poser CM, Paty DW, Scheinberg L, Ebers GC, eds. The Diagnosis of Multiple Sclerosis. New York: Thieme-Stratton, 1984, pp 224–229.
8. Weinshenker BG, Lucchinetti CF. Acute leukoencephalopathies: Differential diagnosis and investigation. Neurologist 1998; 4:148–166.
9. Morrissey SP, Miller DH, Kendall BE, et al. The significance of brain magnetic resonance imaging abnormalities at presentation with clinically isolated syndromes suggestive of multiple sclerosis: A 5-year follow-up study. Brain 1993; 116:135–146.
10. Söderström M, Ya-Ping Jin, Hillert J, Link H. Optic neuritis: Prognosis for multiple sclerosis from MRI, CSF and HLA findings. Neurology 1998; 50(3):708–714.
11. O'Riordan JI, Thompon AJ, Kingsley DP, et al. The prognostic value of brain MRI in clinically isolated syndromes of the CNS: A 10-year follow-up. Brain 1998; 121:495–503.
12. Sailer M, O'Riordan J, Thompson AJ, et al. Quantitative MRI in patients with clinically isolated syndromes suggestive of demyelination. Neurology 1999; 52(3):599–606.
13. Optic Neuritis Study Group. The 5-year risk of MS after optic neuritis. Experience of the optic neuritis treatment trial. Neurology 1997; 49:1404–1413.
14. Lucchinetti CF, Kiers L, O'Duffy A, et al. Risk factors for developing multiple sclerosis after childhood optic neuritis. Neurology 1997; 49:1413–1418.
15. Miller DH, Newton MR, Van der Poel JC, et al. Magnetic resonance imaging of the optic nerve in optic neuritis. Neurology 1998; 38:175–179.

16. Kapoor R, Miller DH, Jones SJ, et al. Effects of intravenous methylprednisolone on outcome in MRI-based prognostic subgroups in acute optic neuritis. Neurology 1998; 50(1):230–237.

17. Monteiro LM, Correia M. Benign relapsing meningomyelitis. J Neurol Neurosurg Psychiatry 1991; 54:939–940.

18. Tippet DS, Fishman PS, Panitch HS. Relapsing transverse myelitis. Neurology 1991; 41:703–706.

19. Jeffrey DR, Mandler RN, Davis LE. Transverse myelitis—Retrospective analysis of 33 cases, with differentiation of cases associated with multiple sclerosis and parainfectious events. Arch of Neurol 1993; 50:532–535.

20. Scott TF, Bhagavatula K, Snyder PJ, Chieffe C. Transverse myelitis: Comparison with spinal cord presentations of multiple sclerosis. Neurology 1998; 50(2):429–433.

21. Lipton HL, Teasdall RD. Acute transverse myelopathy in adults: A follow-up study. Arch Neurol 1973; 28:252–257.

22. Campi A, Filippi M, Comi G, et al. Acute transverse myelopathy: Spinal and cranial MR study with clinical follow-up. AJNR 1995; 16:115–123.

23. Austin SG, Zee CS, Waters C. The role of magnetic resonance imaging in acute transverse myelitis. Can J Neurol Sci 1992; 19:508–511.

24. Choi KH, Lee KS, Chung SO, et al. Idiopathic transverse myelitis: MR charactersistics. AJNR 1996; 17(6):1151–60.

25. Ford B, Tampieri D, Francis G. Long-term follow-up of acute partial transverse myelopathy. Neurology 1992; 42:250–252.

26. Shibasaki H, Kuroda Y, Kuroiwa Y. Clinical studies of multiple sclerosis in Japan: Classical multiple sclerosis and Devic's disease. J Neurol Sci 1974; 23:215–222.

27. O'Riordan JI, Gallagher HL, Thompson AJ, et al. Clinical, CSF and MRI findings in Devic's neuromyelitis optica. J Neurol Neurosurg Psychiatry 1996; 60:382–387.

28. Wingerchuk DM, Hogencamp WF, O'Brien PS, Weinshenker BG. The clinical course of neuromyelitis optica (Devic's syndrome). Neurology 1999; 53:1107–1114.

29. Weinshenker BG, O'Brian PC, Petterson TM, et al. A randomized trial of plasma exchange in acute central nervous system inflammatory demyelinating disease. Ann Neurol 1999; 46(6): 878–886.

30. Weiner HL, Dau PC, Khatri BO, et al. Double-blind study of true vs. sham plasma exchange in patients treated with immunosuppression for acute attacks of multiple sclerosis. Neurology 1989; 39(9): 1143–1149.

31. Johnson MD, Lavin P, Whetsell WO, Jr. Fulminant monophasic multiple sclerosis, Marburg's type. J Neurol Neurosurg Psychiatry 1990; 53:918–921.

32. Giubilei F, Sarrantonio A, Tisei P, et al. Four-year follow-up of a case of acute multiple sclerosis of the Marburg type. Ital J Neurol Sci 1997; 18:163–166.

33. Kesselring J, Miller DH, Robb SA, et al. Acute disseminated encephalomyelitis. MRI findings and the distinction from multiple sclerosis. Brain 1990; 113:291–302.

34. Revel MP, Valiente E, Gray F, et al. Concentric MR patterns in multiple sclerosis: Report of two cases. J Neuroradiol 1993; 20(4):252–7.

35. Bolay H, Karabudak R, Tacal T et al. Balo's concentric sclerosis: Report of two patients. J Neuroimaging 1996; 6:98–103.

36. Kepes JJ. Large focal tumor-like demyelinating lesions of the brain: Intermediate entity between multiple sclerosis and acute disseminated encephalomyelitis—A study of 31 patients. Ann Neurol 1993; 33:18–27.

37. Thompson AJ. Differences between primary and secondary progressive multiple sclerosis. In: Siva A, Kesselring J, Thompson A, eds. Frontiers in Multiple Sclerosis, vol II. London: Martin Dunitz, 1999, pp 29–36.

38. Olerup O, Hillert J. HLA class II associated genetic susceptibility in multiple sclerosis: A critical evaluation. Tissue Antigens 1991; 38:1–15.

39. Weinshenker B, Santrach P, Bissonet AS, et al. Major histocompatibility complex class II

alleles and the course and outcome of MS: A population-based study. Neurology 1998; 51: 742–747.

40. Sadovnick AD, Eisen K, Ebers GC, Paty DW. Cause of death in patients attending multiple sclerosis clinics. Neurology 1991; 41:1193–96.

41. Bronnum-Hansen H, Koch Henriksen N, Hyllested K. Survival of patients with multiple sclerosis in Denmark: A nationwide, long-term epidemiologic survey. Neurology 1994; 44:1901–1907.

42. Levic ZM, Dujmovic I, Pekmezovic T, et al. Prognostic factors for survival in multiple sclerosis. Mult Scler 5(3):171–178, 1999.

43. Kurtzke JF. Rating neurological impairment in MS: an Expanded Disability Status Scale (EDSS). Neurology 1983; 33:1444–1452.

44. Weinshenker BG. The natural history of multiple sclerosis. Neurol Clin North Amer 1995; 13(1):119–146.

45. Kurtzke JF, Beebe GW, Nagler B, et al. Studies on the natural history of multiple sclerosis: Early prognostic features of the later course of the illness. J Chronic Dis 1977; 30:819–830.

46. Confavreux C, Aimared G, Devic M. Course and prognosis of multiple sclerosis assessed by computerized data processing of 349 patients. Brain 1980; 103:281–300.

47. Phadke JG. Clinical aspects of multiple sclerosis in north-east Scotland with particular reference to its course and prognosis. Brain 1990; 113:1597–1628.

48. Weinshenker BG, Rice GPA, Noseworthy JH, et al. The natural history of multiple sclerosis: A geographically based study—III. Multivariate analysis of predictive factors and models of outcome. Brain 1991; 114:1045–1056.

49. Riise T, Gronning M, Fernandez O, et al. Early prognostic factors for disability in multiple sclerosis: A European multicenter study. Acta Neurol Scand 1992; 85:212–218.

50. Runmarker B, Andersson O. Prognostic factors in a multiple sclerosis incidence cohort with 25 years follow-up. Brain 1993; 116:117–134.

51. Rodriguez M, Siva A, Ward J, Stolp-Smith K, O'Brian PC, Kurland LT. Impairment, disability and handicap in multiple sclerosis: A population based study in Olmsted County, Minnesota. Neurology 1994; 44:28–33.

52. Kantarci O, Siva A, Eraksoy M, et al. Survival and predictors of disability in Turkish MS patients. Neurology 1998; 51:765–772.

53. Thompson AJ. Benign multiple sclerosis (editorial; comment). J Neurology Neurosurg Psychiatry 1999; 67(2):138.

54. Confavreux C. Clinical predictive factors in multiple sclerosis. In: Siva A, Kesselring J, Thompson A, eds. Frontiers in Multiple Sclerosis, vol II. London: Martin Dunitz, 1999, pp 63–66.

55. Lublin FD, Reingold SC. The National Multiple Sclerosis Society (USA; Advisory Commitee on Clinical Trials of New Agents in Multiple Sclerosis). Defining the clinical course of multiple sclerosis: results of an international survey. Neurology 1996; 46:907–991.

56. Confavreux C. Presentation at the 13th Congress of the European Committee for Treatment and Research in Multiple Sclerosis. ECTRIMS. Istanbul. Turkey, 1997

57. Revesz T, Kidd D, Thompson A, Barnard R. A comparison of the pathology of primary and secondary progressive multiple sclerosis. Brain 1994; 117:759–765.

58. Miller DH, Grossman RI, Reingold SC, McFarland HF. The role of magnetic resonance techniques in understanding and managing multiple sclerosis. Brain 1998; 121:3–24.

59. Keiper MD, Grossman RI, Hirsch JA, et al. MR identification of white matter abnormalities in multiple sclerosis: A comparison between 1.5 T and T. AJNR 1998; 19:1489–1493.

60. Filippi M, Rocca MA, Rizzo G, et al. Magnetization transfer ratios in multiple sclerosis lesions enhancing after different doses of gadolinium. Neurology 1998; 50(5):1289–1293.

61. Lynch SG, Rose JW, Smoker W, Petajan JH. MRI in familial multiple sclerosis. Neurology 1990; 40:900–903.

62. Filippi M. Magnetization transfer imaging to monitor the evolution of individual multiple sclerosis lesions. Neurology 1999; 53(5 suppl 3):S18–S22.

63. Matthews PM, Francis G, Antel J, Arnold DL. Proton magnetic resonance spectroscopy for metabolic characterization of plaques in multiple sclerosis. Neurology 1991; 41:1251–1256.

64. Davie CA, Barker GJ, Thompson AJ, Tofts PS, McDonal WI, Miller DH. [1]H magnetic resonance spectroscopy of chronic cerebral white matter lesions and normal appearing white matter in multiple sclerosis. J Neurol Neurosurg Psychiatry 1997; 63:736–742.

65. Leary SM, Davie CA, Parker GJM, MacManus DG, Miller DH, Thompson AJ. [1]H magnetic resonance spectroscopy of normal appearing white matter in primary multiple sclerosis. Ann Neurol 1998; 44:464.

66. Losseff N, Webb S, O'Riordan J, et al. Spinal cord atrophy and disability in multiple sclerosis: A new reproducible and sensitive MRI method with potential to monitor disease progression. Brain 1996; 119:701–708.

67. Losseff N, Wang L, Lai H, Yoo D, et al. Progressive cerebral atrophy in multiple sclerosis: A serial MRI study. Brain 1996; 119:2009–2019.

68. Trapp BD, Peterson J, Ransohoff RM, Rudick R, Mork S, Bo L. Axonal transection in the lesions of multiple sclerosis. N Engl J Med 1998; 338:278–285.

69. Fu L, Matthews PM, De Stefano N, et al. Imaging axonal damage of normal-appearing white matter in multiple sclerosis. Brain 1998; 121:103–113.

70. Filippi M, Rocca MA, Minicucci L, et al. Magnetization transfer imaging of patients with definite MS and negative conventional MRI. Neurology 1999; 52:845–848.

71. Stevenson VL, Miller DH, Rovaris M, et al. Primary and transitional progressive MS. A clinical and MRI cross-sectional study. Neurology 1999; 52:839–845.

72. Kappos L, Moeri D, Radue EW, et al. Predictive value of gadolinium-enhancing magnetic resonance imaging for relapse rate and changes in disability or impairment in multiple sclerosis: A meta-analysis. Gadolinium MRI Meta-analysis Group. Lancet 1999; 353(9157): 964–9.

73. Robertson NP, Compston AS. Prognosis in multiple sclerosis: genetic factors. In Siva A, Kesselring J, Thompson A, eds., Frontiers in Multiple Sclerosis, vol II. London: Martin Dunitz, 1999, pp 51–61.

74. Weinshenker BG, Bulman D, Carriere W, Baskerville J, Ebers GC. A comparison of sporadic and familial multiple sclerosis. Neurology 1990; 40:1354–1358.

75. Robertson NP, Clayton D, Fraser M, Deans J, Compston DAS. Clinical concordance in sibling pairs with multiple sclerosis. Neurology 1996; 47:347–352.

76. Brassat D, Azais-Vuillemin C, Yaouanq J, et al. Familial factors influence disability in MS multiplex families. Neurology 1999; 52:1632–1636.

77. Weinshenker B, Santrach P, Bissonet AS, et al. Major histocompatibility complex class II alleles and the course and outcome of MS. A population-based study. Neurology 1998; 51: 742–747.

78. De la Concha EG, Arroyo R, Crusius JBA, et al. Combined effect of HLA-DRB1*1501 and interleukin-1 receptor antagonist gene allele-2 in susceptibility to relapsing/remitting multiple sclerosis. J Neuroimmunol 1997; 80:172–178.

79. Schrijver HM, Crusius JBA, Uitdehaag BMJ, et al. Association of interleukin-1 beta and interleukin-1 receptor antagonist genes with disease severity in MS. Neurology 1999; 52(3): 595–599.

80. Kantarci O, Atkinson EJ, Hebrink DD, McMurray CT, Weinshenker BG. Association of two variants in IL-1β and IL-1receptor antagonist genes with multiple sclerosis. J Neuroimmunol 2000; 106:220–227.

81. Sciacca FL, Ferri C, Vandenbroeck K, et al. Relevance of interleukin 1 receptor antagonist intron 2 polymorphism in Italian MS patients. Neurology 1999; 52:1896–1898.

82. Evangelou N, Jackson M, Beeson D, Palace J. Association of the APOE epsilon 4 allele with disease activity in multiple sclerosis. Neurol Neurosurg Psychiatry 1999; 67(2):203–205.

83. Sylantiev C, Chapman J, Chilkevich O, Nisipeanu P, Chistik V, Korczyn AD. The APOE 4 allele and progression of disability in multiple sclerosis. Neurology 1998; 50(4 suppl. 4): A150.
84. Myhr KM, Raknes G, Nyland H, Vedeler C. Immunoglobulin G Fc-receptor (FCgR) IIA and IIIB polymorphisms related to disability in MS. Neurology 1999; 52:1771–1776.
85. Weinshenker BG, Wingerchuk DM, Liu Q, Bissonet AS, Schaid DJ, Sommer SS. Genetic variation in the tumor necrosis factor alpha gene and the outcome of multiple sclerosis. Neurology 1997; 49(2):378–85.
86. Weinshenker BG, Hebrink D, Wingerchuk DM, Klein CJ, Atkinson E, O'Brien PC, McMurray CT. Genetic variants in the tumor necrosis factor receptor 1gene in patients with MS. Neurology 1999; 52(7):1500–1503.

19

Therapeutic Considerations: Rating Scales

RICHARD RUDICK

Cleveland Clinic Foundation, Cleveland, Ohio

BRIAN G. WEINSHENKER

Mayo Clinic and Foundation, Rochester, Minnesota

GARY CUTTER

AMC Cancer Institute, Denver, Colorado

I. INTRODUCTION

Quantifying the clinical impact of multiple sclerosis (MS) is necessary for a number of reasons. Clinical assessment tools are needed for patient care. If not for clinical outcome assessments, how would a neurologist determine disease severity or the effect of treatment? Clinical assessment tools are also indispensable for judging experimental therapies. If not for clinical assessment tools, how would investigators measure the effectiveness of an intervention?

This chapter focuses on clinical outcome assessments that have been proposed for MS. Generic instruments—e.g. the Functional Independence Measure, the Sickness Impact Profile—are mentioned but not discussed extensively. Optimal assessment methods for patient care and for clinical trials may differ, as pointed out previously (1). This chapter focuses on the use of clinical outcome measures for controlled clinical trials. The patient's history and neurological exam, and the experienced neurologist opinion are considered the principal outcome methods for clinical practice.

No single measure has emerged as the ideal outcome measure, and it seems unlikely that a single assessment strategy will work for all purposes in all MS trials. The reasons for this are listed in Table 1. First, the clinical manifestations of MS are extremely hetero-

Table 1 Complexities in Clinical Outcomes Assessment in Multiple Sclerosis

Problem	Implication for Assessment Tools
Clinical manifestations are heterogeneous	Multidimensional outcome measures are necessary.
Disease activity is subclinical in many patients during the early stages of disease.	Disease activity surrogates are needed during the RR-MS stage; Disability measures may be more useful in the later stages of disease.
Target of clinical trial determines the required outcome measure.	Disease modifying drugs require different measurement tools than symptomatic drugs.

geneous, even within an individual over time. In a clinical trial we wish to know whether a *group* of MS patients has changed compared with another *group* of MS patients. This presents difficulty because different patients within the group may have predominantly cognitive impairment, cerebellar dysfunction, spastic paraparesis, sensory ataxia, visual impairment, or various combinations of these manifestations (2). Treatment arms will therefore contain mixtures of patients with various combinations of motor, sensory, visual, cognitive, affective, bowel, bladder, and sexual dysfunction, each with varying levels of severity. Because of the heterogeneity between patients, disease severity ratings for MS have been developed to apply to patient populations with numerous clinical manifestations. The most widely applied disease severity scales rate different clinical dimensions of the disease process and then combine these measurements in various ways to create composite scores.

A major problem in developing a satisfactory clinical outcome measure relates to the paucity of clinical symptoms in the early stages of MS. Magnetic resonance imaging (MRI) scans have demonstrated that clinical manifestations bear only a loose relationship with the ongoing pathologic process during the relapsing remitting stage of MS. Some patients are entirely stable clinically but have active and progressive disease documented by serial MRI scans. Other patients have only an occasional relapse. Assuming that MRI disease activity and progression is meaningful, this suggests that a sensitive and meaningful *surrogate marker* for the disease process will be required, and most efforts to date have focused on the use of MRI for this purpose. Clinical manifestations may be more apparent at a later stage of the disease, after a threshold of disease severity has been exceeded. Therefore, outcome assessment strategies may differ at different stages of the MS disease process. It may be unrealistic to expect a clinical outcome measure to reflect disease severity or activity during the early stages of MS, when much of the disease activity is subclinical and patients have very little disability. That same outcome measure may work very well during a more advanced stage of the disease.

The optimal outcome assessment strategy for a clinical trial will also vary depending on the specific question being tested. For example, a trial to modify the disease course will require a different outcome measure than a trial for spasticity.

II. THE NATIONAL MS SOCIETY CLINICAL OUTCOME ASSESSMENT INITIATIVE

Because of the complexities and importance of clinical outcomes assessments, the NMSS sponsored an international workshop titled "Outcomes Assessment in Multiple Sclerosis

Clinical Trials: A Critical Analysis'' in Charleston, South Carolina, in February 1994. Participants at the workshop identified desirable attributes for clinical measurements, endorsed a multidimensional assessment measure containing the relatively independent clinical dimensions of MS, including cognitive function, and agreed that no existing clinical scale was optimal (3). The report from the Charleston meeting included the following statement:

> There is a clear need for development of new assessment systems, probably based upon the best aspects of the EDSS scales [Kurtzke Expanded Disability Status Scale]. Any new system must be multidimensional and quantitative. Preferentially, its scoring should be automated to speed the process and to improve consistency from assessment to assessment, between raters and among centers. It should have adequate evaluation of cognition for which there are many validated, though not currently practical, systems. (3)

As an outgrowth from the Charleston meeting, the Multiple Sclerosis Clinical Outcomes Assessment Task Force was convened by the NMSS Advisory Committee on Clinical Trials of New Agents in Multiple Sclerosis. The task force was charged with recommending optimal clinical assessment measures for use in future MS clinical trials. The task force described desirable measurement characteristics in detail, explored the complexities of multivariate composite scoring systems, and evaluated a pooled data set consisting of recently completed clinical trials and natural history studies (1,4). As a result of that analysis, the task force recommended quantitative functional composites, consisting of measures of walking, arm function, and cognition (see below) (5).

III. MEASUREMENT CHARACTERISTICS

The task force recognized that measurement characteristics (Table 2) will significantly influence the effectiveness of outcome measures when applied in the clinical setting. Potential outcome assessment methods need to be evaluated with respect to these considerations. Key characteristics are the type of measurement and its reliability, sensitivity, and validity. Practical considerations include cost, acceptance by patients and neurologists, and safety. These characteristics are described here, to create a context for descriptions of the MS clinical measurement approaches that follow.

A. Type of Measurement

Measures are used to order individual scores within scales (6). The scales themselves can be categorized as nominal, ordinal, interval (discrete), or ratio (continuous) scales. Nominal scales group individual cases without rational quantitative relationships among the categories, e.g. males or females, African Americans or Caucasians. These are often referred to as classifications. Nominal classifications are relevant to this discussion in an overall sense, and are often used to label patients and their severity rather than assess it (e.g., relapsing remitting MS, progressive MS, alive, dead, etc.). Ordinal scales are classifications in which scores represent groupings based on some underlying measurement (e.g., mild, moderate, severe). Ordinal scales are used in two ways. First, the ordinal scale may represent a grouping of scores derived using an explicit continuous scale, e.g. 75 to 100% of normal function is grouped as normal; 50 to 75% as minimal impairment; 25 to 50% as moderate; and 0 to 25% as severe. Second, the ordinal scale may be used when the phenomenon in question cannot be measured using a continuous scale. In that setting, the ordered classification represents an attempt to approximate the continuous

Table 2   Desirable Characteristics of Clinical Outcome Measures[a] in MS

Performance characteristics	Explanation
Type of measurement[b]	The score should be quantitative to the extent possible, and the distance between points on the scale should be known. Interval (continuous) measures are generally preferred over ordinal measures, because they contain a greater amount of information about disease severity.
Reliability	The score should have a high intra- and interrater reliability or, for self-report measure, should have high test-retest reproducibility.
Sensitivity	The measure should be sensitive to clinical change over a relatively short time interval.
Validity	The clinical outcome measure should measure what it is intended to measure (i.e., have demonstrable validity as discussed below).

Practical advantages	Explanation
Easy to administer	The test measure should be easy and quick to administer.
Acceptable to patients and health care professionals	The measurement technique should be consistent with comfort, safety, and compliance.
Resource-efficient	The test measure should conserve time and resources.

[a] A ''measure'' is a set of rules designed to assign numbers to relevant phenomena, e.g., leg or visual function. In MS, demographic measures—e.g., age, gender—are straightforward and do not require complex rules; ''disease measures'' are used to measure constructs (our hypotheses about the ways the MS disease process affects the individual—e.g., sensory dysfunction, ataxia). Disease measures are more complicated and require a more elaborate set of rules.

[b] Scores from clinical measures are used to place an individual along a scale. Scales can be nominal, ordinal, or interval scales, which have varying characteristics, as discussed in the text.

scale by a cruder scale that can be described, but is often a gestalt of numerous assessments and thus is the best one can do at the time. The EDSS is an example of this type of an ordinal scale. The quantitative distance between steps on ordinal scales in this circumstance is unknown, and it is generally inappropriate to use arithmetic operations and parametric statistical tests to analyze change on ordinal scales or to interpret them numerically. Interval or continuous scales are also ordered, but with an indication of how far apart the objects are from one another. For ratio scales, scores are also assigned with respect to the distance from an absolute zero. Examples of interval or continuous scales are timed tests of neurological function. Interval scales offer the potential advantage that arithmetic operations, such as taking differences between the end and beginning of the trial, are meaningful. This makes statistical analysis of change and its interpretation relatively straightforward. Interval scales also provide more information than ordinal scales. *For these reasons, interval scales are generally preferred when they are available.* The principal limitation of interval scales is that the clinical relevance of the changes may be uncertain, either because the underlying test has an unclear relationship to daily function or because a clinically significant change is undefined.

B.   Reliability

Variability in the study population derives from two factors. The first is the biological variability related to MS. Capturing this variability is the principal goal of an assessment instrument. The second source of variability relates to imprecision in the measurement instrument or in the measurement process itself. *Reliability* refers to the reproducibility of an outcome measure, and is the main determinant of the second source of variability. Standard methods can be used to assess reliability, including repeated measurements made by the same rater in the same session or over short time intervals such as successive days (termed intrarater or test-retest reliability), and repeated measurements made on the same subject by different raters (termed interrater reliability). When variability in the test instrument is high relative to biological variability, the outcome measure will not be very useful in demonstrating disease changes. Under those circumstances, measurement variability will obscure biological changes or will require excessive sample sizes.

C. Sensitivity

Sensitivity of a clinical outcome measure to disease progression is also called measurement responsiveness (7). This refers to the ability of an outcome measure to demonstrate change with time in the test population. This is an important clinical measurement attribute because an insensitive measure will be generally uninformative. If the clinical measure does not change during the course of the trial as disease progresses in a control or treatment group, it may fail to demonstrate a difference in the active treatment arm unless there is significant improvement in the treated group. Adequately sensitive measures are critical, since clinical trials are conducted over a 2 to 3-year time frame while populations of MS patients experience clinically obvious deterioration over time frames approximating 10 years.

Using a placebo control group and EDSS, it has been possible to demonstrate statistically significant therapeutic effects with approximately 150 patients per treatment arm using a study duration of 2 to 3 years. More sensitive outcome measures would theoretically reduce the required sample size or length of study, thereby conserving resources. Table 3 shows sample size calculations for two clinical trials using the EDSS as the primary outcome. The first clinical trial is placebo-controlled. The sample size calculation assumes that 40% of placebo recipients will experience the clinical endpoint in 3 years. It is assumed that the active therapy will have 60% of the outcome events that the placebo group experiences (i.e. therapy is 40% effective so that only 24% of patients in the active treatment group will reach the clinical endpoint). Such a trial would require 133 subjects per arm, or a total of 266 subjects. Further assuming a 20% dropout rate, for whom the outcome is unknown, the study would require 334 patients to achieve a power of 80% to show the therapeutic effect at the required significance level of $p \leq 0.05$. The second study in the Table 3 incorporates an active arm comparison, assuming the availability of

Table 3 Increased Sample Size Required for Active-Arm Comparison Trial

	Placebo-controlled trial	Active arm comparison trial
Primary comparison	Treatment 1 vs. Placebo	Treatment 2 vs. Treatment 1
Rate of worsening for placebo	40%	N/A
Rate of worsening for treatment[a]	24%[a]	24%
Rate of worsening for treatment[b]	N/A	14.4%[a]
Sample size for 3-year study[b]	334 subjects required	660 subjects required

[a] Assumes a 40% treatment effect.
[b] Calculation uses a two-tailed test of significance with $\alpha = 0.05$, $1-\beta = 0.80$, and a 20% dropout rate.
Source: From Rudick et al. (1).

a partially effective therapy. In the table, treatment 1 is assumed to be partially effective, and the second study is designed as a follow-up to compare a newer promising therapy to the "standard." For such an active arm comparison study, 528 patients would be required to show a further 40% improvement in the number of patients on treatment 1 who reach the clinical endpoint, assuming that the outcome measure and all other assumptions remain unchanged. With a 20% dropout rate, the active arm comparison study would require 660 patients. This example illustrates a problem that has already arisen with the advent of partially effective interventions. As partially effective therapies are developed, demonstrating superior effectiveness will require longer trials, larger sample sizes, more sensitive clinical outcome measures, or all three.

D. Validity

Validity is defined as measuring what one intends to measure and in laboratory settings is called accuracy. Various types of validity have been defined and discussed in detail-e.g., see Refs. 8 and 9. *Criterion validity* refers to cross-validation of the outcome measure with another relevant measure, or criterion. For example, a urine Dextrostix for assessing glucose can be compared to a blood sample measured in a standard laboratory. *Predictive validity* refers to the ability of a measure to predict future clinical status. Predictive validity is particularly important in making short-term measures of a slow, chronic process. For example, the level of systemic blood pressure correlates with the risk of myocardial infarction 10 or 20 years subsequent to the measurement. The systemic blood pressure itself has no clear clinical significance except in terms of its predictive validity. In the MS context, clinical outcome measures (e.g., the relapse number in 2 years, a quantitative assessment of upper extremity function, or the EDSS score) may predict subsequent behavior on a criterion variable (e.g., ability to walk, dress, or feed oneself 10 or 20 years subsequent to the measurement). Establishing predictive validity is one of the key challenges in assessing the value of clinical outcomes in a chronic disease such as MS (10). Measures that possess a high level predictive validity can be classified as surrogate measures because they can be substituted for clinically relevant change that occurs later in time.

E. Practical Considerations

Costs relate to personnel, equipment, space, and time requirements. Optimally, the time to administer a clinical outcome assessment measure should be brief. The clinical assessment measure should also be acceptable to both neurologists and patients. Testing should be comfortable for the patient and safe. Instrumentation must be highly reliable, easily used and observers easily trained, and usable over a wide range of patient disability status (11).

IV. MULTIVARIATE CLINICAL OUTCOME MEASURES

Clinical heterogeneity of MS expression prompted investigators to propose multidimensional outcome measures (12). However, the manifestations of MS are so protean that it becomes impractical to measure every clinical manifestation. Furthermore, it turns out that measuring too many manifestations may actually reduce the power of an outcome measure to show change. The simple explanation for this is that the outcome measure may be weighed down with so many measures that do not change that it becomes insensitive. An example would be to include a measure of dystonic spasms in the multivariate

MS composite measure. Dystonic spasms affect approximately 1% of MS patients. When they occur, they are very disabling, and one might be tempted to include them in the composite measure because they can be so important to an individual patient. However, the vast majority of patients in a trial will not demonstrate a change on a theoretical "dystonic spasm scale." For reasons discussed below, including this in the composite will reduce the power of the composite to demonstrate drug effects. Simply stated, it will add measurement variability and little information about the disease process in the group.

What clinical dimensions should be included in a composite measure? Two possible approaches are factor analysis and expert opinion (e.g., derived from neurologists or patients). Factor analysis is a statistical method that groups variables or tests by their relatedness to other variables or tests and by their ability to explain the variability in test results among patients (13). Factor analysis has been applied to a number of data sets from MS clinical trials that include subjects with relapsing remitting as well as chronic progressive MS (14). Consistent factors have been identified across data sets, including (a) leg dysfunction; (b) arm dysfunction; (c) sensory dysfunction (superficial touch, position sense, and possibly vibration threshold); (d) visual dysfunction; (e) mental or cognitive dysfunction; and (f) bowel/bladder/sexual dysfunction. Quantitative motor testing, neuropsychological testing, elements from the standard neurological examination, the EDSS and functional system scores (FSS), and patient self-report measures cluster appropriately in these clinical dimensions using factor analysis. Clinicians on the NMSS task force reviewed these results and endorsed the validity of these clinical dimensions.

Roberts (15) provides a succinct discussion of the advantages and disadvantages of composite measures. A multivariate outcome measure is a type of composite in which individual dimensions of the process are measured—e.g., ambulation, arm function, vision, cognitive function. Each of these measures retains its identity as an individual component. There are ways of handling multivariate outcome measures, but for comparing groups, most involve combining them into a single testable (statistical) measure. When individual assessments are combined into a single variable, this is called a composite measure. A multivariate outcome measure is a tool that uses each separate measurement to represent a patient; however, it is difficult to use these measures as a single clinical outcome measure. Thus, we usually combine multivariate measures into a single measure in some manner. Clinically, we use true multivariate outcome measures in assessing patients. For example, consider time as one variable and ambulation as another. We commonly consider how well the patient walked at the past visit and how he or she walks today. Clinically, we are able to "deal" with the time separation and understand its importance (e.g., if you have not seen a patient in 4 years, a decline of 10 seconds on a timed walk would probably mean something very different than if you saw the patient 3 months ago). As an outcome measure for a study, we often make a composite variable of these two dimensions to use statistically, a simple change in the ability to walk. We lose the time dimension but try to control for this in an experimental study by making the visits equally spaced in time or at least the same between the two groups, thereby implicitly letting us know the time.

Each component of a multivariate outcome measure could itself be a composite measure based on a number of measures of that same clinical dimension; e.g., a "cognitive" score could represent the sum of three separate individual test scores. In this case, the individual component measures of the multidimensional outcome measure can be combined into a single score, termed a *multivariate* or *multivariable composite outcome*. Combining scores from the separate components into a single score entails statistical complexities that have been addressed elsewhere (16). However, the implications of these complexities relate primarily to power, sample sizes and for the clinician, and interpretation. For example, adding an additional component to a multidimensional outcome measure may reduce the sensitivity of the outcome measure. This can occur if the additional component is not correlated with other components of the multidimensional measure and does not change or show a treatment effect during the trial. For example, the addition of four component measures that showed no treatment effect might increase the required sample size of a trial by 50% by making the means of the two groups closer together and adding variability to the outcome measure. In contrast, the addition of uncorrelated component measures that do show treatment effects results in improved power or reduced sample sizes required to achieve the same statistical power. The overall conclusion of this is that there is significant disadvantage to including component measures that do not show a treatment effect or change over time in a multivariate test measure but considerable benefit in including multiple independent component measures that are sensitive to change. Unfortunately, one is more likely to want to include measures that are correlated than measures that are uncorrelated, because more is known about the correlated type, since it is easier to satisfy conditions of validity discussed above. Petkau (16) provides a more detailed discussion of these complexities, including comparisons with other statistical approaches.

Table 4 provides the implications of using a multivariate outcome measure for MS studies: (a) There are both risks and benefits in using a multivariate outcome measure for MS studies. In particular, caution should be used to avoid including multiple dimensions that do not change with treatment as they bring the groups closer together, making the detection of change more difficult. Caution should also be used to avoid including multiple highly correlated measures because they add little new information about change while increasing the measurement error, again making assessing change more difficult because of the larger variation. (b) All components of a multidimensional outcome measures should have optimal performance characteristics—e.g., they should have high reliability, validity, and sensitivity. (c) To the extent possible, the inclusion of various measures of the principal clinical dimensions should be based both on expert opinion and careful empirical investigations in which available data on candidate outcome assessments are analyzed to determine their variability and sensitivity to change over time.

Table 4   Attributes of a Multivariate Clinical Outcome Measure for MS Trials

Measure attribute	Explanation
Multidimensional	The outcome measure is based on components that measure different key dimensions of the disease.
Individual components change over time	The individual components of the outcome measure change in a significant proportion of the population who experience change.
Components change independently	Change in the individual components is relatively independent from other components.
Applicable to range of MS severity most often included in MS trials	Available scores should allow classification of all patients to avoid ceiling effects.

V. QUANTIFYING NEUROLOGIC FUNCTION

The World Health Organization (WHO) (17) distinguished impairment from disability and handicap. According to this classification, *impairment* is caused by the underlying disease process and results in abnormalities evident on the neurological exam. Functional consequences of these impairments resulting in problems with activities of daily living are termed *disabilities*. These can be quantified by standardized timed tests of neurological function or by patient self-report related to disability. The vocational, social, or role limitations resulting from the interaction between disability and the environment are termed *handicap*, which can be measured by patient self-report. Generally, impairment is graded using categorical clinical ratings, while disability is measured using quantitative functional assessments. These measures are supplemented with patient self-reports. The utility of this classification for outcome measures in MS clinical trials, however, is unclear.

VI. CLINICAL OUTCOME MEASURES FOR MULTIPLE SCLEROSIS

Clinical outcome measures for MS trials can be divided into three categories (Table 5).

1. In one class of measures, information about disease severity is provided by the patient or designate such as a family member. Examples in this category include the incapacity status scale (ISS), the environmental status scale (ESS) [both part of the Minimal Record of Disability (MRD)], the Fatigue Severity Scale (FSS), the MS Quality of Life Index (MSQLI), and the Guy's Neurologic Disability Scale (GNDS). Information for this type of measure can be obtained by the

Table 5 Clinical Outcome Measures Proposed for Multiple Sclerosis

Type of measure	Name of measure	Abbreviation
Patient self-report	Incapacity Status Scale	ISS
	Environmental Status Scale	ESS
	Fatigue Severity Scale	FSS
	Fatigue Impact Scale	FIS
	MS Quality of Life Index	MSQLI
	Guy's Neurologic Disability Score	GNDS
Ratings based on neurological examination	Expanded Disability Status and Functional System Scales	EDSS, FSS
	Ambulation Index	AI
	Scripps Neurologic Rating Scale	SNRS
	MS Impairment Scale	MSIS
	Troiano Scale	TS
	Cambridge Multiple Sclerosis Basic Score	CMSBS
Quantitative functional assessment	Quantitative Evaluation of Neurologic Function	QENF
	Quantitative Motor Testing	QMT
	9-Hole Peg Test, Box and Blocks Test	9-HPT, BBT
	Quantitative Ambulation	T8, D_{max}
	Multiple Sclerosis Functional Composite	MSFC
Mixed	Relapses	

patient completing a questionnaire with or without assistance or by the rater interviewing the patient.

2. The second category of measures involves the neurologist making clinical ratings, commonly based on the standardized neurological examination. Examples in this category include the Kurtzke Expanded Disability Status Scale (EDSS), the Scripps Neurologic Rating Scale (SNRS), and the MS Impairment Scale (MSIS).

3. In the third category, quantitative measures of neurological function (e.g., cognitive, visual, motor, and sensory function) are obtained by a standardized test procedure, often by a trained technician. Examples in this category include the Quantitative Evaluation of Neurologic Function (QENF), the nine-Hole Peg Test (9HPT), or the Multiple Sclerosis Functional Composite (MSFC). There are some measures that have features of more than one category [e.g., the Ambulation Index (AI) or counting relapses].

There are advantages and disadvantages to these different types of measures (Table 6). Self-report measures provide information that is relevant to the patient. However, these measures can be influenced by the patient's perception of disease severity at the time of measurement and over the recent past and often lack the perspective of the range of problems that could arise now and in the future. These deficiencies may relate to personality factors, affective disturbance, or even to events in the patient's life that have nothing to do with the disease. These problems limit the utility of self-report instruments as primary outcome measures in clinical trials. They remain important nonetheless because of their obvious relevance to the patient. Neurological ratings are more objective, and all neurologists are able to perform these ratings through the neurological exam. Measures in this

Table 6   Advantages and Disadvantages of Types of Measures

Type of measure	Main advantages	Main disadvantages
Patient self-report	1. Clinically relevant	1. Heavily influenced by patient perception, premorbid personality 2. May be related to factors other than disease severity
Ratings based on neurological examination	1. More objective than patient self report. 2. Dependent on known neurologic manifestations	1. Ratings imprecise, insensitive (particularly related to neuropsychological impairments) and may vary substantially by observer 2. Ordinal scales based on neurologic ratings insensitive to change
Quantitative functional assessment	1. Strong psychometric properties 2. Cost effective (can be performed by technicians) 3. Data on a continuous scale may be more sensitive to change	1. Clinical relevance of change may not be apparent 2. Measures not familiar to most neurologists

category have achieved widespread acceptance as primary outcome measures in MS clinical trials but have been criticized as having poor measurement characteristics. Specifically, they are poorly reproducible and generally utilize ordinal scales. This reduces the sensitivity of this type of measure. Quantitative ratings of neurological function are felt to be most objective and reproducible, but they have been criticized as having an unclear relationship to daily function.

A. Self-Report Measures

Minimal Record of Disability (Incapacity Status Scale (ISS) and Environmental Status Scale (ESS)

The International Federation of Multiple Sclerosis Societies developed a Minimal Record of Disability (MRD) based on the WHO definitions of impairment, disability, and handicap (18). In the MRD, impairment is measured with the EDSS (see below). Disability is measured by the ISS, which was developed by Kurtzke and Granger. The ISS is based on the physical condition, upper limb function, lower limb function, sensory function, excretory functions, support factors (e.g., psychological and financial) (19), and the Barthel Index. Scoring is based on interview and is determined according to the patient's actual level of function and not presumed abilities. Therefore, it may be affected by coexisting disease, which is a limitation in its use in a clinical trial as a primary outcome. The ISS evaluates the following 16 items: stair climbing, ambulation, transfers, bowel function, bladder function, bathing, dressing, grooming, feeding, vision, speech and hearing, medical problems (either MS- or not MS-related), mood and thought disturbance, mentation, fatigability, and sexual function. Each is scored from 0 (no dysfunction) to 4 (worst dysfunction); therefore the maximum possible score is 64.

The ESS, developed by an international group chaired by Mellerup and Fog, assesses social dysfunction appropriate to one's cultural setting (18). It consists of seven items, each rated from 0 (no dysfunction) to 5 (greatest dysfunction). Again, the rating is based on performance. For example, someone capable of working but unemployed would be given the worst score (5) for actual work status if the evaluator deems that the "customary" role for that individual in his or her social background would be full-time employment. Other items rated are financial/economic status, personal residence, personal assistance requirements, transportation, community services, and social activities.

Granger et al. (20) evaluated a number of measurements of disability and handicap—including the ISS, ESS, and the functional independence measure (FIM)—in 24 patients. The FIM (21) is an updated version of the Barthel Index and the brief symptom inventory (BSI) (22), a measure of psychological distress. The FIM includes items for toileting and better distinguishes degrees of bladder and bowel involvement. The FIM also separates transferring from bed or chairs, from tub or showers, and from a toilet. Theoretically, this provides improved precision and sensitivity compared to the ISS. There have been more extensive evaluations of inter rater agreement, redundancy, and predictive value of the FIM compared with the ISS, albeit not for MS specifically. Each of these measures and their component domains were evaluated as predictors for the minutes per day of required help by MS patients and for their self-expressed general life satisfaction. The FIM and ISS were each satisfactory in explaining approximately 75% of the variability among patients (20). A multiple regression analysis revealed that the predictors most likely associated with the need for help were transfers from tub and shower (FIM), vision (ISS), and "walk or wheelchair" (FIM). With the effect of vision removed, multiple FIM items were predictive, including transfers from a chair or bed, memory, "walk or wheelchair," dressing lower body, bladder management, and eating. The items associated with general life satisfaction differed from those associated with the need for help and included items from the BSI (interpersonal, sensitivity, and hostility), ESS (transportation and social activity), and the FIM (toileting, dressing lower body, and climbing stairs).

Cohen et al. (23) found that the ability to accomplish activities of daily living worsened exponentially once the EDSS score exceeded 5. The predictive value of the EDSS on activities of daily living was primarily due to its assessment of mobility. The EDSS did not, however, explain adequately the variability between individuals in activities of daily living.

The usefulness of the ISS or ESS as a clinical trial outcome measure has not been determined. They may have greatest application as secondary outcome measures to provide relevant patient information related to disability and handicap. The data can be used to explore the significance of changes observed using impairment or quantitative disability measures in the same trial.

Fatigue Scales (FSS)

Fatigue is a common disabling symptom in MS patients and is only weakly correlated with other aspects of physical, cognitive, or emotional impairment. Krupp et al. used a fatigue severity scale (24), in which fatigue was quantified by means of a visual analogue scale, to study 32 consecutive MS patients. Patients were asked to place a mark on a 10-cm line ranging from "no fatigue" to "severe fatigue" appropriate to the point that best described their fatigue. In this study, fatigue predated other symptoms in 31% and was the most troublesome symptom in 28%. The Pearson correlation coefficient between EDSS and fatigue was not statistically significant. A number of factors distinguished MS-associated fatigue from fatigue in normal controls: MS-related fatigue prevented sustained physical functioning, was aggravated by heat, interfered with home and work responsibilities, came on easily, interfered with physical functioning, and caused frequent problems.

Fisk et al. used the Fatigue Impact Scale (25) to analyze 85 MS patients and 20 patients with hypertension. MS patients reported significantly higher fatigue impact than hypertensive patients, and 55% of MS patients reported that fatigue was one of their worst symptoms. The Fatigue Impact Scale also demonstrated that fatigue has a significant effect on the mental health and general health the status of MS patients.

Fatigue seems to be distinguishable from depression, but subjectivity and lack of association with other objective measurable dysfunction make it a poor choice for a primary outcome measure in a clinical trial. However, its frequency and strong impact on quality of life make it an important secondary outcome measure.

Multiple Sclerosis Quality of Life Inventory

The MSQLI was developed by a research group under the auspices of the Consortium of Multiple Sclerosis Centers. It is composed of the SF-36 plus either established scales or ones developed for this purpose that assess disease specific aspects of MS. This approach allows comparison with the general population and other illness groups using the generic instrument and comparison with other illnesses that share the same symptoms. The scales comprised by the MSQLI include the following. General well being is assessed with the generic HRQoL measure, the Medical Outcomes Study Short Form 36 (SF-36) (26). Fatigue assessment utilizes the 21-item Modified Fatigue Impact Scale (M-FIS) (27). Pain and disturbing sensations are quantified using the six-item MOS Pain Effects Scale (28).

Assessment of sexual functioning (four-item scale) is based on the work of Shover and colleagues (29). Subscales for assessing bladder function (four-items) and bowel function (five items) were developed for the MSQLI. Perceived visual function (five-item scale) was adapted from the Functional Capacities Assessment that was developed by the Michigan Commission for the Blind. Assessment of perceived cognitive functioning (20 items) utilzes the Perceived Deficits Questionnaire (PDQ) (30). Emotional status assessment is made with the 18-item Mental Health Inventory (MHI-18) (31). Finally, social functioning is measured using the 18-item MOS Social Support Survey (SSS) (32).

Details of the development process included two phases, (a) instrument selection and content validation and (b) reliability assessment, construct validation and item reduction (33). The instrument selection and content validation phase of this study began with a definition of the conceptual framework that is based on the WHO's scheme of impairment, disability, and handicap and then a review of the literature for established measures that assessed those domains. Where developed measures were not available, scales were developed. The adequacy of the model and the measures that operationalized it were confirmed during a content validation process that included review by three expert panels comprised of neurologists specializing in MS care, allied health professionals specializing in MS care, and patients and their family caregivers. The reliability, construct validation, and item reduction phase included a pilot test of 15 subjects and a field test of 300 subjects from 4 MS clinics in the United States and Canada who were stratified by gender and disability. The instruments were administered in the clinic setting and objective measures of physical and cognitive disability were completed on all subjects. Scale reliability was demonstrated for the SF-36 and all disease-specific scales. Content validity was established for the SF-36 when correlations among its subscale scores performed in the predicted manner as did the disease-specific scales for bladder, bowel, sexual, and visual function. Generally, construct validation was supported for the MSQLI. The MSQLI has been used in a cross-sectional study of the burden of illness of MS (34) and is included in an ongoing longitudinal randomized, controlled trial of rehabilitation after relapse (personal communication, D. Miller).

Guys Neurologic Disability Scale (GNDS)

The GNDS (35) was developed in response to an international postal survey of neurologists involved with MS research. The survey results suggested that currently existing outcome measures for MS were inadequate. The GNDS assesses 12 separate categories including cognition, mood, vision, speech, swallowing, upper limb function, lower limb function, bladder function, bowel function, sexual function, fatigue, and "others." The GNDS is based primarily on patient self-report, although there are some required neurologist observations. For example, to assess cognitive disability the examiner asks the MS patient "Do you have any problems with your memory or your ability to concentrate and work things out?" A second question is posed: "Do your family or friends think that you have such a problem?" If the answer to either question is yes, a third questions is asked: "Do you need help from other people for planning your normal daily affairs, handling money, or making decisions?" If the answer to this is yes, the examiner determines if the patient is fully oriented, partially oriented, or totally disoriented. The scoring ranges from 0 (no cognitive problems) through 5 (patient is completely disoriented in time, place, and person). Each of the 12 dimensions is scored on an ordinal subscale based on a variable combination of patient self-report and examiner observation. The mood, visual, swallowing, lower limb, bladder, bowel, sexual, and fatigue scales are entirely patient self-report. The overall scale ranges from 0 (no disability) to 60 (maximal disability score).

The GNDS was tested at the Guy's Hospital in London. Face validity was determined by repeat survey of the same neurologists who participated in the initial survey. Of 33 neurologists who returned the follow-up survey, 82% expressed general approval. 50 MS patients were studied serially at the Guy's Hospital to evaluate the GNDS. Factor analysis suggested a four-factor model that accounted for 58.7% of the total variance. Factors that were identified included a "spinal factor" that was correlated with the lower limb, bladder, bowel, and sexual function sub-scales; a "mental factor" that correlated with the cognition, mood, and fatigue subscales; a "bulbar factor" that correlated with speech and swallowing subscales; and a fourth factor that correlated with the upper limb, vision, and other disabilities subscales.

Interrater reliability was assessed in these 50 MS patients. Each patient was interviewed independently by two neurologists who applied the GNDS. Agreement was 100% when defined as ≤ 3 point difference, and the intra class correlation coefficient was 0.98. Scale responsiveness was determined by follow-up examination of the same 50 patients with assessments every 3 months for 9 months. For patients judged clinically to be stable, the GDNS scores changed by ≤ 5 points. The effect size was reported to be 0.58 for patients who were classified clinically as better or worse, indicating "moderate responsiveness." GNDS correlated with SNRS ($r = -0.78$); EDSS ($r = -0.75$); London Handicap Scale ($r = 0.52$); the Functional Independence Measure ($r = -0.81$); and the physical domain of the SF-36 ($r = -0.81$).

The GNDS appears promising as a patient oriented measure of MS-related disability. As with other self-report measures, it can be largely scored by the patient independently or by telephone interview. It would seem to be most appropriate as a secondary outcome measure for MS clinical trials.

B. Ratings Based on the Neurological Examination

Counting Relapses

Relapse frequency is a seemingly straightforward clinical outcome measure. Relapses in MS patients are defined as new or worsening symptoms attributable to MS lasting greater than 24 h. The requirement for symptoms to last at least 24 h is intended to eliminate "pseudoexacerbations," which are episodes of deterioration in neurological function precipitated by heat exposure, fever, or fatigue that are reversible within hours. Relapse frequency in the first 2 years from onset has been inversely associated with the time to reach DSS 6 in some (36) but not all studies (37). Parametric statistical tests can be used to compare mean relapse rates in the treatment arms of a clinical trial. This is a more powerful method than nonparametric tests used to compare change in EDSS. Despite this advantage, there are several drawbacks to the use of relapse frequency as a primary outcome. First, relapses decrease in frequency with time in all MS patients. This phenomenon is often exaggerated in clinical trials in which patients selected for relatively high relapse frequency tend to "regress to the mean" (38). Also, relapses vary in severity and degree of recovery and these factors are hard to compare between patients. For example, it is difficult to say how a severe optic neuritis, with an excellent chance for full recovery, should be compared with a more insidious relapse in a patient with chronic myelopathy, with a lesser chance for full recovery. Furthermore, while there is an association between relapse frequency and time to DSS 6, the association is weak (36). An additional concern about relapses as an outcome measure is the subjective element of this outcome measure. The patient must report worsening to the neurologist to be considered for a relapse. Particularly for more mild relapses, patients may vary considerably in what they report. This can be a problem in a trial where the patients are not totally blinded to treatment arm. Many neurologists argue that sustained change in neurological functional status is a more relevant outcome in MS clinical trials.

Expanded Disability Status Scale (EDSS) and Functional System Scales (FSS)

Kurtzke developed a set of scales that has gained wide acceptance for quantifying disability resulting from MS (12,39,40). Kurtzke's original disability status scale (DSS) and functional system (FS) scores were subsequently expanded (Expanded Disability Status Scale, EDSS) and modifications in the guidelines for scoring were made over the years. The FS scores are based primarily on the neurological examination. The DSS is an ordinal composite measure of neurological impairment with scores ranging from zero (normal neurologic examination) to 10 (death). The DSS score is determined by the FS scores at the lower range of the scale and by an assessment of ambulation, ability to transfer, upper extremity function and bulbar function at successively higher levels.

The DSS and its successors, the EDSS and FS, have been extensively field-tested over the last 20 years. Kurtzke's initial observation that patients are distributed normally over the range of DSS disability (12) has been disputed by a number of studies that show the distribution to be bimodal. Prospective longitudinal studies reveal that staying times at different levels of the DSS vary sufficiently to alter the probability of worsening by one DSS point during a 2- or 3-year clinical trial, depending on the entry DSS level (41,42).

Kurtzke introduced the DSS in 1955 (43), and the FS in 1961 (12). These scales were designed to capture the degree of impairment on independent measures of neurological function felt to be relevant to patients with MS. The scores are determined by the neurological examination with the exception of bladder and bowel scores, which are based on self reports. The FS scores are based upon a neurological assessment of the following systems: pyramidal, cerebellar, sensory, brainstem, bowel and bladder, cerebral, visual, and other. Kurtzke classified the FS as major (pyramidal, cerebellar, sensory, and brainstem) and minor (bowel and bladder, visual, cerebral, and other) based on the frequency with which these systems were affected. Kurtzke (44) pointed out that only a fraction of the possible permutations and combinations of theoretical FS involvement are actually represented in MS population samples. The DSS was left as the composite measure of impairment because the FS usually "peaked" at scores lower than the maximum impairment for a given subscale and because a summed score did not adequately represent the patient's impairment.

The DSS was later expanded (EDSS) by adding 0.5 points to all levels except 0.0 to generate a 20-point scale with finer steps (40). The scoring of the EDSS was clearly designed to reflect the pattern of worsening of MS. Initially, patients experience one or more neurological impairments reflected on the FS but do not have impaired mobility or upper extremity dysfunction. The EDSS scores 1.0 to 4.0 were designed to reflect the FS scores, especially the severity on individual FS. Minor additional weighting is given for the number of systems involved. For example, a score of 3.0 on two FS rather than on one FS elevates the score from 3.0 to 3.5. From EDSS scores 4.0 to 8.0, the scale was designed to reflect difficulty with ambulation, the most common problem encountered by

MS patients. These scores are based on the distance a patient can reasonably walk without having to stop for rest. Beginning with EDSS score 6.0, the scale measures both distance and required ambulation aids. Assessments are based on the physician's assessment of a patient's best reasonable performance without requiring supramaximal performance. All scores are rated according to the principle of "closest" to the most appropriate score (45). At EDSS score 7.5, the ability to walk is essentially lost, and worsening from scores 8.0 to 9.0 is based primarily on upper extremity dysfunction. From EDSS scores 9.0 to 9.5, rating is based on bulbar dysfunction. An EDSS score of 10 indicates that a patient's death was due to MS.

The EDSS is an ordinal scale, so a change from 2.0 to 3.0 is not equivalent to change from 3.0 to 4.0. A 4-point deterioration is not necessarily "twice as bad" as a 2-point deterioration. Kurtzke found that a cross section of MS patients were distributed in a normal (Gaussian) distribution according to the scale, but this has not been the experience of other cross-sectional population-based studies (12). There is a relative dearth of patients at EDSS 4.0 to 5.5, which is likely due to the fact that the staying time at these levels is significantly shorter, as has been discovered in both combined retrospective and prospective longitudinal studies (41) and in entirely prospective series (42). Kurtzke has argued that this may be an artifact of misuse of the EDSS, wherein patients are assigned a score of 6.0 if they use a cane, without assessing their ability to walk the distance that must be observed without walking aids for grades 4.0 to 5.5. This point of contention has not been formally resolved, but this clearly indicates a potential source of interrater variability based on the observer's perceptions of a patient's ability.

The EDSS and FS have been extensively investigated for interrater agreement at both the upper range and at the lower range (46–48,49,50). Although interrater agreement is not perfect, it is greater than 80% when perfect agreement is defined as $+/-$ 0.5 EDSS points or $+/-$ 1.0 FS points (49). The interrater agreement in the EDSS range 1.0 to 3.5 is only 60 to 70% when perfect agreement is defined as $+/-$ 1.0 EDSS point (48).

While the EDSS has achieved widespread use as a primary clinical rating scale in recent years, it has well recognized shortcomings (51). The main problems with the EDSS can be summarized as follows: (a) In the lower range of EDSS, the definitions for the functional system scales gradations are vague and subjective, limiting the reproducibility of the functional system scales. Some of the FS scores are not objectively verifiable, such as bladder and bowel involvement. Additionally at the low end of the scale the definition of EDSS using the various functional system scores is somewhat arbitrary. (b) In the mid range of the scale, the EDSS is almost entirely an ambulation instrument, yet the information is truncated into a small number of discrete categories, discarding important information about change. For example, an individual patient may remain at the 6.5-level for several years during which walking becomes increasingly limited. The patient changes, but the EDSS score does not reflect it, contributing to unequal staying times at various EDSS levels. For this reason, it has been argued that the EDSS is inadequately sensitive to change for the purposes of controlled clinical trials. (c) In the upper range, EDSS steps represent such large changes as to be almost useless as a rating scale for clinical trials because of poor sensitivity. (d) At any range of the scale, there are no cognitive assessments, even though cognitive impairments are common in MS patients. (e) At the range from 4.0 to 6.5, the EDSS is insensitive to arm impairment.

The ordinal nature of the EDSS must be accounted for in the choice of instruments used for statistical analyses. Mean change in EDSS is unacceptable as an endpoint for clinical trials. A treatment failure endpoint is more acceptable, wherein a degree of broadly accepted change indicative of unequivocal deterioration is defined a priori. However, even with this approach, the probability of treatment failure is dependent on the baseline EDSS score. One approach to bypass the nonlinear nature of this scale without modifying the scale itself is to adapt the use of this scale based on the results of field-testing. Based on the work of several groups, it has been suggested that a buffer of $+/-$ 0.5 points should be allowed for baseline EDSS less than or equal to 5.5 without declaring treatment failure, but for EDSS greater than or equal to 6.0, 0.5 EDSS worsening should be accepted as meeting the criterion for failure. This recommendation is based on differences in the observed staying times at different levels of the EDSS. This approach may have successfully bypassed some of the difficulties posed by differing probabilities for treatment failure according to entry EDSS level. It has also substantially improved the sensitivity of the EDSS in a clinical trial by allowing less stringent treatment failure criteria at higher EDSS levels. Goodkin et al. (52) utilized this approach in defining one of several secondary outcome measures in a clinical trial of azathioprine in relapsing remitting MS; he based this approach on his own observations of interrater reliability at different levels of the EDSS as well as those of others. At approximately the same time, in studies of the natural history of MS, Weinshenker et al. (41) observed that staying times were roughly two to three times longer at DSS 6 and 7 than at DSS 4 and 5. In a metanalysis of four large randomized clinical trials of progressive MS, Weinshenker et al. (53) found that the proportion of treatment failures using different definitions varied considerably. Over 2 to 3 years follow-up, the proportion of treatment failures increased from 30 to 50% when allowance was made for a modified definition of treatment failure, with 0.5 EDSS point being the criterion for treatment failure with baseline EDSS greater than or equal to 6.0.

A variation on the use of EDSS was introduced by Liu and colleagues (54). This method calculates an area under the curve generated from all EDSS scores collected during the course of a clinical trial. The resulting number, which has been termed the Integrated Disability Status Scale (IDSS), is said to capture information about both disability and relapse. The IDSS has been applied to recently completed clinical trials in post-hoc analyses.

Ambulation Index (AI)

The AI (55) was developed by Hauser et al. (55) for use as an outcome measure in a clinical trial of cyclophosphamide, plasma exchange, and ACTH in progressive MS. It is based only on ambulation and was used as an adjunct to the EDSS in the context of that trial. Some elements are subjective (e.g. level 1 requires patient-reported fatigue with demanding activity, while level 2 requires a gait disorder "noted by family and friends"). However, timed walking of 25 ft is used for most levels of the 10-step scale, making it a hybrid scale with elements of subjective self-report, neurological impairment, and quantitative neuroperformance. The timed 25-ft walk is a significant advantage, as assessment of time to walk 25 ft is more practical than observing the patient walk 500 m, as is necessary to score the EDSS at some levels. Francis et al. (47) found the kappa statistic for interrater agreement to be better for the AI than for the EDSS. Although somewhat limited by an exclusive focus on ambulation, the AI appears to be a useful adjunct for improving sensitivity and interrater reliability of the EDSS in the range of 4.0 to 7.0.

Scripps Neurologic Rating Scale (NRS)

The NRS is an impairment scale developed by Sipe et al. (56) for use in a trial of alpha interferon conducted at the Scripps Clinic. It is a direct translation of the scoring on standard neurological examination. It rates abnormalities in the following dimensions: mentation and mood (10 points), cranial nerves of vision (21 points), lower cranial nerves (5 points), strength (20 points), deep tendon reflexes (8 points), Babinski signs (4 points), sensory function rated for each limb (12 points), cerebellar function rated separately for upper and lower extremities (10 points), and gait and balance (10 points). The maximum score for a normal individual is 100. Abnormalities lower the score. Up to a further 10 points can be deducted for various combinations of bowel, bladder, and sexual dysfunction. The principal advantages are its ready derivation from the neurological examination and added sensitivity by virtue of a much greater range of scores than the EDSS. Other advantages include the fact that each limb is separately rated as to motor and sensory function on a scale of 1 to 5, and it is more sensitive to vision than the EDSS. Disadvantages include lack of guidelines on scoring severity, retention of imprecise descriptions, such as "mild, moderate, and severe" impairment, and somewhat arbitrary weighting of various neurological functions, albeit this was done with due regard to the frequency with which these findings are seen in MS and their impact on neurological function (i.e. strength has more points than reflexes). It is insensitive to mental status change and relatively insensitive to ambulation.

The added sensitivity of this scale resulted in its being chosen to arbitrate the severity of relapses in the IFNβ-1b pivotal trial (57). In this study, a decline of less than or equal to 7 points was regarded as a mild relapse, 8 to 14 points moderate, and greater than or equal to 15 points severe. Using this classification, the annualized relapse rate in the control (placebo) group was 0.55 mild attacks/year and 0.45 moderate and severe attacks/year over the first 2 years. There was imperfect agreement between this "objective" criterion of relapse severity and the subjective evaluation of the investigators, although Goodkin et al. (58) previously expressed reservation about the impact of imprecise descriptive terms in determining relapse severity.

The MS Impairment Scale (MSIS)

The MSIS (59) was developed by Ravnborg and colleagues in the Copenhagen MS Clinic at the University Hospital in Copenhagen Denmark. Conceptually, the MSIS is quite similar to the NRS except that the MSIS contains more standardized neuropsychological tests. The score is computed following a standardized neurologic examination supplemented by a brief battery of cognitive tests. The theoretical range for the scale is from 0 (best result) through 204 (worst result). Twelve (6%) of 204 "impairment points" can be accrued through the neuropsychological tests; 15 (7%) of the 204 impairment points through visual or oculomotor tests; 8 (4%) through speech disorder or facial weakness; 94 (46%) through extremity weakness spasticity or plantar responses; 48 (24%) through sensory testing; and 27 (13%) for problems with gait, stance, or axial stability. A total of 210 MS patients were rated using the MSIS, EDSS, and AI by a single neurologist. The relationship between MSIS and EDSS was described best as an exponential function, with a nonlinear correlation coefficient of 0.87. A second neurologist reexamined 62 patients and the interrater reliability of the MSIS was found to be excellent, comparable to the interrater reliability of the EDSS and AI.

The first 66 patients examined in this study were evaluated again after 1 year. Intrarater variability was used to determine the amount of change that could be explained by test variability. Of the total, 24 (36%) of the patients had deteriorated beyond that level after 1 year. In comparison, 15 (23%) of the patients had worsened by at least 1 point on the EDSS. By this measure, the MSIS appears more sensitive to change than the EDSS.

Potential weakness of the MSIS relate to its structure and the somewhat arbitrary weighting. It consists of a number of individual ordinal rating scales that are added together to create an impairment score. The definitions are somewhat more clear than in the EDSS, FSS, or NRS. However it is likely that interrater reliability would remain a problem in the context of a multicenter study because definitions of some of the steps in the individual components remain vague. Also, 83% of the MSIS impairment points are assigned to motor function, sensory function, and gait, compared with 13% assigned to cognitive function and visual function. This distribution may improve the correlations with EDSS and AI but may underestimate important aspects of MS. As a neurologist-based rating scale, the MSIS is considered an interesting alternative to EDSS and NRS. It has not yet been tested in the context of a controlled clinical trial.

Troiano Scale (60)

The TS was designed for use in a clinical trial of total lymphoid irradiation in chronically progressive MS (60). The TS is a 12-point hybrid impairment and disability scale scored in three subscales: gait, activities of daily living, and transfers. The gait scale is substantially similar to the AI but abbreviated to a 6-point scale. The transfer scale is a 4-point scale, of which only the last two steps refer to a significant requirement for assistance in transfers. The ADL subscale is a 5-point disability scale. Its major advantage is simplicity. The drawbacks are insensitivity and lack of assessment of vision, sphincter, brainstem, and mental function. As acknowledged by the authors, it is designed primarily to assess progressive MS and not relapses. Work by the authors suggests that scores are unimodal. It is difficult to accept the independence of the three measures and the assertion that it is more sensitive than the EDSS. For example, there is no attempt to grade ambulation according to either distance or speed but only on requirement for walking aids, with the inherent subjectivity of this observation.

Cambridge Multiple Sclerosis Basic Score

The CAMBS was proposed by Mumford and Compston (61) of the University of Cambridge. This score is a shorthand method to express disability and impairment, relapse status and severity, degree of progression, and patient perceived handicap using a visual analog scale. Each of these dimensions is graded on an abbreviated 5-point scale, and expressed as a four digit score. Reproducibility is claimed to be good but given its inherent insensitivity, this is not surprising. The authors point out that it is not designed to be an outcome measure for clinical trials. Recording relapse and progression status removes the restriction of other rating scales to assessment when the disease is in a relatively stable state. Its advantages are simplicity and wide applicability. Otherwise, it offers no unique advantages.

C. Quantitative Assessments of Function

Quantitative Evaluation of Neurological Function

Quantitative evaluation of neurological function (QENF), developed by Tourtellotte et al. (62,63), is a battery of tests that can be timed and expressed as parametric data, often as a percentage of normal function. These measurements are not MS-specific but are designed to be objective measures that are sensitive to change in function. The battery of tests includes the following: symbol digit modality test (cognitive); finger tapping, Purdue pegboard, foot tapping, standing/balance (two legs and one leg), tandem walking, and simulated activities of daily living (e.g., dressing, buttoning, zipping, tying a bow, cutting with knife, etc). Testing is administered by a trained technician and can be completed in approximately 1 hour. In longitudinal studies, each testing session is preferably administered at the same time of day.

Syndulko et al reviewed the results of a neuroperformance battery administered in the context of a controlled trial of cyclosporine in chronic progressive MS (64). They found that these tests were reproducible over multiple baseline examinations and that changes over time correlated with changes on the EDSS and AI. The neuroperformance tests detected favorable treatment effects that were not detected by the EDSS or other standard clinical rating scales at the Los Angeles site. Interestingly, treatment effects detected by the QENF reflected similar benefits detected with the EDSS for the overall study (65), which led the investigators to conclude that QENF was more sensitive than EDSS. These investigators noted that the magnitude of change and the difference between the placebo and active treatment groups were such that a smaller sample size would be necessary to detect a treatment effect if the neuroperformance battery were used as the primary outcome measure rather than the EDSS. Proponents of this approach acknowledge that practice effects are problematic in some of the subtests.

Conclusions based on the QENF are conceptually difficult. It is unappealing to conclude a treatment effect when a single or composite neuroperformance score changes by a small, albeit statistically significant amount. The issue of predictive criterion validity is especially important for these quantitative tests. The QENF approach was critical in subsequent development of the Multiple Sclerosis Functional Composite (see below).

Quantitative Motor Power Testing

Noseworthy found that quantitative isometric strength assessment in a biomechanics laboratory was more sensitive than assessment of muscle weakness by two blinded neurologists in a pilot trial of IVIg (66). The reliability of isometric muscle testing was adequate with 73 and 80% reproducibility for markedly ($> 50\%$) and mildly ($< 25\%$) weak muscle on repeated studies separated by at least to 2 weeks. Of 432 muscles with less than 50% normal power by isometric testing, two neurologists rated strength as normal in 41% and mildly reduced in 15% of muscles. The investigators concluded that the clinical neurological examination underestimates the degree of MS-associated weakness, and quantitative isometric testing might significantly enhance the sensitivity with good reliability.

Box and Blocks Test (BBT) and 9-Hole Peg Test (9HPT)

Goodkin et al. assessed the BBT and 9HPT as quantitative measures of upper extremity function (58). This group investigated the frequency of impairment, stability of the results over serial studies, and the potential to use these tests as more sensitive measures that correlate with subjective deterioration in MS. The tests were administered by an occupational therapist who was masked to the neurologist assessment of stability. Some 60 to 90% of patients were impaired (scores $<10\%$ of age- and sex-matched normal controls). Among 68 MS patients who were stable by EDSS over 6 months, 22.2% showed deterioration of 10% on the BBT and 16.3% showed deterioration of 10% on the 9HPT. Of the MS patients, 8.2% showed 20% deterioration on the BBT and 7.1% on the 9HPT. These results suggested that the BBT and 9HPT were more sensitive in showing deterioration than the EDSS. Reproducibility was high for controls who were assessed on several occasions at baseline, but substantially larger variations were encountered in MS patients who were followed over 6 months. Whether the greater variation was truly due to a change in function or to the greater interval between testing and repeat testing is uncertain. The authors concluded that these tests were more sensitive than the EDSS in detecting upper extremity function change.

These upper extremity functional tests were encorporated into a composite outcome measure by Goodkin et al. (67) in a randomized clinical trial of oral methotrexate in 60 ambulatory and chronically progressive MS patients. The greatest difference in favor of treatment benefit were seen in measures of upper extremity function, while less significant benefit was detected in ambulation or EDSS.

Goodkin and colleagues measured 9HPT, BBT, and timed 25-ft walk in patients participating in the IFNβ-1a (Avonex) phase III trial (68). Treatment failure for individual measures was defined as sustained ($\geq$6 months) worsening by 20% or more from baseline 9HPT or BBT, or slowing of 3s or more on timed 25-ft walk. EDSS worsening was defined as $\geq$1.0 point worsening from baseline sustained for $\geq$6 months. A composite of the non-physician-based measures (9HPT, BBT, and timed walk) was compared with the EDSS in showing treatment effects. The sensitivity of the non-physician based measures was comparable to the EDSS, based on analysis of time-to-failure survival curves using the log rank test. The combined use of the EDSS together with the timed tests of neurologic function appeared slightly more sensitive than the EDSS alone.

Timed Ambulation and Maximal Distance Walk

Schwid and colleagues measured a timed 8-m walk and a maximal distance walk up to 500 m (D_{max}) in 237 ambulatory MS patients. Results were compared with EDSS and AI scores (69). The D_{max} and walk times were strongly correlated with EDSS scores, but there was considerable variability within each EDSS or AI step. Most of the variability occurred at EDSS levels 6.0 to 7.0 and AI levels 3 to 6. Interestingly, use of a specific walking aid, which defines EDSS 6.0 and 6.5, was not closely correlated with the walk time or D_{max}. The authors concluded that considerable variability exists within the discrete EDSS and AI levels, and suggested that quantitative funcitonal testing would be a more sensitive method for following ambulatory function in MS patients.

Multiple Sclerosis Functional Composite (MSFC)

This measure was recommended by the NMSS Task Force as most closely meeting the desirable measurement characteristics in Table 2 (5). Particular emphasis was placed on reproducibility and sensitivity to change, which may be greater with quantitative functional testing compared with neurologist clinical ratings. The task force analyzed a pooled data set to arrive at its recommendation of the MSFC. The use of multiple data sets during development ensured that the MSFC was not biased. A detailed account of the development of this measure is provided elsewhere (70).

The recommended MSFC is a unified score representing the combination of results from three performance tests: (a) the 9 Hole Peg Test (9HPT), (b) the timed 25-foot walk, and (c) The 3-s Paced Auditory Serial Addition Test (PASAT3). These performance tests are combined to form a single score. The MSFC scores are generated as follows: (a) The scores from 4 trials on the 9-HPT—two trials of the left hand and two trials of the right hand—are transformed and averaged. (b) Scores from two trials of the timed 25-ft walk are averaged. (c) The number of correct answers from the PASAT3 test is used. The

MSFC score thus incorporates three clinical dimensions representing arm, leg, and cognitive function to create a single score that can be used to detect change over time in a group of MS patients.

Since the underlying measurement variables differ between these tests (time for the 9HPT and timed 25-ft walk compared with the number of correct answers for the PASAT3), a Z-score was selected as a common metric. The Z-score is a standardized number representing how close a test result is to the mean of a standard or reference population to which the result is compared. The Z-score is expressed in units of standard deviation and usually ranges from -3 to $+3$, although there are no restrictions on its values. The standard deviation of a measure is, on average, how far an observation is from the mean in the original units of measurement, whereas the Z-score is a relative measure (e.g., a Z-score of 2 always implies an observation is 2 standard deviations from the mean, whereas in the original units of measurement, the meaning of a standard deviation of 2 depends on what is being measured: seconds, minutes, number correct, etc., which would need to be known before the value could be considered as large or small). The Z-score is obtained by subtracting the mean of the all the measurements from the test result and then dividing by the standard deviation of the these values. When a sample is considered to come from some reference population, the mean and standard deviation of this reference population are used to create the Z-scores. *Because the Z-score is a relative measure indicating how many standard deviation units the current observation is from the mean of the reference population, the units are the same irrespective of the underlying measurement scale.* For example, the number of seconds required to perform a test can be represented on the same Z-score scale as the number of correct responses on the PASAT3. This allows the results from tests using different metrics (e.g., seconds and number correct) to be combined. The three components of the MSFC are combined by creating a Z-score for each component, after which the Z-scores are averaged to generate the overall MSFC score. Patients who deteriorate or improve on all three component measures will have an overall larger change than patients who change on only one of the three measures. Also, patients who deteriorate in one area but improve in another may show no change on the MSFC, because the MSFC represents the *average* change in the three tests.

The validity of the MSFC is of great interest in the face of the NMSS Task Force recommendations. From its pooled data set, the MSFC was validated using the Kurtzke EDSS as the criterion variable. Concurrent validity was defined as the relationship between the MSFC change and EDSS change during the same time interval. Predictive validity was defined as the relationship between MSFC change in the initial year of observation with EDSS change in the subsequent year of observation (i.e., patients change in the composite was used to predict who would have a 3-month sustained change in their EDSS among patients not found to change in the first year on their EDSS). Using these definitions, the MSFC was found to have both concurrent and predictive validity with respect to the EDSS.

In a separate prospective study, the MSFC was found to have moderate to strong correlations with a number of self-report measures of quality of life (71). In particular, there were moderately strong correlations between the MSFC and the physical component of the Sickness Impact Profile and between MSFC and the physical component of the SF-36. These correlations between MSFC scores and Multiple Sclerosis Quality of Life (MSQLI) measures for the total study population in this study indicated that the MSFC reflects the severity of MS as perceived by patients. MSFC scores best reflect general physical well being, as indicated by strong correlations with the SIP physical scores. However, the study also demonstrated significant correlations with measures of psycho-social functioning, suggesting that MSFC scores capture important psychosocial consequence of physical impairments. Finally, this study demonstrated moderate correlations between MSFC scores and employment status, indicating that the MSFC assesses dimensions relevant to everyday functioning.

Results of this study could direct future improvements in the MSFC measurement method in several ways. As an example, lack of correlation with a disease specific measure of fatigue used in this study suggested that including a fatigue measure in the MSFC might improve overall correlation with disease as perceived by the patients. However, as a treatment for this long term condition, the lack of influence on the MSQLI of transient fatigue, may be seen as a strength. Furthermore, correlations between MSFC and MSQLI measures were lower in the high-disability subgroup. This may be explained by inability of the patients in this sub-group to perform the walking task that is included in the MSFC. Each patient unable to perform this task because of MS was assigned a constant severe score for the walking component of the MSFC. This had the effect of truncating biological variability relating to leg function in this subgroup. This may have accounted for the lower correlations. Finally, as noted by the task force, it may be useful to include a visual score (5).

This study does not resolve the relative value of the MSFC scores compared with other disease measures in actually quantifying the disease severity. Rather, it demonstrates significant correlations with between MSQLI measures and MSFC, and it shows significant residual correlations between MSQLI and MSFC after controlling for EDSS scores. These findings dcmonstrate clinical relevance of the MSFC scores across the range of MS disease severity. In this regard, the study strongly supports the use of the MSFC as a clinical trials outcome measure because of the robust correlations with physician- and patient-derived comparison measures. Further validation of the MSFC using longitudinal methods will clarify the significance of MSFC changes, and determine its utility as a primary outcome measure in clinical trials.

VII. CONCLUSION

There is no single clinical outcome measure for MS that will serve all purposes. For studies related to specific symptoms of MS (e.g., depression, spasticity, bladder control), the outcome instrument must be specifically tied to the target question. For studies of disease-modifying agents, the outcome measure may relate to the stage of the disease being studied. Subjective self-report instruments for MS clinical studies have been increasingly refined, and the MSQLI and the GNDS appear promising. It is most appealing to use these measures as secondary outcomes in clinical trials, where they can be invaluable in assessing the clinical relevance of any observed therapeutic effect.

The Kurtzke EDSS remains the most widely accepted neurologist rating scale, although the SNRS and the MSIS have added precision and range. The latter might provide improved responsiveness compared with the EDSS, but this improvement may not be sufficient in this time of partially effective therapies.

Quantitative tests of neurological function were pioneered by Tourtellotte and Syndulko, simplified by Goodkin and Schwid, and a particular three-part composite was recommended for use by the National MS Society Task Force on Clinical Outcomes Assessment. A major factor in that recommendation was the observation that MSFC change could be observed in advance of EDSS change in the Task Force metanalysis. This finding was consistent the outcome of neuroperformance testing in the cyclosporine study and with the use of upper extremity testing in the methotrexate study. Added sensitivity of the MSFC might serve to shorten clinical trials or reduce required sample sizes. The MSFC is currently being tested as an outcome measure in a number of controlled clinical trials, and its performance relative to other assessment methods should soon be clarified.

References

1. Rudick R, Antel J, Confavreux C, Cutter G, Ellison G, Fischer J, Lublin F, Miller A, Petkau J, Rao S, Reingold S, Syndulko K, Thompson A, Wallenberg J, Weinshenker B, Willoughby E. Clinical outcomes assessment in multiple sclerosis. Ann Neurol 1996; 40:469–479.
2. Poser S, Wikstrom J, Bauer HJ. Clinical data and the identification of special forms of multiple sclerosis in 1271 cases studied with a standardized documentation system. J Neurol Sci. 1979; 40:159–168.
3. Whitaker JN, McFarland HF, Rudge P, Reingold SC. Outcomes assessment in multiple sclerosis clinical trials: A critical analysis. Mult Scler 1995; 1:37–47.
4. Cutter GR, Baier ML, Rudick RA, et al. Development of a multiple sclerosis functional composite as a clinical trial outcome measure. Brain 1999; 122:871–882.
5. Rudick R, Antel J, Confavreux C, et al. Recommendations from the National Multiple Sclerosis Society Clinical Outcomes Assessment Task Force. Ann Neur 1997; 42:379–382.
6. Nunnally JC. Psychometric Theory. New York, McGraw-Hill, 1967.
7. Fitzpatrick R, Ziebland S, Jenkinson C, Mowat A. Importance of sensitivity to change as a criterion for selecting health status measures. Quality Health Care 1992; 1:89–93.
8. Stewart AL, Hays RD, Ware JE Jr. Methods of validating MOS health measures. In: Stewart AL, Ware JE Jr., eds. Measuring Functioning and Well-Being. The Medical Outcomes Study Approach. Durham, NC: Duke University Press, 1993; pp 309–325.
9. Hays RD, Steward AL. Construct validity of MOS health measures. In: Stewart AL, Ware JE Jr, eds. Measuring Functioning and Well-Being. The Medical Outcomes Study Approach. Durham, NC: Duke University Press; 1993, pp 325–345.
10. Weinshenker BG. Clinical outcome measures for multiple sclerosis. In: Goodkin DE, Rudick RA, eds. Multiple Sclerosis: Advances In Clinical Trial Design, Treatment, And Future Perspectives, 2nd ed. London: Springer-Verlag, 1996; pp 105–122.
11. Albert MS. Criteria for the choice of neuropsychological tests in clinical trials. In: Mohr E, Brouwers P, eds. Handbook of Clinical Trials. The Neurobehavioral Approach. Berwyn, PA: Swets & Zeitlinger, 1991, pp 131–139.
12. Kurtzke JF. On the evaluation of disability evaluation in multiple sclerosis. Neurology. 1961; 11:686–694.
13. Henderson WG, Fisher SG, Cohen N, Waltzman S, Weber L. Use of principal components analysis to develop a composite score as a primary outcome variable in a clinical trial. The VA Cooperative Study Group on Cochlear Implantation. Contr Clin Trials 1990; 11:199–214.
14. Syndulko K, Ke D, Ellison GW, et al. Comparative evaluations of neuroperformance and clinical outcome assessments inmultiple sclerosis. I. Primary dimensions, construct validation and sensitivity to disease progression. Mult Scler 1996; 2:142–156.
15. Roberts RS. Pooled outcome measures in arthritis: The pros and cons. J Rheumatol. 1993; 20:566–567.
16. Petkau AJ. Statistical and design considerations for multiple sclerosis clinical trials. In: Goodkin DE, Rudick RA, eds. Multiple sclerosis: Advances in Clinical Trial Design, Treatment, and Future Perspectives. London: Springer-Verlag, 1996.
17. World Health Organization, 1980.
18. International Federation of Multiple Sclerosis Societies. Minimal Record of Disability for Multiple Sclerosis. New York: National Multiple Sclerosis Society, 1985.

19. Granger CV, Albrecht GL, Hamilton BB. Outcome of comprehensive medical rehabilitation: measurement by PULSES profile and the Barthel Index. Arch Phy Med Rehabil. 1979; 60: 145–154.

20. Granger CV, Cotter AC, Hamilton BB, Fiedler RC, Hens MM. Functional assessment scales: A study of persons with multiple sclerosis. Arch Phys Med Rehabil. 1990; 71:870–875.

21. Keith RAGCV, Hamilton BB, Sherwin FS. The functional independence measure: A new tool for rehabilitation. In: Eisenberg MG, Grzesiak RD, eds. Advances in Clinical Rehabilitation, vol 1. New York: Springer-Verlag, 1987, pp 6–18.

22. Derogatis LR, Melisaratos N. The Brief Symptom Inventory: an introductory report. Psychol Med. 1983; 13:595–605.

23. Cohen RA, Kessler HR, Fischer M. The Extended Disability Status Scale (EDSS) as a predictor of impairments of functional activities of daily living in multiple sclerosis. J Neurol Sci. 1993; 115:132–135.

24. Krupp LB, LaRocca NG, Muir-Nash J, Steinberg AD. The fatigue severity scale: Application to patients with multiple sclerosis and systemic lupus erythematosus. Arch Neurol 1989; 46: 1121–1123.

25. Fisk JD, Pontefract A, Ritvo PG, Archibald CJ, Murray TJ. The impact of fatigue on patients with multiple sclerosis (see comments). Can J Neurol Sci 1994; 21:9–14.

26. Ware JEJ, Snow KK, Kosinski M, Gandek B. SF-36 Health Survey: Users Manual and Interpertation Guide. Boston: The Health Institute, New England Medical Center, 1993.

27. Fisk JD, Ritvo PG, Ross L, Haase DA, Marrie TJ, Schlech WF. Measuring the functional impact of fatigue: initial validation of the fatigue impact scale. Clin Infect Dis. 1994; 18 (suppl 1):S79–S83.

28. Stewart AL, Ware JJ. Measuring functioning and well-being: The Medical Outcomes Study Approach. Durham, NC: Duke University Press, 1992.

29. Schover LR, Friedman JM, Weiler SJ, Heinman JR, LoPiccolo J. Multiaxial problem-oriented system for sexual dysfunctions. Arch Gen Psychiatry. 1982; 39:614–619.

30. Sullivan MJL, Edgley K, Dehoux E. A survey of multiple sclerosis: Part 1. Perceived cognitive problems and compensatory strategy use. Can J Rehabil 1990; 4:99–105.

31. Veit CT, Ware JEJ. The structure of psychological distress and well-being in general populations. J Consult Clin Psychol. 1983; 51:730–742.

32. Sherbourne CD, Stewart AL. The MOS Social Support Survey. Soc Sci Med 1991; 32:472–480.

33. Fischer JS, LaRocca NG, Miller DM, Ritvo PG, Andrews H, Paty D. Recent developments in the assessment of quality of life in multiple sclerosis (MS). Mult Scler 1999; 5:251–259.

34. Burden of illness of multiple sclerosis: Part I: Cost of illness. The Canadian Burden of Illness Study Group. Can J Neurol Sci 1998; 25:23–30.

35. Sharrack B, Hughes RAC. The Guy's Neurological Disability Scale (GNDS): A new disability measure for multiple sclerosis. Mult Scler Clin Lab Res 1999; 5:223–234.

36. Weinshenker BG, Bass B, Rice GP, et al. The natural history of multiple sclerosis: a geographically based study: I. Clinical course and disability. Brain 1989; 112:133–146.

37. Runmarker B, Andersen O, Anderson O. Prognostic factors in a multiple sclerosis incidence cohort with twenty-five years of follow-up. Brain 1993;116: 117–134.

38. Weinshenker BG. The natural history of multiple sclerosis. Neurol Clin 1995; 13:119–146.

39. Kurtzke JF. Neurological impairment in multiple sclerosis and the disability status scale. Acta Neurol Scand 1970; 46:493–512.

40. Kurtzke JF. Rating neurologic impairment in multiple sclerosis: An expanded disability status scale (EDSS). Neurology 1983; 33:1444–1452.

41. Weinshenker BG, Rice GP, Noseworthy JH, Carriere W, Baskerville J, Ebers GC. The natural history of multiple sclerosis: a geographically based study: 4. Applications to planning and interpretation of clinical therapeutic trials. Brain 1991; 114:1057–1067.

42. Ellison GW, Myers LW, Leake BD, et al. Design strategies in multiple sclerosis clinical trials. Ann Neurol. 1994; 36:S108–S112.

43. Kurtzke JF. A new scale for evaluating disability in multiple sclerosis. Neurology. 1955; 5: 580–583.

44. Kurtzke JF. Patterns of neurologic involvement in multiple sclerosis. Neurology 1989; 39: 1235–1238.

45. Kurtzke JF. The disability status scale for multiple sclerosis: Apologia pro DSS sua. Neurology 1989; 39:291–302.

46. Amato MP, Fratiglioni L, Groppi C, Siracusa G, Amaducci. Interrater reliability in assessing functional systems and disability on the Kurtzke scale in multiple sclerosis. Arch Neurol 1988; 45:746–748.

47. Francis DA, Bain P, Swan AV, Hughes RA. An assessment of disability rating scales used in multiple sclerosis. Arch Neurol 1991; 48:299–301.

48. Goodkin DE, Cookfair D, Wende K, et al. Inter- and intrarater scoring agreement using grades 1.0 to 3.5 of the Kurtzke Expanded Disability Status Scale (EDSS): Multiple Sclerosis Collaborative Research Group. Arch Neurol 1992; 42:859–863.

49. Noseworthy JH, Vandervoort MK, Wong CJ, Ebers GC. Interrater variability with the Expanded Disability Status Scale (EDSS) and Functional Systems (FS) in a multiple sclerosis clinical trial. The Canadian Cooperation MS Study Group. Neurology 1990; 40:971–975.

50. Verdier-Taillefer MH, Zuber M, Lyon C, et al. Observer disagreement in rating neurologic impairment in multiple sclerosis: facts and consequences. Eur Neurol. 1991; 31:117–119.

51. Willoughby EW, Paty DW. Scales for rating impairment in multiple sclerosis: A critique. Neurology 1988; 38:1793–1798.

52. Goodkin DE, Bailly RC, Teetzen ML, Hertsgaard D, Beatty W. The efficacy of azathioprine in relapsing remitting multiple sclerosis. Neurology 1991; 41:20–25.

53. Weinshenker BG, Issa M, Baskerville J. Meta-analysis of the placebo-treated groups in clinical trials of progressive MS. Neurology 1996; 46:1613–1619.

54. Liu C, Li WP, Blumhardt LD. "Summary measure" statistic for assessing the outcome of treatment trials in relapsing-remitting multiple sclerosis (see comments). (Review). J Neurol Neurosurg & Psychiatry 1998; 64:726–729.

55. Hauser SL, Dawson DM, Lehrich JR, et al. Intensive immunosuppression in progressive multiple sclerosis. A randomized, three-arm study of high-dose intravenous cyclophosphamide, plasma exchange, and ACTH. N Engl J Med 1983; 308:173–180.

56. Sipe JC, Knobler RL, Braheny SL, Rice GP, Panitch HS, Oldstone MB. A neurologic rating scale (NRS) for use in multiple sclerosis. Neurology 1984; 34:1368–1372.

57. The IFN-b Multiple Sclerosis Study Group T. Interferon beta-1b is effective in relapsing-remitting multiple sclerosis: I. Clinical results of a multicenter, randomized, double-blind, placebo-controlled trial. Neurology 1993; 43:656–661.

58. Goodkin DE, Hertsgaard D, Seminary J. Upper extremity function in multiple sclerosis: Improving assessment sensitivity with box-and-block and nine-hole peg tests. Arch Phys Med Rehabil 1988; 69:850–854.

59. Ravnborg M, Gronbech-Jensen M, Jonsson A. The MS Impairment Scale: A pragmatic approach to the assessment of impairment in patients with multiple sclerosis. Mult Scler 1997; 3:31–42.

60. Cook SD, Devereux C, Troiano R, et al. Effect of total lymphoid irradiation in chronic progressive multiple sclerosis. Lancet 1986; 1:1405–1409.

61. Mumford CJ, Compston A. Problems with rating scales for multiple sclerosis: A novel approach—the CAMBS score. J Neurol 1993; 240:209–215.

62. Tourtellotte WW, Haerer AF, Simpson JF, Kuzma JW, Sikorski J. Quantitative clinical neurological testing: I. A study of a battery of tests designed to evaluate in part the neurologic function of patients with multiple sclerosis and its use in a therapeutic trial. Ann NY Acad Sci 1965; 122:480–505.

63. Kuzma JW, Tourtellotte WW, Remington RD. Quantitative clinical neurological testing. II. Some statistical considerations of a battery oftests. J Chronic Dis 1965; 18:303–311.

64. Leaf RC, DiGiuseppe R, Mass R, Alington DE. Statistical methods for analyses of incomplete clinical service records: Concurrent use of longitudinal and cross-sectional data. J Consul Clin Psych 1993; 61:495–505.

65. The Multiple Sclerosis Study Group. Efficacy and toxicity of cyclosporine in chronic progressive multiple sclerosis: A randomized, double-blinded, placebo-controlled clinical trial. Ann Neurol 1996;27:591–605.

66. Noseworthy JH, Rodrigues M, An K-N, et al. IVIg treatment in multiple sclerosis: Pilot study results and design of a placebo-controlled, double-blind clinical trial. Ann Neurol 1994; 36: 325–325.

67. Goodkin DE, Rudick RA, Medendorp SV, et al. Low-dose (7.5 mg) oral methotrexate reduces the rate of pregression in chronic progressive multiple sclerosis. Ann Neurol 1995; 37:30–40.

68. Goodkin DE, Priore RL, Wende KE, et al. Comparing the ability of various compositive outcomes to discriminate treatment effects in MS clinical trials. The Multiple Sclerosis Collaborative Research Group (MSCRG). Mult Scler 1998; 4:480–486.

69. Schwid SR, Goodman AD, Mattson DH, et al. The measurement of ambulatory impairment in multiple sclerosis. Neurology 1997; 49:1419–1424.

70. Cutter GC, Baier ML, Rudick RA, et al. Development of a multiple sclerosis functional composite as a clinical trial outcome measure. Brain 1999; 122:871–882.

71. Miller DM, Rudick RA, Cutter G, Baier M, Fischer JS. Clinical significance of the multiple sclerosis functional composite: Relationship to patient-reported quality of life. Arch Neurol 2000; 57:1319–1324.

20

Therapeutic Considerations: Treatment of the Acute Exacerbation

RAYMOND TROIANO

University of Medicine and Dentistry of New Jersey and New Jersey Medical School, Newark, New Jersey

I. INTRODUCTION

After a clinical relapse, most multiple sclerosis (MS) patients will improve to a variable extent without treatment. However, many will be left with clinically detectable residual neurological impairment. In addition, substantial functional disability may accumulate after one or a series of recurrent relapses.

Several studies have shown that MS patients in acute clinical relapse who are treated with corticosteroids will recover more rapidly than similar patients who are not treated. In addition, corticosteroid treatment causes rapid improvement of abnormal cerebrospinal fluid (CSF) parameters, such as IgG synthesis rate and myelin basic protein (MBP) levels, as well as a reduction of MS plaque contrast enhancement seen on diagnostic imaging studies. Rapid clinical recovery, improvement of abnormal diagnostic imaging studies, and improvement of CSF parameters are compelling therapeutic results, and in current neurological practice, corticosteroids are commonly used as the primary treatment for acute MS relapses.

However, there has never been a study adequately designed to determine the ultimate effect of corticosteroid treatment in relapsing MS. It is not known if treatment reduces the incremental functional disability that may accumulate after multiple recurrent relapses in some patients or if treatment changes the number of relapses that ultimately occur.

II. CLINICAL STUDIES

Because of the potent anti-inflammatory and immunosuppressive properties of ACTH and corticosteroids, there has been sustained interest in their effects when used in MS patients ever since these medications first became available for clinical studies over 45 years ago. The earliest studies were encumbered by methodological deficiencies. These studies were inadequately randomized and controlled, and they frequently used small numbers of patients. Also, patients with relapsing and chronic forms of MS were frequently mixed indiscriminately. The results of these studies were conflicting and unconvincing.

In the first randomized, placebo-controlled study in 1961 (1), MS patients treated with a 3-week tapering course of intramuscular ACTH within 14 days of an acute relapse improved significantly more frequently than well-matched placebo-treated control patients. Ten years later, the results of this study were confirmed in a large multicenter trial in which MS patients, treated with a 2-week tapering course of intramuscular ACTH within 8 weeks of an acute relapse, showed significantly more improvement during treatment than placebo-treated, well-matched, randomized control patients (2). After this study, a 2-week course of ACTH became an accepted therapy for acute exacerbations of MS.

During this period, there were several reports of beneficial effects of very high dose pulsed intravenous methylprednisolone therapy in patients with acute renal transplant rejections (3,4). Consequently, very high dose intravenous methylprednisolone therapy was attempted in MS patients in acute relapse (5). In several uncontrolled trials, this treatment was associated with rapid improvement in a high proportion of MS patients in acute relapse (6–8). These open trials were soon followed by several controlled studies. In two such studies, MS patients in acute relapse for less than 8 weeks improved more frequently when treated with short courses of high doses of intravenous methylprednisolone when compared with randomized, placebo-treated control patients (9,10).

In two further randomized studies, intravenous methylprednisolone was directly compared with ACTH (11,12). In both studies, MS patients in acute relapse who were treated with courses of high-dose intravenous methylprednisolone improved more rapidly than randomized ACTH-treated patients.

The results of these studies indicate that MS patients in acute relapse improve more rapidly when treated with short-term courses of high-dose corticosteroid or ACTH therapy when compared with placebo treated controls. The results further indicate that the onset of improvement is more rapid with high dose corticosteroid treatment compared with ACTH. The rapid onset of improvement with high-dose corticosteroid treatment will be especially beneficial to patients with severe and rapidly progressive exacerbations. All of these studies have evaluated patients only for short-term periods of follow-up and few studies have evaluated the effect of brief courses of corticosteroid treatment on the long-term course of MS.

In a recent prospective, randomized, partially blinded multicenter trial, 457 patients with new-onset, acute, unilateral, monosymptomatic optic neuritis were treated within 8 days of clinical onset (13). Visual function improved more rapidly in patients treated with IV methylprednisolone (250 mg q6h for 3 days, followed by 11 days of oral prednisone, 1 mg/kg in a single morning dose) when compared with patients treated with 14 days of oral prednisone (1 mg/kg) or oral placebo. At 6 months follow-up, visual fields, contrast sensitivity, and color vision remained slightly better in the IV methylprednisolone group. The most convincing advantage of IV methylprednisolone (percentage of patients with normal vision at 6 months) was seen in patients who had visual acuity of 20/200 or worse at the start of therapy.

After excluding patients with known MS, the remaining 389 patients were followed for 2 to 4 years. Definite MS developed in 7.5% of the IV methylprednisolone group, 14% of the oral prednisone group and 16.7% of the oral placebo group (14). Benefit was most apparent in patients with abnormal brain magnetic resonance imaging (MRI) scans at entry. The beneficial effect was lessened after 2 years of follow-up. The results of this study provide evidence that a brief course of IV methylprednisolone therapy may have a long-term effect on the evolution of MS.

These findings have been viewed with caution because the physiological effects of corticosteroids are not known to be prolonged. It is possible that pulsed corticosteroid therapy introduced during a critical phase of an immune reaction may have effects that persist long after observable physiological effects.

III. EFFECT OF CORTICOSTEROIDS ON DIAGNOSTIC IMAGING

Contrast enhancement of MS plaques is seen on computed tomography (CT) scans in approximately 60% of patients who are in acute exacerbation and in pathological studies is associated with an alteration of the blood brain barrier (BBB) within regions of inflammatory demyelination. Intravenous methylprednisolone (1 to 1.5 g) substantially reduces the enhancement of MS lesions within a period as brief as 8 h after treatment (15). Oral maintenance treatment with high dose (60 to 120 mg/day) prednisone also substantially reduces the enhancement of MS plaques, whereas lower doses are less effective, especially if taken on alternate days (16).

These findings have been corroborated by more recent studies using magnetic resonance imaging (MRI) scans with gadolinium enhancement. In one study with IV methylprednisolone (1 g/day for 3 days) in 10 patients, plaque enhancement was attenuated in 96% of the lesions during treatment. However, many plaques reenhanced within a few days after stopping therapy (17). In another study with IV methylprednisolone (1 g/day for 1 to 4 days), repeat MRI scans performed within 1 to 4 days after treatment showed complete or substantial suppression of enhancement of all the lesions in seven patients treated (18). In a further study with IV methylprednisolone (1 g/day for 10 days) 80% of enhancing plaques lost enhancement on repeat scans performed 2.6 +/- 2.5 days after treatment in 12 patients (19). However, in all of these studies, all of the plaques that ceased to enhance remained visible on nonenhaced MR images.

If the passage of immunocompetent cells and serum factors into brain tissue is an obligatory step in the pathogenesis of MS lesions, then early and rapid normalization of the BBB by corticosteroids could be of critical importance in attenuating demyelination.

IV. EFFECT OF CORTICOSTEROIDS ON CEREBROSPINAL FLUID
IMMUNOLOGICAL PROFILE

A. Immunoglobulin G

De novo synthesis of IgG within the CNS occurs in over 90% of patients with clinically definite MS and most have elevated levels of CSF IgG. Treatment with methylprednisolone, dexamethasone, or prednisone causes a significant reduction in the CSF IgG synthesis rate that may persist after treatment is discontinued, although a rebound increase in IgG synthesis rate has been noted with prolonged follow-up in some patients (10,20–22). In general, high-dose IV treatment has been more effective than low-dose oral therapy in lowering abnormal IgG levels. Intravenous methylprednisolone causes the most rapid fall in IgG synthesis rate. In one report, this treatment (15 mg/kg/day) caused the IgG synthesis rate to become normal or nearly normal in all five patients with acute MS who had measurements taken within 3 to 6 days from the onset of treatment (10). In another study, treatment with methylprednisolone (2 g/day IV) brought patients' CSF IgG synthesis rates to the near normal range after 10 days of treatment, whereas infusion of smaller amounts of methylprednisolone (160 mg/day IV for 10 days) caused a less dramatic 40% fall in CSF IgG during acute relapse (22).

B. Myelin Basic Protein

CSF levels of MBP are transiently increased in 90% of patients during acute exacerbations. Treatment with IV methylprednisolone (either 160 mg or 2 g daily for 10 days) significantly reduced CSF MBP levels in 40 patients treated during an acute exacerbation (22). In addition, the level of CSF antibody to MBP was also significantly reduced by treatment with IV methylprednisolone (22). In another study, 40 patients with relapsing progressive or chronic progressive MS were treated with prednisone (total of 3940 mg administered over 54 days starting at 200 mg daily) (23). A significant reduction in CSF anti-MBP antibodies was reported. In 30% of patients in this series, circulating immune complexes were also found in the CSF. As with MBP and anti-MBP antibodies, the level of immune complexes in CSF was also significantly reduced by high-dose prednisone treatment. In a further study, the number of MR-enhancing plaques correlated significantly with the CSF MBP level in 16 relapsing MS patients. After treatment with IV methylprednisolone (1 g/day for 10 days), there was a significant reduction in the number of MR-enhancing lesions, intrathecal IgG synthesis rate, and CSF MBP levels (24).

C. Oligoclonal Bands

Oligoclonal IgG bands are a characteristic finding in the CSF and are thought to remain relatively constant in individual MS patients throughout the duration of the disease. In two studies, these bands have been noted to disappear in some MS patients in association with reduction of the IgG synthesis rate after treatment with methylprednisalone pulses (1 g/day IV) (10,20).

D. Cytokines

The mechanisms by which corticosteroids normalize CSF parameters of immune activation and inflammation are unknown. A variety of cytokines, including interleukin-1 and 2 (IL-1, IL-2), tumor necrosis factor (TNF), and interferon gamma have been found within MS plaques. In addition, TNF, IL-1, and IL-2 have been found in the CSF of MS patients. Cytokines may generate focal brain edema and increase the entry of soluble immunocompetent mediators by opening the BBB, increase the traffic of lymphocytes by upregulating endothelial adhesion molecules, activate lymphocytes, and upregulate MHC expression. Of particular note, TNF induces injury to oligodendrocytes in a time and concentration dependent manner (25).

Many of the cytokine genes have a glucocorticoid response element in their regulatory region that binds the heterodimeric complex formed by corticosteroids and the intracellular glucocorticoid receptor protein. Corticosteroids inhibit the expression of the genes for the cytokines IL-1, IL-2, IL-6, TNF, and interferon gamma and decrease the production of these cytokines by leukocytes (26). These mechanisms of corticosteroid activity provide a plausible basis for the normalization of CSF parameters associated with corticosteroid therapy in MS patients.

E. Summary

In summary, all of these studies indicate that corticosteroid treatment will normalize or significantly improve abnormal CSF parameters such as IgG synthesis rate, MBP, antibodies to MBP, and circulating immune complexes in patients with MS. However the most rapid improvement in abnormal CSF IgG synthesis rate has been reported with high-dose IV corticosteroid therapy. The improvement of all these pathological findings in MS could be a nonspecific effect of corticosteroid treatment, because a cause-effect relation between normalized laboratory values and clinical improvement has never been established. However, taken together, the rapid and simultaneous improvement of so many laboratory abnormalities is highly consistent with the rapid and favorable clinical outcome observed in relapsing MS patients treated with high doses of corticosteroids.

V. CORTICOSTEROID DOSAGE

There are no exact experimental models of most inflammatory diseases of putative autoimmune mediated etiology including MS; therefore clinical methods of corticosteroid administration have been developed empirically by clinical trials in patients with these disorders.

The anti-inflammatory and immunosuppressive actions of corticosteroids are not at maximum potency at physiological concentrations. To assure maximum anti-inflammatory and immunosuppressive effects during the acute phase of inflammatory, immune-mediated diseases, initial daily high-dose supraphysiologic corticosteroid treatment is generally recommended. For example, transplant recipient patients may develop acute transplant rejection crises while receiving low-dose corticosteroid maintenance therapy. These rejection crises are frequently treated with favorable results with intravenous corticosteroids in high doses (10 to 15 mg/kg/day methylprednisolone or equivalents) (4).

In MS patients, corticosteroids have been used in a variety of dosage schedules to treat patients during relapsing phases of illness. Rapid clinical improvement has been seen in MS patients in acute relapse who have been treated with starting doses of intravenous methylprednisolone ranging from 250 mg daily to 20 mg/kg daily for 2 to 7 days, followed by abrupt withdrawal or tapering doses (5–12). Methylprednisolone 1g IV slowly over 1 to 4 h daily for 3 to 5 days is a commonly prescribed regimen.

In addition, in MS patients, high doses of corticosteroids have been more effective than lower doses in normalizing abnormal CSF parameters and also in normalizing the BBB dysfunction seen in MS plaques on contrast MRI and CT scans (15–24).

In situations in which IV access is a problem, oral methylprednisolone in doses as high as 500 mg have been clinically effective and well tolerated (27).

With regard to ACTH, further studies in MS and other patients have shown that the cortisol response to ACTH injection is not consistently reproducible, may not be prompt, may be markedly variable between individual patients and even within the same patient from day to day, and may never reach the range generally recommended for treatment of inflammatory autoimmune diseases (28–31). Notably, ACTH is not currently used as the preferred treatment for any diseases of presumed autoimmune etiology.

VI. DURATION OF TREATMENT

By definition, MS relapses are transient; however, the average relapse duration has never been established. This is important, because if relapses are prolonged in some patients, then short courses of coticosteroid treatment may not be sufficient.

There are several lines of evidence indicating that MS relapses are prolonged in a proportion of patients, including patients who manifest early improvement during corticosteroid treatment. It should be noted that many clinical studies have been designed to administer high doses of ACTH or corticosteroids for short periods, generally 3 days to 2 weeks, followed by rather rapid or abrupt withdrawal. From the earliest clinical studies, it has been observed repeatedly that after short courses of ACTH or corticosteroid treatment, even when used in high doses, a proportion of relapsing MS patients regress clinically as treatment is withdrawn, despite initial favorable response during treatment.

Radiological studies corroborate these clinical observations concerning the duration of MS relapses. In a study of MS patients during clinical relapse, CT-enhancing lesions were found in 60% of patients. In patients with multiple enhancing lesions, the average interval between the clinical onset of relapses and the performance of the CT scans was 5.6 weeks, with a range of 2 to 16 weeks (16). Both CT and MRI contrast-enhancing lesions in MS patients have been correlated with regions of acute inflammatory demyelination on pathological studies. The finding of enhancing lesions 2 to 16 weeks after the clinical onset of relapses implies that, in a proportion of patients, the duration of disease activity during a relapse may be prolonged. In further studies, using serial contrast-enhancing MRI scans in relapsing MS patients, enhancement persisted beyond 4 weeks in approximately 20 to 30% of lesions (32–34). In addition, CT and MRI scan enhancement of MS plaques may be diminished or eliminated by high-dose corticosteroid treatment; however, as corticosteroids are withdrawn, CT and MRI scan enhancement may recur in the same patients (15,17). Similarly, in acutely relapsing MS patients, increased CSF IgG synthesis rate may be diminished or normalized by high-dose corticosteroid treatment; however, an increased CSF IgG synthesis rate may recur as corticosteroids are withdrawn from the same patients (10).

Patients in acute MS relapse must be monitored closely during corticosteroid withdrawal. The optimal rate of corticosteroid withdrawal must be determined for each individual patient by clinical trial. Patients who regress clinically during corticosteroid withdrawal should be treated with corticosteroids in doses that effectively maintain clinical improvement during tapered withdrawal until a stable course can be sustained without corticosteroids.

VII. COMPLICATIONS

The metabolic actions, pharmacology, side effects, and complications of corticosteroid therapy are well known and have been thoroughly reviewed elsewhere (35,36). In all of the reported studies of short-term, high-dose corticosteroid treatment of MS patients, serious side effects have seldom been observed (37). However, in these studies, most patients have received only one, two, or three short courses of high-dose treatment; the incidence of serious long-term complications of multiple courses of high-dose corticosteroid treatment in MS patients has not been well documented. If a protracted course of tapering of oral corticosteroids is required, then an increased incidence of complications may be expected. Many of the serious complications of corticosteroid therapy—such as hypertension, diabetes mellitus, infections, osteoporosis, atherosclerosis, hypokalemia, and peptic ulcers—are potentially treatable. Many of these complications are also, to a certain extent, preventable if prudent prophylactic measures such as restricted caloric and salt intake, calcium and vitamin D supplements, biphosphonates or calcitonin, antacids and inhibitors of gastric acid secretion, potassium supplements, and cholesterol-lowering drugs are initiated early in the course of treatment when indicated. The most effective way to prevent complications is to make the course of corticosteroid treatment as brief as possible, depending on the patient's response to treatment and tolerance of side effects and corticosteroid withdrawal.

VIII. SUMMARY

Several studies have demonstrated that short-course, high-dose corticosteroid treatment improves the rate of recovery from acute MS exacerbations. Until more effective and specific treatments are available, it is reasonable to treat acute exacerbations of MS with high-dose corticosteroids in patients who can tolerate the side effects. The most rapid improvements in clinical condition, diagnostic imaging, and CSF parameters have been observed with very high dose intravenous corticosteroid therapy (10 to 20 mg/kg/day of methylprednisolone for 3 to 5 days being a common regimen). This form of therapy would be most advantageous for patients with severe and rapidly progressive exacerbations.

Although extremely short, intensive courses of high-dose corticosteroid treatment are ideal, a period of tapered treatment with oral corticosteroids may be required following the high-dose treatment. Close clinical monitoring is required during the course of tapering and therapy must be individualized. Ultimately, the duration of treatment depends on the patient's response to treatment and tolerance of corticosteroid withdrawal as well as the occurrence of significant complications of therapy.

REFERENCES

1. Miller H, Newell DJ, Ridley A. Multiple sclerosis: Treatment of acute exacerbations with corticotrophin (ACTH). Lancet 1961; 2:1120–1122.
2. Rose AS, Kuzma JW, Kurtzke JF, et al. Cooperative study in the evaluation of therapy in multiple sclerosis: ACTH vs. placebo. Final report. Neurology 1970; 20 (suppl):1–159.
3. Coburg AJ, Gray SH, Katz FH, Penn I, Halgrimson C, Starzl TE. Disappearance rates and immunosuppression of intermittent intravenously administered prednisolone in rabbits and human beings. Surg Gynecol Obstet 1970; 131:933–942.
4. Gray D, Shepherd H, Daar A, Oliver DO, Morris PJ. Oral versus intravenous high dose steroid treatment of renal allograft rejection. Lancet 1978; 1:117–118.
5. Dowling PC, Bosch VV, Cook SD. Possible beneficial effect of high dose intravenous steroid therapy in acute demyelinating disease and transverse myelitis. Neurology 1980; 30:33–36.
6. Buckley C, Kennard C, Swash M. Treatment of acute exacerbations of multiple sclerosis with intravenous methylprednisolone. J Neurol Neurosurg Psychiatry 1982; 45:179–181.
7. Goas JY, Marion JL, Missoum A. High dose intravenous methylprednisolone in acute exacerbations of multiple sclerosis. J Neurol Neurosurg Psychiatry 1983; 46:99.

8. Newman PK, Saunders M, Tilley PJ. Methylprednisolone therapy in multiple sclerosis. J Neurol Neurosurg Psychiatry 1983; 46:941–942.

9. Milligan NM, Newcombe R, Compston DAS. A double blind controlled trial of high dose methylprednisolone in patients with multiple sclerosis: 1. Clinical effects. J Neurol Neurosurg Psychiatry 1987; 50:511–516.

10. Durelli L, Cocito D, Riccio A, et al. High dose intravenous methylprednisolone in the treatment of multiple sclerosis: Clinical immunologic correlation. Neurology 1986; 36:238–243.

11. Abbruzzese G, Gandolfo C, Loeb C. Bolus methylprednisolone versus ACTH in the treatment of multiple sclerosis. Ital J Neurol Sci 1983; 2:169–172.

12. Barnes MP, Bateman DE, Cleland PG, et al. Intravenous methylprednisolone for multiple sclerosis in relapse. J Neurol Neurosurg Psychiatry 1985; 48:157–159.

13. Beck R, Cleary P, Anderson M, et al. A randomized, controlled trial of corticosteroids in the treatment of acute optic neuritis. N Engl J Med 1992; 326:581–588.

14. Beck R, Cleary P, Trobe S, et al. The effect of corticosteroids for acute optic neuritis on the subsequent development of multiple sclerosis. N Engl J Med 1993; 329:1764–1769.

15. Troiano R, Hafstein M, Ruderman M, et al. Effect of high dose intravenous steroid administration on contrast enhancing computed tomographic scan lesions in multiple sclerosis. Ann Neurol 1984; 15:257–263.

16. Troiano R, Hafstein M, Zito G, et al. The effect of oral corticosteroid dosage on CT enhancing MS plaques. J Neurol Sci 1985; 70:67–72.

17. Miller D, Thompson A, Morrissey S, et al. High dose steroids in acute relapses of multiple sclerosis: MRI evidence for a possible mechanism of therapeutic effect. J Neurol Neurosurg Psychiatry 1992; 55:450–453.

18. Burnham T, Wright R, Dreisbach T, Murray R. The effect of high dose steroids on MRI gadolinium enhancement in acute demyelinating lesions. Neurology 1991; 41:1349–1354.

19. Barkhof F, Hommes O, Scheltens P, Valk T. Quantitative MRI changes in gadolinium-DTPH enhancement after high-dose intravenous methylprednisolone in multiple sclerosis. Neurology 1991; 41:1219–1222.

20. Trotter JL, Garvey WF. Prolonged effects of large dose methylprednisolone infusion in multiple sclerosis. Neurology 1980; 30:702–708.

21. Tourtellotte WW, Baumhefner RW, Porvin AR, et al. Multiple sclerosis de novo CNS IgG synthesis: Effect of ACTH and corticosteroids. Neurology 1980; 30:1155–1162.

22. Warren KG, Catz I, Verona MJ, Carroll DJ. Effect of methylprednisolone on CSF IgG parameters, myelin basic protein and anti-myelin basic protein in multiple sclerosis exacerbations. Can J Neurol Sci 1986; 13:25–30.

23. Wajgt A, Gorny M, Jenek R. The influence of high dose prednisone medication on autoantibody specific activity and on circulating immune complex level in cerebrospinal fluid of multiple sclerosis patients. Acta Neurol Scand 1983; 68:378–385.

24. Barkhof F, Frequin S, Hommes O, et al. A correlative triad of gadolinium-DTPA MRI, EDSS and CSF-MBP in relapsing multiple sclerosis patients treated with high dose intravenous methylprednisolone. Neurology 1992; 42:63–67.

25. Selmas K, Raine C, Farooq M, Norton W, Brosnan C. Cytokine cytotoxicity against oligodendrocytes, apoptosis induced by lymphotoxin. J Immunol 1991; 147:1522–1529.

26. Suthanthiran M, Strom T. Renal transplantation. N Engl J Med 1994; 331:365–375.

27. Sellebjerg F, Fredericksen JL, Nielson PM, Olesen J. Double blind, randomized, placebo controlled study of oral, high dose methylprednisolone in attacks of MS. Neurology 1998; 51:529–534.

28. Renold A, Jenkins D, Forsham PH, Thorn GW. The use of intravenous ACTH: A study in quantitative adrenocortical stimulation. J Clin Endocrinol Metab 1952; 12:763–797.

29. Alexander L, Cass LJ. The present status of ACTH therapy in multiple sclerosis. Ann Intern Med 1963; 58:454–471.

30. Maida E, Summer K. Serum cortisol levels in multiple sclerosis patients during ACTH treatment. J Neurol 1979; 220:143–148.

31. Snyder BD, Lakatua DJ, Doe RP. ACTH induced cortisol production in multiple sclerosis. Ann Neurol 1981; 10:388–389.

32. Miller DH, Rudge P, Johnson G, et al. Serial gadolinium enhanced magnetic resonance imaging in multiple sclerosis. Brain 1988; 111:927–939.

33. Bastianello S, Pozzilli C, Bernardi S, et al. Serial study of gadolinium-DTPA MRI enhancement in multiple sclerosis. Neurology 1990; 40:591–595.

34. Harris TO, Frank JA, Patronas N, McFarlin DE, McFarland HF. Serial gadolinium enhanced magnetic resonance imaging scans in patients with early, relapsing remitting multiple sclerosis: Implications for clinical trials and natural history. Ann Neurol 1991; 29:548–555.

35. Katz P. Glucocorticosteroids in relation to inflammatory diseases. In: Bannett JC, Plum F. eds. Cecil Textbook of Medicine, 20th ed. Philadelphia: Saunders, 1996, pp 108–110.

36. Williams GH, Dluhy RG. Diseases of the adrenal cortex. In: Fauci AS, Braunwald E, Isselbacher KJ, Wilson JD, Martin JB, Kasper DL, Hauser SL, Longo DD, eds. Harrison's Principles of Internal Medicine, 14th ed. New York: McGraw Hill, 1998, pp 2035–2056.

37. Lyons PR, Newman PK, Saunders M. Methylprednisolone therapy in multiple sclerosis: A profile of adverse effects. J Neurol Neurosurg Psychiatry 1988; 51:285–287.

21

Interferon-β-1b: Prophylactic Therapy in Multiple Sclerosis

KENNETH P. JOHNSON and PETER A. CALABRESI

University of Maryland Medical Center, Baltimore, Maryland

I. INTRODUCTION

Multiple sclerosis (MS) has intrigued, baffled, and challenged neurologists since it was first described by Charcot. Its typically episodic, relapsing, remitting, but eventually progressive clinical course initially suggested an infectious (in particular, viral) etiology. However, a specific virus has never been convincingly related to MS, despite a diligent and ongoing search for a causative agent. Although the etiology of MS is still not conclusively established, the preponderance of evidence suggests that it is an immune-mediated disease characterized by localization of several types of inflammatory cell types in MS lesions with altered levels of inflammatory cytokines in the serum, cerebrospinal fluid, and central nervous system (CNS) (1,2).

For most of the twentieth century treatment of patients with MS was limited primarily to the management of associated symptoms and, subsequently, to the use of corticosteroids during relapses. The second half of the century saw an accelerating search for immunosuppressive or immunomodulating therapies. Although clinical studies with immunosuppressive agents began in the 1970s and continued into the 1990s, the focus of interest by this time had shifted to immunomodulating agents, particularly the interferons (IFNs) and glatiramer acetate.

The IFNs are a family of cytokines that possess antiviral, antiproliferative, and immunomodulating properties. The multiple actions of the IFNs suggested that they may be beneficial in controlling the MS disease process. Although the initial premise for studying the therapeutic use of IFNs in MS was as an antiviral agent, the focus subsequently shifted to their immunomodulating actions. These natural human proteins are divided into 2 groups: type 1, (which includes IFN-α and IFN-β) and type 2 (consisting only of IFN-γ). All three human IFNs have been cloned by recombinant DNA technology, and the resulting preparations have all been tested in clinical trials in patients with MS using various routes of administration, at widely varying doses, and during different stages of MS (3,4). Clinical studies began in the late 1970s when California investigators began testing natural IFN-α administered subcutaneously (SC) (5,6) and New York investigators explored the use of natural IFN-β administered intrathecally (5,7). Although reductions in exacerbation rates were noted with the intrathecal route of administration, this technique was later abandoned as too toxic. In 1986 Panitch et al. observed that IFN-γ markedly worsened MS, which ended further testing of type 2 IFN as a therapeutic agent (8). However, this later prompted studies that explored the potential pathophysiological roles of IFN-γ in MS.

The approval of IFN-β-1b (Betaseron) by the U.S. Food and Drug Administration in the summer of 1993 marked a turning point in the treatment of MS. IFN-β-1b was the first IFN to be approved for the treatment of MS and has now been prescribed for more than 68,000 patients with MS in the United States. The approval of IFN-β-1b for RR MS was based on the results of a double-blind, placebo-controlled, multicenter study which showed that it reduced the exacerbation rate in patients with RR MS and decreased MS activity in the brain based on magnetic resonance imaging (MRI) (9,10). As a result of this pivotal study, the Quality Standards Subcommittee of the American Academy of Neurology issued a practice advisory in which they broadened their recommendations for the use of IFN-β-1b to include any patient with MS who experienced "true" exacerbations (11). Published in 1994, these revised guidelines made IFN-β-1b available to a wide range of patients with MS, including patients over the age of 50, those with SP MS associated with relapses, and nonambulatory patients with an Expanded Disability Status Seale (EDSS) score ≤6.0.

This chapter provides an in-depth review of the clinical and MRI experience with IFN-β-1b in patients with RR and SP MS, including a discussion of the proposed mechanisms of action of IFN-β in MS and the still controversial role of neutralizing antibodies in the treatment response.

II. PROPOSED MECHANISMS OF ACTION OF IFN-β IN MS

Despite more than a decade of clinical experience with IFN-β, its mechanisms of action in the treatment of MS remain unclear. Nonetheless, numerous studies now suggest that IFN-β has multiple biological activities that enable it to create an anti-inflammatory "milieu," both systemically and within the CNS. Table 1 lists the various immunomodulating effects attributed to IFN-β. By inhibiting lymphocyte proliferation, affecting antigen processing, modulating the production of proinflammatory cytokines, and reducing T-cell migration into the CNS, IFN-β appears to produce an overall reduction in immune reactivity.

A. Effects on Inflammatory Cell Activation, Proliferation, and Antigen Processing

Considerable evidence supports the hypothesis that MS is an immune-mediated disease and that IFN-β has multiple immunomodulating activities in this setting (12,13). Noronha

Table 1 Proposed Mechanisms of Action of IFN-β[a]

Inhibits or attenuates proliferation and activation of inflammatory cells, including T_H1
lymphocytes
Enhances T_H2 suppressor function
Downregulates IFN-γ and TNF-α production
Affects antigen presentation in systemic and CNS compartments
Shifts the overall "cytokine milieu" toward an anti-inflammatory environment
Reduces entry of leukocytes into the CNS through effects on adhesion molecules, chemokines,
and MMPs

---

[a] TNF indicates tumor necrosis factor; CNS, central nervous system; MMPs, matrix metalloproteinases.
Source: Ref. 13.

et al. found that IFN-β inhibited T-cell proliferation and reduced their production of IFN-γ, a cytokine with multiple proinflammatory effects, including activation of monocytes and upregulation of adhesion molecules on endothelial cells (14).

IFN-β also may affect antigen presentation and processing, a critical event in the immune response. Two signals are necessary to fully activate T-cells: (a) the binding of accessory molecules on antigen-presenting cells (APCs) to appropriate T-cell ligands and (b) the binding of major histocompatibility complex (MHC) haplotypes on APCs to T-cell receptors. Since IFN-γ is known to promote MHC class 2 expression, IFN-β could theoretically inhibit antigen presentation by counteracting the effects of IFN-γ. However, the available data have not been consistently positive (13,15). It has also been postulated that IFN-β may indirectly affect antigen presentation by inhibiting the expression of accessory molecules that serve as the costimulatory signals for T-cell activation. One study reported that IFN-β-1b reversed the increased expression of one such accessory molecule, B7–1 (CD80), on B lymphocytes from patients with MS as compared with control subjects [16].

B. Effects on T_H1 and T_H2 Cytokine Production

CD4$^+$ T lymphocytes can be divided into T_H1 and T_H2 populations, which are associated with distinct but interacting, cytokine profiles (17). The T_H1 subset secretes proinflammatory cytokines, including interleukin (IL)-2, tumor necrosis factor (TNF)-β, and IFN-γ. The T_H2 subset produces anti-inflammatory cytokines, including IL-4, IL-5, IL-6, IL-10, and IL-13. It has been hypothesized that the balance between the T_H1 and T_H2 cytokine phenotypes may influence disease activity in patients with MS. Although somewhat conflicting, the results of recent studies suggest that IFN-β causes a shift of the cytokine profile toward the T_H2-like anti-inflammatory phenotype (18–23).

C. Effects on Transmigration of T Cells Across the Blood-Brain Barrier

The infiltration of T cells across the blood-brain barrier (BBB) and into the CNS is considered to be an important event in the pathogenesis of MS. This transmigration of leukocytes across the vascular endothelium is a sequential and multistepped process (24). First, vascular or leukocyte adhesion molecules are expressed or upregulated, resulting in an increase in adhesive interaction and the "roll and capture" of leukocytes. The parenchymal expression of chemotactic cytokines (chemokines) is the second factor involved in transmigration. These chemokines arrest lymphocyte rolling and provide direction to their migration. The third governing factor in the transmigration process is the degradation of the endothelial basement membrane by matrix metalloproteinases (MMPs) produced by leukocytes, which allows them to intravasate into the CNS parenchyma.

Available data suggest that IFN-β-1b attenuates the entry of T cells at the level of the BBB into the CNS by altering the expression or function of adhesion molecules and/or by inhibition of MMP production (13). The results of several studies suggest that IFN-β-1b may downregulate the expression of adhesion molecules. Calabresi et al. found increased levels of soluble VCAM-1 in the sera of patients with MS who were treated with IFN-β, and these elevations correlated with decreases in gadolinium-enhanced MRI activity (25). Since soluble VCAM-1 is produced by cleavage of its tissue-bound form, such elevations may reflect a decrease in endothelial VCAM-1 expression in IFN-β-1b–treated patients. Corsini et al. found that monocytes or lymphocytes obtained from patients with MS who were treated with IFN-β-1b for 6 months exhibited less adherence to endothelial cells in vitro when compared with monocytes or lymphocytes obtained from the same patients prior to treatment (26). Trojano et al. followed 36 patients with MS during 24 months of treatment with IFN-β-1b by periodic assessment of serum levels of soluble ICAM-1 and MMP-9, MRI scans (enhanced and T2), and changes in the integrated area under the Kurtzke Expanded Disability Status Scale (EDSS) time curve (ΔEDSS AUC) (27). They found that IFN-β-1b increased soluble ICAM-1 levels and reduced MMP-9 levels and that these changes correlated with significant decreases in enhanced MRI lesions and ΔEDSS AUC.

III. CLINICAL STUDIES OF IFN-β-1b IN MS

A. Pilot Study

In 1986 a pilot study was conducted at three sites in the United States to determine the optimal dose of recombinant human IFN-β-1b to use in the treatment of patients with RR MS (28). A total of 31 ambulatory patients with RR MS were randomized to receive placebo or one of four doses of IFN-β-1b [0.8, 4, 8, or 16 million international units (MIU)] given by SC injection every other day for 6 months. A relatively clear dose response was apparent at 6 months, at which time the annualized exacerbation rate was 1.8 in the placebo group as compared with 0.9 in the IFN-β-1b 8-MIU group and 0.0 in the IFN-β-1b 16-MIU group. Although patients receiving the highest dose of IFN-β-1b (16 MIU) had the greatest reduction in the relapse rate, the incidence of adverse effects, particularly flu-like reactions, was considered too high to be clinically acceptable. As a result, all patients were switched to IFN-β-1b 8 MIU at the end of 6 months of treatment. However, it should be noted that in this early trial treatment with all regimens was initiated at full doses, in contrast to the common current practice of gradual dose escalation during the first few months of therapy.

B. Phase 3 Trial in Patients with Relapsing-Remitting MS

The approval of IFN-β-1b for use in the treatment of MS was based on the results of a 2-year, multicenter, double-blind, placebo-controlled clinical study conducted at 11 sites in Canada and the United States in which two doses of IFN-β-1b were tested against placebo (9). Patients were eligible for study entry if they were between 18 and 50 years of age, had active RR disease (≥2 attacks in the past 2 years), were ambulatory, and had an EDSS score ≤5.5.

A total of 372 patients were randomized to one of three treatment groups: (a) IFN-β-1b 1.6 MIU (125 patients); (b) IFN-β-1b 8 MIU (124 patients); or (c) placebo (123 patients). All treatments were injected SC every other day. This study was initially designed to last 2 years but was ultimately extended for up to 5 years to provide long-term efficacy data (29). The primary efficacy endpoints were the annual exacerbation rate and the proportion of exacerbation-free patients. In addition, annual nonenhanced magnetic resonance imaging (MRI) scans were performed on all patients to measure changes in lesion size and number (i.e., disease burden). A subset of 52 patients at one center underwent frequent MRIs (1 every 6 weeks) (10). Subsequent trials in patients with MS have used gadolinium-enhanced scans in addition to T2-weighted MRIs, but the former technology was not widely available at the time of study initiation. Other secondary endpoints included exacerbation severity, exacerbation duration, and disability. Progression of disability was assessed by time to worsening by ≥1 point on the EDSS and mean change in confirmed EDSS from baseline.

The results at the end of 2 years showed that high-dose IFN-β-1b reduced the exacerbation rate by about 34%, a statistically significant ($p = 0.0001$) difference as compared with placebo. In addition, significantly ($p = 0.007$) more patients in the high-dose IFN-β-1b group than in the placebo group remained exacerbation-free (31% versus 16%, respectively). The median time to first exacerbation was also longer in the high-dose IFN-β-1b group than in the placebo group (9.8 versus 5.1 months, respectively). Moderate and severe exacerbations were significantly ($p = 0.002$) lower in the high-dose IFN-β-1b group as compared with the placebo group, which was reflected in a significant ($p = 0.046$) reduction in the number of hospitalizations in the high-dose IFN-β-1b group. These positive clinical results were supported by both the annual and "frequent" MRI findings, which showed significant reductions in disease activity in the high-dose IFN-β-1b group as compared with the placebo group based on new, recurrent, and enlarging lesions. As in the pilot study, this trial also demonstrated a strong dose effect in that the 8-MIU dose produced a significantly superior treatment effect on all clinical and MRI measures.

Among the patients who remained in the study for up to 5 years, the annual exacerbation rates continued to decline in all three treatment groups. The decrease in exacerbation rates in the high-dose IFN-β-1b group as compared with the placebo group was maintained at approximately 30% per year. However, the differences were not statistically significant beyond 2 years (Fig. 1) (29). There are two possible explanations for this observation. First, the study was statistically powered to be a 2-year trial and did not take into account the possibility that some patients might continue on treatment for 5 years. Second, too few patients may have remained in the study beyond 2 years to discern a clear treatment effect.

Over the course of the study, fewer patients in the high-dose IFN-β-1b group (35%) than in the placebo group (46%) satisfied the criterion for progression of disability (≥1 point increase on the EDSS), but this difference was not statistically significant. Again, this could have been because the study was not designed or powered to detect a significant difference in this endpoint. However, a clear trend is apparent by the continuing separation of the Kaplan-Meier curves.

The clinical data from patients remaining in the extension phase of the study were once again supported by the MRI findings from 217 patients who had a year 4 or 5 scan (29). Significant increases in lesion burden of the placebo group compared to the high-dose

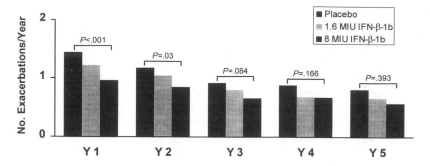

Figure 1 Annual exacerbation rates by year of study. (From Ref. 29.)

IFN-β-1b group were seen up until year 5 (Fig. 2). There was no significant progression of lesion burden in the high-dose IFN-β-1b group when compared with baseline at any year. In contrast, there was a highly significant (*p* ranging from 0.003 to 0.0001) increase in lesion area in the placebo group at each interval. The mean percentage increase in lesion burden in the placebo group was approximately three times greater than that of either IFN-β-1b group.

C. European Trial of IFN-β-1b in Patients with Secondary-Progressive MS

One of the major concerns in treating patients with MS is that the vast majority of patients with RR disease ultimately develop SP disease. Once this progression begins to occur, neurological deficits and related disability develop at a more rapid rate. Therefore a multicenter, double-blind, placebo-controlled study was conducted in Europe to evaluate the efficacy and safety of IFN-β-1b 8 MIU SC every other day in patients with SP MS (30). This dose was chosen on the basis of the significantly superior results of the higher dose in the pivotal trial in patients with RR MS (9). At the time of its inception, this was the largest clinical trial of its kind ever conducted in patients with MS. The study partici-

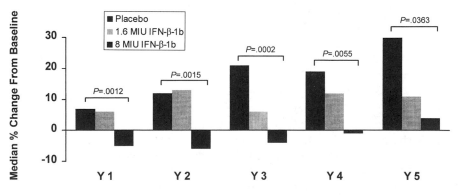

Figure 2 Change from baseline in cumulative MRI lesion burden in 217 patients having at least a year 4 annual scan. (From Ref. 29.)

pants were required to be between the ages of 18 and 55 years, have EDSS scores between 3.0 and 6.5 inclusive, and have a definite diagnosis of MS based on clinical or laboratory findings. SP MS was defined as a sustained (lasting ≥6 months) period of deterioration, independent of relapses, following a period of RR MS. Patients had to have at least two relapses or a ≥1 point increase on the EDSS documented in the 2 years prior to entering the study. The primary outcome measure in this study was time to confirmed disease progression based on a 1-point increase on the EDSS (which was sustained for at least 3 months) or a 0.5-point increase in patients whose baseline EDSS was ≥6.0. EDSS values obtained during relapses were not included in the analyses. Additional EDSS-related outcome variables included time to reach an EDSS score ≥7.0 (i.e., wheelchair-bound), proportion of patients who became wheelchair-bound, proportion of patients with confirmed progression, and endpoint EDSS. Relapse-related outcome variables included the annual relapse rate, time to first relapse, and percentage of patients with moderate or severe relapses.

Annual proton density/T2-weighted MRI scans were conducted in all patients to assess total lesion volume, as well as the number of new and enlarging lesions. In addition, a subgroup of patients (i.e., the ''frequent MRI'' group) underwent monthly gadolinium-enhanced T1-weighted and proton density/T2-weighted MRIs at months 1 through 6 and again at months 18 through 24 to determine disease activity based on new enhancing lesions and new or enlarging nonenhancing T2 lesions.

A total of 768 patients were screened at 32 centers in 12 countries in Europe. Not surprisingly, the patients enrolled in this trial were generally older and had more advanced disease than the patients with RR MS who participated in previous immunotherapy trials. Of the 718 patients randomized to treatment with either IFN-β-1b 8 MIU (360 patients) every other day or placebo (358 patients), 26 patients in the IFN-β-1b group and 31 patients in the placebo group withdrew prematurely and were lost to follow-up, while 64 patients in the IFN-β-1b group and 66 patients in the placebo group discontinued treatment early but were still included in the intent-to-treat analysis. Therefore, 270 patients in the IFN-β-1b group and 261 patients in the placebo group completed treatment and were followed up as planned. As described earlier, a cohort of 125 patients underwent frequent MRIs.

The two groups were similar with respect to their major demographic characteristics, except for a slight but not statistically significant preponderance of females in the placebo group. The patients' mean age at the time of study enrollment was 41 years; their mean duration of disease was slightly more than 13 years. The mean time since the first evidence of progressive deterioration was about 4 years, while the mean time since a diagnosis of SP MS was 2.15 years. Approximately 84% of the patients had mean EDSS scores ranging from 4.0 to 6.5 at baseline, indicating moderate to severe disability. Approximately 94% of the patients in this study completed 2 years of treatment, at which time a prospectively planned interim analysis of efficacy and safety was performed. Because of the highly significant difference in the primary endpoint, the study was terminated early—at 2 years instead of the planned 3 years—and all patients in the placebo group were offered continuing treatment with IFN-β-1b.

The results showed a highly significant ($p = 0.0008$) difference in the time to confirmed disease progression in the IFN-β-1b group as compared with the placebo group (Fig. 3). Approximately half of placebo-treated patients had confirmed progression, as compared with only about 39% of patients receiving IFN-β-1b. The delay in progression in the IFN-β-1b group was apparent within 9 months of treatment and was significantly

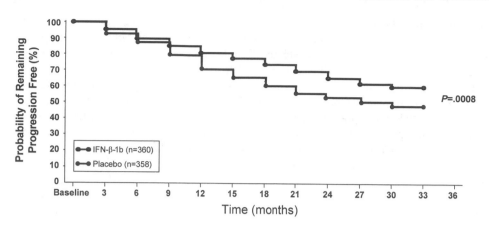

Figure 3   Life-table estimate of time to confirmed progression. (From Ref. 30.)

($p \leq .0031$) greater than that of the placebo group from month 10 onward. Overall, the proportion of patients who progressed over the entire study period was reduced by about 22% in the IFN-β-1b group as compared with the placebo group—once again, a statistically significant ($p = 0.0048$) difference between groups. The time to becoming wheel-chair-bound (i.e., reaching an EDSS score of 7.0) was also significantly ($p = 0.0133$) delayed in the IFN-β-1b group. Only 17% of patients in the IFN-β-1b group became severely disabled (i.e., wheelchair-bound) as compared with about 25% of patients in the placebo group, a statistically significant ($p = 0.0277$) difference between groups representing a reduction of 32%. The mean annual relapse rate was reduced by about 30% ($p = 0.002$), and the proportion of patients with moderate or severe relapses was also reduced ($p = 0.0083$). As was the case in the pivotal study in RR MS, IFN-β-1b significantly reduced MS-related steroid use ($p < 0.0001$) and the number of MS-related hospitalizations ($p = 0.0003$), two pharmacoeconomic endpoints of the study.

One of the questions that arose during the inception of this study was whether patients with SP MS who still had relapses might actually have RR MS. Since IFN-β-1b reduces the relapse rate and lesion burden in patients with RR MS, one of the goals of the study was to determine that the drug was also effective specifically in the population with SP disease. Therefore, the data were analyzed separately based on whether or not patients had relapses before or during the study. The proportion of patients who progressed during treatment with IFN-β-1b was similar, independent of whether or not the patients had "on-study" relapses (Fig. 4). A similar pattern emerged with regard to relapse activity during the 2 years prior to study entry. Namely, the proportion of patients with confirmed progression who had relapse activity before the study was virtually identical to that of patients who did not have any relapse activity.

There was also concern during the planning stages of the study that the positive effects of IFN-β-1b in terms of slowing the rate of disability might be correlated with the patient's baseline level of disability. In other words, it seemed plausible that patients with a low EDSS (e.g., relatively minimal disability) might benefit from treatment to a greater extent than those with a high EDSS (e.g., severe disability). However, the results showed a consistent treatment effect independent of the patient's baseline EDSS (Fig. 5).

As was the case in the RR MS trial, the MRI findings in patients with SP MS add strong support for the clinical efficacy of IFN-β-1b (31). There was a highly significant

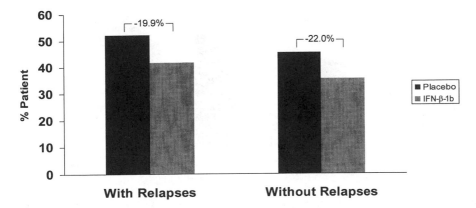

Figure 4 Relative reductions in confirmed progression, with and without relapse activity on study. (From Ref. 30.)

($p < 0.0001$) difference in the percent change in total annual lesion volume during years 1 through 3: the placebo group showed a 15% increase from baseline to last scan while the IFN-β-1b group showed a 2% reduction. There also was a highly significant ($p < 0.0001$) reduction in the number of new or enlarging lesions in the IFN-β-1b group at all annual time points as compared with baseline (Fig. 6).

Since previous studies had suggested that IFN-β-1b suppresses new lesion formation as early as 2 weeks after the onset of treatment, the investigators sought to determine whether this effect was sustained over time. The results from the ''frequent MRI'' subgroup showed a significant ($p = 0.0001$) reduction in the cumulative numbers of new (i.e., 65% mean decrease) and persistent (i.e., 67% mean decrease) active lesions in the IFN-β-1b group at months 1 through 6 as compared with the placebo group (Figs. 7 and 8). The significant treatment effects were apparent at every monthly time point and were already significant at the first month. These findings were equally dramatic during months 19 through 24, by which time there were approximately four times more new and persistently active lesions in the placebo group as compared with the IFN-β-1b group.

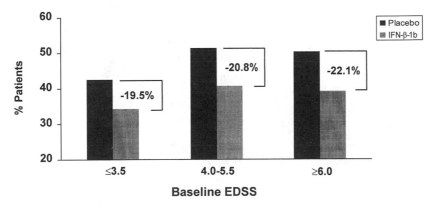

Figure 5 Relative reductions in confirmed progression by baseline Expanded Disability Status Scale score. (From Ref. 30.)

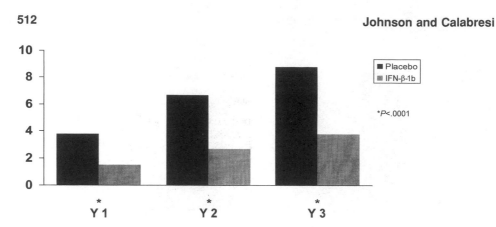

Figure 6   Cumulative number of active lesions (mean) from annual-MRI analysis during years 1 to 3. (From Ref. 31.)

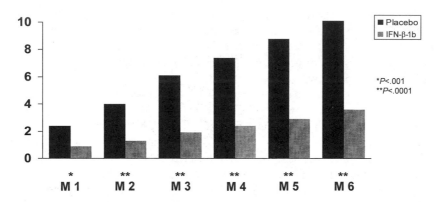

Figure 7   Cumulative number of newly active lesions (mean) in frequent-MRI subgroup: lesion activity during months 1 to 6. (From Ref. 31.)

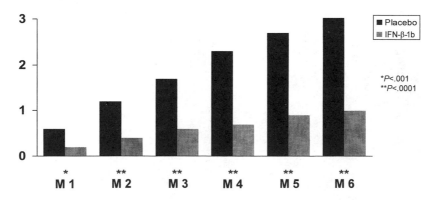

Figure 8   Cumulative number of persistently active lesions (mean) in frequent-MRI subgroup: lesion activity during months 1 to 6. (From Ref. 31.)

An additional large, multicenter, placebo-controlled trial of IFN-β-1b in patients with SP MS was initiated in the United States and Canada after the European trial began. The design of this North American study differed from that of the European trial primarily by the inclusion of three treatment arms: (a) placebo, (b) IFN-β-1b 8 MIU SC, and (c) IFN-β-1b dose adjusted for body size. The results of this trial were not available at the time of this publication.

D. Adverse Effects of IFN-β-1b

The adverse-effect profile of IFN-β-1b is consistent with that of all type 1 IFNs. The most common adverse effects associated with IFN-β-1b therapy are a flu-like syndrome (e.g., fever, chills, myalgia, malaise, and sweating) and injection-site reactions (e.g., erythema, inflammation, and pain). These adverse effects are generally manageable and usually abate after the first few months of treatment. The general rule for managing the adverse effects of IFN-βs is to start at a low (e.g., one-quarter or one-half) dose and titrate up gradually. If treatment-related adverse effects occur, concomitant drug therapy may be used for symptomatic relief. This, in turn, will enhance patient compliance. Patients tend to tolerate IFN-β-1b better when it is injected at bedtime. In rare cases the use of a drug holiday will permit patients to resume use of IFN-β-1b. The following recommendations are specific for the most common adverse effects associated with IFN-β-1b therapy.

Flu-like Symptoms

Flu-like symptoms are among the most common adverse effects of IFN-β therapy but typically occur within hours of starting therapy and dissipate within several months. The intensity of these and other treatment-related adverse effects may be correlated with female gender and a low body mass (32). However, there is no evidence of any age-related toxicity with IFN-β, and older patients appear to tolerate flu-like symptoms better than younger patients.

Various strategies can be used to lessen the severity and duration of flu-like symptoms. As noted earlier, one recommendation is to administer IFN-β-1b at bedtime and to increase the dose gradually, starting with half a dose given for 4 to 6 weeks. Patients should also be encouraged to premedicate with a nonsteroidal anti-inflammatory agent, acetaminophen, or even a low-dose oral steroid (e.g., oral prednisone 10 mg/day), although some authorities in the field recommend ibuprofen over acetylsalicylic acid or acetaminophen (33). A recent study designed to evaluate the effects of ibuprofen and/or gradual dose escalation of IFN-β-1b in patients with MS showed that the use of either ibuprofen alone or a combination of ibuprofen and gradual introduction of IFN-β-1b significantly reduced the incidence of flu-like symptoms to a rate comparable to that observed with placebo (34).

Injection-Site Reactions

In the pivotal study of IFN-β-1b in patients with RR MS, injection-site reactions were the most common adverse effect reported (9,29). These reactions typically occur in patients who inject themselves at the same site several times each week, which underscores the importance of training patients to rotate the injection sites. In rare instances skin necrosis may complicate a severe injection-site reaction and may require discontinuation of IFN-β-1b therapy.

Numerous strategies can be used to prevent injection-site reactions (32,33). Many patients do not inject themselves correctly, and every effort should be made to ensure that the patient is using an optimal injection technique. One of the first steps is for the patient to identify the skin sites that are most sensitive and to avoid these whenever possible. Patients should also rotate the injection site and avoid areas that cover bony surfaces. The medication should be brought up to room temperature and a small-gauge (and sufficiently long) needle should be used. The use of separate needles for drawing up the medication and for injection helps to eliminate skin irritation. Applying ice or a topical steroid (e.g., 1% hydrocortisone cream/ointment) to the injection site before and after injecting can reduce pain at the injection site. Premedicating with oral steroids or antihistamines may also be beneficial, although a recent report suggests that the use of ibuprofen may slightly exacerbate injection-site reactions during the first month of therapy (34). Patients should also avoid excessive exposure of recent injection sites to sunlight or ultraviolet rays. In some cases a ''drug holiday'' may help to relieve the discomfort.

Depression

The exact relationship between IFN-β use and clinical depression remains unclear. In the pivotal trial of IFN-β-1b in RR MS, depressive symptoms and suicide attempts were reported more frequently in patients receiving the higher dose of IFN-β-1b as compared with those receiving placebo (29). However, it remains to be determined whether this reflects the patients' unrealistic expectations regarding the potential benefits of therapy or whether this is a true treatment response (35). A recent study monitored depression levels of patients with MS both before and after treatment with IFN-β1-a. Findings revealed that levels of depression dropped prior to initiation of treatment—possibly in anticipation of receiving therapy—and increased to pretreatment levels after 8 weeks (35). Thus, reported increases in depression following IFN-β treatment may actually represent a return to pretreatment levels of depression rather than an adverse effect of the therapy. The issue of depression and IFN-β-1b therapy must be considered in light of the fact that a large proportion of patients with MS experience clinical depression, which is a largely underdiagnosed and undertreated problem in this population and should be considered an independent disease variable (36). Of particular concern is the high rate of suicide among patients with MS, which in one study was approximately 7.5 times that of age-matched individuals in the general population (37).

The question of the possible relationship between depression and IFN-β-1b treatment was specifically addressed in the European SP MS trial (30). The Montgomery Åsberg Depression Rating Scale, an observer rating scale used to assess mood changes and suicidal risk (38), was administered at baseline and at all regular quarterly follow-up visits. There were no differences in the incidence of new or worsened depression among patients receiving IFN-β-1b as compared with those receiving placebo. Suicides or suicide attempts occurred in 5 patients in the placebo group and 3 patients in the IFN-β-1b group.

Given the association between depression and MS, it is important to approach depression as a clinical problem in its own right. Patients at risk should be identified prior to initiating therapy, and their family members should be alerted to this potential problem. Patients should then be monitored closely once they start therapy. Fortunately, depression in patients with MS has been shown to be highly responsive to interventions, such as pharmacological therapy and psychotherapy. Therefore, antidepressants should be prescribed whenever appropriate and patients should be encouraged to seek psychological counseling (33). Severely depressed patients should not receive IFN-β-1b; however, mildly depressed patients who are receiving an antidepressant may be started on low-dose IFN-β-1b therapy, titrating upward gradually and using ''drug holidays'' as necessary.

Spasticity

More than half of the patients with MS experience spasticity, which is associated with exaggerated withdrawal, spasms, clonus, and hyperreflexia. In the European SP MS trial, hypertonia was reported more frequently in the IFN-β-1b group as compared with the placebo group (37.8 versus 27.4%, $p = 0.0032$) (30). Since IFN-β-1b may exacerbate spasticity, patients should be aware of this possible adverse effect. When treatment related, spasticity and other functional deteriorations are usually transient and appear with the flu-like symptom complex during the early weeks of treatment (33). Spasticity has multiple consequences in patients with MS, including impeded movement, pain, disrupted sleep, and trouble performing the activities of daily living. The one positive consequence of spasticity is that it may aid in support or motion. Several factors can cause an abrupt worsening of spasticity, including urinary tract infection, relapse of MS, or the use of serotoninergic medications.

Several approaches may be used to manage spasticity. The most optimal approach is to prevent or treat the triggering factor, although physical measures—such as stretching or standing—can also be useful. Use of an oral antispasmodic agent (e.g., baclofen or tizanidine) as first-line therapy, possibly combined with low-dose diazepam, may be beneficial. Drugs such as gabapentin may be used as second-line therapy, while invasive or surgical procedures (e.g., intrathecal baclofen) should be reserved for severe or refractory cases. It is rarely necessary to reduce the dosage of IFN-β-1b in patients with spasticity even temporarily (33).

Laboratory Abnormalities

The prolonged use of IFN-β-1b may be associated with certain laboratory abnormalities. For example, rare instances of autoimmune thyroid or liver disease have been reported, and caution should be exercised when starting a patient with liver or thyroid disease on IFN-β-1b. Although leukopenia is common in patients receiving IFN-β-1b, it rarely interferes with therapy, and no patients were withdrawn from the pivotal study in RR MS because of this laboratory abnormality (9). Mild anemia and liver function abnormalities (especially elevations in SGPT) are also common but are rarely of any clinical significance. Liver function returns to normal when IFN-β-1b is discontinued. Thrombocytopenia is quite unusual and usually does not require discontinuation of treatment.

It is recommended that patients receiving IFN-β-1b undergo routine monitoring every 3 months or more frequently if laboratory abnormalities are detected. Most laboratory changes can be reversed by lowering the dose of IFN-β-1b or, in rare cases, discontinuing therapy (33).

Treatment may then be reinstated once the laboratory values have returned to the normal range, usually starting at one-half the previous dose for the first month and titrating upward with the patient under careful surveillance. However, a patient should be switched to an alternative treatment if the same laboratory abnormality recurs after IFN-β-1b therapy has been reinstated.

IV. NEUTRALIZING ANTIBODIES

All IFNs induce the production of antibodies. Therefore, it is not surprising that neutralizing antibodies to IFN-β have been detected in the sera of patients with MS receiving this immunotherapy (29,30,39). Although there has been some question as to whether the presence of these antibodies might affect the long-term clinical efficacy of IFN-β-1b

(40,41), the results of a longitudinal analysis based on 5 years of available data from the pivotal IFN-β-1b trial in patients with RR MS who changed from antibody-negative to antibody-positive failed to support any association between diminished efficacy and a change in antibody status (42). Thus, the clinical relevance of neutralizing antibodies is far from clear at present. Indeed, the fact that these antibodies disappear over time in the majority of patients receiving IFN-β-1b therapy suggests that treatment decisions in MS should be based on clinical criteria and that the role of antibodies is less important than was previously believed (41,42).

V. SUMMARY

The National Multiple Sclerosis Society's recommendation that immunomodulating therapy be initiated early in patients with a definite diagnosis of MS and evidence of ongoing disease activity is supported by current clinical experience (9,30,39,43). As the multicenter, double-blind, placebo-controlled studies described in this chapter have illustrated, IFN-β-1b is effective in patients with MS with a wide range of EDSS scores. More than a decade of clinical experience with IFN-β-1b has clearly shown that it is effective in reducing the rate and severity of exacerbations in patients with MS, as well as disability and disease progression as measured by MRI scans. The follow-up data support the long-term use of IFN-β-1b. This is a time for real optimism in the treatment of this challenging and potentially crippling disease. The consensus today is to treat patients with MS at an earlier age based on MRI evidence of disease progression, even though a patient clinically may still be relatively asymptomatic. The rationale for early treatment is that it is difficult to predict when a serious exacerbation associated with significant lesion damage will occur. The role of neutralizing antibodies in response to IFN-β-1b continues to be confusing. Many authorities in the field feel that patients with MS who receive immunotherapy are underdosed and that even more favorable results could be achieved with higher doses of IFN-β-1b. Significant strides have been made in this field, and new challenges are ahead as we "fine tune" our available treatment options.

REFERENCES

1. Stinissen P, Raus J, Zhang J. Autoimmune pathogenesis of multiple sclerosis: Role of autoreactive T lymphocytes and new immunotherapeutic strategies. Crit Rev Immunol 1997; 17:33–75.
2. Hohlfeld R. Biotechnological agents for the immunotherapy of multiple sclerosis: Principles, problems and perspectives. Brain 1997; 120:865–916.
3. Jacobs L, Johnson KP. A brief history of the use of interferons as treatment of multiple sclerosis. Arch Neurol 1994; 51:1245–1252.
4. Arnason BGW. Immunologic therapy of multiple sclerosis. Annu Rev Med 1999; 50:291–302.
5. Johnson KP. The historical development of interferons as multiple sclerosis therapies. J Mol Med 1997; 75:89–94.
6. Knobler RL, Panitch HS, Braheny SL, et al. Clinical trial of natural alpha interferon in multiple sclerosis. Ann NY Acad Sci 1984; 436:382–388.
7. Jacobs L, O'Malley J, Freeman A, Ekes R. Intrathecal interferon reduces exacerbations of multiple sclerosis. Science 1981; 214:1026–1028.
8. Panitch HS, Hirsch RL, Schindler J, Johnson KP. Treatment of multiple sclerosis with gamma

interferon: Exacerbations associated with activation of the immune system. Neurology 1987; 37:1097–1102.

9. The IFNB Multiple Sclerosis Study Group. Interferon beta-1b is effective in relapsing-remitting multiple sclerosis: I. Clinical results of a multicenter, randomized, double-blind, placebo-controlled trial. Neurology 1993; 43:655–661.

10. Paty DW, Li DKB, the UBC MS/MRI Study Group, and the IFNB Multiple Sclerosis Study Group. Interferon beta-1b is effective in relapsing-remitting multiple sclerosis: II. MRI analysis results of a multicenter, randomized, double-blind, placebo-controlled trial. Neurology 1993; 43:662–667.

11. Quality Standards Subcommittee of the American Academy of Neurology. Practice advisory on selection of patients with multiple sclerosis for treatment with Betaseron. Neurology 1994; 44:1537–1540.

12. Weinstock-Guttman B, Ransohoff RM, Kinkel RP, Rudick RA. The interferons: Biological effects, mechanisms of action, and use in multiple sclerosis. Ann Neurol 1995; 37:7–15.

13. Yong VW, Chabot S, Stuve O, Williams G. Interferon beta in the treatment of multiple sclerosis: mechanisms of action. Neurology 1998; 51:682–689.

14. Noronha A, Toscas A, Jensen MA. Interferon β decreases T cell activation and interferon γ production in multiple sclerosis. J Neuroimmunol 1993; 46:145–154.

15. Yong VW, Antel JP. Major histocompatibility complex molecules on glial cells. Semin Neurosci 1992; 4:231–240.

16. Genç K, Dona DL, Reder AT. Increased CD80$^+$ B cells in active multiple sclerosis and reversal by interferon β-1b therapy. J Clin Invest 1997; 99:2664–2671.

17. Romagnani S. The Th1/Th2 paradigm. Immunol Today 1997; 18:263–266.

18. Yasuda CL, Al-Sabbagh A, Oliveira EC, Diaz-Bardales BM, Gracia CAA, Santos LMB. Interferon β modulates experimental antoimmune encephalomyelitis by altering the pattern of cytokine secretion. Immunol Invest 1999; 28:115–126.

19. Kozovska ME, Hong J, Zang YCQ, et al. Interferon beta induces T-helper 2 immune deviation in MS. Neurology 1999; 53:1692–1697.

20. Porrini AM, De Luca G, Gambi D, Reder AT. Effects of anti-IL-10 monoclonal antibody on rIFNβ-1b-mediated immune modulation: Relevance to multiple sclerosis. J Neuroimmunol 1998; 81:109–115.

21. Rep MHG, Hintzen RQ, Polman CH, van Lier RAW. Recombinant interferon-β blocks proliferation but enhances interleukin-10 secretion by activated human T-cells. J Neuroimmunol 1996; 67:111–118.

22. Rudick RA, Ransohoff RM, Peppler R, Medendorp SV, Lehmann P, Alam J. Interferon beta induces interleukin-10 expression: Relevance to multiple sclerosis. Ann Neurol 1996; 40:618–627.

23. McRae BL, Picker LJ, van Seventer GA. Human recombinant interferon-β influences T helper subset differentiation by regulating cytokine secretion pattern and expression of homing receptors. Eur J Immunol 1997; 27:2650–2656.

24. Butcher EC, Picker LJ. Lymphocyte homing and homeostasis. Science 1996; 272:60–66.

25. Calabresi PA, Tranquill LR, Dambrosia JM, et al. Increases in soluble VCAM-1 correlate with a decrease in MRI lesions in multiple sclerosis treated with interferon β-1b. Ann Neurol 1997; 41:669–674.

26. Corsini E. Gelati M, Dufour A, et al. Effects of β-IFN-1b treatment in MS patients on adhesion between PBMNCs, HUVECs and MS-HBECs: an in vivo and in vitro study. J Neuroimmunol 1997; 79:76–83.

27. Trojano M, Avolio C, Liuzzi GM, et al. Changes of serum sICAM-1 and MMP-9 induced by rIFNβ-1b treatment in relapsing-remitting MS. Neurology 1999; 53:1402–1408.

28. Knobler RL, Greenstein JI, Johnson KP, et al. Systemic recombinant human interferon-β treatment of relapsing-remitting multiple sclerosis: Pilot study analysis and six-year follow-up. J Interferon Res 1993; 13:333–340.

29. The IFNB Multiple Sclerosis Study Group and the University of British Columbia MS/MRI Analysis Group. Interferon beta-1b in the treatment of multiple sclerosis: Final outcome of the randomized controlled trial. Neurology 1995; 45:1277–1285.

30. European Study Group on Interferon β-1b in Secondary Progressive MS. Placebo-controlled multicentre randomised trial of interferon β-1b in treatment of secondary progressive multiple sclerosis. Lancet 1998; 352:1491–1497.

31. Miller DH, Molyneux PD, Barker GJ, et al. Effect of interferon-β1b on magnetic resonance imaging outcomes in secondary progressive multiple sclerosis: Results of a European multicenter, randomized, double-blind, placebo-controlled trial. Ann Neurol 1999; 46:850–859.

32. Lublin FD, Whitaker JN, Eidelman BH, et al. Management of patients receiving interferon beta-1b for multiple sclerosis: Report of a consensus conference. Neurology 1996; 46:12–18.

33. Walther EU, Hohlfeld R. Multiple sclerosis: Side effects of interferon beta therapy and their management. Neurology 1999; 53:1622–1627.

34. Rice GPA, Ebers GC, Lublin FD, Knobler RL. Ibuprofen treatment versus gradual introduction of interferon β-1b in patients with MS. Neurology 1999; 52:1893–1895.

35. Mohr DC, Likosky W, Dwyer P, Van Der Wende J, Boudewyn AC, Goodkin DE. Course of depression during the initiation of interferon beta-1a treatment for multiple sclerosis. Arch Neurol 1999; 56:1263–1265.

36. Goodin DS, and the Northern California MS Study Group. Survey of multiple sclerosis in Northern California. Mult Scler 1999; 5:78–88.

37. Sadovnick AD, Eisen K, Ebers GC, Paty DW. Cause of death in patients attending multiple sclerosis clinics. Neurology 1991; 41:1193–1196.

38. Montgomery SA, Åsberg M. A new depression scale designed to be sensitive to change. Br J Psychiatry 1979; 134:382–389.

39. Jacobs LD, Cookfair DL, Rudick RA, et al. Intramuscular interferon beta-1a for disease progression in relapsing multiple sclerosis. Ann Neurol 1996; 39:285–294.

40. The IFNB Multiple Sclerosis Study Group and the University of British Columbia MS/MRI Analysis Group. Neutralizing antibodies during treatment of multiple sclerosis with interferon beta-1b. Experience during the first three years. Neurology 1996; 47:889–894.

41. Rice GPA, Paszner B, Oger J, Lesaux J, Paty D, Ebers G. The evolution of neutralizing antibodies in multiple sclerosis patients treated with interferon β-1b. Neurology 1999; 52:1277–1279.

42. Arnason BG, Dianzani F. Correlation of the appearance of anti-interferon antibodies during treatment and diminution of efficacy: summary of an international workshop on anti-interferon antibodies. J Interferon Cytokine Res 1998; 18:639–644.

43. Johnson KP, Brooks BR, Cohen JA, et al and the Copolymer 1 Multiple Sclerosis Study Group. Extended use of glatiramer acetate (Copaxone) is well tolerated and maintains its clinical effect on multiple sclerosis relapse rate and degree of disability. Neurology 1998; 50:701–708.

22

Therapeutic Considerations: Prophylactic Therapy with Interferon-β-1a

LAWRENCE JACOBS

School of Medicine and Biomedical Services,
State University of New York at Buffalo,
Buffalo, New York

I. INTRODUCTION

The initial rationale for first testing interferon in MS was based on the belief that MS was caused by a persistent or ongoing viral infection in a dysimmune host and interferon had antiviral and immunomodulatory actions (1–5). Multiple sclerosis, rather than some other disease of purported viral and dysimmune etiology (e.g., amyotrophic lateral sclerosis, or ALS), was chosen for study simply because the earliest MS studies were conducted in a northern latitude U.S. city (Buffalo, N.Y., approx. 43 degrees north) where there was an abundant MS population available for study, compared with ALS or other potentially appropriate disease.

Previously, both alpha (α) and beta (β) forms of type I interferons (IFN) had been assessed in early, very small (three to six patients) clinical trials without clinical benefit by Fog and Ververken et al. in Europe before being tested in the United States (6,7). Interferon-β, rather than IFN-α, was tested in the first U.S. trials because, at that time, Roswell Park Cancer Institute in Buffalo was producing natural human IFN-β for early clinical trials in cancer, and some of that natural substance became available to us for our early neurological clinical trials. Thus, many of the earliest U.S. trials were based on the clinical environment—and serendipity.

Mechanistically, it was presumed that type I IFN acted on specific cellular receptors to induce a series of cytoplasmic reactions resulting in transcription factor activation and induced expression of IFN-responsive genes, the products of which mediated specific biological events (8). Subsequently, several further observations provided more specific scientific rationale for testing IFN-β in MS: (1) IFN-β was found to inhibit experimental allergic encephalomyelitis (9–11); (2) IFN-β was found to inhibit T-cell activation (12); (3) IFN-β was found to correct nonspecific T cell–mediated peripheral blood suppressor function in MS patients (13,14); and (4) IFN-β caused a reduction in IFN-γ secretion in vivo and in vitro (5–17). These actions of IFN-β might be of benefit in MS.

II. EARLY STUDIES

The first preliminary systematic trial of IFN-β in MS was conducted from 1977 to 1980 and initially published in 1981 (18,19). In that study, natural human IFN-β was administered intrathecally by serial lumbar puncture over a 6-month period and the patients were observed for the next 18 months. The results suggested that active treatment reduced the number of clinical MS exacerbations. The second systematic study was a much larger, randomized, double-blinded, placebo-controlled, multicenter trial inititally published in 1986 that confirmed the findings of the earlier one (20,21). Intrathecally administered natural human IFN-β caused a significant reduction in exacerbation rate of patients with relapsing disease.

In these early studies, natural IFN-β was administered by intrathecal (IT) injections directly into the cerebrospinal fluid, because it was believed that systemically administered interferon did not effectively cross the blood-brain barrier (BBB). Subsequently, however, it was shown that systemically administered type I interferon provoked the expressions of interferon-inducible genes in the central nervous system (CNS), indicating that it did, indeed, cross the BBB (22,23). Evidence was also presented that activated myelin-reactive lymphocytes were present in the peripheral blood of MS patients, raising the possibility that systemic immunotherapy might be targeted at lymphoid tissue (24).

Subsequently, two small studies of systemically administered natural (n) human IFN-β were conducted. Baumhefner et al. (25) reported a beneficial effect of nIFN-beta administered intravenously (IV) in six chronic-progressive MS patients. The nIFN-beta dosage was 3×10^6IU weekly for 12 weeks. Improvement in weekly coded neurological examinations was observed in four of the six patients. In addition, a transient significant reduction of intrathecal IgG synthesis rates was seen in one patient. No changes in evoked responses, magnetic resonance imaging (MRI) scans, or other laboratory tests were observed. No significant side effects occurred. It was concluded that IV nIFN-β, even at the low dose tested for a three-month period, could provide clinical benefit in some patients with chronic-progressive MS. The authors concluded that higher doses by the IV route should be investigated.

Huber et al. (26) tested nIFN-β administered intravenously to nine patients with chronic-relapsing MS. Patients received 3×10^6IU of nIFN-β twice per week for 4 weeks and then twice per month for the next 5 months. These treatments were well tolerated, but there was no change in exacerbation rates, CSF IgG synthesis, or MRI plaque formation during a total follow-up period of 1.2 years.

In addition to the evidence that systemically administered interferon did effectively cross the BBB, important advances in newer genetic engineering technology had produced a highly purified recombinant human interferon beta (IFN-β-1a) in large quantities, which made systemic administration possible at a reasonable cost. Therefore, the efficacy and tolerability of systemically administered IFN-β-1a in MS could be definitively assessed. To date, there have been several large controlled trials conducted using two different

IFN-β-1a products (Avonex produced by Biogen, Inc., and Rebif produced by Ares-Serono, Inc.), which are described below.

III. STUDIES IN RELAPSING MS

A. The Trial with Avonex for Relapsing MS

This trial was conducted from November 1990 through February 1994. The IFN-β-1a (Avonex) utilized was produced by Biogen, Inc. It is a natural sequence, glycosylated, recombinant Chinese hamster ovary product with a structure basically identical to that of natural human IFN-β. It has been demonstrated that the glycosylation of the molecule is extremely important in terms of pharmacokinetics and antigenicity; deletion of the glycol carbohydrate from the molecule results in significant denigration of biological functions, development of aggregation, and provocation of antibody responses (27).

The treatment regimen for the study was determined by a double-blinded pilot study to establish the most appropriate dose level and interval for MS patients (28). Five relapsing MS patients were given a weekly intramuscular (IM) injection of placebo or varying doses of Avonex in random order, together with acetaminophen (650 mg) taken every 6 h just before and continuing for 24 h after each injection. Avonex doses tested were $3.0 \times 10^6 IU$, $6.0 \times 10^6 IU$, $9.5 \times 10^6 IU$, and $18.0 \times 10^6 IU$. At doses of $9.5 \times 10^6 IU$ and $18.0 \times 10^6 IU$, patients experienced flu-like symptoms that were not adequately suppressed by acetaminophen to ensure blinding. A single dose of $3.0 \times 10^6 IU$ produced elevated serum B_2 microglobulins for 2 days, whereas a single dose of $6.0 \times 10^6 IU$ produced a serum B_2-microglobulin increase that persisted for 6 days. On the basis of these pilot study results, it was concluded that $6.0 \times 10^6 IU$ of IFN-β-1a was the highest dose that could be administered in a blinded fashion and that biological effects of this dose were observable for 6 days, making a weekly dosing interval ideal.

The primary outcome measure of the early intrathecal studies was exacerbations; no definite benefit on clinical physical disability was demonstrated. However, clinicians' experience repeatedly demonstrated that the most important factor affecting the lives of individual MS patients was the degree of physical disability that accumulated over time, and there seemed to be many instances of mismatch between exacerbations and physical disability (e.g., exacerbations decrease or stop, but physical disability increases or worsens). Since physical disability is a more important factor than clinical relapses, it was important that future definitive trials be designed with clinical physical disability as the primary outcome measure.

The primary outcome measure of the Avonex phase III trial was based on the previously determined fact that a 1.0-point change on the Expanded Disability Status Scale (EDSS) of Kurtzke was clinically meaningful in patients with mild- to- moderate disability (EDSS 1.0 to 3.5) and that such a change could be reliably identified on serial examinations by the same blinded examining physician (29). Intrarater agreement on serial examinations was found to be 100% when agreement was defined as a difference of 1.0 point or more on the EDSS. Previous clinical experience had demonstrated the clinical importance of a 1.0-point increase on the EDSS sustained for 6 months. Ninety percent of the time, such a sustained 1.0-point increase represented permanent worsening of physical disability that would not spontaneously improve in the natural course of untreated MS (30).

The study included 301 patients with relapsing MS enrolled at four clinical centers in the U.S. Inclusion criteria were definite MS for at least 1 year, baseline EDSS of 1.0

to 3.5 inclusive, at least two documented exacerbations in the prior 3 years, no exacerbations for at least 2 months at study entry, and age 18 to 55 years (5,31). This patient population was relatively homogeneous, with active relapsing disease and relatively low EDSS scores in a range where disability changes occur more quickly than at higher scores. Patients who received prior therapy with immunosuppressant drugs (e.g., cyclophosphamide, azathioprine), interferon, or ACTH or corticosteroids (within 2 months of study entry) were not eligible for enrollment. Other exclusion criteria included: concurrent infection, the presence of any serious disease other than MS, chronic progressive MS, pregnant women or nursing mothers, and patients unwilling to practice a form of contraception acceptable to the investigator.

The study was a randomized, double-blinded, and placebo-controlled trial (Efron's biased coin) using Kaplan-Meier analysis for sample size and an intent-to-treat design, assuming that 50% of placebo recipients and 33% of Avonex recipients would worsen by at least 1.0 EDSS point within 104 weeks. The expected placebo progression rate was based on the placebo arm progression of a previous clinical trial (32). Sample size estimates also assumed that 25% of Avonex recipients would discontinue treatment prematurely but would still be followed, and that 10% of patients would be lost to follow-up (31).

The 301 patients were randomly assigned to receive placebo ($n = 143$) or Avonex ($n = 158$) administered IM at a dosage of 6 million units (30 μg) once weekly for up to 104 weeks. Patients were reassessed on a scheduled basis every 6 months and on an unscheduled basis as needed to assess for exacerbations. At the discretion of the blinded treating physician, patients in exacerbation received IM ACTH gel, 80 U daily for 10 days or IV methylprednisolone, 1,000 mg daily for 4 days, followed by a brief course of oral prednisone.

On-study exacerbations were defined by the appearance of new neurological symptoms or worsening of preexisting neurological symptoms lasting at least 48 h in a patient who had been neurologically stable or improving for the previous thirty 30 days. Symptoms had to be accompanied by objective change on neurological examination (worsening of 0.5 point on the EDSS or a worsening by $\geq$ 1.0 point on the pyramidal, cerebellar, brainstem, or visual functional system scores as determined by the blinded examining physician). Brain magnetic resonance imaging (MRI) was performed yearly using a standardized protocol (98% at 1.5 T, the remainder at 1.0 T).

There were no significant differences between groups in baseline demographic, clinical disease, or MRI characteristics. In accordance with the study design, patients were treated and followed for variable lengths of time. All patients, regardless of duration of follow-up, were included in the failure-time analyses.

Disability Progression

Time to sustained progression of disability, the primary outcome measure, was significantly greater in Avonex-treated patients than placebo-treated patients ($p = 0.02$). The Kaplan-Meier failure-time curve illustrates the cumulative percentage of patients whose disability progressed at or before a given week while in the study (Fig. 1). The proportion with progression of disability by 104 weeks estimated from Kaplan-Meier curves was 34.9% in patients who received a placebo and 21.9% in patients who received Avonex, representing a 37% reduction in risk of disability progression with Avonex. Of the patients accrued early enough to complete at least 104 weeks of the study, 29 (33.3%) of

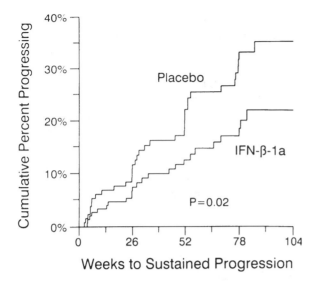

Figure 1 Kaplan-Meier failure-time curve from Avonex phase III trial showing the cumulative percent progressing according to number of weeks to beginning of sustained disability progression (confirmed at 6 months). (From Ref. 31.)

87 placebo recipients patients and 18 (21.2%) of 85 Avonex patients developed disability progression.

There was significantly greater change ($p = 0.02$) in sustained EDSS scores from baseline to week 104 in placebo (mean 0.61, SE 0.18) compared with Avonex (mean 0.02, SE 0.14) recipients. Sustained change in EDSS score was calculated using the lower of the week 104 and week 130 EDSS scores, to ensure that any worsening was sustained for at least 6 months.

Exacerbations

Avonex patients were less likely than placebo patients to have experienced multiple exacerbations. The annual exacerbation rates for patients accrued early enough to complete 104 weeks were 0.90 for placebo patients and 0.61 for Avonex patients ($p = 0.002$), representing a 32% reduction in exacerbation rate with Avonex, A 29% reduction in exacerbation rate by Avonex was observed by the end of the first year of treatment and a 35% reduction was observed by the end of the second year of treatment. The annual exacerbation rate for all patients using all time in the study was 0.82 for placebo patients and 0.67 for Avonex patients ($p = 0.04$). In addition, the number of exacerbations per patient was significantly higher in the patients treated with a placebo than in those treated with the Avonex ($p = 0.03$). More than twice as many placebo as Avonex patients had at least three exacerbations in 104 weeks.

MRI

The proportion of baseline MRI scans showing gadolinium-enhanced lesions did not differ by treatment group. By year 1, the proportion of positive scans among patients treated with Avonex had dropped to 29.9%, while the proportion of positive scans in placebo-treated patients was 42.3% ($p = 0.05$). This group difference persisted at year 2.

Avonex significantly reduced the number of gadolinium-enhanced lesions compared with placebo at year 1 (1.0 versus 1.6, $p = 0.02$) as demonstrated by MRI scans; these differences were maintained at year 2 (0.8 versus 1.6, $p = 0.05$). There also were significant differences in favor of Avonex regarding the volume ($p = 0.02$) of gadolinium-enhanced lesions per patient. The median within-patient percent change in T2 lesion volume from baseline to year 1 was -3.3% in placebo patients and -13.1% in Avonex patients ($p = 0.02$), representing a 75% reduction in lesion volume with Avonex. From baseline to year 2, Avonex produced a 51% reduction in lesion volume compared with placebo; the median within-patient percent change in T2 lesion volume from baseline to year 2 was -6.5% in placebo patients and -13.2% in the Avonex patients (not significantly statistically different).

Blinding and Tolerance

Blinding analyses questionnaires completed at weeks 6, 52, and 104 indicated that the site personnel had remained blinded throughout the study. In particular, at all time points at least 99% of examining physicians (who tested for the primary outcome measure) completing the form reported that they did not know the patients' treatment assignment.

The Avonex was well tolerated, and 93% of patients completed treatment as scheduled. Symptoms reported more frequently ($p < 0.10$) by Avonex patients were restricted to flu-like symptoms, muscle aches, asthenia, chills, and fever. Injection-site reactions occurred rarely and with equal frequency in Avonex and placebo patients.

Comment

This was the first study to show that treatment with intramuscularly administered IFN-β-1a could significantly slow the accumulation of physical disability that characterizes the natural course of untreated relapsing MS. This was in addition to a prophylactic benefit on relapses similar to that previously shown with intrathecal administration of natural human IFN-β. The positive effects on MRI lesions were also new.

B. The Trial with Rebif for Relapsing MS

This trial was conducted from May 1994 through February 1995 by the Prevention of Relapses and Disability by Interferon β-1a Subcutaneously in Multiple Sclerosis (PRISMS) Study Group (33). The IFN-β-1a utilized (Rebif, Ares-Serono) was produced in Chinese hamster ovary cells, was glycosylated, and identical structurally to native human IFN-β. While structurally the same as Avonex, the Rebif formulation process is different, with Rebif having mannitol as an additional excipient. Furthermore, Rebif is formulated in an acetate buffer at pH 3.8, whereas Avonex is less acidic, being formulated in a phosphate buffer at pH 7.2.

The study included 560 patients enrolled from 22 centers in nine countries (seven European, one Canadian, one Australian) who had clinically definite or laboratory-supported definite relapsing MS of at least 1 year's duration (33). Patients had at least two relapses during the previous 2 years and had a Kurtzke EDSS score of 0 to 5.0. Exclusion criteria included prior systemic IFN treatment, lymphoid irradiation, cyclophosphamide, or immunomodulatory or immunosuppressive treatment during the prior 12 months.

Patients were randomly assigned to receive Rebif 22 μg ($n = 189$), Rebif 44 μg ($n = 184$), or placebo ($n = 187$) administered (usually self-administered) subcutaneously (SC) three times weekly for up to 104 weeks. Rebif doses were based on prior pilot studies (34).

The primary outcome measure was relapse count, with relapse defined as the appearance of a new symptom or worsening of an old symptom over at least 24 h that could be attributed to MS and was preceded by stability or improvement for at least 30 days. Investigators requested a visit to the study center within 7 days of relapse for confirmation and assessment of severity by the assessing neurologist (compliance with this request was not stated). The severity of the relapses was also assessed by the Scripps method. Secondary outcome measures included times to first and second relapse, proportion of relapse-free patients, progression in disability (an increase in EDSS of at least one point sustained over 3 months), ambulation index, arm-function index, need for steroid administration and hospitalization, and disease activity and burden of disease by MRI.

The study was randomized, double-blinded, and placebo-controlled. Equal allocation of the three treatment groups was used with a block size of 6. Analysis was by intent to treat and powered at 80% to detect a mean difference of 0.64 in the mean number of relapses between the 44-μg group and the placebo group. A generalized linear model with a log link and variance proportional to the mean was used to analyze relapse count. Cox proportional hazards were used to analyze time-to-event endpoints. Other tests performed were analysis of variance (ANOVA) on rank data for other endpoints and x^2 tests for counts of patients with certain adverse events. The main comparison of interest was that between the high-dose group (44 μg) and the placebo group. Also a new analysis, the integrated disability status scale was used; this is the area under a time/EDSS curve.

Patients were assessed by separate "treating" and "assessing" neurologists. The injection sites were covered at neurological examinations to assure that masking was not compromised because of local reactions. Relapses could be treated with IV methylprednisolone. Patients were reassessed on a scheduled basis every three months or as needed on an unscheduled basis for relapses.

There were no significant group differences in demographics or baseline clinical characteristics among the three groups. The median age of patients was 34.9 years and 69% of patients were female. Patients had a mean of 3.0 ± 1.2 relapses in the 2 years prior to enrollment and a mean EDSS score of 2.5 ± 1.2 at baseline. Of 560 patients randomized to treatment, 533 (95%) completed 1 year of treatment and 502 (90%) completed 2 years of treatment. A total of 58 patients discontinued treatment early, 17 due to adverse events.

Relapses

The relapse rate was significantly lower (29 to 32%) during the 2 years of treatment with both doses of Rebif compared with placebo ($p < 0.005$); the mean number of relapses per patient was 1.82 for the 22-μg group, 1.73 for the 44-μg group, and 2.56 for the placebo group. The proportion of relapse-free patients was significantly increased in the two Rebif groups compared with placebo ($p < 0.005$), and the mean number of moderate-to-severe relapses was significantly lower in both Rebif groups than in the placebo group ($p < 0.005$). No significant differences were observed between the two Rebif doses, indicating a lack of a dose-response effect on relapse rate between Rebif 22 μg and Rebif 44 μg SC three times weekly.

Disability Progression

Time to sustained disability progression was significantly longer ($p < 0.05$) in both Rebif treatment groups than in the placebo group (Fig. 2). Sustained disability progression (confirmed at 3 months) was 39% in patients who received placebo, 30% in patients receiving 22 µg (23% reduction in risk of disability progression) and 27% in patients receiving 44 µg (30.3% reduction in risk of disability progression). It was suggested that a dose-effect was observed on the delay in disability progression for patients with EDSS scores >3.5; however, the effect was not statistically significant and the number of patients included for the 2-year assessment in this group was too small to make a convincing argument.

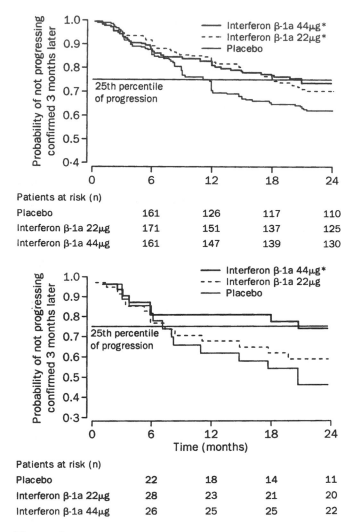

Patients at risk (n)

Placebo	161	126	117	110
Interferon β-1a 22µg	171	151	137	125
Interferon β-1a 44µg	161	147	139	130

Patients at risk (n)

Placebo	22	18	14	11
Interferon β-1a 22µg	28	23	21	20
Interferon β-1a 44µg	26	25	25	22

Figure 2 Time to confirmed progression in disability after 3 months in whole study group (*top*) and in patients with baseline EDSS >3 to 5. *$p < 0.05$ compared with placebo. (From Ref. 33.)

MRI

The T2 burden of disease showed a progressive median increase of 10.9% in the placebo patients, a median decrease of 1.2% in the 22 µg Rebif group and a median decrease of 3.8% in the 44 µg Rebif group ($p < 0.0001$ compared with placebo for both doses). The number of T2 active lesions was also significantly lower (67 and 78% lower in the 22 µg and 44 µg groups, respectively) for both doses compared with the placebo group ($p < 0.0001$). A dose effect in favor of the 44 µg dose was only observed for the number of T2 active lesions ($p < 0.0003$).

Adverse Events

Headache and flu-like symptoms as well as injection-site reactions (redness, inflammation, pain, skin necrosis) occurred more frequently with both Rebif doses than with placebo. In addition, significant asymptomatic decreases in white cells, neutrophils, and lymphocytes, and increased alanine aminotransferase levels were observed in patients who received Rebif compared with placebo ($p \leq 0.05$); these effects were more pronounced in the 44 µg group. After 2 years of treatment, neutralizing antibodies were identified in 23.8% of patients receiving Rebif 22 µg and 12.5% receiving Rebif 44 µg.

Comment

For all of the major outcome measures—relapse rate, sustained disability progression at 3 months, and MRI measures of disease burden and T2 active lesions—Rebif at either dose yielded benefit compared with placebo. Only the number of T2 active lesions demonstrated a dose effect in favor of the 44 µg dose. The suggestion of a dose-effect benefit on disability progression confirmed after 3 months for patients with baseline scores of 3.5 to 5.0 could not be substantiated because of the small subgroup analysis.

C. The Trial with Rebif Once Weekly for Relapsing MS (OWIMS)

Recently, the Once Weekly Interferon for MS (OWIMS) Study Group reported the results of a study comparing the efficacy of once weekly SC administration of Rebif 22 µg and 44 µg with placebo (35). This was a multicenter (11 centers in Europe and Canada) randomized, double-blind, placebo-controlled study conducted between March 1995 and November 1996 that included 293 relapsing-remitting MS patients. The basis of the trial was the fact that many MS patients were being treated with once weekly administration of Avonex, with advantages of less frequent injections and side effects than three times weekly administration, and the perceived need to test Rebif administered in a similar fashion.

Patients in this study had clinically definite or laboratory supported definite relapsing-remitting MS of at least 1 year duration, EDSS score of 0 to 5.0, at least one relapse in the prior 24 months, and at least three MS lesions on MRI. Exclusion criteria included a relapse during the prior 8 weeks, prior IFN, cyclophosphamide, lymphoid irradiation, immunosuppressive treatment or experimental therapies in the prior 12 months, or corticosteroid treatment during the prior 8 weeks.

The primary outcome measure was the number of combined unique active lesions (T1-Gd enhanced and PD/T2) at 24 weeks on MRI. Secondary MRI outcome measures included the proportion of scans showing combined active lesions; the percentage change in burden of disease, and T2 lesion activity. Clinical outcome measures included exacerbations and need for steroid therapy and hospitalizations related to MS (35).

Patients were randomized in a 1 : 1 : 1 ratio and stratified by study center to receive placebo, Rebif 22 µg, or Rebif 44 µg administered SC once weekly for an initial period of 24 weeks. Two physicians at each center assessed each patient. The "treating" physician supervised drug administration, recorded and treated adverse events, and monitored safety assessments. The "evaluating" physician performed neurological assessments at scheduled visits and during exacerbations

Patient demographic and baseline clinical characteristics were similar in all treatment groups.

MRI

There was a significant reduction in the median number of combined active lesions compared to placebo in patients who received Rebif 44 µg (53, $p = 0.002$), but not in patients who received Rebif 22 µg (29, $p = 0.08$); there was no significant difference between the two doses ($p = 0.20$). For T2 active lesions alone and T1-Gd enhancing lesions alone, Rebif 44 µg produced a statistically significant reduction in activity ($p < 0.01$); however, there was no significant difference between doses. PD/T2 lesion activity at 24 weeks was reduced in both Rebif groups, with a significant reduction for the 44 µg dose ($p = 0.02$). No significant differences were observed between the two doses on the proportion of active scans and PD/T2 lesion activity at 24 and 48 weeks.

Exacerbations

Neither Rebif dose resulted in significant clinical improvement compared to placebo as measured by mean exacerbation count, percentage of exacerbation-free patients, median days to first exacerbation, and percentage of patients with moderate/severe exacerbations. Rebif 44 µg did produce a significant reduction in the mean number of steroid treatments per patient during the study ($p = 0.014$). No significant difference in steroid use was observed between the two Rebif doses (35).

Adverse Events

Five adverse events in the Rebif 44 µg group and one in the Rebif 22 µg group led to discontinuation of therapy. Significantly higher incidences of flu-like symptoms, headache, fever, chills and injection-site inflammation occurred in the Rebif 44 µg group compared with placebo ($p < 0.05$) and significantly higher incidences of headache and injection-site inflammation were observed in the Rebif 22 µg group compared with placebo ($p < 0.05$).

Comment

This study showed that Rebif significantly reduced the number of active lesions and the accumulation of burden of disease as measured by MRI. For all MRI measures, Rebif 44 µg was statistically better than placebo, whereas Rebif 22 µg was statistically better than placebo on two of the MRI measures. No significant differences on MRI parameters were observed between the two Rebif doses. Neither Rebif dose produced significant clinical improvements compared to placebo on multiple exacerbation parameters. However, the mean number of steroid treatments per patient was significantly affected by Rebif 44 µg compared with placebo. No significant differences between doses were observed for any of the other clinical efficacy measures. It was hypothesized that the lack of a treatment difference between doses may have been due to an underpowering of the study for the outcome measure, insufficient change in the variable to be detected, or insufficient differ-ence in total dose within the study.

The OWIMS Study Group felt that their observations indicated efficacy of SC, once-weekly low-dose Rebif treatment on MRI activity in MS (35). They also suggest that the low dose has only limited clinical activity. Despite the fact that they did not observe any clinical benefit during their study, the authors still compared the 1-year relapse rate data from the Avonex 30 μg IM once-per-week trial, the Rebif-OWIMS trial at 22 μg SC once per week, and 44 μg SC per week, and the Rebif-PRISMS trial at 22 μg SC three times per week and 44 μg SC three times per week. The comparison was interpreted as showing a dose-response effect on relapse rates favoring the 22 μg SC three-times-per-week and 44 μg SC three-times-per-week doses, which showed significant reduction in exacerbation counts. However, there were several problems with these comparisons making interpreta-tion difficult.

1. The OWIMS trial made direct comparisons of relapse rates at 1 year across three different studies, which had different designs, study lengths, primary and secondary endpoints, and different definitions of endpoints. In particular, the Avonex study utilized a different definition for relapse than did the Rebif study.
2. The OWIMS trial made direct comparisons between IFN-β-1a administered IM and IFN-β-1a administered SC, but there is considerable evidence that the bio-availability of interferon is quite different after administration by the two routes. Some data have shown a three-fold greater bioavailability of IFN-β-1a adminis-tered IM compared to SC. Serum levels of IFN are probably not directly corre-lated with clinical efficacy in MS. It has been shown that biological response markers remain elevated for 6 days after a single administration of an IFN-β-1a dose (28). The cytokine IL-10 remained elevated for 7 days after a single IM injection of IFN-β-1a in MS patients (36). It is likely that the cascade of events triggered by IFN-β-1a rather than the level of IFN-β-1a itself produce the clinical responses to treatment.
3. The OWIMS was a 1-year study; the Avonex pivotal trial with which it was compared was a 2-year study. The statistical powering of the two studies was different because of their prospectively determined durations, which differed. In the final analysis, only head-to-head comparative trials can provide com-pletely valid data comparing two drugs in terms of doses, frequency, route of administration, and clinical and MRI efficacy.

IV. FOLLOW-UP OBSERVATIONS

Further post-hoc analyses of the data from the phase III Avonex trial were conducted. In addition to a positive survival analysis on the primary outcome measure—effect on dis-ability in MS, the study's secondary outcome measures further corroborated the primary outcome measure result. A robust clinical benefit from Avonex treatment was seen, in that the clinical efficacy did not depend on the disability endpoint and significantly higher proportions of placebo patients than IFN-β-1a patients reached clinically important EDSS milestones of 4.0 (relatively severe disability; still walking independently) and 6.0 (unilat-eral assist with cane/crutch) (37).

Other analyses showed the beneficial effect of IFN-β-1a treatment on MRI measures of brain lesions, including a significant effect in decreasing the development of new and enlarging T2 lesions (38). Recently, measures more specific to destructive changes in the brain were evaluated. It was shown that Avonex treatment reduced the development over 2 years of the T1-hypointense lesion burden. It was also shown that brain atrophy based on ventricle and corpus callosum measures progressed over 1- and 2-year intervals in untreated patients and that, using refined techniques for measuring whole-brain atrophy (brain parenchymal fraction or BPF), treatment with IFN-β-1a significantly reduced the progression of atrophy after the first year of treatment. (Fig. 3, top, bottom) (39,40). At baseline, BPF was found to be lower in MS patients than the healthy control group ($p <$ 0.0001). The BPF in MS patients was more than 5 SD below the mean of the healthy control group. Ninety-six percent of the MS patients had baseline BPFs at least two standard deviations below the mean of the healthy controls. BPF in placebo and IFN-β-1a patients was not different. There were no significant correlations between baseline BPF and

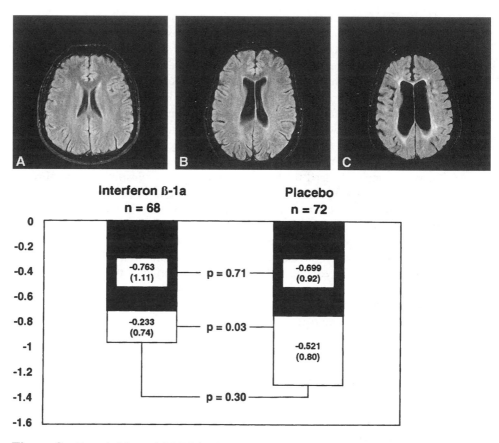

Figure 3 *Top*: Axial cranial MRI in three individuals shows increasing ventricular size with decreasing brain parenchymal fractions (BPF). A. A 31-year-old healthy man, BPF 0.87. B. A 36-year-old woman with relapsing remitting MS, 2 years' disease duration, BPF 0.85 (Z score = −2.6). C. A 43-year-old woman with secondary progressive MS, 19 years disease duration. BPF 0.71 (Z score = −20.8). *Bottom*: Change in brain parenchymal fraction (BPF) according to treatment arm in the Avonex phase III clinical trial. The rate of brain atrophy in year 1 (*solid bars*) was not affected by treatment arm, but there was significantly less brain atrophy in Avonex patients during the second year (*open bars*). (From Ref. 40.)

prestudy relapse rate, number, or volume of gadolinium-enhancing lesions, cerebrospinal fluid (CSF) free kappa light chains, or CSF leukocyte counts. The percent change in BPF was similar during the first year in the IFN-β-1a group and the placebo group. In the second year, change was less ($p = 0.03$) in the IFN-β-1a group (-0.233 ± 0.74) compared with the placebo group (-0.521 ± 0.80). This represented a 55% reduction in the rate of brain atrophy during the second year in the IFN-β-1a group compared with the placebo group.

Other post-hoc analyses demonstrated that reduced CSF pleocytosis and increased CSF expression of IL-10 significantly correlated with favorable clinical response to IFN-β-1a treatment, providing new potential measures of efficacy in future trials (36,41). Additionally, methodology to assess the clinical relevance of neutralizing antibodies to IFN in patients undergoing treatment was published (42).

It was also shown that neuropsychological deterioration (the most sensitive functions being memory and information processing) could be identified in low- to moderate- disability relapsing MS patients, and that treatment with IFN-β-1a slowed or prevented the deterioration (43).

The Avonex trial for relapsing MS ultimately served as the phase III pivotal trial for U.S. FDA purposes, and the recombinant IFN-β-1a utilized (Avonex, Biogen, Inc.) was approved by the FDA for treatment of physical disability in relapsing MS in May 1996. Based in part on recent findings of axonal pathology, including transections in MS brains and data indicating the clinically silent evolution of cerebral atrophy in patients with early or mild- to- moderate relapsing MS (44), the National Multiple Sclerosis Advisory Board officially recommended that immunomodulatory therapy with IFN-β-1a (Avonex), IFN-β-1b (Betaseron) or Copaxone be considered as soon as possible after certain diagnosis in patients with relapsing MS (45).

Recently, data from the Avonex study was used by a National Multiple Sclerosis Society committee of experts (46) to design a new outcome measure for MS clinical trials, the Multiple Sclerosis Functional Composite (MSFC). This composite could substantially simplify the performance of and shorten the time required for clinical MS therapeutic trials in the future.

An open-label, safety-extension study of the phase III pivotal trial of Avonex is being conducted to determine the long-term safety and tolerability (>2 years of use) of Avonex 30 μg IM once weekly in patients with relapsing MS (47). A total of 382 patients were enrolled and the extension study was conducted for in excess of 4.5 years.

The adverse events profile in the extension study was similar to that observed in the phase III trial. Ninety percent of injections were administered at home and the majority of injections were self-administered by patients. A total of 53 of 382 patients (14%) discontinued participation in the study; the mean time on study for these patients was 60 weeks. Of the 382 patients, 18 (5%) discontinued the study because of their physician's or their own perception that therapy was ineffective. Other reasons for patient discontinuation included inconvenience (2%); alternative therapy (1%), dislike of injections (1%), noncompliance (1%), unspecified (1%), and other (1%). The percentage of patients who discontinued treatment due to adverse events was 2% (7 of 382).

The definition of a patient testing positive for neutralizing antibodies to Avonex (NABs) in the open-label, safety extension study was a single serum sample at the designated time point with a titer of ≥ 5 or ≥ 20. After 6 months of Avonex treatment, few patients developed NABs. The incidence of NABs plateaued around 12 months, and at 24 months, the percentage of patients with NAB titers ≥ 5 or ≥ 20 was approximately 5% (47).

Steroid use for exacerbations in the phase III trial was compared with steroid use for exacerbations in the open-label extension study for patients who participated in the phase III trial. There was a 47% reduction in the number of IV steroid courses per year in placebo patients who had been switched to Avonex during the open-label study ($p < 0.001$). In contrast, patients who received Avonex in the phase III trial and remained on it in the open-label study, showed no change in the number of steroid courses per patient per year ($p < 0.10$).

Comment

These long-term data are important because MS is a chronic disease that will probably require ongoing, chronic treatment. To date, long-term treatment appears to be safe, and the associated side effects and inconveniences are acceptable for the benefits achieved.

V. STUDIES IN SECONDARY PROGRESSIVE MS

A. The Rebif Trial for Secondary Progressive MS (SPECTRIMS)

The SPECTRIMS study included 618 patients with secondary-progressive MS (SPMS) (48). It was a multicenter (22 clinical centers in Europe, Australia, and Canada), randomized, double-blind, placebo-controlled phase III study conducted between 1996 and 1999. Two doses of Rebif (22 and 44-μg) were compared against placebo. Active drug or placebo was self-administered subcutaneously three times weekly for up to 3 years.

Patients aged 18 to 55 years with clinically definite secondary progressive MS were included. Secondary progressive MS was defined as progressive deterioration of disability for ≥6 months with an EDSS increase of ≥1 point during the previous 2 years (or 0.5 point between EDSS 6.0 and 6.5), with or without superimposed exacerbations. Patients had to have an EDSS score of 3 to 6.5, a pyramidal functional score ≥2, and no relapses during the prior 2 months.

The primary outcome variable was progression in physical disability, defined as the time to progression by 1.0 point on the EDSS (0.5 point for baseline EDSS ≥5.5) sustained for 3 months. Secondary outcome measures included relapse frequency, severity, and time to first relapse, the number and activity of brain lesions on MRI, and the need for treatment with steroids and MS-related hospitalization.

There were no significant differences between the treatment arms at baseline. Median EDSS was 6.0, relapse rate was 0.9 (all groups), and duration of MS was 13.3 years (SPMS, 4.0 years). Three-year data were available on 571 (92.4%) of 618 patients. The results of the study were announced on June 7, 1999.

Disability Progression

Time to sustained progression was not significantly delayed in either of the Rebif groups compared with placebo.

Relapses

Relapse rates were significantly lower in both Rebif groups compared with placebo during the 3 years of the study; the mean number of relapses was reduced by approximately 31% in both treatment groups ($p < 0.001$). No treatment dose-effects on relapses were observed.

MRI

Over 3 years, burden of disease measured with proton density T2 MRI showed a median decrease of 0.5% in patients treated with Rebif 22 µg, a median decrease of 1.3% in patients treated with Rebif 44 µg, and a progressive median increase of 10% in patients treated with placebo ($p < 0.0001$). The number of T2 active lesions was significantly lower ($p = 0.0001$), and significantly more patients had no activity ($p = 0.01$), in both active treatment groups compared with placebo. Both doses significantly decreased combined unique activity in a subset of patients with monthly T2 and gadolinium-enhanced MRI; a dose effect was observed in favor of the 44 µg dose for this measure.

Adverse Events

Significantly higher incidences of adverse events (injection site reactions, lymphopenia, and elevated levels of alanine aminotransferase (ALT) and neutralizing antibodies) were observed in both the 22 µg and 44 µg Rebif groups compared with placebo ($p < 0.05$). Rebif 44 µg was associated with significantly more episodes of lymphopenia than 22 µg (48).

Comment

It was suggested that the negative results with regard to disability progression may have been due to the fact that the trial's secondary progressive patients had relatively high levels of disability to begin with and had the disease relatively longer than in previous studies of relapsing disease. Nevertheless, the beneficial effects on relapses and MRI in this secondary progressive study were similar to those observed in the previous relapsing-remitting MS trials with Rebif.

B. The Avonex Trial in Secondary Progressive MS (IMPACT)

This phase III study, currently being conducted at 44 centers in the United States and Canada, has enrolled approximately 440 patients with secondary-progressive MS. To be included, patients must have had EDSS scores between 3.5 and 6.5 inclusive, and experienced progression of disease during the past 12 months. Patients were randomly assigned to receive weekly IM injections of placebo or 60 µg of Avonex for up to 24 months under double-blind conditions. The primary outcome measure of the study was change in the Multiple Sclerosis Functional Composite (MSFC) (46), a composite outcome measure consisting of timed 25-ft walk, 9-hole peg test (9HPT), and paced auditory serial addition test 3 (PSAT3). Secondary objectives of the study include the effect of treatment on Gd-enhancing lesions and new and enlarging T2 lesions on brain MRIs conducted on Avonex-treated versus placebo-treated patients and confirmed change from baseline EDSS score for subjects treated with Avonex compared with placebo. The study began in March 1998 and is now fully enrolled.

The dosage of Avonex in this study is higher than that used in the pivotal phase III trial in relapsing MS. The rationale for this dosage was that although it had been previously shown that Avonex 30 µg administered once weekly was effective in relapsing MS, the effect of and optimal dose of Avonex in secondary progressive MS was unknown. Determination of dose for this study was based on a tolerability and safety study that demonstrated that both Avonex doses of 30 and 60 µg IM once weekly were well tolerated in subjects with EDSS scores between 4.0 and 6.5 and favorable observations made on pooled safety data from a dose-comparison study of 30 versus 60 µg IM once weekly in patients with relapsing MS.

VI. STUDIES IN PRIMARY PROGRESSIVE MS

A. The Avonex Trial in Primary Progressive MS

A small pilot study of Avonex treatment in primary progressive MS is under way at the National Hospital, Queens Square, London, UK. Both 30 μg and 60 μg IM doses of Avonex are being compared with placebo IM injections. Fifty patients with primary progressive disease were enrolled. The primary outcome measure was sustained physical disability and the secondary outcome measure was based on MRI parameters. None of the patients showed clinical benefit from taking Avonex; those using the standard dose (30 μg) showed a reduction in size of brain lesions detected by MRI (National MS Society, Res. Update, 9/15/00).

VII. STUDIES IN PATIENTS AT RISK FOR MS IN THE FUTURE

A. The Avonex Trial to Prevent MS in Patients at High-Risk (CHAMPS)

This randomized, double-blind, placebo-controlled phase III study of Avonex for the treatment of subjects at high risk for the development of MS following the first onset of an isolated demyelinating event was begun in 1996 and concluded March 2000. The rationale for the study is that subjects who have a first-isolated, well-defined neurological event consistent with MS—i.e., either monosymptomatic optic neuritis, or a spinal cord syndrome, or a brainstem/cerebellar syndrome and then experience clearing of symptoms (complete, incomplete)—are at higher risk than the normal population for subsequent conversion to clinically definite MS (CDMS) (manifest by a second episode involving another portion of the central nervous system). Approximately half of such patients have MS lesions of the brain visualized by MRI that are already present, but "clinically silent" at the time of the first episode, and such patients are at even higher risk for subsequent conversion to CDMS than the ones whose MRIs are normal. The purpose of this study was to determine if treatment with IM weekly Avonex at 30 μg per dose would significantly reduce or prevent the development, compared to placebo, of CDMS in a series of patients with first onset of monosymptomatic event connected with MS.

   The patients had to be treated within 27 days of onset. A total of 383 patients were randomized to the study: Fifty percent had optic neuritis, 28% had brainstem/cerebellar syndrome, and 22% had spinal cord syndrome. Compliance with study requirements was excellent. Fifty centers in the U.S. and Canada participated. During three years of follow-up, the cumulative probability of the development of CDMS was significantly lower in the Avonex group than in the placebo group (rate ratio, 0.56; 95 percent confidence interval, 0.38 to 0.81; $P = 0.002$) (Fig. 4) (49). As compared with the patients in the placebo group, patients in the Avonex group had a relative reduction in the volume of brain lesions ($P < 0.001$), fewer new or enlarged lesions ($P < 0.001$), and fewer gadolinium-enhancing lesions ($P < 0.001$) at 18 months. This study indicated that initiating treatment with Avonex at the time of a first demyelinating event is beneficial for patients with brain lesions on MRI that indicate a high risk of CDMS.

B. The Rebif Early Treatment of MS (ETOMS) Study of Patients at Risk

This was a double-blinded, randomized, placebo-controlled study conducted at multiple centers in Europe over 2 years. A total of 311 patients were studied, having been enrolled

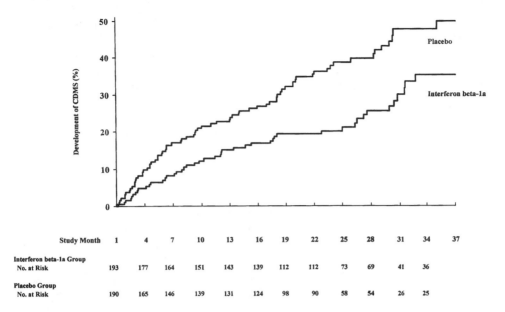

Figure 4   Kaplan-Meier estimates of the cumulative probability of the development of clinically definite multiple sclerosis (CDMS) according to treatment group. The cumulative probability of the development of CDMS during the three-year follow-up period was significantly lower in the interferon beta 1-a group than in the placebo group (P = 0.002 by the Mantel log-rank test). The numbers of patients at risk are the numbers in whom CDMS had not developed at the beginning of each three-month period. Data were censored at the time of a patient's last completed neurologic examination. (From Ref. 49.)

within 3 months of a first attack that suggested demyelinating disease (i.e., optic neuritis, brainstem/cerebellar syndrome, spinal cord syndrome). They were randomly assigned to receive either placebo or Rebif 22 μg SC once per week. Certain baseline results were presented at the 1999 ECTRIMS/ACTRIMS meeting in Switzerland (50). Efficacy results were presented at the American Academy of Neurology Meeting, 2000 (San Diego). The conversion to CDMS was reduced by 31% in the Rebif group compared with placebo (rate ratio 0.69, P = 0.047). Active MRI brain lesions were also reduced significantly by Rebif treatment compared to placebo (P = 0.002).

VIII.   INCIDENCE OF ANTIBODY FORMATION TO RECOMBINANT IFN-β-1a

Studies of formation of neutralizing antibodies (NAB) to Avonex and Rebif have been reported in association with the clinical trials (33,42). The incidence for Avonex at 30 μg week was 5%; that for Rebif was 24% for the 22 μg dose three times per week and 13% for the 44 μg dose three times per week. Structurally, the two IFN-β-1a molecules appear to be identical. Thus, the disparity in antibody formation between the two preparations may be due to the route of their administration. In this regard it is well recognized that protein administered intradermally or subcutaneously is more antigenic than protein administered intramuscularly (51,52). The lower NAB incidence at the higher dose of Rebif was considered by the authors to be due possibly to high-zone tolerance. Antibody levels were determined by cytopathic effect after enzyme-linked immunosorbent assay (ELISA) determination of binding. It is likely that the development of neutralizing antibodies is associated with some reduction of efficacy of IFN-β-1a. However, the detection of neutralizing antibodies should not be the sole reason to discontinue treatment with IFN-β-1a. The patient's disease status is of paramount importance. There is clear evidence that treatment may continue to be effective in some of the patients who have developed neutralizing antibodies. At present there is not enough information regarding the interpretation of the results of existing IFN-β assays to warrant routine testing outside the research setting. However, knowledge of the neutralizing antibody status can be helpful for making a decision about stopping the drug.

IX. DISCUSSION

These studies have clearly demonstrated that treatment with systemically administered IFN-β-1a can have a major beneficial effect in relapsing MS. These treatments have been shown not only to benefit relapses (as did the earliest studies in which natural IFN-β was administered intrathecally), but also to favorably influence the accumulation of physical disability over time, which is the most important factor affecting the lives of MS patients. The data in this regard were more impressive for Avonex (31), with a 37% reduction in risk of disability progression confirmed at 6 months, compared to the 30.3% reduction in risk of disability progression confirmed at 3 months in the Rebif study (33). Still, for the first time we have a treatment that can delay or prevent the accumulation of physical disability in a prophylactic fashion in relapsing MS patients.

MRI has revealed that IFN-β-1a treatment favorably influences multiple parameters of MS lesions of the brain, including the earliest stages of lesion development, where there is an active breakdown of the BBB (31,38,39). Most recently, it has been discovered that treatment with one of the IFN-β-1a preparations (Avonex) can significantly slow the development of brain atrophy that occurs during the natural course of untreated MS (40, 44). The beneficial effect on the atrophy could be discerned after the second year of treatment with weekly IM injection of 30 μg (6 MIU) (40). Possibly, the atrophy could be prevented altogether if treatment was started early enough. These findings and other considerations have led the National Multiple Sclerosis Society of the United States to formally recommend that basically all patients with relapsing-remitting MS should be considered for treatment with one of three new immunomodulatory agents (of which IFN-β-1a is one) as soon as possible after certain diagnosis unless there are contraindications (45). These occurrences have revolutionized the modern treatment of MS; as of December 1999 it was estimated that approximately 112,200 MS patients were receiving one of these IFN-β-1a treatments (Avonex, 83,000 patients; Rebif, 18,000 patients). Certain aspects of the cited studies are difficult to compare and reconcile because of some differences in method of drug production—preservation, study designs, primary endpoints, definitions of events and treatment regimens, including administration route. Despite these variances, there is no doubt that treatment with both preparations of IFN-β-1a produce such significant benefit in relapsing MS that they are clearly the most important prophylactic treatment measures for this disease.

In general, the treatments with both products are well tolerated and side effects are clearly acceptable for the benefits achieved. However, the once per week treatment schedule for Avonex would seem more desirable than the three times per week regimen for Rebif if the benefits were comparable. In this regard, suggestion of a Rebif dose-effect with higher doses administered more frequently providing increased benefit have not been convincingly demonstrated (35). Although Avonex and Rebif appear to be structurally identical, the differences in their modes of preparation and preservation may be important. The incidence of development of neutralizing antibodies is lower for Avonex than for Rebif. In this regard, the route of administration may also be important; it is known that SC injections used for Rebif are more antigenic than IM injections used for Avonex (51,52).

The findings of the Rebif trial in secondary progressive MS were disappointing (48). No significant benefit on physical disability was discerned at either the 22 μg or 44 μg dose, compared with placebo even when the disability increase had to be confirmed after only three months rather than six months. Moreover, no dose-effect was seen for relapses or MRI measures. It is possible that the disability measurements in secondary progressive disease will be more difficult to make than in relapsing disease because, in general, secondary progressive patients have higher baseline disabilities than relapsing patients. It is also possible that a longer treatment period will be required to identify disability changes in the secondary progressive group. The use of the new composite measurement may be helpful in this regard (46). Hopefully, these early negative results of IFN-β-1a treatment in secondary progressive disease will not persist in future trials. There is considerable evidence that secondary progressive MS is a later stage in the continuum of the same disease that begins as relapsing MS, where both forms of recombinant IFN-β-1a have been shown to be effective. The Avonex trial in secondary progressive disease (in which the new composite outgoing measure (46) is being used) is still ongoing; the results should be known within the next 2 years.

Two studies designed to assess the efficacy of IFN β 1a at the other end of the MS disease continuum—namely patients at-risk for MS, have recently been completed (49,50). These studies included patients who experienced their first clinical episode of demyelinating symptoms and were found to have "clinically silent" MS lesions of the brain revealed by MRI examination. Such patients are known to be at high-risk for a second clinical attack and the diagnosis of clinically definite MS within 1 to 4 years.

They are also at risk for repeated bouts of "clinically silent" CNS inflammation, demyelination, axonopathy, and even brain atrophy before the second attack occurs. Active treatment significantly reduced the occurrence of the second clinical attack (relapse) compared to the placebo in both studies, but the magnitude of the reduction was greater in the CHAMPS study (44% reduction; rate ratio 0.56, 95 percent confidence interval = 0.38 to 0.81; $p = 0.002$) than in the ETOMS study (31% reduction; rate ratio 0.69, $p = 0.047$). The magnitude of the beneficial effect on MRI lesions was also greater in the CHAMPS study ($p = 0.0001$ at 18 months) than in the ETOMS study ($p = 0.002$) (49,50). The reasons for the differences in the magnitude of benefits in the two studies (CHAMPS—383 patients; ETOMS—308 patients) are not yet clear and will require further analyses. However, these studies provide important rationale for early treatment of such patients even before they have received the diagnosis of clinically definite MS by conventional criteria.

REFERENCES

1. Cook SD, Dowling PC. Multiple sclerosis and viruses: an overview. Neurology 1980; 20: 80–91.
2. Leibowitz S. The immunology of multiple sclerosis. In: Hallpike JF, Adams CWM, Tourtellotte WW, eds. Multiple Sclerosis. Baltimore: Williams & Wilkins, 1983, pp 379–412.

3. Stewart WE II. The Interferon System. New York: Springer-Verlag, 1979.

4. Ter Meulen V, Stephenson JR. The possible role of viral infections in multiple sclerosis and other related demyelinating diseases. In: Hallpike JF, Adams CWM, Tourtellotte WW, eds. Multiple Sclerosis. Baltimore: Williams & Wilkins, 1983, pp 241–274.

5. Jacobs L, Cookfair DL, Rudick RA, et al. A phase III trial of intramuscular recombinant interferon beta for exacerbating-remitting multiple sclerosis: Design and conduct of study; baseline characteristics of patients. Multiple Sclerosis 1995; 1:118–135.

6. Fog T. Interferon treatment of multiple sclerosis patients: A pilot study. In: Boese A, ed. Search for the Cause of Multiple Sclerosis and Other Chronic Diseases of the Nervous System. Weinheim: Verlag Chemie, 1980, pp 491–493.

7. Ververken D, Carton H, Billiau A, et al. Intrathecal administration of interferon in MS patients. In: Karcher D, Lowenthal A, Strosberg AD, eds. Humoral Immunity in Neurological Disease. New York: Plenum, 1979, pp 625–627.

8. Weinstock-Guttman B, Ransohoff RM, Kinkel RP, Rudick RA, et al. The interferons: biologic effects, mechanisms of action, and use in multiple sclerosis. Ann Neurol 1995; 37:7–15.

9. Abreu SL. Suppression of experimental allergic encephalomyelitis by interferon. Immunol Invest 1982; 11:1–7.

10. Abreu SL, Tondreau J, Levine S, Sowinski R. Inhibition of passive localized allergic encephalomyelitis by interferon. Int Arch Allergy Appl Immunol 1983; 72:30–33.

11. Hertz F, Deghenghi R. Effect of rat and beta human interferon on hyperacute experimental allergic encephalomyelitis in rats. Agents Actions 1985; 16:397–403.

12. Rudick RA, Carpenter CS, Cookfair DL, et al. *In vitro* and *in vivo* inhibition of mitogen-driven T-cell activation by recombinant interferon beta. Neurology 1993; 43:2080–2087.

13. Noronha A, Toscas A, Jensen MA. Interferon beta augments suppressor cell function in multiple sclerosis. Ann Neurol 1990; 27:207–210.

14. Schapner HW, Aune TM, Pierce CW. Suppressor T cell activation by human leukocyte interferon. J Immunol 1983; 131:2301–2306.

15. Barna BP, Chou SM, Jacobs B, et al. Interferon-beta impairs induction of HLA-DR antigen expression in cultured adult human astrocytes. J Neuroimmunol 1989; 23:45–53.

16. Inaba K, Kitaura M, Kato T, et al. Contrasting effects of alpha/beta and gamma-interferons on expression of macrophage Ia antigens. J Exp Med 1986; 163:1030–1035.

17. Ling PD, Warren MK, Vogel SN. Antagonistic effect of interferon-beta on the interferon-gamma-induced expression of Ia antigen in murine macrophages. J Immunol 1985; 135:1857–1864.

18. Jacobs L, O'Malley J, Freeman A, Ekes R. Intrathecal interferon reduces exacerbations of multiple sclerosis. Science 1981; 214:1026–1028.

19. Jacobs L, O'Malley J, Freeman A, Ekes R. Intrathecal interferon in multiple sclerosis. Arch Neurol 1982; 39:609–615.

20. Jacobs L, Salazar AM, Herndon R, et al. Multicenter double-blind study of effect of intrathecally administered natural human fibroblast interferon on exacerbations of multiple sclerosis. Lancet 1986; 2:1411–1414.

21. Jacobs L, Salazar AM, Herndon R, et al. Intrathecally administered natural human fibroblast interferon reduces exacerbations of multiple sclerosis: Results of a multicenter double-blind study. Arch Neurol 1987; 44:589–595.

22. Flenniken AM, Galabru J, Rutherford MN, et al. Expression of interferon-induced genes in different tissues of mice. J Virol 1988; 62:3077–3083.

23. Wong GHW, Bartlett PF, Clark-Lewis I, et al. Inducible expression of H-2 and Ia antigens on brain cells. Nature 1984; 310:688–691.

24. Ransohoff RM, Tuohy V, Lehmann P. The immunology of multiple sclerosis: new intricacies and new insights. Curr Opin Neurol 1994; 7:242–249.

25. Baumhefner RW, Tourtellotte WW, Syndulkok, et al. Effect of intravenous natural beta-interferon on clinical neurofunction, magnetic resonance imaging plaque burden, intrablood-brain

barrier IgG synthesis, blood and cerebrospinal fluid cellular immunology and visual evoked responses. Ann Neurol 1987; 22:171.

26. Huber M, Bamborschke S, Assheuer J, Heiss WD. Intravenous natural beta interferon treatment of chronic exacerbating-remitting multiple sclerosis: clinical response and MRI/CSF findings. J Neurol 1988; 235:171–173.

27. Runkel L, Meier W, Pepinsky RB, et al. Structural and functional differences between glycosylated and non-glycosylated forms of human interferon-β (IFN-β). Pharm Res 1998; 15:641–649.

28. Jacobs L, Munschauer FE. Treatment of multiple sclerosis with interferons. In: Rudick RA, Goodkin DE, eds. Treatment of Multiple Sclerosis: Trial Design, Results and Future Perspectives. London: Springer Verlag, 1992, pp 223–250.

29. Goodkin DE, Cookfair D, Wende K, et al., and the Multiple Sclerosis Collaborative Research Group. Inter-rater and intra-rater scoring agreement using grades 1.0 to 3.5 of the Kurtzke Expanded Disability Status Scale (EDSS). Neurology 1992; 42:859–863.

30. Ellison GW, Myers LW, Leake BD, et al. Design strategies in multiple sclerosis clinical trials. Ann Neurol 1994; 36:S108-S112.

31. Jacobs L, Cookfair D, Rudick R, et al. Intramuscular interferon beta-1a for disease progression in relapsing multiple sclerosis. Ann Neurol 1996; 39:285–294.

32. Bornstein MB, Miller A, Slagle S, et al. A pilot trial of COP 1 in exacerbating-remitting multiple sclerosis. N Engl J Med 1987; 317:408–414.

33. PRISMS (Prevention of Relapses and Disability by Interferon β-1a Subcutaneously in Multiple Sclerosis) Study Group. Randomized double-blind placebo-controlled study of interferon β-1a in relapsing/remitting multiple sclerosis. Lancet 1998; 352:1498–1504.

34. Johnson KP, Knobler RL, Greenstein JI, et al. Recombinant human beta interferon treatment of relapsing-remitting multiple sclerosis: Pilot study results. Neurology 1990; 40 (suppl 1): 261.

35. The Once Weekly Interferon for MS Study Group (OWIMS). Evidence of interferon β-1a dose response in relapsing-remitting MS. Neurology 1999, 53.679–686.

36. Rudick RA, Ransohoff RM, Peppler R, et al. Interferon beta induces interleukin-10 expression: Relevance to multiple sclerosis. Ann Neurol 1996; 40:618–627.

37. Rudick R, Goodkin D, Jacobs L, et al. The impact of interferon beta-1a on neurologic disability in relapsing multiple sclerosis. Neurology 1997; 49:358–363.

38. Simon J, Jacobs L, Campion M, et al., and the Multiple Sclerosis Collaborative Research Group. Magnetic resonance studies of intramuscular interferon β-1a for relapsing multiple sclerosis. Ann Neurol 1998; 43:79–87.

39. Simon JH, Jacobs LD, Campion MS, et al., and the Multiple Sclerosis Collaborative Research Group. A longitudinal study of brain atrophy in relapsing multiple sclerosis. Neurology 1999; 53:139–148.

40. Rudick RA, Fisher E, Lee JC, et al., and the Multiple Sclerosis Collaborative Research Group. Use of the brain parenchymal fraction to measure whole brain atrophy in relapsing remitting MS. Neurology 1999; 53:1698–1704.

41. Rudick RA, Cookfair DL, Simonian NA, et al., and the Multiple Sclerosis Collaborative Research Group. Cerebrospinal fluid abnormalities in a phase III trial of Avonex (IFNβ-1a) for relapsing multiple sclerosis. J Neuroimmunol 1999; 93:8–14.

42. Rudick RA, Simonian NA, Alam JA, et al., and the Multiple Sclerosis Collaborative Research Group. Incidence and significance of neutralizing antibodies to interferon beta-1a in multiple sclerosis. Neurology 1998; 50:1266–1272.

43. Fischer J, Priore R, Jacobs L, et al., and the Multiple Sclerosis Collaborative Research Group. Neuropsychological effects of interferon beta-1a in relapsing multiple sclerosis. Ann Neurol 2000 (in press).

44. Trapp BD, Peterson J, Ransohoff RM, Rudick R, Mörks Bö L. Axonal transection in the lesions of multiple sclerosis. N Engl J Med 1998; 338:278–285.

45. Disease Management Consensus Statement, October 23, 1998. Clinical bulletin. National Multiple Sclerosis Society.

46. Fischer JS, Rudick RA, Cutter GR, et al. The Multiple Sclerosis Functional Composite measure (MSFC): an integrated approach to MS clinical outcome assessment. Mult Scler 1999; 5:244–250.

47. Herndon RM, Jacobs LD, Coats ME, et al. Results of an ongoing, open-label, safety-extension study of interferon beta-1a (Avonex) treatment in multiple sclerosis. Int J MS Care (serial online) December 15, 1999. Available at http://mscare.com/Dec_99/ dec_99.html.

48. SPECTRIMS data presented at the 9th European Neurological Society Meeting; June 1999; Milan, Italy.

49. Jacobs LD, Beck RW, Simon JH, et al., and the CHAMPS Study Group. The effect of interferon beta-1a treatment initiated at the time of a first acute demyelinating event on the rate of development of clinically definite multiple sclerosis. N Engl J Med 2000; 343:898–904.

50. Comi G, Filippi M, Barkhof F, et al. and the ETOMS Study Group. Interferon beta 1a (Rebif) in patients with acute neurological syndromes suggestive of multiple sclerosis: a multi-center, randomized, double-blind, placebo-controlled study. Neurology 2000; 54(No. 7, Suppl 3): A85–A86.

51. Male D, Cooke A, Owen M, et al. Immunoregulation. In: Advanced Immunology, 3rd ed. London: Mosby, 1996, pp 11.1–11.17.

52. Janeway CA, Travers P, Walport M, Capra JD. The induction, measurement, and manipulation of the immune reponse. In: Immunobiology, 4th ed. London: Current Biology Publications, Elsevier Science London, 1999, p 37.

23

Prophylactic Therapy—Glatiramer Acetate (Copaxone)

HILLEL PANITCH

University of Maryland School of Medicine, Baltimore, Maryland

I. INTRODUCTION

The "Decade of the Brain" (1990–2000) could not have been more aptly named, as it produced a revolution in the understanding and management of many neurological diseases, including multiple sclerosis (MS). Since publication of the previous edition of this handbook, glatiramer acetate (Copaxone, copolymer 1) was approved by the U.S. Food and Drug Administration and has come into widespread use for treatment of relapsing-remitting MS. Approval was granted on the basis of two pivotal double-blind, placebo-controlled clinical trials (1,2) that demonstrated convincingly the ability of glatiramer acetate to reduce relapse rates in MS and, to a lesser extent, to slow the progression of neurological disability. Treatment with glatiramer acetate, Betaseron (IFN-β-1b), or Avonex (IFN-β-1a) has become the standard of care for patients with relapsing-remitting MS. In addition, their clinical success has generated a wealth of basic research and clinical trials that have helped to elucidate their mechanisms of action and extend their clinical applications. The purpose of this chapter will therefore be to review (a) the pivotal trials that led to the approval of glatiramer acetate, (b) subsequent studies that established its effect on MRI activity in MS, (c) ongoing clinical trials of glatiramer acetate for new indications and in a novel oral formulation, (d) new insights into the immunological mechanism of action of the drug, and (e) current thinking about the appropriate place of glatiramer acetate in the MS therapeutic armamentarium.

It should be noted that confusion may arise because different names have been used to describe this product over the past 30 years. The original name, copolymer 1 or cop 1, was replaced after FDA approval by the generic name glatiramer acetate and the trade name Copaxone. However, some authors continue to refer to it as copolymer 1 or cop 1 in their publications. In this review, the generic name is used unless otherwise specified.

II. CLINICAL STUDIES OF GLATIRAMER ACETATE

A. Phase II Pilot Study in Relapsing-Remitting MS

Following an open-label dose-finding study in 16 patients, in which glatiramer acetate was shown to be safe and the standard dose of 20 mg/day established (3), Bornstein et al. undertook a randomized, double-blind, placebo-controlled phase II trial in 50 patients with relapsing-remitting MS (1). The principal outcome measures were relapse rate and proportion of relapse-free patients. Patients were enrolled as matched pairs, stratified by age, sex, relapse rate, and Kurtzke DSS score and were followed at regular intervals by blinded examiners. The results were remarkably supportive of a treatment effect with 62 confirmed attacks in the placebo group, vs. only 16 in the glatiramer acetate–treated group over 2 years, corresponding to a reduction in annualized relapse rate from 1.35 to 0.30—a highly significant result. In addition, the proportion of relapse-free patients was twice as great in the glatiramer acetate group as in the placebo group. Notably, patients with the lowest disability scores (0 to 2) responded best, with 27 attacks in the placebo-treated patients but only 4 among those treated with glatiramer acetate, suggesting that treatment should be initiated as early as possible. A beneficial effect was also found for progression of disease, with significant differences between the active drug and placebo groups' proportion of progression-free patients and time to confirmed progression. This trial also established the tolerability of glatiramer acetate, which has been confirmed in all later trials. The only adverse events of importance were local injection site reactions and, in two patients, a transient reaction immediately after injection of glatiramer acetate consisting of flushing, sweating, palpitations, a sensation of chest tightness, shortness of breath, and anxiety lasting for minutes and resolving spontaneously. This has been seen in all subsequent studies and remains an enigma. It does not appear to be allergic in nature, since most patients experience the syndrome only once or twice, have no symptoms after rechallenge with the drug, and have no detectable IgE antibody or other immune markers of allergy. Attempts to study the reaction have been futile because of its unpredictable occurrence and brief duration and because the reaction cannot be reproduced in animals treated with glatiramer acetate.

B. Phase II Pilot Study in Chronic Progressive MS

A study of glatiramer acetate in patients with chronic progressive MS was conducted at two MS centers in the mid-1980s (4). Although carefully designed and controlled, this study was marred by problems of insufficient statistical power and intersite variation. Patients with scores of 2.0 to 6.5 on the Kurtzke EDSS and a progressive course in the previous 2 years were followed in a pretrial observation period to confirm progression. A Total of 106 patients (mean age 42 years, mean EDSS score 5.6) were then randomized to receive either glatiramer acetate 15 mg subcutaneously twice a day or a placebo administered in the same way. The primary endpoint was time to confirmed progression, defined as worsening by 1.0 point for patients with EDSS ≥ 5.0 and 1.5 points for EDSS < 5.0 maintained for at least 3 months. Despite the unusual pretrial observation period and stringent progression criteria, the effect of glatiramer acetate on progression was not statistically significant, although all outcome measures showed favorable trends. When the data from the two centers were analyzed individually, there was a significant treatment effect at one center but not the other, which could be attributed to failure of placebo-treated patients at that site to progress as expected. Although a larger multicenter study may have resulted in a different outcome, the study tended to support the findings of the relapsing-remitting trial, described above (1), that glatiramer acetate is most effective in early, mild, relapsing MS and less effective in more disabled patients. As in the earlier trial, side effects were confined to injection site reactions and the transient systemic reaction, which occurred in 12 of the 51 glatiramer acetate-treated patients (Table 1).

This study was important in another respect as well, because on reanalysis 30 of the patients were found to have primary progressive MS, and to be divided almost evenly between glatiramer acetate and placebo groups (data on file, Teva Pharmaceuticals Ltd.). They responded favorably to glatiramer acetate in terms of progression after 12 and 24 months of treatment, suggesting that a more extensive trial of glatiramer acetate in patients with primary progressive MS was warranted. Indeed, such a trial (the PROMiSe study) was recently undertaken, and is described more fully below.

C. Phase III Pivotal Trial, Extension, and Open-Label Study in Relapsing-Remitting MS

In order to undertake a definitive clinical trial, it was first necessary to standardize the preparation of the drug and to produce it in large enough quantities to perform a phase III multicenter study. Glatiramer acetate used in previous studies had been prepared in small batches that, despite their constant amino acid composition (Table 2), varied widely in molecular weight and ability to suppress experimental allergic encephalomyelitis (EAE). In 1987, development of glatiramer acetate was undertaken by Teva Pharmaceutical Industries Ltd, Petah Tiqva, Israel, but not until 1991 did the company succeed in standardizing the manufacturing process to produce large batches of consistently active drug that were acceptable to the FDA for use in a pivotal trial. The formulated product, known as Copaxone, contained 20 mg/mL of glatiramer acetate with an average molecular weight of 4700 to 13,000 Da and 40 mg/mL of mannitol to increase stability and solubility. Each batch of the commercial product was tested for uniformity by chromatographic and amino acid analysis and was capable of suppressing EAE.

The trial, conducted in the United States from 1991 to 1994 (2,5), included 251 patients 18 to 45 years of age with clinically definite relapsing-remitting MS, EDSS scores from 0 to 5.0, and a history of two or more relapses in the 2 years prior to entry. They were randomized to receive either 20 mg of glatiramer acetate or a placebo by daily subcutaneous injection for 24 months. The primary outcome measure was a comparison of relapse rates in the two groups, with relapses being carefully defined as appearance of a neurologic abnormality persisting at least 48 h following a period of stability or improvement lasting at least 30 days. Only relapses confirmed by objective changes on neurological examination were used in the analysis. Secondary outcome measures included proportion of relapse-free patients, time to first relapse, sustained progression (defined as an increase of one or more points on the EDSS persisting for at least 3 months), and mean EDSS change in the two groups. Patients were instructed in self-injection of the drug and were examined at 3-month intervals by a blinded examininer and a blinded treating neurologist who was responsible for steroid treatment, if necessary, for confirmed relapses. Magnetic resonance imaging (MRI) was performed in a small cohort of patients at a single center (6,7).

Table 1 Principal Trials of Glatiramer Acetate in Multiple Sclerosis

Study	Patients	Clinical Type	Dose	Duration	Outcome
Bornstein et al. (1987), DB, PC	48	RR DSS 0–6	20 mg/day SC	2 years	Reduction in relapse rate (75%) and progression
Bornstein et al. (1991), DB, PC (two centers)	106	SP and CP EDSS 2–6.5	15 mg SC bid	2 years	Decreased time to progression, inter-center differences
Johnson et al. (1995), DB, PC, multicenter	251	RR EDSS 0–5	20 mg/day SC	2 years	Reduction in relapse rate, trend to slowing progression
Johnson et al. (1998), extension of above	251	RR EDSS 0–5.5	20 mg/day SC	2–3 years	Continued efficacy on relapse rate and disability
Mancardi et al. (1998) Baseline vs. treatment	10	RR DSS 3.8 ± 1.3	20 mg/day SC	9–27 months	57% reduction in Gd-enhancing lesions
Comi et al. (in press), DB, PC, crossover	239	RR EDSS 0–5	20 mg/day SC	18 months	35% reduction in Gd-enhancing lesions, delayed effect on MRI and relapses
Wolinsky et al., DB, PC multicenter	947	PP EDSS 3–6.5	20 mg/day SC	3 years	In progress "PROMiSe" trial
Comi et al., DB, PC, multinational	1650	RR EDSS 0–5	5 mg vs. 50 mg/day vs placebo PO	15 months	In progress "CORAL" trial
Lublin et al., glatiramer plus IFN beta-1a	33	RR EDSS 0–5.5	20 mg/day SC plus IFN beta-1a (Avonex)	15 months	In progress "Combi-Rx" trial

Key: SP, secondary progressive; CP, chronic progressive; RR, relapsing-remitting; PP, primary progressive; IM, intramuscular; SC, subcutaneous; (E)DSS, (Expanded) Disability Status Scale; DB, double-blind; PC, placebo-controlled; Gd, gadolinium; IFN, interferon.

Table 2 Composition of Glatiramer Acetate

Amino Acid	Molar Ratio
L-alanine	4.2
L-glutamic acid	1.4
L-lysine	3.4
L-tyrosine	1.0
Mean molecular weight 4.7–13 kDa	

Source: From Ref. 28.

The placebo and active drug groups were well matched except for mean EDSS, which was slightly higher in the glatiramer acetate–treated patients (Table 3). Approximately equal numbers of patients withdrew from both groups over 2 years, which did not appreciably affect the intention-to-treat analysis. The principal outcome of the study was a 29% reduction ($p = 0.007$) in the mean 2-year relapse rate from 1.68 in the placebo group to 1.19 in the glatiramer acetate group (2). Additional supporting relapse data are shown in Table 4. Patients in both groups with higher EDSS scores at entry had more relapses during the trial, but the therapeutic effect was greatest in patients with EDSS scores of 0 to 2.0, who showed a 33% reduction in relapse rate, while those with higher scores had only a 22% reduction.

Table 3 Demographics of Patients in Phase III Glatiramer Acetate Trial

Characteristic (mean ± SD)	Cop 1 ($n = 125$)	Placebo ($n = 126$)
Age	34.6 ± 6.0	34.3 ± 6.5
Prior 2-year relapse rate	2.9 ± 1.3	2.9 ± 1.1
EDSS at entry	2.8 ± 1.2	2.4 ± 1.3
Duration of MS (years)	7.3 ± 4.9	6.6 ± 5.1

Source: From Ref. 28.

Table 4 Effects of Glatiramer Acetate and Placebo on Relapse Rates

	Copolymer 1 ($n = 125$)	Placebo ($n = 126$)	Significance
Number of relapses	161	210	
Two-year relapse rate	1.19	1.68	$p = 0.007$
Annualized relapse rate	0.59	0.84	
Relapse-free patients	33.6%	27.0%	$p = 0.098$
Days to first relapse (median)	287	198	$p = 0.097$
Relapses per patient			
0	42	34	
1–2	60	55	$p = 0.023$
≥3	23	37	

Source: Adapted from Ref. 28.

The effect of glatiramer acetate on progression was significant as measured by the proportion of patients who improved or worsened by one or more EDSS points compared to patients treated with placebo (Table 5). More patients on glatiramer acetate improved and more on placebo worsened over the 24 study months. Mean change in EDSS from baseline was also statistically better in the glatiramer acetate–treated group, although the difference was numerically small and of dubious clinical significance. However, there was no effect on the proportion of progression free patients, defined as those having a 1-point change in EDSS sustained for at least 3 months. MRI analysis of a small cohort of patients at one of the clinical centers (6) revealed a trend toward benefit with glatiramer acetate in terms of reduced numbers of gadolinium-enhancing lesions. Later reanalysis of the same data was reported to show an effect on brain atrophy as well (7). However, the patient population was too small to provide definitive results, and the methodology of the brain atrophy study is questionable.

Adverse events were numerous but relatively mild. Local injection-site reactions consisting of erythema with or without induration occurred in 90% of glatiramer acetate–treated patients and were sometimes painful but never resulted in skin necrosis. An immediate postinjection reaction—consisting of variable combinations of flushing, chest tightness, shortness of breath, palpitations, and anxiety—was again seen, as in previous studies. The symptoms were sporadic, beginning seconds to minutes after injection, lasting up to 30 min, and resolving spontaneously. They occurred in 19 (15.2%) of the patients taking glatiramer acetate as well as a few taking placebo. Most patients had only one or two such reactions over the course of the study, although five patients discontinued treatment because of it, including one in whom the reaction persisted for over an hour. Occasional true allergic reactions with skin rash and urticaria were seen but were much less frequent than the postinjection reaction. No significant laboratory abnormalities were found, nor were neutralizing antibodies detected. The possible occurrence of neutralizing antibodies

Table 5   Effects of Glatiramer Acetate and Placebo on Progression

	Glatiramer	Placebo	Significance
Core study			
Progression-free patients	78.4%	75.4%	NS
(EDSS confirmed at 3 months)			
EDSS change from baseline			
Improved	24.8%	15.2%	
Unchanged	54.4%	56.0%	$p = 0.037$
Worse	20.8%	28.8%	
Mean EDSS change from baseline	−0.05	0.21	$p = 0.023$
Extension			
Progression-free patients	70.6%	76.8%	NS
EDSS change from baseline			
Improved	27.2%	12.0%	
Unchanged	54.4%	56.8%	$p = 0.024$
Worse	18.4%	31.2%	
Mean EDSS change from baseline	−0.11	0.34	$p = 0.02$
Progression ≥ 1.5 EDSS points by Kaplan-Meier analysis	21.6%	41.6%	$p = 0.001$

Sources: From Refs. 28 and 54.

was a matter of interest because of a compelling, though controversial, body of evidence suggesting that neutralization of IFN-β is important in determining loss of clinical and MRI efficacy (8–10). Nearly all patients receiving glatiramer acetate developed binding antibodies detectable by enzyme-linked immunosorbent assay (ELISA) (11,12), with antibody levels peaking at 3 to 4 months and then declining to a level slightly above baseline. However, no evidence of neutralization could be detected, and no correlations were found between glatiramer acetate antibody titer and the occurrence of relapses or postinjection reactions.

After 2 years, subjects were given the option of continuing on blinded treatment. Over 80 percent of patients (99 on glatiramer acetate and 104 on placebo) elected to do so, the glatiramer acetate patients continuing for a mean of 5.2 months, and the placebo patients for 5.9 months. Some patients continued for up to 35 months. This extension (Table 5) permitted the collection of additional data that confirmed and strengthened the results of the core study (5). Final relapse rates, recalculated for the entire trial period, showed a 32% reduction in favor of glatiramer acetate ($p = 0.002$). The proportion of relapse-free patients, and median time to first relapse also became statistically significant. All patients who had been relapse-free in the original study remained so in the extension. When proportions of patients who improved on glatiramer acetate and worsened on placebo by one or more EDSS points were tested, the significant differences favoring glatiramer acetate were maintained, although the comparison of patients with progression sustained for 3 months still did not attain significance (29.4% of placebo patients versus 23.2% of glatiramer acetate patients, $p = 0.199$). However, Kaplan-Meier curves generated for patients who progressed by 1.5 EDSS points did show a significant treatment effect on slowing of disability progression (5). In the placebo group, 41.6% of patients worsened by 1.5 points or more, whereas in the glatiramer acetate group only 21.6% worsened ($p = 0.001$). The result was not complicated by intercurrent relapses, since EDSS scores obtained during relapses and for 30 days afterward were excluded from the survival analysis. Significant results were also obtained for progression by ≥ 1.0 EDSS point (placebo 59.2% versus glatiramer acetate 42.4%, $p = 0.008$), but the data for a 1.5-point change were considered more robust and less subject to examiner variability (13). When a somewhat different data analysis, the integrated disability status score (IDSS) or area under the curve (14) was applied, this combined measure of relapes and progression over time also showed a positive effect of the drug (15). Thus the therapeutic effects of glatiramer acetate were maintained for up to 35 months, and most of the outcome measures suggested that its clinical efficacy persisted and improved with time.

The patients were then permitted to continue on open-label treatment. Of the original 251 patients, 208 chose to continue on active drug. Data are now available for 5 to 7 years of follow-up, including the double-blind phase of approximately 30 months and the open-label phase of over 36 months (16). The subjects were approximately evenly divided between those originally assigned to glatiramer acetate or placebo. Patients were examined every 6 months, using the same outcome measures as in the blinded portion of the study, and in most cases by the same examiners. Admittedly, there are problems in interpreting such a study without a placebo control group. Various attempts have been made to use natural history controls with questionable success. Nevertheless, at this time some conclusions can be drawn: The majority of patients (152 of 208 or 73%) remain on treatment, continue to experience extremely low rates of relapse and progression, and tolerate the drug well. The overall annualized relapse rate for patients on active drug throughout the study (median time on drug, 5.83 years) was 0.42 attacks per year, and for year 6 the relapse rate was 0.23—i.e., one relapse every 4 to 5 years. Similar rates of decline were seen in the group originally randomized to placebo, although their annualized relapse rate was higher. Meanwhile, the majority showed no evidence of EDSS progression, indicating that cessation of relapses did not signal conversion to secondary progressive MS. Patients who left the study were surveyed by questionnaire. As expected, they reported more frequent relapses and greater disability than those remaining in the study, indicating a certain amount of selection bias. However the majority continued to take an immunomodulator, including 10 patients who remained on treatment with glatiramer acetate.

In addition, a limited magnetic resonance imaging (MRI) component was belatedly added to the open-label trial (17). Gadolinium-enhanced and T2-weighted MRI scans were performed in 135 patients, distributed evenly between those originally randomized to glatiramer acetate (mean 6.7 years on treatment) or to placebo (mean 4.0 years on treatment). Surprisingly, significant differences, favoring early initiation of therapy, were found in terms of gadolinium-enhancing lesions, brain atrophy, and a composite score that included those two variables as well as T2 lesion volumes and T1 hypointense lesion volumes. Admittedly, the clinical significance of these findings is problematic in this mixed and selected population followed in the absence of a control group. However, there are no comparable long-term follow-up data for any other immunomodulator. Therefore, plans have been made to continue the open-label study, including additional MRI scans, for a full 10 years from original study enrollment.

D. European-Canadian MRI Study of Glatiramer Acetate in Relapsing-Remitting MS

MRI studies were not included in the phase III pivotal trial except for those done at a single site (6), which showed a trend toward reduction in enhancing and T2 lesions. In another small study (18), Mancardi and colleagues followed 10 patients with monthly gadolinium-enhanced scans for 9 to 27 months before and 10 to 14 months during treatment with glatiramer acetate. The mean number of new contrast-enhancing lesions was reduced by 57% during the treatment period; there were significant reductions in number of new enhancing lesions per patient and proportion of scans with new enhancing lesions as well as a trend toward reduction of mean lesion area. Relapses were also greatly reduced, from 2.5 per year in the pretreatment period to 0.3 in the treatment phase of the study.

In 1997 a multinational randomized, double-blind, placebo-controlled MRI trial was begun in patients with relapsing-remitting MS and EDSS scores of 0 to 5 to determine the magnitude and time course of the effect of glatiramer acetate (19,20). The study population was enriched for patients with active disease by requiring one or more relapses in the 2 years prior to entry, and one or more contrast-enhancing lesions on baseline MRI scan. A total of 239 eligible patients were randomized to treatment with either placebo or 20 mg/day of glatiramer acetate and followed clinically and with monthly scans for 9 months. The placebo-treated patients were then crossed over to active drug and all participants were followed for an additional 9 months, with scans every 3 months. All MRI scans were analyzed at a central reading facility utilizing semiautomated techniques. Except for the inclusion of MRI, the study design was very similar to the U.S. pivotal trial, and the patients populations were also comparable in terms of age, disease duration, prestudy relapse rate, and EDSS score. In addition, the treatment and placebo groups were well matched within the study for both clinical and MRI parameters. Nearly all patients completed the study, and approximately 95% of the planned MRI scans were available for analysis.

In the double-blind portion of the study, there was a statistically significant 29% reduction ($p = 0.003$) in the primary outcome measure, mean total number of gadolinium-enhancing lesions, with glatiramer acetate treatment. Similar results were found for nearly all secondary outcome measures, including new enhancing lesions ($p < 0.003$), enhancing lesion volumes ($p = 0.01$), new T2 lesions ($p < 0.003$), and change in T2 lesion volumes from baseline to month 9 ($p = 0.006$). The most striking feature of the study was the time course of the response to glatiramer acetate.

Treatment effects for all outcome variables could be expressed as a series of diverging curves (Fig. 1), with differences between placebo and treatment groups first becoming apparent at 3 months, and statistically significant at 6 to 7 months. Although enhancing lesions and T2 volumes accumulated in both groups, the rate of accumulation was consistently lower in glatiramer acetate–than in placebo-treated patients. In addition, the mean relapse rate was 33% lower in the glatiramer acetate group ($p = 0.012$), with nearly all of the difference coming in the third trimester. The drug was well tolerated, with the most severe adverse events being immediate postinjection reactions in 37.8 percent of the drug-treated group—a surprisingly high number compared to previous trials.

After 9 months, all patients were crossed over to open-label treatment with glatiramer acetate and were examined every 3 months. Of the original 239 patients, 225 entered the open-label phase and over 95% completed it, showing that the drug was extremely well tolerated. The robust effects on MRI were maintained in the group originally treated with active drug, and their relapse rates continued to decline as well. The group that switched from placebo to glatiramer acetate responded positively to treatment and showed significantly fewer enhancing lesions ($p = 0.0001$) than during the placebo-treatment

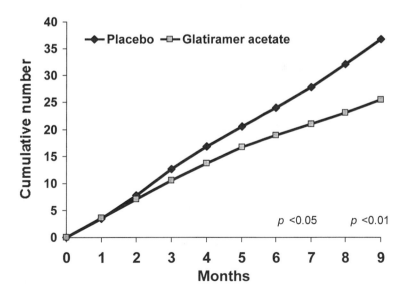

Figure 1 Cumulative number of enhancing lesions over 9 months in the European/Canadian MRI trial of glatiramer acetate. This curve is representative of the time course for nearly all MRI parameters. Slowing in accumulation of lesions was first apparent at month 3 and became statistically significant after 6 months.

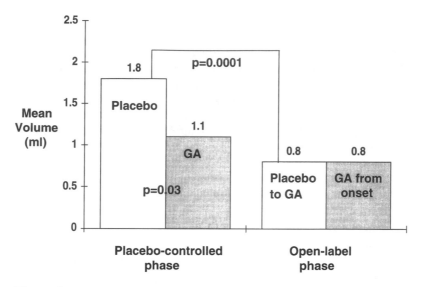

Figure 2 Total enhancing lesion volume in the placebo-controlled and open-label phases of the European/Canadian MRI trial. For this analysis, data obtained at 3-month intervals during both phases were used. There was a significant reduction in lesion volume ($p = 0.03$) during the initial phase and an even more significant reduction ($p = 0.0001$) during the second phase for subjects who were switched from placebo to glatiramer acetate. Subjects maintained on glatiramer acetate from onset showed a further reduction in lesion volume during the open-label phase.

phase. Similar effects were seen for enhancing lesion volume (Fig. 2), change in T2 lesion volume, and relapse rate. Thus the clinical and MRI benefits of glatiramer acetate treatment seen in the placebo-controlled trial were confirmed in the open-label phase and in fact continued to improve with increasing time on active treatment.

The results of this trial indicate a highly significant effect on MRI measures of disease activity but one that is delayed by 3 to 6 months in contrast to the effect of INF-β, which is almost immediate (21,22). This is thought to be consistent with the mechanism of action of glatiramer acetate, which involves generation of activated Th2 lymphocytes that cross the blood-brain barrier, become restimulated by myelin antigens within MS lesions, and secrete suppressive cytokines that downregulate the inflammatory autoimmune response (23). As described below, this process leads to gradual induction of immune tolerance but requires several months to take effect and is thus highly consistent with the changes seen on MRI. Effects on blood-brain barrier permeability, as detected by gadolinium-enhanced MRI, are probably secondary to reduced disease activity and therefore may take months to appear. Furthermore, the MRI effects of glatiramer acetate are consistent with its degree of clinical efficacy, in contrast the the beta interferons, which reduce MRI activity by 70 to 90% but reduce relapse rates or slow progression by only about 30%.

E. Studies of Glatiramer Acetate Currently in Progress

Three studies of interest are mentioned briefly here. The first is the PROMiSe trial of glatiramer acetate in primary progressive MS. Primary progressive disease afflicts 12 to 15% of all MS patients and has a relatively poor prognosis, usually leading to ambulatory disability in 10 years or less. The trial is based on a retrospective analysis of an earlier study in progressive MS (4), which showed an effect on a subgroup of 30 subjects with primary progressive disease. In addition, there is relatively little evidence of inflammation on MRI in primary progressive MS, suggesting that an agent such as glatiramer acetate, whose mechanism of action does not primarily involve blood-brain barrier integrity, may be potentially beneficial. In the PROMiSe trial, 947 patients with progressive spastic paraparesis, EDSS scores of 3.0 to 6.5 inclusive, and oligoclonal bands or elevated IgG index in the cerebrospinal fluid (CSF) were randomized at over 50 centers in the United States and Canada to receive either 20 mg of glatiramer acetate or placebo by daily subcutaneous injection for a period of 3 years. Two-thirds of the patients receive active drug and one-third placebo. The primary efficacy endpoint is time to confirmed disease progression as measured by defined incremental changes in EDSS scores. Patients are evaluated every 3 months by blinded examiners. A number of secondary outcome measures, including measurement of brain atrophy and T1 hypointense lesions (''black holes'') on MRI, will also be assessed. Currently the study is fully enrolled, which is encouraging considering the rarity of the condition. However, results are not anticipated for several years.

A large multinational trial of oral glatiramer acetate, given the acronym CORAL, has also recently begun. It is based on observations in experimental animals (rats, mice, and monkeys) showing that glatiramer acetate can prevent or suppress EAE when administered orally and apparently does so by inducing suppressive Th2 cytokines, similar to its mechanism of action when given parenterally (24). Although induction of oral tolerance with whole myelin did not succeed in suppressing disease activity in MS (25,26), glatiramer acetate may be more effective because it is not encephalitogenic in animals and its efficacy in MS by the parenteral route has already been established (27). CORAL is designed as a global study including 1650 patients with clinically definite relapsing-remitting MS, one or more attacks in the year prior to entry, and EDSS scores of 0 to 5.0. They have been randomized to either 5 mg or 50 mg of glatiramer acetate or matched placebo tablets taken daily for 56 weeks and will be evaluated clinically every 2 months. MRI scans will be done on all patients at baseline and study completion and a subset of one-third of the patients will have gadolinium-enhanced scans every 2 months. The primary outcome measure, selected to establish efficacy comparable to that shown by parenteral glatiramer acetate, is total number of documented relapses per group. Numerous clinical and MRI-based secondary outcome variables will be evaluated as well. In designing this study, there was concern about the ethics of performing a placebo-controlled trial in relapsing-remitting MS now that at least three approved products are readily available. However, a study of brief duration was considered acceptable provided that subjects were fully informed and aware of the alternatives. A preliminary safety study in MS patients given doses up to 300 mg of oral glatiramer acetate for 10 days revealed only mild adverse events; however, two interim analyses were built into the protocol to permit the committee monitoring data and safety to stop the study in the event of unacceptable toxicity. If successful, this study could revolutionize the treatment of relapsing-remitting MS. Despite the encouraging preclinical data and plausible immunological rationale, however, it remains an uncertain and risky undertaking.

The third study of current interest is a combination trial of glatiramer acetate and IFN-β-1a in relapsing-remitting MS called CombiRx. This is a small multicenter study to determine whether adding daily injections of glatiramer acetate to weekly IFN-β-1a (Avonex) is safe or results in increased clinical or MRI activity. The study is based on two conflicting sets of observations: a study in vitro demonstrating additive and synergistic suppression of myelin basic protein (MBP)–specific T cell lines by combined treatment with IFN-β and glatiramer acetate (28) and a study in vivo showing that combination therapy with glatiramer acetate and IFN-α resulted in worsening of EAE in mice (29). Although type I interferons and glatiramer acetate both suppress EAE, they work by different mechanisms. The beneficial effect of IFN-β in MS is partially related to its ability to inhibit matrix metalloproteinase secretion by activated T cells, reducing their ability to penetrate the blood-brain barrier (30,31). Glatiramer acetate's mechanism of action, on the other hand, probably requires migration of activated T cells into the CNS, where they produce Th2 type cytokines that act via bystander suppression (23,32,33). Its effects on blood-brain barrier permeability appear to be indirect (34). Thus treatment with IFN-β could theoretically impede access of glatiramer acetate-activated cells to sites of inflammation in the CNS. The CombiRx study is nearing completion, and the results should be available early in 2001. If successful, it could serve as the prototype for a larger controlled trial of the IFN-β/glatiramer acetate combination as well as other potential combinations of immunoactive agents.

III. IMMUNOLOGICAL ACTIVITY OF GLATIRAMER ACETATE

A. Studies in EAE

Glatiramer acetate is a synthetic mixture of polypeptides composed of four amino acids, L-alanine, L-glutamic acid, L-lysine, and L-tyrosine (Table 2) synthesized in the 1960s by Drs. Sela, Arnon, and Teitelbaum and their colleagues at the Weizmann Institute of Science in Israel as one of several copolymers developed to resemble MBP (35). These copolymers were originally designed to investigate the interaction of myelin proteins and lipids thought to be responsible for induction of EAE, a T cell–mediated autoimmune disease of the central nervous system and the best available animal model of MS. EAE can be induced by sensitization with encephalitogenic peptide fragments of the MBP molecule and prevented or modified by many antigen-specific and nonspecific manipulations, including treatment with nonencephalitogenic fragments of MBP (36). When the copolymers were initially tested, animals challenged with them failed to develop EAE but were protected when rechallenged with MBP or spinal cord emulsion (37). Glatiramer acetate was the most effective of these substances in preventing EAE in rodents and was found to be effective in other species as well (38).

Perhaps the most intriguing observations from the point of view of MS therapy were those on chronic relapsing EAE, which closely mimics the human disease in terms of clinical activity and pathology (39). Pretreatment with glatiramer acetate reduced or delayed relapses of clinical signs, and administration of glatiramer acetate after onset of disease modified the duration and intensity of relapses. These early observations showed that glatiramer acetate could suppress an ongoing autoimmune response after establishment of disease—an obvious requirement for treatment of MS. Glatiramer acetate was also remarkably nontoxic, producing no significant adverse reactions in treated animals. Moreover, it did not appear to interfere with systemic immunity to nonneural antigens.

B. Proposed Mechanisms of Action

The two principal mechanisms proposed for glatiramer acetate activity in EAE and MS are (a) interference with T-cell activation by competition with MBP for the MHC class

II binding site involved in antigen presentation and (b) induction of glatiramer acetate-specific CD4+ T cells that produce regulatory cytokines and downregulate the disease process via the process of bystander suppression. Early studies of cellular and humoral immune responses indicated that glatiramer acetate has at least partial cross-reactivity with MBP and reacts with monoclonal antibodies raised against MBP as well as with T cells or T-cell lines sensitized to MBP (40–43). Other investigators, however, have disputed the claims that glatiramer acetate and MBP are antigenically cross-reactive in the strict sense (44–46). Teitelbaum and coworkers reported that glatiramer acetate could specifically inhibit proliferation and IL-2 secretion by murine (42) and human (43) MBP-specific T-cell lines and clones in vitro through competition with MBP for binding to MHC class II molecules on antigen-presenting cells. More recently, direct "promiscuous" binding of glatiramer acetate to human antigen-presenting cells and purified HLA-DR molecules was shown (47,48). Furthermore, glatiramer acetate can inhibit binding of MBP or the MBP peptide p84-102 to these cells through competition for MHC class II surface molecules. Thus, it may be more appropriate to characterize glatiramer acetate and MBP as mutually inhibitory rather than cross-reactive in the classic sense.

Evidence for suppressor activity has evolved more recently, especially since the Th1/Th2 paradigm of T-cell regulation (49) has become more widely appreciated and demonstrated in humans as well as mice. The early observation that spleen cells from mice treated with glatiramer acetate could transfer protection against EAE but that the effect was abrogated by cyclophosphamide suggested that the protection was mediated by regulatory cells (50). This was later confirmed by showing that T-cell hybridomas and T-cell lines induced with glatiramer acetate could inhibit the response of MBP-specific T cell lines and prevent active induction of EAE (51). Subsequently, a number of additional studies were reported supporting the finding that glatiramer acetate induces and activates CD4+ cells of the Th2/Th3 phenotype, which secrete suppressive cytokines such as IL-4, IL-6, IL-10, and TGF-β, but not the Th1 cytokines IFN-γ or TNF-α (32,33). In these studies, the Th2 response arose slowly, beginning after 6 weeks in culture, and was not fully developed until 6 months of restimulation with antigen. Treatment of MS patients with glatiramer acetate for 1 year was recently reported (23) to upregulate cytokine mRNA expression of IL-4 and TGF-β, reduce expression of TNF-α mRNA, and increase serum levels of IL-10. The most striking feature of these findings was their slow development over 3 to 6 months, which corresponds to the delay in generation of MBP cross-reactive Th2 cells seen in vitro (33) and to the delay in clinical and MRI efficacy noted in the recent European/Canadian MRI study (19,20). These findings are all consistent with the proposed mechanism of action of the drug. However, the cytokine study was confined to a small number of patients, utilized methods that are not quite state-of-the-art, and has not yet been confirmed. Thus the mechanism of action of glatiramer acetate in humans remains semihypothetical, although evidence for real and reproducible regulatory effects on the immune system is undeniable.

The relative specificity of glatiramer acetate for MBP may seem paradoxical in view of its random molecular structure and striking lack of specificity for species, MBP epitope, or MHC restriction. Alternatively, the specificity of glatiramer acetate for MBP may be a function of limited testing, as suggested by Racke et al. (52), who found that glatiramer acetate inhibited in vitro responses of T-cell hybridomas specific for ovalbumin and insulin. Other investigators have shown that ovalbumin, a nonneural protein, can inhibit activation of MBP-specific T cells (53). As additional antigens are investigated, it may become clear why immune responses to some are inhibited by glatiramer acetate while responses to others are not. Furthermore, glatiramer acetate can inhibit binding of myelin proteolipid protein (PLP) and myelin-oligodendrocyte glycoprotein (MOG), both of which are encephalitogenic, to MHC molecules on antigen-presenting cells (54), and it can suppress EAE induced in mice by PLP (55) and MOG (56). Since there is essentially no sequence homology between MBP and PLP or MOG, the suppressive effect may be attributed to induction of Th2 cytokines and bystander suppression.

Other immunological mechanisms may also be involved. Glatiramer acetate has long been known to induce proliferation of naive normal T cells (57). Furthermore, glatiramer acetate–reactive T-cell lines can easily be generated from normal individuals (28, 43,45). These observations were recently confirmed by Hafler and colleagues (58), who characterized glatiramer acetate as a "universal antigen" that induces proliferation in T-cell lines from normal or MS subjects independent of any prior exposure. In MS patients treated with glatiramer acetate, the proliferative response declined gradually; after several months, it could not be restored with IL-2, suggesting the development of tolerance by activation-induced cell death (59). Glatiramer acetate-reactive T cell lines secreted the Th2 cytokines IL-5 and IL-13. They were also shown to cross-react rather broadly with a combinatorial peptide library based on the immunodominant epitope of MBP, indicating "degeneracy" of the the T-cell receptor and suggesting that glatiramer acetate may act as an altered peptide ligand to induce Th2 cells in response to itself or to MBP peptides. It has been shown that a single amino acid substitution can convert an encephalitogenic MBP peptide to a protective one (60). This mechanism has also been applied to reactivity of human T-cell lines, in which substitution of individual MBP contact residues (amino acids at specific positions in the dominant epitope, critical for contact with the T-cell receptor) can convert inflammatory Th1-type cells to regulatory Th2-type cells that secrete suppressive cytokines (61). Although the structure of glatiramer acetate is random, particular sequences may be present in adequate quantity to act as altered peptide ligands for MBP and possibly other myelin antigens. These would resemble the native peptides sufficiently to bind avidly to MHC class II molecules and react with the MBP-specific T-cell receptors but induce tolerance or a regulatory cytokine profile rather than an autoimmune attack on CNS myelin. This scenario would account for many of the features of glatiramer acetate described above. It would also bring together the observations on competitive MHC binding and suppressor cell induction as parts of the same immunoregulatory process.

One additional issue must be mentioned, namely oral tolerance induced by glatiramer acetate. The mechanism by which this occurs is not entirely understood, but the available evidence suggests it may be remarkably similar to the mechanism of action of the parenterally administered agent (27). Oral glatiramer acetate can suppress EAE in rats and mice, and suppression can be adoptively transferred by antigen-specific T cells obtained from treated animals (24). It induces the suppressive cytokines IL-10 and TGF-β (but not IL-4) and inhibits secretion of IFN-γ. Furthermore, it is nonencephalitogenic in animals and already proven to reduce MS activity in humans. Thus it appears to be a very promising treatment modality and much more acceptable to patients than the daily injections required currently. In addition, the availability of an effective oral therapy for MS would greatly facilitate trials in combination with other drugs.

In summary, the mechanism of action of glatiramer acetate has become much more clearly defined in the past few years, although many details remain to be clarified. It may be briefly summarized as follows: Glatiramer acetate is a universal antigen that binds readily to multiple MHC types in both normal individuals and MS patients, induces proliferation, and acts as an altered peptide ligand to activate antigen-specific CD4+ T cells, polarizing them toward the Th2 phenotype. These activated cells cross the relatively intact blood-brain barrier, react with certain epitopes of MBP, and secrete regulatory cytokines such as IL-4, IL-10, IL-13, and TGF-β, which downregulate the synthesis of proinflammatory cytokines within active MS plaques, leading to suppression of the ongoing autoimmune response to multiple myelin antigens, including PLP and MOG, and ultimately to amelioration of the inflammatory, demyelinating, and neurodegenerative process.

IV. THE PLACE OF GLATIRAMER ACETATE IN MS THERAPY

Comparisons between glatiramer acetate (Copaxone) and the beta interferons (Avonex, Betaseron, and Rebif) are potentially hazardous because each agent was tested in separate studies, under different conditions, and in patient populations with different prestudy demographics, relapse rates, and levels of disability. IFN-β-1b was originally shown to have no convincing clinical effect on progression of MS, even though the trial was continued for up to 5 years in a subgroup of patients (62,63). Nevertheless, its effect on relapse rate and prevention of new MRI lesions was dramatic (64), suggesting that slowing of sustained neurological impairment might ultimately be expected. This was recently confirmed in the European study of IFN-β-1b in secondary progressive MS (65), but a similar North American study failed to show an effect on progression (66). IFN-β-1a (Avonex) was reported to slow progression (67), although it was tested in a much shorter clinical trial. The population studied was one with early relapsing-remitting disease and EDSS scores of 3.5 or less, raising questions as to whether 1-point changes at the lowest levels of the EDSS reflect genuine disability. Other studies of IFN-β-1a (Rebif) have given conflicting results, showing highly significant effects on relapses and MRI activity but no appreciable slowing of progression.

Glatiramer acetate was shown to have a definite and statistically significant effect on relapses and disability scores in a patient population with mild to moderate disability and an effect on MRI activity that was consistent with its clinical efficacy. Any attempt to compare glatiramer acetate with the various IFN-β products is subject to bias; however, in a recent review (68), we have attempted to give a fair appraisal of their strengths and weaknesses.

In the opinion of most neurologists, prevention or retardation of disability is the ''gold standard'' for MS treatment; however, agents that reduce the relapse rate may have substantial long-term benefit as well. The episodes of incapacity caused by MS attacks often result in time lost from work or other activities of daily living, increased medical expenses, and emotional distress. Thus agents that prevent even one-third of relapses, provided that they are easily administered and free of toxicity, represent substantial progress in the management of MS. Furthermore, prevention of acute attacks and of subclinical disease activity may have a long-term beneficial effect on the risk of future disability, as implied by epidemiological studies (69) and recent reports of frequent MRI scanning of MS patients (70–72). It is likely that this will prove to be true with all of the currently approved agents.

Other variables such as cost, frequency of dosing, and route of administration may favor one agent over another, but none of these is likely to be the determining factor in deciding which drug to recommend for a given patient (73). A major advantage of glatiramer acetate over IFN-β-1b and to a lesser extent IFN-β-1a is its favorable side-effect profile, consisting of relatively mild injection-site reactions and the transient systemic postinjection reaction of flushing, chest tightness, shortness of breath, palpitations, and anxiety that immediately follows a small percentage of injections. Nearly all patients who experience such a reaction quickly realize that it is not hazardous and accept the possibility of another one as a minor inconvenience. In contrast, patients beginning treatment with IFN-β-1b are subject to more severe injection-site reactions, an annoying flu-like syndrome that often (but not always) diminishes after the first few weeks or months, and a variety of other less common symptoms, including the worrisome risk of severe depression (62,63). In addition, up to 38% of patients taking IFN-β-1b for 18 to 24 months develop neutralizing antibodies, and many then cease to respond to the drug (63). The frequency of neutralizing antibody in patients treated with IFNβ-1a (Avonex) was reported to be somewhat less, 23% after 2 years (67), possibly because of the lower dose and the fact that IFN-β-1a resembles native human IFN-β more closely than IFN-β-1b does. In subsequent studies, the incidence was even lower (approximately 5%). Glatiramer acetate, by contrast, induces binding antibodies in all or nearly all patients, but thus far no evidence of neutralizing activity has been detected (11,12). In fact, its efficacy seems to increase with prolongation of treatment (5,16). Finally, although none of these agents should be taken during pregnancy, the risk appears to be least with glatiramer acetate (2).

V. SUMMARY

Glatiramer acetate is an unique noninterferon nonsteroidal therapy for MS that may be considered at least partially immunospecific. It has been extensively studied, and its mechanism of action is relatively well understood in the light of current immunological concepts. Not only has it been shown in randomized controlled clinical trials to be at least as effective as the beta interferons but its efficacy appears to increase with time. Furthermore, it has the most favorable side effect profile of all agents available to treat MS. Therefore it should be considered as first-line therapy for ambulatory patients with clinically definite or laboratory-supported definite relapsing-remitting MS, and treatment should be started as soon as possible after the diagnosis is established. In addition, it is suitable as alternative therapy for patients treated with IFN-β-1b who are unable to tolerate the drug or who are able to take it only at reduced dosage because of persistent side effects or laboratory abnormalities and in patients treated successfully with IFN-β-1b who, after a period of time, resume an unacceptable rate of relapses or progression associated with the development of neutralizing antibodies. In the future, glatiramer acetate in the oral formulation, and in combination with interferons or other drugs may prove to be useful in primary progressive MS. These ongoing studies, as well as the individual experience of neurologists and patients, will help to define further the role of this novel therapeutic agent.

REFERENCES

1. Bornstein MB, Miller A, Slagle S, Weitzman M, Crystal H, Drexler E, et al. A pilot trial of Cop 1 in exacerbating-remitting multiple sclerosis. N Engl J Med 1987; 317:408–414.
2. Johnson KP, Brooks BR, Cohen JA, Ford CC, Goldstein J, Lisak RP, et al. Copolymer 1 reduces relapse rate and improves disability in relapsing-remitting multiple sclerosis: Results of a phase III multicenter, double-blind, placebo-controlled trial. Neurology 1995; 45:1268–1276.

3. Bornstein MB, Miller AI, Teitelbaum D, Arnon R, Sela M. Multiple sclerosis: Trial of a synthetic polypeptide. Ann Neurol 1982; 11:317–319.

4. Bornstein MB, Miller A, Slagle S, Weitzman M, Drexler E, Keilson M, et al. A placebo-controlled, double-blind, randomized, two-center, pilot trial of cop 1 in chronic progressive multiple sclerosis. Neurology 1991; 41:533–539.

5. Johnson K, Brooks B, Cohen J, Ford C, Goldstein J, Lisak R et al. Extended use of glatiramer acetate (Copaxone) is well tolerated and maintains its clinical effect on multiple sclerosis relapse rate and degree of disability. Neurology 1998; 50:701–708.

6. Cohen JA, Grossman RI, Udupa JK et al. Assessment of the efficacy of copolymer-1 in the treatment of multiple sclerosis by quantitative MRI (abstr). Neurology 1995; 45(suppl 4): A418.

7. Ge Y, Grossman R, Udupa J, Fulton J, Constantinescu C, Gonzales-Scarano F, et al. Glatiramer acetate (Copaxone) treatment in relapsing-remitting MS. Quantitative MR assessment. Neurology 2000; 54:813–817.

8. The IFNB Multiple Sclerosis Study Group and the University of British Columbia MS/MRI Analysis Group. Neutralizing antibodies during treatment of multiple sclerosis with interferon beta-1b: Experience during the first three years. Neurology 1996; 47:889–894.

9. Rudick R, Simonian N, Alam J, Campion M, Scaramucci J, Jones W, et al. Incidence and significance of neutralizing antibodies to interferon beta-1a in multiple sclerosis. Neurology 1998; 50:1266–1272.

10. Paszner B, Petkau J, Oger J. Neutralising antibodies to interferon-beta in the treatment of multiple sclerosis. Cause for concern? CNS Drugs 1999;11:225–243.

11. Johnson KP, Teitelbaum D, Arnon R. Antibodies to copolymer 1 do not interfere with its clinical effect (abstr). Ann Neurol 1995; 38:973.

12. Brenner T, Meiner Z, Abramsky O, Steinitz M, Sicsic C, Wirguin I, et al. Humoral responses to copolymer 1 in multiple sclerosis patients: Preferential production of IgG1 over IgG2 (abstr). Ann Neurol 1996; 40:518.

13. Sharrack B, Hughes R. Clinical scales for multiple sclerosis. J Neurol Sci 1996; 135:1–9.

14. Liu C, Li Wan Po A. "Summary measure" statistic for assessing the outcome of treatment trials in relapsing-remitting multiple sclerosis. J Neurol Neurosurg Psychiatry 1998; 64:726–729.

15. Johnson K and the Copolymer 1 Study Group. Efficacy of glatiramer acetate (Copaxone) on multiple sclerosis disability is confirmed by analysis with the integrated disability status scale (IDSS). Neurology 1998; 50(suppl 4):A62–A63.

16. Johnson K, Brooks B, Ford C, Goodman A, Guarnaccia J, Lisak R, et al. Sustained clinical benefits of glatiramer acetate in relapsing multiple sclerosis patients observed for six years. Multiple Sclerosis 2000; 6:255–266.

17. Wolinsky J, Narayana P. Magnetic resonance imaging and clinical correlation in a cross-sectional analysis of patients in the open-label extension of the US pivotal trial of glatiramer acetate (Copaxone) in relapsing multiple sclerosis (abstr). Ann Neurol 1999; 46:471.

18. Mancardi G, Sardanelli F, Parodi R, Melani E, Capello E, Inglese M, et al. Effect of copolymer-1 on serial gadolinium-enhanced MRI in relapsing remitting multiple sclerosis. Neurology 1998; 50:1127–1133.

19. Comi G, Filippi M, for the Copaxone MRI Study Group. The effect of glatiramer acetate (Copaxone) on disease activity as measured by cerebral MRI in patients with relapsing-remitting multiple sclerosis (RRMS): A multi-center, randomized, double-blind, placebo-controlled study extended by open-label treatment (abstr). Neurology 1999; 52(suppl 2):A289

20. Comi G, Filippi M, and the European/Canadian Glatiramer Acetate Study Group. The European/Canadian multicenter, double blind, placebo controlled study of the effects of Glatiramer Acetate on magnetic resonance imaging-measured disease activity and burden in patients with relapsing multiple sclerosis. Ann Neurol. In press.

21. Stone LA, Frank JA, Albert PS, Bash C, Smith ME, Maloni H, et al. The effect of interferon-β on blood-brain barrier disruptions demonstrated by contrast-enhanced magnetic resonance imaging in relapsing-remitting multiple sclerosis. Ann Neurol 1995; 37:611–619.

22. Calabresi P, Stone L, Bash C, Frank J, McFarland H. Interferon beta results in immediate reduction of contrast-enhanced MRI lesions in multiple sclerosis patients followed by weekly MRI. Neurology 1997; 48:1446–1448.

23. Miller A, Shapiro S, Gershtein R, Kinarty A, Rawashdeh H, Honigman S, et al. Treatment of multiple sclerosis with copolymer-1 (Copaxone): Implicating mechanisms of Th1 to Th2/Th3 immune deviation. J Neuroimmunol 1998; 92:113–121.

24. Teitelbaum D, Arnon R, Sela M. Immunomodulation of experimental autoimmune encephalomyelitis by oral administration of copolymer 1. Proc Natl Acad Sci USA 1999; 96:3842–3847.

25. Weiner HL, Mackin GA, Matsui M, Orav EJ, Khoury SJ, Dawson DM, et al. Double-blind pilot trial of oral tolerization with myelin antigens in multiple sclerosis. Science 1993; 259:1321–1324.

26. Panitch H, Francis G and the Oral Myelin Study Group. Clinical results of a phase III trial of oral myelin in relapsing-remitting multiple sclerosis (abstr). Ann Neurol 1997; 42:459.

27. Weiner H. Commentary: Oral tolerance with copolymer 1 for the treatment of multiple sclerosis. Proc Natl Acad Sci USA 1999; 96:3333–3335.

28. Milo R, Panitch H. Additive effects of copolymer-1 and interferon beta-1b on the immune response to myelin basic protein. J Neuroimmunol 1995; 61:185–193.

29. Brod S, Lindsey J, Wolinsky J. Combination therapy with glatiramer acetate (copolymer-1) and a type I interferon (IFN-α) does not improve experimental autoimmune encephalomyelitis. Ann Neurol 2000; 47:127–131.

30. Stüve O, Dooley N, Uhm J, Antel J, Francis G, Williams G. Interferon β-1b decreases the migration of T lymphocytes in vitro: Effects on matrix metalloproteinase-9. Ann Neurol 1996; 40:853–863.

31. Yong V, Chabot S, Stuve O, Williams G. Interferon beta in the treatment of multiple sclerosis: Mechanism of action. Neurology 1998; 51:682–689.

32. Aharoni R, Teitelbaum D, Sela M, Arnon R. Bystander suppression of experimental autoimmune encephalomyelitis by T cell lines and clones of the Th2 type induced by copolymer 1. J Neuroimmunol 1998; 91:135–146.

33. Aharoni R, Teitelbaum D, Sela M, Arnon R. Copolymer 1 induces T cells of the T helper type 2 that crossreact with myelin basic protein and suppress experimental autoimmune encephalomyelitis. Proc Natl Acad Sci USA 1997; 94:10821–10826.

34. Prat A, Al-Asmi A, Duquette P, Antel J. Lymphocyte migration and multiple sclerosis: Relation with disease course and therapy. Ann Neurol 1999; 46:253–256.

35. Arnon R. The development of cop 1 (Copaxone), an innovative drug for the treatment of multiple sclerosis: Personal reflections. Immunol Lett 1996; 50:1–15.

36. Paterson PY. Autoimmune neurological disease: experimental animal systems and implications for multiple sclerosis. In: Talal N, ed. Autoimmunity: Genetic Immunologic, Virologic and Clinical Aspects. New York: Academic Press, 1977, pp 643–692.

37. Teitelbaum D, Meshorer A, Hirshfeld T, Arnon R, Sela M. Suppression of experimental allergic encephalomyelitis by a synthetic polypeptide. Eur J Immunol 1971; 1:242–248.

38. Arnon R, Teitelbaum D. Desensitization of experimental allergic encephalomyelitis with synthetic peptide analogues. In: Davison AN, Cuzner ML, eds. The Suppression of Experimental Allergic Encephalomyelitis and Multiple Sclerosis. New York: Academic Press, 1980, pp 105–117.

39. Keith AB, Arnon R, Teitelbaum D, Caspary EA, Wisniewski HM. The effect of cop 1, a synthetic polypeptide, on chronic relapsing experimental allergic encephalomyelitis in guinea pigs. J Neurol Sci 1979; 42:267–274.

40. Webb C, Teitelbaum D, Arnon R, Sela M. In vivo and in vitro immunological cross-reactions between basic encephalitogen and synthetic basic polypeptides capable of suppressing experimental allergic encepyalomyelitis. Eur J Immunol 1973; 3:279–286.

41. Teitelbaum D, Aharoni R, Sela M, Arnon R. Cross-reactions and specificities of monoclonal antibodies against myelin basic protein and against the synthetic copolymer 1. Proc Natl Acad Sci USA 1991; 88:9528–9532.

42. Teitelbaum D, Aharoni R, Arnon R, Sela M. Specific inhibition of the T-cell response to myelin basic protein by the synthetic copolymer cop 1. Proc Natl Acad Sci USA 1988; 85: 9724–9728.

43. Teitelbaum D, Milo R, Arnon R, Sela M. Synthetic copolymer 1 inhibits human T-cell lines specific for myelin basic protein. Proc Natl Acad Sci USA 1992; 89:137–141.

44. Lisak RP, Sweiman B, Blanchard N, Rorke LB. Effect of treatment with copolymer 1 (cop 1) on the in vivo and in vitro manifestations of experimental allergic encephalomyelitis. J Neurol Sci 1983; 62:281–293.

45. Burns J, Krasner J, Guerrero F. Human cellular immune response to copolymer 1 and myelin basic protein. Neurology 1986; 36:92–94.

46. Burns J, Littlefield J. Failure of copolymer 1 to inhibit the human T-cell response to myelin basic protein. Neurology 1991; 41:1317–1319.

47. Fridkis-Hareli M, Teitelbaum D, Gurevitch E, Pecht I, Brautbar H, Kwon OJ, et al. Direct binding of myelin basic protein and synthetic copolymer 1 to class II major histocompatibility complex molecules on living antigen presenting cells-specificity and promiscuity. Proc Natl Acad Sci USA 1994; 91:4872–4876.

48. Fridkis-Hareli M, Strominger J. Promiscuous binding of synthetic copolymer 1 to purified HLA-DR molecules. J Immunol 1998; 160:4386–4397.

49. Mosmann T, Coffman R. Two types of mouse helper T cell clone: Implications for immune regulation. Immunol Today 1987; 8:223–227.

50. Lando Z, Teitelbaum D, Arnon R. Effect of cyclophosphamide on suppressor cell activity in mice unresponsive to EAE. J Immunol 1979; 123:2156–2160.

51. Aharoni R, Teitelbaum D, Arnon R. T suppressor hybridomas and interleukin-2–dependent lines induced by copolymer 1 or by spinal cord homogenate down-regulate experimental allergic encephalomyelitis. Eur J Immunol 1993; 23:17–25.

52. Racke MK, Martin R, McFarland H, Fritz RB. Copolymer-1-induced inhibition of antigen-specific T cell activation: interference with antigen presentation. J Neuroimmunol 1992; 37: 75–84.

53. Gautam AM, Glynn P. Competition between foreign and self proteins in antigen presentation: Ovalbumin can inhibit activation of myelin basic protein-specific T cells. J Immunol 1990; 144:1177–1180.

54. Fridkis-Hareli M, Teitelbaum D, Kerlero de Rosbo N, Arnon R, Sela M. Synthetic copolymer 1 inhibits the binding of MBP, PLP, and MOG peptides to class II major histocompatibility complex molecules on antigen presenting cells. J Neurochem 1994; 63 (suppl 1):S61D.

55. Teitelbaum D, Fridkis-Hareli M, Arnon R, Sela M. Copolymer 1 inhibits the onset of chronic relapsing experimental allergic encephalomyelitis induced by proteolipid protein (PLP) peptides in mice and interferes with PLP-specific T-cell responses. J Neuroimmunol 1996; 64: 209–217.

56. Ben-Nun A, Mendel I, Bakimer R, Fridkis-Hareli M, Teitelbaum D, Arnon R, et al. The autoimmune reactivity against myelin oligodendrocyte glycoprotein (MOG) in multiple sclerosis is potentially pathogenic: Effect of copolymer-1 on MOG-induced disease. J Neurol 1996; 243(suppl):S14–S22.

57. Brosnan CF, Litwak M, Neighbour A, Lyman WD, Carter TH, Bornstein MB, et al. Immunogenic potentials of copolymer 1 in normal human lymphocytes. Neurology 1985; 35:1754–1759, 1985

58. Duda P, Schmied M, Cook S, Krieger J, Hafler D. Glatiramer acetate (Copaxone) induces

degenerate, Th2-polarized immune responses in patients with multiple sclerosis. J Clin Invest 2000; 105:967–976.

59. Schmied M, Duda P, Krieger J, Trollmo T, Hafler D. Subcutaneous administration of glatiramer acetate induces antigen specific CD4 T cell tolerance. Neurology 2000; 54(suppl 3): A149.

60. Smilek DE, Wraith DC, Hodgkinson S, Dwivedy S, Steinman L, McDevitt HO. A single amino acid change in a myelin basic protein peptide confers the capacity to prevent rather than induce experimental autoimmune encephalomyelitis. Proc Natl Acad Sci USA 1991; 88: 9633–9637.

61. Hafler DA, Weiner HL. Immunologic mechanisms and therapy in multiple sclerosis. Immunol Rev 1995; 144:75–105.

62. IFNB Multiple Sclerosis Study Group. Interferon beta-1b is effective in relapsing-remitting multiple sclerosis: I. Clinical results of a multicenter, randomized, double-blind, placebo-controlled trial. Neurology 1993; 43:655–661.

63. IFNB Multiple Sclerosis Study Group and University of British Columbia MS/MRI Analysis Group. Interferon beta-1b in the treatment of multiple sclerosis: Final outcome of the randomized controlled trial. Neurology 1995; 45:1277–1285.

64. Paty DW, Li DKB, UBC MS/MRI Study Group and IFNB Multiple Sclerosis Study Group. Interferon beta-1b is effective in relapsing-remitting multiple sclerosis: II. MRI analysis results of a multicenter, randomized, double-blind, placebo-controlled trial. Neurology 1993; 43:662–667.

65. European Study Group on Interferon β-1b in Secondary Progressive MS. Placebo-controlled multicentre randomised trial of interferon β-1b in treatment of secondary progressive multiple sclerosis. Lancet 1998; 352:1491–1497.

66. Goodkin DE and the North American Study Group on Interferon beta-1b in Secondary Progressive MS. Interferon beta-1b in secondary progressive MS: Clinical and MRI results of a 3-year randomized controlled trial. Presented at American Academy of Neurology, May 2000.

67. Jacobs L, Cookfair D, Rudick R, Herndon R, Richert J, Salazar A et al. Intramuscular interferon beta-1a for disease progression in relapsing multiple sclerosis. Ann Neurol 1996; 39: 285–294.

68. Milo R, Panitch H. Glatiramer acetate or interferon-β for multiple sclerosis? A guide to drug choice. CNS Drugs 1999; 4:289–306.

69. Weinshenker BG, Bass B, Rice G, Noseworthy JX. The natural history of multiple sclerosis: A geographically based study: 2. Predictive value of the early clinical course. Brain 1989; 112:1419–1428.

70. Barkhof F, Filippi M. Can MRI be a predictor of long-term clinical outcome? Int MSJ 1995; 2:4–9.

71. Filippi M, Horsfield MA, Morrissey SP, MacManus DG, Rudge P, McDonald WI, et al. Quantitative brain MRI lesion load predicts the course of clinically isolated syndromes suggestive of multiple sclerosis. Neurology 1994; 44:635–641.

72. Khoury SJ, Guttmann CRG, Orav EJ, Hohol MJ, Ahn SS, Hsu L, et al. Longitudinal MRI in multiple sclerosis: correlation between disability and lesion burden. Neurology 1994; 44: 2120–2124.

73. Wolinsky J. Copolymer 1: A most reasonable alternative therapy for early relapsing-remitting multiple sclerosis with mild disability. Neurology 1995; 45:1245–1247.

24

Treatment of Multiple Sclerosis with Intravenous Immunoglobulin

PETER RUDGE

The National Hospital for Neurology and Neurosurgery, London, England

I. INTRODUCTION

For the past 50 years clinicians have attempted to alter the course of multiple sclerosis (MS) by injecting blood or blood products. The rationale for such therapy is twofold. First, many clinicians believe that an infective agent plays a part in the disease and that patients are unable to eradicate this agent. In contrast, blood from subjects who do not have MS contains products that are effective (i.e., antibodies). Second, some investigators believe that immune mechanisms are important in causing damage to the central nervous system (CNS) and that blood products, especially immunoglobulins, will abrogate this potentially damaging process. The second rationale has tended to replace the first over the past 30 years, although the two hypotheses are not mutually exclusive. The recent burgeoning of trials of immunoglobulin therapy (IVG) for a wide variety of disorders stems from the success of using specific antibodies prophylactically to prevent hemolytic disease of the newborn, a process that is clearly immunologically based. Subsequently, nonspecific immunoglobulin therapy has been used in patients with diseases that are thought to be immunologically based or could conceivably be of viral origin. This empirical approach has been particularly successful in Kawasaki disease, in which such treatment certainly reduces coronary aneurysm development (1), and in childhood idiopathic thrombocytopenic purpura (ITP) (2). In diseases of the nervous system, IVG therapy is clearly effective in patients with multifocal conduction block motor neuropathy (3), and there is some evidence that immunoglobulin administration is beneficial in myasthenia gravis (4), Guillain-Barré syndrome (5,6), chronic demyelinating inflammatory polyneuropathy (7–10), polymyositis (11), Rasmussen's encephalitis (12), and a variety of other neurological

561

syndromes with an autoimmune component. This chapter is concerned with the use of immunoglobulins in MS. Only papers published in definitive form in peer review journals are quoted.

II. CLINICAL TRIALS OF IMMUNOGLOBULIN IN MULTIPLE SCLEROSIS

A. Early Trials

One of the earliest trials of immunoglobulin administration in MS was conducted by Alexander and colleagues (13). These authors proposed that the disease was of viral origin and that blood or blood products from normal subjects would contain antibodies to that agent—antibodies that were deficient in quality or quantity in the patients. The first part of their trial recruited 50 patients with MS who received 500 mL of blood by transfusion every 4 to 7 days for 6 weeks; 8 additional patients received saline infusions twice a week for 3 weeks. Assessment was limited to full neurological examination and follow-up by nonneurologists: 46% of the patients improved, 32% were unchanged, 12% were worse. In the control group, 1 of the 8 patients improved. Because of the primitive design of this trial, it is not possible to decide if blood transfusion had any effects on the disease. Interestingly, full recovery occurred in 3 patients receiving blood, and all would have been classified by present standards as having had a recent relapse—i.e., their improvement could well have been spontaneous. The authors also studied 10 patients who received immunoglobulin therapy comprising 12 mL of immunoglobulin given intramuscularly at weekly intervals for 6 weeks; only 8 of the patients completed the full course. There was no effect of this treatment on the disease. Of importance is the small amount of immunoglobulin given in this trial.

In 1963, Miller and colleagues (14) conducted a trial of immunoglobulin therapy that was remarkable for its essentially sound design and the recognition of the importance of power calculation. Twenty-one patients were recruited into a therapeutic and a control group; they were allotted to these two groups by a restricted randomization. The groups were, as expected, well matched for age, duration of disease, and disability as assessed by the Alexander score. Immunoglobulin was given intramuscularly in a dose of 500 mg every 2 weeks for 6 months to the treated group, and the control group received saline injections. There were three dropouts. No difference between the two groups was seen after 6 months; it was calculated that the trial should have detected a true 30% difference between these groups. Again, of importance is the small amounts of immunoglobulin given. Subsequently, there have been several trials, but none until recently has attained this trial's quality of design.

With improvement in IgG production technology in the 1980s, there was a resurgence of interest concerning its use in MS; these trials were all uncontrolled and all were conducted in continental Europe. Rothfelder and colleagues reported their experience in 20 patients with relapsing-remitting MS in giving intravenous (IV) IgG 500 mg at 2-monthly intervals for 1 year (15). There were 12 females in this study and the patients' ages ranged from 18 to 42 years. There was a significant reduction in disability assessed by the Fog score; this reduction was most marked in the first 6 months. The investigators claim that the brainstem auditory evoked potential improved in 3 of the 9 patients in whom it was initially abnormal and that those patients with clinical evidence of a brainstem abnormality had the greatest improvement.

Schuler and Govaerts studied 31 patients with MS to determine if immunoglobulin had any effect on the progression of the disease (16). The mean age of the patients was 39.9 years (range 21 to 55 years); they had had their disease for a mean of 9.8 years (range 1 to 33 years) and had a mean disability of 3.8 (range 1 to 7) on the Kurtzke disability status scale (KDSS). Intravenous immunoglobulin was given in a dose of 5 g at weekly intervals for 3 weeks, and the dose was then reduced to 3 g/week for 1 year. Unfortunately, there was no simultaneous control group, and the study was not blinded. The authors compared the effect on the group receiving intravenous immunoglobulin with that of 164 control subjects receiving different (unspecified) therapy. Although the control subjects ages and disabilities were similar to those of the immunoglobulin-treated patients, it is not possible to determine from the paper if the latter patients did better or worse than the whole of the control group—although the authors, in a rather selective analysis, claimed they did. Soukop and Tschabitscher conducted a small unblinded trial in 27 patients using IVG (7 S) in a dose of approximately 50 mg/kg, which was repeated after 2 or 3 weeks in 23 of the patients (17). The age and sex of the patients is not given, but they had had their disease for a mean of 7.5 years and the Kurtzke extended disability status score (EDSS) was 4.2. Five of the patients had chronic progressive disease. It is unclear in the paper what the temporal relation of the infusion to a relapse was; however, in the summary, it is stated that the best results were obtained if the treatment was given shortly after a new relapse. Of the total, 16 of the patients 1 of whom had chronic progressive disease, were said to benefit, whereas 11 were unresponsive. Not surprisingly, the mean duration of disease and disability in nonresponders was greater than that in those who responded (10 versus 5 years; 4.5 versus 4.0 EDSS score respectively). The beneficial effect was short-lived. The authors claimed that the T-helper/T-suppressor cell ratio fell significantly after therapy. One interpretation of these data is that the investigators were reporting the normal spontaneous recovery after relapse.

Unfortunately, none of these three papers provides good evidence of the efficacy of IVG in MS because none included a suitable control group or blind assessment.

B.   Trials Conducted Since 1990

In 1992, Cook and coworkers reported their experience in a pilot study using 500 mg/kg to 2 g/kg IVG at monthly intervals in patients with relapsing and remitting disease (18). All patients received pulsed methylprednisolone and some were given oral prednisolone. The IVG was given for a mean of 7.8 months to 14 patients, of whom 11 had a total of 17 exacerbations. The design of the trial meant that patients who had severe relapses received higher doses of immunoglobulin. It is not possible to draw any definite conclusions from this study on the clinical efficacy of IVG; however, as the authors point out, exacerbations were not stopped, and there was little evidence that the dose of oral steroids was reduced, although there is no good evidence that steroids alone are beneficial in the long term. Of theoretical interest was the reduction of free light chains in the urine, which might mean a modulation of plasma cell function in a favorable direction.

In 1992, Achiron and colleagues reported the first properly designed controlled trial of IVG in MS, in which a restricted randomization procedure was used (19). The authors selected 36 patients with relapsing and remitting disease out of a population of 120 subjects in whom there had been at least two relapses per year in the 2 years before the study and who had an EDSS score of less than 6. From these 36 patients they matched 10 pairs on age, disease duration, and number of exacerbations, the last variable being the most important. Having obtained two groups, they then randomly assigned one to active therapy and one to placebo. Not surprisingly there was no significant difference the two groups in the variables by which they were selected; the control subjects were 2 years older than those assigned to active treatment but had had the disease for 18 months less and were less disabled by nearly 1 point on the Kurtzke scale. The relapse rate at baseline in the control subjects was 3.3 ± 1.4/year, compared with 3.7 ± 1.2/year for the treated subjects; both rates are at the upper extreme for MS. Interestingly, the sex ratios were not given. The treatment regimen comprised IVG 0.4 g/kg/day for 5 consecutive days, then a similar dose every 2 months for 1 year. It is unclear what the control subjects were given.

In the year following entry into the trial, there was a significant difference ($p <$ 0.001) in the relapse rate in favor of the IVG; the relapse rate in the treated patients was 1.0 ± 0.7 (mean ± SD) and in the control patients 3.0 ± 1.6. A total of 30 relapses occurred in the control group, compared with 10 in the treated group. An analysis of the severity of the relapses using the Kurtzke score at the nadir of the relapse as a measure showed that the relapses were significantly ($p < 0.001$) less severe in the treated group. The authors also claim that the frequency of exacerbation was significantly less ($p <$ 0.001) in the treated group if those who had one or no relapses are compared with those who had two or more. This type of calculation is critically dependent on the cutoff; more usually a comparison is made between the number of patients without an exacerbation with those with one or more. If this is done in the present study, there was no difference between the groups. It is, however, one of the most stringent criteria used in any MS trial. In contrast with the benefit seen in terms of relapse rate, there was no significant effect of the treatment on the increase in the long-term disability, although there was a minor trend in favor of the therapy (decrease in the EDSS score of 0.3 points in the treated group compared with an increase of 0.2 points in the control patients).

Subsequently, the same authors have published a follow-up study of what appears to be the same cohort of patients (20); in this publication, all the data at baseline and at 1 year are identical with the original publication except for a small difference in the exacerbation rate standard deviation in the control group and a minor variation in the significance value for decline in exacerbation rate at 1 year. The follow-up study confirms a significant reduction in relapse rate over 2 to 3 years, reaching 0.5 ± 0.5 for the treated group and 1.7 ± 0.7 for the control population. The fact that the control group had such a large reduction in relapse rate is typical of therapeutic trials in MS, and presumably reflects a regression to the mean, patients having been selected for a high initial relapse rate, as in this trial. A second point of interest in the follow-up study is the rapid decline in the relapse rate in the first year in the treated group, followed by a slowing of the rate at years 2 and 3. It is this rapid decline that contributes to the highly significant results seen in a trial with such small numbers; a similar effect has been observed in other trials of immunosuppression, as with cyclosporine (21). Analysis of disability showed that by the third year the increase of EDSS score was significantly less ($p < 0.001$) in the treated group (0.35) than the control patients (1.7). Data are not given concerning the absolute EDSS at 3 years, but presumably there was no significant difference between the two groups, as this is a less sensitive measure with which to detect the efficacy of therapy.

In the past 3 years three further controlled trials have been published, in two of which MRI assessment was also done (Table 1).

Fazekas and colleagues (22) conducted the largest randomized placebo-controlled study to date. Monthly IVG (0.15 to 0.2 mg/kg) was given to a group of relapsing and remitting (two relapses in the previous 2 years) patients without secondary progression.

Table 1 Randomized Blinded Controlled Trials of IVIG in MS

Study	Number of Patients	Type of MS	Age (years)	EDSS at Baseline (range)	Duration (years)	Total Dose of IV IgG (g/kg)	Relapse Rate Reduction (%)	EDSS Change	MRI
Ref. 23	40	RR	34[†]	2.85 (0–6.0)*	2	6.8	63	0	0
Ref. 22	148	RR	37[†]	3.3 (2.9–3.7)	2	1.8–2.4	59	+	ND
Ref. 27	26	RR/SP	31/39[xx]	3.5/4.5 (2.0–7.0)	0.5 × 2	12.0	27–42[++]	0	+

[†] Rounded figures.
* Range given in selection criteria.
[xx] Age in RR and SP respectively.
[++] Not significant.
0 = No change.
+ = Improvement.
ND = Not done.

Saline was used as a placebo. The trial lasted 2 years. Patients were between 15 and 64 years old with a disability assessed by the EDSS of 1 to 6.0. A total of 243 patients were screened, of which 150 were selected. Half of these received the active treatment. The patients were assessed at 6-monthly intervals by a neurologist blinded to the treatment; another physician administered the therapy and was aware of the allocation. Patients were seen at a nonscheduled visit if their condition changed; occurrence of relapse was determined at the time and the patient treated with steroids if indicated. The study medication was temporarily stopped if a relapse had occurred, but the total number of infusions was adjusted (not specified how) so that all patients received the same amount of IVG or placebo. Primary outcome measures were absolute change in the EDSS and proportion of patients who were better, the same, or worse ($\geq$ than 1 Kurtzke point change) was determined. Secondary outcomes were number of relapses, annual relapse rate, proportion of patients free of relapses, and time to first relapse.

Two patients assigned placebo decided not to take part in the study after randomization. They were not included in the intention-to-treat analysis, which comprised 75 patients receiving IVG and 73 patients receiving placebo. There was no significant difference between the IVG- and placebo-treated groups in age (36.7 versus 37.3 years), male-to-female sex ratio (18 of 56 versus 19 of 54), duration of disease (6.8 versus 7.3 years), previous annual relapse rate (1.3 versus 1.4), disability at baseline (EDSS 3.3 versus 3.3) or time from last relapse (151 versus 185 days). In all, 64 patients in the IVG group and 56 patients in the placebo group completed 2 years on study.

Of those patients having had at least two EDSS measurements during the trial, 31% improved by at least one Kurtzke point in the treated group and 14% in the placebo; conversely, deterioration occurred in 16% of the immunoglobulin group compared with 23% in the placebo group. These figures are marginally significant ($p = 0.04$). A similar outcome was found in those patients who strictly followed protocol, 33% of the treated group improving compared with 14% of the controls. The mean change in EDSS was small; the actively treated patients had an improvement of -0.23 and the control group a worsening of $+0.12$. This small difference was highly significant ($p = 0.008$) in the intention-to-treat analysis. Analysis of the smaller group who completed the protocol gave essentially similar results but with wider confidence limits and therefore a larger p value (0.02).

The annual relapse rate in the actively treated group was about half that of the placebo group (0.52 versus 1.26, $p = 0.004$). As expected, the relapse rate in the placebo group declined during the study. Among the control patients, 36% were relapse-free over the entire follow-up period compared with 53% of the actively treated group ($p = 0.03$); the total number of relapses in the control patients was nearly twice that of the treated group. The time to first relapse was longer in the treated patients (237 days versus 151 days; not significant) and the severity of the relapse, using the EDSS change at the nadir of the relapse, was significantly less in the treated group.

The major criticism of this trial is the acceptance of a change of EDSS that was not confirmed at 3 or 6 months in order to assess permanent progression. As relapses were more frequent in the placebo group, there will be more patients in whom the EDSS is temporarily depressed because of the proximity of a relapse. If this occurred at the final assessment, the effect of the therapy will have been overestimated. It would be interesting to know if those patients who were relapse-free also showed a beneficial effect of the therapy on progression of EDSS, but the numbers would be too small to reach a definite conclusion. Another criticism concerns the adequacy of the blinding of the observers, as no data were given on the proportion of correct guesses as to which patients received therapy, and one of the neurologists who was assessing adverse events but not scoring the neurological change was unblinded. Nevertheless, this study is consistent with earlier smaller ones and remains the largest randomized controlled study of IVG published to date.

Achiron et al. (23) have published the results of a new series of relapsing and remitting patients in 1998 and included some MRI measurement of disease activity. A total of 40 patients were selected from a cohort of 164. The criteria for entry were 0.5 to 3.0 relapses per year in the preceding 2 years, EDSS of 0 to 6.0 and age 18 to 60 years. Secondary progressive patients were excluded. The dosage regimen was 0.4 g/kg IVG daily for 5 days, then 0.4 g/kg every 2 months for 2 years. Saline was used as the placebo. Neurological assessment was done by two neurologists at monthly intervals and each scored the patients on the EDSS. To be accepted, a relapse had to be accompanied by a change in neurological signs assessed by a blinded neurologist. The severity of the relapse was scored as mild, moderate, or severe using the functional scores of the EDSS, not the disability score. Neuropsychiatric evaluation was assessed at yearly intervals using an anxiety, depression, cognition, and general psychopathology score, but these scales were not defined.

The 40 patients were equally divided into active and placebo groups. The two groups were matched for age (35.4 and 33.8 years), for active versus placebo therapy, disease duration (4.1 versus 3.95 years), exacerbation rate (1.85 versus 1.55) and baseline EDSS (2.9 versus 2.82). The major analyses were done on the patients who completed 2 years of therapy. It is unclear how many patients completed the trial per protocol, but it is stated that two patients (one in each arm) withdrew in the first year. It is stated that 630 infusions were given in all, indicating that about 7% of the infusions were missed, but the distribution of patients receiving these infusions is unclear. The only intention-to-treat data given are the relapse rate in the second year of 0.4 in the treated group and 1.54 in the placebo group ($p = < 0.001$). In the 30 patients who were not withdrawn, there was a highly significant difference in the relapse rate in the first and second years in favor of the treated group. Thus, at the end of the first year, the relapse rate was 0.75 in the treated patients and 1.8 in the placebo group. During the second year, the corresponding figures were 0.42 and 1.42. Over the whole trial, the relapse rate difference was 1.02. Oddly, the relapse rate did not decline significantly in the placebo group; indeed, it rose in the first year from 1.55 to 1.8. After 2 years, 15% of the treated patients had not had a relapse, whereas all the placebo group had; a life-table analysis of the probability of being relapse-free just reached the conventional levels of significance ($p < 0.05$). The time to first exacerbation was significantly ($p = 0.003$) longer (233 days versus 82 days) in the treated group. Relapse severity did not significantly differ between the two groups. The mean change of EDSS at the end of the study was not significantly different between the two groups (-0.3 versus $+0.15$ in the treated and control groups, respectively). The psychometric variables did not differ between the two groups.

This study again shows an impressive reduction of relapse rate in the treated patients, but on this occasion, Achiron et al. did not find an effect on disability. It is odd that the analysis was not a true intention-to-treat one given the extremely low dropout rate (5%) and the apparent high proportion of treatments given per protocol (92%). A further unusual feature was the maintenance—indeed, increase in the first year—of the exacerbation rate in the placebo group. This would accentuate the apparent effect of IVG; it has not been the finding in other studies and was not predicted from natural history databases. This paper generated an acrimonious correspondence concerning blinding, since the placebo and IVG vials were apparently recognizable (24). However, the authors shielded the vials so they could not be seen by the physician giving the drug, and there was no evidence that the patients knew which preparation they were receiving. Unfortunately, however, no data were given on guesses by the physicians. The editor of the publishing journal accepted that the study was truly blinded. Finally, yet again, confirmed progression was not assessed, although in this study there was no difference between the final EDSS scores in the two groups.

C. Magnetic Resonance Scanning

Most recent trials of therapy of MS have included MRI measures, since in parallel-design placebo-controlled study of relapses, it is known that there are 8 to 10 clinically silent new lesions detected on MRI for each clinical relapse, thereby greatly increasing the power of a trial. Further, with MRI, it is possible to be more certain of the blinding and to obtain more objective quantitative data on disease activity. But there are difficulties in using MRI as a surrogate for clinical activity. First, although there is evidence that pathology is reflected in the images, the correlation between some aspects of the clinical course and a given MRI parameter is rather poor. Thus, T2 lesion load has a low correlation ($r = 0.2$ to 0.3) with disability as assessed on the Kurtzke scale (25). T1 black holes correlate better ($r =$ approximately 0.7) (26), and it is thought that gadolinium enhancement reflects early features of new lesions, with breakdown of the blood-brain barrier (27). Second, techniques used in MRI are rapidly improving, such that during a long trial, suboptimal measures by contemporary standards are obtained and comparison between trials may be difficult. In particular, new sequences for obtaining MRI images are being developed all the time—e.g., MTR, diffusion, and new methods for measuring lesion load and activity are being devised. Finally, certain measures of MRI activity, such as gadolinium enhancement and new lesion accumulation, are not randomly distributed between patients. Thus, in all studies in which MRI has been used as a surrogate, there has been extreme variability of T2 lesion load, new T2 lesions, and gadolinium enhancement; some patients have no activity at all and others having hundreds of new lesions. This renders analysis difficult.

The most extensive MRI study in a trial of IVG is that of Sorenson et al. (28). This was a crossover study in 21 relapsing and remitting and 5 secondary progressive patients. There is great potential power in such a study and to some extent this overcomes the interindividual variation that one finds on MRI parameters of activity. Of the 26 patients included, half received IVG first and placebo second. As expected with such small numbers, there were significant differences at baseline between those receiving IVG first and those receiving placebo first. Thus, the first group were younger (mean age 31 versus 39 years), had significantly shorter disease duration (34 versus 81 months), and—interestingly—were less disabled when assessed by the EDSS (3.5 versus 4.5). Of relevance to the study was the fact that the MRI parameters were not significantly different, in that the mean number of gadolinium-enhancing lesions was the same (4.1 ± 9.1 versus 3.2 ± 5.1) for those who received IVG first [median 1 (0 to 4) and 1 (0 to 18)] and for the T2 lesion burden assessed by area in square millimeters [1721 (699 to 13,546) versus 2583 (140 to 32,291)]. These baseline figures immediately highlight the extreme variation in the MRI measures of disease between patients.

The trial design was for 24 weeks with IVG or placebo, followed by a 12-week washout period; then the therapy was reversed. IVG was given in a dose of 1 g/kg/day for 2 days followed by monthly infusions for the next 24 weeks—i.e., 7 g/kg in total. The active preparation started with a Gammagard, but this was changed to Gammagard S/D. The placebo group received a 2% albumin solution. The study was blinded.

Using the EDSS and Scripps scale, clinical assessment was made at baseline and at monthly intervals or when an exacerbation was reported. MRI was obtained at this time. When an exacerbation was reported, an MRI was obtained, preferably before steroid therapy. If it was not obtained or steroids were given, an MRI was obtained at least 3 weeks later. All MRIs were obtained on a 1.5 Tesla machine, in the horizontal plane, with adjacent slices 4 mm thick. T2, proton-density, and gadolinium-enhanced images were obtained. The images were assessed blindly by two neuroradiologists and the area of abnormal tissue determined by a computerized system (coefficient of variation not given). Finally, multimodal evoked potentials were obtained at the beginning and end of each period.

The primary endpoint of this trial was the total number of lesions and of new enhancing lesions. Additional secondary endpoints were proportion of patients with active scans, total lesion load (T2), and alteration in the evoked potential parameters.

A total of 18 patients completed the crossover (4 withdrew in each group). An intention-to-treat analysis differed little from those patients who followed the protocol. The number of enhancing lesions were 60% less in the IVG group ($p < 0.05$). There was a mean of 1.1 and a median of 0.4 new lesions in the treated group, compared with 2.2 and 0.9, respectively, in the placebo group of patients. In the treated group, 22% of the patients had no new lesions, whereas all of the placebo group had at least one enhancing lesion. The effect of IVG appeared at 1 month. Active scans were found in 37% of the IVG-treated patients and 68% of the placebo group ($p = 0.01$). There was no change in the T2 lesion load in either group. Clinical variables and individual evoked potential studies were similar in the two groups, but the central motor conduction time did demonstrate a difference in favor of the actively treated group.

Crossover studies such as this have great power if there is no carryover effect and the dropout is low. While the former did not occur, the dropout rate was surprisingly high—a factor that would have reduced the power substantially. Nevertheless, the study did demonstrate a reduction in gadolinium-enhancing lesions in those patients receiving IVG. A change of lesion load on T2 scanning was not seen, but the study did not have sufficient power to show this; it would need many more patients treated for a much longer period.

Two other studies of the effect of IVG upon the MRI have been published. In the latest trial by Achiron et al. (see above) (23), T1- and T2-weighted scans using a 0.5-tesla machine and 5-mm noncontiguous slices (1-mm gap) at baseline, 1 and 2 years, showed no difference between the treated and untreated patients. The authors base their evidence on a peculiar MRI score of lesion load, in which the average diameter of the lesion was multiplied by the number of lesions to give a score between zero (no lesions) and 10 (maximum number of lesions). At 1 year, the score had increased by 12% in the treated group and by 30% in the placebo patients, but no data are given on the raw score. Calculation of these data from those in the publication show that the IVG group increased their score from 3.21 to about 3.60 and the placebo group from 3.04 to about 3.95. In the second year, only the score is given, not the percentage increase; but 10 patients were not scanned. The results show that in the IVG group the mean score was 3.82 and in the placebo group 3.20. No conclusions can be drawn from these data and they cannot be compared with any other series, as parameters such as number of lesions or lesion load were not reported.

Francis et al. (29) reported that IVG given to a group of severely disabled patients in a dose of 0.4 g/kg/day for 3 consecutive days, then single monthly injections of 0.4 g/kg for 1 year had no effect on MRI activity as determined by new or expanding lesions detected on T2-weighted scans. This trial was uncontrolled and unblinded. Only nine patients with different forms of the disease (relapsing remitting, secondary progressive, and primary progressive) were studied. No conclusions can be drawn from a study designed like this.

D. Other Studies

There are a number of other studies that are inadequately designed to give answers to the questions posed. One of these involves a combination of IVG given in conventional dosage (loading dose of 0.4 g/kg/day for 5 days, then a maintenance dose of 0.2 g/kg at monthly intervals) and azathioprine at a high dose (2.5 to 3 mg/kg/day) (30). All the patients had relapsing and remitting MS. Of 34 patients, 24 improved on the EDSS (0.5 to 1.0) during the 3 years of this trial, but no data are given concerning relapse rate. Trials such as this are impossible to assess as there is no control group, the results are inadequately documented, and there is the confounding of two potentially effective drugs. At best, such trials can be classified as anecdotal.

One interesting study, so far published only in abstract, concerns the effect of IVG on relapse rate and pregnancy (31). It is known that pregnancy is associated with a low risk of relapse and the puerperium a period of higher risk (32). Karageorglou and colleagues treated 10 women who were pregnant with 0.4 g/kg/day for 7 days during the final month of pregnancy, then gave a similar course 5 days after delivery and subsequently 5 more sessions at monthly intervals. The patients were followed for 1 year after delivery. The investigators compared the results in this treated group with those in 18 women with relapsing and remitting MS who did not receive any treatment. This control group was assessed retrospectively. Of the untreated control group, 10 had a relapse in the following year, 6 of them in the first 3 months after delivery. This contrasted with only 1 patient in the treated group, who had a relapse 5 months after delivery.

This study is remarkable in that IVG was given to pregnant women, usually considered a contraindication to entering any trial. The results are striking. In a group of patients with active relapsing and remitting disease, a relapse rate of 0.5 relapses per year would be expected, and that is what was observed in the control group. While one might find the relapse rate dropping to 0.1 relapse per year by chance these data are quite suggestive of a beneficial effect of IVG. The problem is whether it would be possible to do a proper double-blind controlled trial, particularly in relation to the potential adverse effects of immunoglobulins given in this manner to pregnant women. One would need to know more about the final outcome in this small trial before considering whether the potential risks are worth taking in a much larger trial, so that a definitive answer can be obtained.

III. POTENTIAL MECHANISMS OF ACTION

A. Effects on the Immune System

If IVG administration is effective in altering the natural history of MS, the question arises of what mechanisms might be involved. They broadly fall into two groups: namely, a direct antibody effect on an infective agent and immunomodulation. As far as the first mechanism is concerned, there is no proof that an infective agent is involved in the genesis of the disease. Nevertheless, it was with such a mechanism in mind that IVG was initially given. Similar reasoning was instrumental in the initiation of the trials of interferon therapy. Several potential mechanisms of immunomodulation are possible—namely, alteration in the immunological response by anti-idiotypes, interaction with Fc receptors, and control of feedback loops. These mechanisms are not mutually exclusive.

The concept of idiotypic networks was brilliantly developed by the Nobel laureate Jerne. Central to this model is the idea that the great diversity of antigens map to idiotypic antibodies that, in turn, map to anti-idiotypic antibodies in a potentially infinite but degenerate regression. The recognition of idiotypes by anti-idiotypes is dependent on the hypervariable loops of the immunoglobulin molecules—i.e., the $F(ab)_2$ region. Such a network can provide a series of feedback loops between the cells of the immune system involving the various T-cell subsets as well as B cells. It has been suggested that this type of network is responsible for preventing autoreactivity in normal subjects. Cohen and Young have proposed that the network encodes an immunological homunculus (analogous to the cortical sensory homunculus) by which a continuous attack on self-proteins is controlled (33). A breakdown of the network would cause an autoimmune attack. Theoretically, it might be possible to reset the disordered network by adding the appropriate (unknown) anti-idiotypes in the form of pooled immunoglobulins containing tens of thousands of idiotypic molecules. Direct evidence that recovery from autoimmune disease can depend on anti-idiotypic antibodies was first obtained by Rossi and colleagues (34) in a patient with a bleeding diathesis caused by circulating autoantibodies against factor VIII. After recovery, the antifactor VIII antibody present in the blood before recovery had disappeared, and this coincided with the appearance of anti-idiotypic antibodies to the factor VIII antibody present initially. The activity resided in the $F(ab)_2$ fraction. These workers also demonstrated a similar phenomenon in a patient recovering from inflammatory demyelinating polyneuropathy (35).

Alternatively, it has been argued that Fc receptor saturation by immunoglobulin is crucial to the beneficial effect of administered IVG. The Fc receptors for IgG (FcγR) are part of the immunoglobulin superfamily and are all encoded by genes on chromosome 1 in humans (36). They are divided into three groups (I to III), and all are constitutively expressed on monocytes and macrophages. Binding to IgG to these receptors induces a variety of functional changes, including phagocytosis, antibody-dependent cytotoxicity, enhancement of antigen presentation, and cytokine release. The beneficial effects of IVG could conceivably be due to binding of the IgG to the FcγR, thereby blocking further stimulation. Such a mechanism has been suggested in patients with ITP; binding of the FcγR to macrophages might decrease platelet destruction. However, this cannot be the sole mechanism, even in ITP, since $F(ab)_2$ fragments are also beneficial.

The importance of humoral mechanisms in MS has always been unclear. Although abnormal or excessive antibody production is a feature of MS, most notably in the CSF compartment with the production of oligoclonal bands, the immunopathogenesis of the disease has traditionally been attributed to cellular immune processes. Therefore, it is of some interest that the FcγRs are also induced on activated T cells (37). These receptors are closely connected with the T-cell receptor (TCR), suggesting the possibility of modulation of the latter by FcγR stimulation. Conceivably IVG could modify this modulation, and there is some evidence that T-cell function is altered by IVG. Thus, IVG given in a dose of 800 mg/kg/day for 2 consecutive days to patients with MS, causes decrease in peripheral blood T lymphocytes (CD3$^+$, CD4$^+$, CD8$^+$, CD45+, RA+) and B lymphocytes, as well as NK cells for up to 5 weeks (38).

There have been a number of papers recently describing alteration of cytokine production and the balance between TH_1 and TH_2 activity in humans and experimental allergic encephalomyelitis (EAE) (39). Van Schaik and colleagues (40), in their review of in vitro work, suggested that polyclonal IVG can inhibit TH_1 activity thought to be important in cellular damage in MS, an effect that is partially reversed by administration of TH_1 cytokines (IL-2, TNF-α, IFN-γ). Conversely, immunoglobulin has a synergistic effect upon TH_2 responses concerned with antibody production. Such work does not, however, fully specify the mechanisms of the beneficial effects of immunoglobulins in demyelinating diseases; the alterations observed are merely the proximate cause of the effect.

A unifying hypothesis of the beneficial effects of immunoglobulins in antibody-mediated autoimmune diseases has been proposed by Yu and Lennon (41). These workers point out that the fractional metabolism of IgG is proportional to its plasma concentration. Recent experiments in which the beta-microglobulin gene was deleted in mice resulted in virtual IgG agammaglobulinemia; these mice did not produce IgG antibodies when immunized with antigens but had a normal IgM response. The reason for the low immunoglobulin levels was the greatly increased catabolism of immunoglobulin. When IgG enters a cell, it is rapidly destroyed. In the normal cell, a receptor for IgG is FcRn (Fc receptors of the neonate initially found in neonatal intestinal epithelium). This receptor has a beta-microglobulin component. Binding of IgG to beta microglobulin protects it from catabolic breakdown. The concept proposed by Yu and Lennon is that saturating the FcRn receptor with exogenous IgG leads to increased metabolism of unprotected endogenous IgG and thus removes the damaging immunoglobulin. This process would account for the beneficial effects of IgG in a wide variety of disorders in which it is used. Whether this is indeed the mechanism by which IVG works awaits further elucidation.

B. Effects on Experimental Demyelination

Few experiments have been done on the effect of IVG in animal models of demyelination. Achiron and colleagues (20) have reported a remarkable series of experiments in Lewis rats in which experimental allergic encephalomyelitis (EAE) was induced actively and passively; they have shown that IVG alters the course of the actively induced disease but not the passively induced one. Human IgG in a dose of 0.4 g/kg/day, starting on the day of inoculation, reduced the severity and mortality from induced EAE but did not alter the time to onset of the disease. The animals were resistant to EAE if they were later reinoculated with myelin basic protein (MBP). In contrast, passive induction of EAE by adoptive transfer of lymphocytes from affected animals was not altered by IVG. Finally, in vitro T-cell proliferation to MBP was increased in the IVG-treated animals. From these experiments, it can be concluded that IVG alters the immune response if given before T cells are activated; it has no effect on T-cell proliferation. Such a pattern of response is consistent with alteration of TCR modulation by induced FcγR, as described earlier.

C. Effects on Remyelination

Although the EAE model provides some evidence of prevention of demyelination, there are data in mice suggesting that remyelination may also be affected by IVG. Theiler's virus infection in mice causes a biphasic neurological disorder (42). Within 9 to 20 days of intracerebral inoculation, over 85% of animals developed a polioclastic encephalomyelitis, and virus can be isolated. Many of these animals die, but after 1 to 5 months, the survivors and those animals not initially affected develop a demyelinating disorder. This is thought to be immune-mediated, and immune suppression prevents its occurrence (43). It is obviously tempting to compare this disease with MS, particularly as it can be a relapsing and remitting disorder in some strains of mouse and, with variation of the virus and under certain conditions, remyelination by Schwann cells and oligodendrocytes occurs (44). Rodriguez and colleagues (45) have conducted some intriguing experiments using the Theiler's virus model of demyelination and have shown that IVG enhances remyelination by progenitor cells sixfold. They showed that antibody to spinal cord homogenate is the important immunoglobulin and, more recently, Noseworthy's group have shown that commercially prepared IgG contains appropriate antibodies (46). These animal studies are important if they are confirmed, as they indicate that enhancement of repair is a possible action of IVG in addition to the prevention of demyelination. No other immunomodulating therapy has shown the former effect.

Evidence for a similar effect in patients with MS is lacking, but two observations are consistent with a similar phenomenon. First, van Engelen et al. (47) showed that IVG in a dose of 0.4 g/kg for 5 days, then given fortnightly for 3 months, resulted in an unexpected and sustained (for 3 months) improvement in visual acuity in 3 of 5 patients (5 of 8 eyes) with optic neuritis as a result of MS in whom in visual acuity had remained stable for 6 months. As the patients were stable and the effect seemed to persist for 3 months after treatment began, alteration of cytokine production seems an unlikely explanation for the effect, and remyelination was postulated by the authors. Oddly, different functions recovered in different patients; for example, improvement in visual acuity did not parallel recovery of color vision.

A second piece of evidence comes from the follow-up of Fazekas' trial, where analysis of the course of improvement in the EDSS shows that the placebo and treated groups diverge within 6 months, then remain parallel (48). This is consistent with a direct effect on remyelination but is equally consistent with a concept of relapse-rate reduction, enabling spontaneous remyelination to occur.

Overall, there is no convincing evidence in MS of remyelination enhancement due to IVG, but it does remain a possibility.

IV. PREPARATION OF IMMUNOGLOBULIN G

The World Health Organization (WHO) has laid down guidelines for the preparation and use of immunoglobulins (49,50). Intravenous IgG is prepared for clinical use from a pool of at least 1000 donors (usually 4000 to 10,000), who should be screened for hepatitis virus B and C (HBV, HCV), human immunodeficiency virus (HIV) 1 and 2, and syphilis, and they should have normal liver function tests. They should be unpaid (51). The proportion of the various immunoglobulin classes should be approximately those found in the normal subjects. All IVG is prepared by a modified Cohn fractionation procedure, involving cold ethanol precipitation at low pH (52). To prevent aggregation of protein, a phenomenon that is associated with adverse reactions, a small amount of proteolytic enzyme is added. There is virtually no risk of transmitting HIV-1, HIV-2, or HBV in IgG prepared according to these standards, and the risk of transmission of HCV and nonenvelope DNA viruses is extremely low now that screening has been implemented.

Finally immunoglobulin from blood donors in the UK or from people who have resided in the UK in the previous five years is not available for therapeutic use because of the perceived risk of transmission of prion disease in a population thought to be at risk of contracting variant Creutzfeldt-Jakob disease. There is no scientific evidence for this action and the reason for it is opaque.

V. SAFETY

Adverse events are in general infrequent in patients receiving IVG (53,54). Minor side effects such as headache, myalgia, fever, back and chest pain, and nausea occur in up to 5% of patients, particularly if the rate of infusion is high. Most commercial preparations of IVG contain 2 to 6% of protein in a weak maltose, sucrose, or glucose solution. If the infusion contains 5% IgG, it is recommended that it be given at a rate of 30 mL/h for the first 15 min and then increased to 150 mL/h subsequently. Giving the agent at this rate results in few adverse effects, and the systemic events can easily be controlled with analgesics. Minor alterations of liver enzymes and occasional cases of aseptic meningitis do occur; the latter may be avoided by altering the product being given. Rarely, an encephalopathy occurs. All these adverse events are reversible.

More serious adverse events include anaphylactic reactions, especially in those with IgA deficiency, in whom IgG and IgE antibodies against donor IgA occurs. Some clinicians advise assessing the IgA status of a patient before giving IgG, but the incidence of anaphylactic reaction seems to be less than that of IgA deficiency in the community.

Theoretically, the increased viscosity of the blood can cause thromboembolism and the increased volume of the vascular compartment may lead to cardiac failure, but the risk is low. Minor alterations in hematological parameters can occur, particularly lymphopenia. These effects are transient and of no significance.

In all the MS studies except one, adverse events have been of little concern. The exception is the study of Sorenson (28) in which a relatively large dose (1 to 2 g/kg/day) were given rapidly (3 to 5 h) resulting in high plasma IgG concentration. The systemic side effects of headache and fever were reduced by giving the IVG at a lower rate. However, eczema occurred in 11 patients (out of a total of 26) and was prolonged. One patient developed hepatitis C while receiving a product prior to the introduction of virus inactivation. It appears that the unusually severe and frequent adverse events in this trial were related to the infusion rate (except hepatitis C) and are not due to a peculiarity of patients with MS.

There is no evidence that IVG-induced immunosuppression is a problem, but the theoretical risk of infection and even long-term neoplasia have not been assessed.

VI. CONCLUSION

The studies of IVG to date have been small in scale but are suggestive of a beneficial effect upon relapse rate and perhaps on accumulation of disability. The effects seem to be of the same order as those seen with other therapies, such as interferons. There are several large-scale studies in progress at the present time that should give a definitive answer as to the efficacy of this type of therapy. The data from MRI studies are too fragmentary to allow a definite conclusion as to the effects upon lesion accumulation or on the blood-brain barrier, but such studies are of secondary significance compared with determining the effect upon the progression of the disease clinically. Adverse events seem to be of little importance provided that infusion rates are not rapid. Dosage regimens have not been standardized and will have to be investigated if the results of the trials being conducted at present are positive.

REFERENCES

1. Newberger, JW, Takehashi M, Burns JC, et al. The treatment of Kawasaki syndrome with intravenous gammaglobulin. N Engl J Med 1986; 315:341–347.
2. Imbach P, D'Apuzzo V, Hirt A, et al. High dose intravenous gammaglobulin for idiopathic thrombocytopenic purpura in childhood. Lancet 1981; 1:1228–1231.
3. Chaudhry V, Corse AM, Cornblath DR, et al. Multifocal motor neuropathy: Response to human immune globulin. Ann Neurol 1993; 33:237–242.
4. Cosi V, Lombardi M, Piccolo G, Erbetta A. Treatment of myasthenia gravis with high dose intravenous immunoglobulin. Acta Neurol Scand 1991; 84:81–84.
5. Plasma exchange/sandoglobulin Guillain-Barré Trial Group. Randomised trial of plasma exchange, intravenous immunoglobulin and combined treatment in Guillain-Barré syndrome. Lancet 1997; 349:225–230.
6. Van der Meché FGA, Schmitz PIM, The Dutch Guillain-Barré Study Group. A randomised trial comparing intravenous immunoglobulin and plasma exchange in Guillain-Barré syndrome. N Engl J Med 1992; 326:1123–1129.
7. Vermeulen M, van Doorn PA, Brand A et al. Intravenous immunoglobulin treatment in patients with chronic inflammatory demyelinating polyneuropathy. J Neurol Neurosurg Psychiatry 1993; 56:36–39.
8. Dyck PJ, Litchy WJ, Ktraz KM, et al. A plasma exchange versus immune globulin infusion trial in chronic inflammatory demyelinating polyradiculo neuropathy Ann Neuro 1994; 36: 838–845.
9. Hahn AF, Bolton CF, Zochodne D, Feasby TE. Intravenous immunoglobulin treatment in chronic inflammatory demyelinating polyneuropathy: A double-blind, placebo-controlled, cross-over study. Brain 1996; 119:1067–1077.
10. Van Doorn PA, et al. High dose intravenous immunoglobulin treatment in chronic inflammatory polyneuropathy: a double-blind, placebo-controlled, cross-over study. Neurology 1990; 40:209–212.
11. Gyerin P, Herson S, Wechsler B, et al. Efficacy of intravenous gammaglobulin therapy in chronic refractory polymyositis and dermatomyositis: An open study with 20 adult patients. Am J Med 1991; 91:162–168.
12. Hart YM, Cortez M, Andermann F et al. Medical treatment of Rasmussen's syndrome (chronic encephalitis with epilepsy): Effect of high dose steroids or immunoglobulins in 19 patients. Neurology 1994; 44:1030–1036.
13. Alexander L, Loman J, Lesser MF, Green I. Blood and plasma transfusions in multiple sclerosis. Association for Research in Nervous and Mental Disease 1950; 28:178–206.
14. Miller HG, Foster JR, Newell DR, Barwick DD, Brewis RAL. Multiple sclerosis therapeutic trials of chloroquine, soluble aspirin and gammaglobulin. BMJ 1963; 2:1436–1439.
15. Rothfelder V, Neu I, Pelka R. Therapie der Multiplen Sklerose mit Immunglobulin G Munch Med Wochenschr 1982; 124:74–78.
16. Schuller E, Govaerts A. First results of immunotherapy with immunoglobulin G in multiple sclerosis patients. Eur J Neurol 1983; 22:205–212.
17. Soukop W, Tschabitscher H. Gammaglobulintherapie bei Multipler Sklerose (MS) Wien Med Wochenschr 1986; 18:477–480.
18. Cook SD, Troiano R, Romowsky-Kochin C, et al. Intravenous gammaglobulin in progressive MS. Acta Neurol Scand 1992; 86:171–175.
19. Achiron A, Pras E, Gilad R, et al. Open controlled therapeutic trial of intravenous immune globulin in relapsing-remitting multiple sclerosis. Arch Neurol 1992; 49:1233–1236.

20. Achiron A, Gilad R, Margaltt R, et al. Intravenous gammaglobulin treatment in multiple sclerosis and experimental auto-imune encephalomyelitis: Delineation of usage and mode of action, J Neurol, Neurosurg Psychiatry 1994; 57(suppl):57–61.

21. Rudge P, Koetsier JC, Mertin J, et al. Randomised double blind controlled trial of cyclosporine in multiple sclerosis. J Neurol Neurosurg Psychiatry 1989; 52:559–565.

22. Fazekas F, Deisenhammer F, Strasser-Fuchs S, Nahler G, Mamoli B for the Austrian Immunoglobulin in Multiple Sclerosis Study Group. Randomised placebo-controlled trial of monthly intravenous immunoglobulin therapy in relasping-remitting multiple sclerosis. Lancet 1997; 349:589–593.

23. Achiron A, Gabbay U, Gllad R, et al. Intravenous immunoglobulin treatment in multiple sclerosis: Effect on relapses. Neurology 1998; 50:398–402.

24. Gadoth N, Melamed E, Muller A, Steiner I, Abramsky O. Correspondence: intravenous immunoglobulin treatment in multiple sclerosis. Neurology 1999; 52:214–215.

25. Filippi M, Camp IA, Martinella V et al. Correlations between change in disability and T_2 weighted brain MRI activity in multiple sclerosis. Neurology 1995; 45:255–260.

26. Van Walderveen MA, Barkhof F, Hommes OR, et al. Correlating MRI and clinical disease activity in multiple sclerosis: Relevance of hypo-intense lesions on short TR/short TE (T_1 weighted spin echo images. Neurology 1995; 45:1684–1690.

27. Miller DH, Rudge P, Johnson G et al. Serial gadolinium enhanced magnetic resonance imaging in multiple sclerosis Brain 1988; 111:927–939.

28. Sorenson PS, Wanscher B, Jensen CV, et al. Intravenous immunoglobulin G reduces MRI activity in relapsing multiple sclerosis. Neurology 1998; 50:1273–1281.

29. Francis GS, Freedman MS, Antel JP. Failure of intravenous immunglobulin to correct progression of multiple sclerosis: a clinical and MRI based study. Mult Scler 1997; 3:370–376.

30. Kelanie H, Tabatabai SS. Combined immunoglobulin and azathioprine in multiple sclerosis. European Neurology 1998; 39:178–181.

31. Karageorgiou CE, Tagaris G, Terzoudi G, Cheilakos G, Panagopoulos. Intravenous immunoglobulin in childbirth-related exacerbation of multiple sclerosis. Mult Scler 1999; 5(suppl): 571.

32. Confavreux C, Hutchinson M, Houts MM, et al. Rate of pregnancy related relapse in multiple sclerosis. New Engl J Med 1998; 339:285–291.

33. Cohen IR, Young DB. Autoimmunity, microbial immunity and the immunological homunculus. Immunol Today 1991; 12:105.

34. Rossi F, Dietrich G, Kazatchkine D. Anti-idiotype against autoantibodies in normal immunoglobulins: Evidence for network regulation of human autoimmune response. Immunol Rev 1989; 110:135–149.

35. Van Doorn PA, Rossi F, Brand A, va Lint M, Vermolzem M, Kazatchkine MD. On the mechanism of high dose intravenous immunoglobulin treatment of patients with chronic inflammatory demyelinating polyneuropathy with high dose intravenous immunoglobulins. J Neuroimmunol 1990; 29:57.

36. van de Winkel JGJ, Capel PJA. Human IgG Fc receptor heterogeneity: Molecular aspects and clinical implications. Immunol Today 1993; 14:215–221.

37. Sandor M, Lynch RG. Lymphocyte Fc receptors: the special case of T cells. Immunol Today 1993; 14:227–231.

38. Tenser RB, May KA, Aberg JS. Immunoglobulin G immunosuppression of multiple sclerosis. Arch Neurol 1993; 50:417–420.

39. Pashov A, Bellon B, Kaveri SV, Kazatchkine MD. A shift in encephalitogenic T cell cytokine pattern is associated with suppression of EAE by intravenous immunoglobulins (IVIg). Mult Scler 1997; 3:153–156.

40. Van Schaik IN, Vermeulen M, Brand A. Immunoglobulin and remyelination: two aspects of human polyclonal immunoglobulin treatment in immune mediated neuropathies. Mult Scl 1997; 3:98–104.

41. Yu Z, Lennon VA. Mechanism of intravenous immunoglobulin therapy in antibody-mediated autoimmune diseases. New Engl J Med 1999; 340:227–228.

42. Lipton HL. Theiler's virus infection in mice: An unusual biphasic disease process leading to demyelination. Infect Immun 1975; 11:1147–1155.

43. Lipton HL, Del Canto MC. Contrasting effects of immunosuppression on Theiler virus infection in mice. Infect Immun 1977; 15:903–909.

44. Del Canto MC, Barbano RL. Remyelination during remission in Theiler's virus infection. Am J Pathol 1984; 116:30–45.

45. Rodriguez M, Lennon VA. Immunoglobulins promote remyelination in the central nervous system. Ann Neurol 1990; 27:12–17.

46. Noseworthy JM, O'Brien PC, van Engalen BGM, Rodriguez M. Intravenous immunoglobulin therapy in multiple sclerosis: Progress from remyelination in Theiler's virus model to a randomised, double-blind placebo controlled clinical trial. J Neurol Neurosurg Psychiatry 1994; 57(suppl):11–14.

47. van Engelen BGM, Hommes OR, Pinckers A, Cruysberg JRM, Barkof F, Ridriguez M. Improved vision after intravenous immunoglobulin in stable demyelinating optic neuritis. Ann Neurol 1992; 32:834.

48. Fazekas F, Deisenhammer F, Strasser-Fuchs S, Nahler G, Mamoli B. Treatment effects of monthly intravenous immunoglobulin in patients with relapsing-remitting multiple sclerosis: further analysis of the Austrian immunoglobulin MS Study Mul Scler 1997; 3:137–141.

49. World Health Organisation. Appropriate uses of human immunoglobulin in clinical practice Memorandum from an IQIS/WHO meeting. WHO Bull 1982; 60:43–47.

50. Rutter GH. Requirements for safety and quality of intravenous immunoglobulin G preparations. J Neurol, Neurosurg Psychiatry 1994; 57(suppl):2–5.

51. Council Directive. EEC 1989; 381.

52. Cohn EJ, Strong LE, Hughes WL, et al. Preparation and properties of serum and plasma proteins: a system for the separation into fractions of the protein and lipoprotein components of biological tissues and fluids. J Am Chem Soc 1946; 68:459–475.

53. Stangel M, Hartung HP, Marx P, Gold R. Side effects of high-dose intravenous immunoglobulins. Clinical Neuropharmacology 1997; 20:385–393.

54. Dubhelm C, Dicato MA, Ries F. Side effects of intravenous immunoglobulins Clin Exp Immunol 1994; 97(suppl):79–83.

25

Immunosuppressive Drugs

MARIKO KITA and DONALD E. GOODKIN

UCSF/Mt. Zion MS Center, San Francisco, California

I. INTRODUCTION

Disease-modifying therapies that target the immune cascade in MS can be divided into two main types of therapies. Directed immunotherapies can effect immunomodulation in an antigen-specific fashion in the case of glatiramer acetate or T-cell vaccination, or in an antigen-nonspecific fashion as with IVIg, interferon beta-la, or interferon beta-lb. Alternatively, immunotherapies can produce global nonspecific immunosuppression. The treatment of relapsing forms of MS with the immunomodulators interferon beta-la, interferon beta-lb, and glatiramer acetate has become relatively standard and patients who are not on disease-modifying therapy of some kind appear to be in a diminishing minority. What is less standarized is the treatment of patients with atypical relapsing forms of MS, aggressive early MS, and progressive MS. It is often the case that clinicians turn to immunosuppressive agents for more aggressive or difficult cases of MS that either do not seem to be appropriate for treatment with the currently approved disease-modifying therapies or have exhibited an inadequate response to therapy. It is often difficult to apply results of clinical trials to clinical practice. Ideally, our treatment decisions are data-driven, but in reality the choice of therapy for patients reflects a clinician's clinical judgment, his or her breadth of experience with various agents, the patient's preference, as well as the patient's expectations.

This chapter reviews several nonspecific immunosuppressant drugs that have been studied in multiple sclerosis. The review focuses on methotrexate, cyclical pulses of methylprednisolone, cyclophosphamide, mitoxantrone, azathioprine, Cladribine, and cyclosporine.

II. METHOTREXATE

Methotrexate, a competitive inhibitor of dihydrofolate reductase, interferes with the production of reduced cofactors necessary for the synthesis of DNA and RNA (1). Low-dose weekly oral methotrexate (MTX) remains a standard, effective, and relatively safe regimen in the treatment of rheumatoid arthritis (RA) (2). While the exact mechanism of action in RA is unclear (3), low-dose MTX has immunosuppressive activity (4–6), anti-inflammatory activity (7–11), and immunoregulatory effects (12,13).

Several observations suggest that MTX exerts an immunosuppressive effect. Immunoglobulin (Ig) M-rheumatoid factor levels have been found to be significantly decreased in MTX-treated RA patients who showed clinical improvement (4). Serial assessments of T-cell subsets in MTX-treated RA patients have demonstrated a significant increase in suppressor-effect (CD8+CD11+) cell numbers and a trend for increases in suppressor-inducer (CD4+2H4+) cells that paralleled clinical improvement (5). Peripheral blood lymphocytes from RA patients receiving MTX that are grown in low folate culture conditions show in vitro proliferation indices that are lower than those from normal individuals and from RA patients not being treated with MTX (6).

In 1995, Goodkin et al. reported the results from the first double-blind, placebo-controlled phase II trial of low-dose, weekly oral MTX in 60 chronic progressive MS patients (42 with SPMS, 18 with PPMS) (14). Patients enrolled in the study met the following entry criteria: (a) age 21 to 60 years, (b) disease duration of greater than 1 year, and (c) an EDSS (15) score of 3.0 to 6.5. Participants were stratified by their ability to walk without (EDSS < 6.0) or with (EDSS $\geq$ 6.0) assistance and then randomized to receive 7.5 mg oral MTX or placebo one day per week. The primary outcome measure for the study was the proportion of patients experiencing "treatment failure" on methotrexate versus placebo using a composite outcome measure of disability. Patients could meet requirements for sustained treatment failure by experiencing change in any of the following parameters sustained for a minimum of 2 months.

1. Worsening of the entry Expanded Disability Status Scale score (EDSS) by $\geq$ 1.0 point for patients with an entry score of 3.0 to 5.0 or by $\geq$ 0.5 point for those patients with entry EDSS score of 5.5 to 6.5
2. Worsening of the entry ambulation index (AI) (15a) score of 2–6 by $\geq$ 1.0 point
3. Worsening of $\geq$ 20% from baseline value on best performance of 2 consecutive performances of Box and Block test (BBT) (16) scores obtained with either hand
4. Worsening of $\geq$ 20% from baseline value on best performance of two consecutive performances of the 9-Hole Peg Test (9HPT) (16) scores obtained with either hand

Treatment with methotrexate had a favorable effect on sustained progression compared to placebo (MTX = 51.6% and placebo = 82.8%; $p = 0.011$). Analysis of each of the components of the composite showed the effect was strongest for 9HPT ($p = 0.007$) and was seen to a lesser extent in the BBT ($p = 0.068$) and the EDSS ($p = 0.205$). Sustained treatment failure as defined by change in AI did not differ between groups. The time elapsed before 50% of patients achieved sustained treatment failure was 74.4 weeks in the MTX-treated group compared to 23.4 weeks in the placebo group. The difference between overall sustained treatment failure distributions for these groups was highly significant ($p \leq 0.001$).

Forty-two of the 60 patients entered into this study had secondary progressive MS. MTX had a statistically significant treatment effect on the rates of sustained treatment failure measured with the composite outcome variable for secondary progressive patients ($p = 0.005$) but not for primary progressive patients ($p = 0.630$). However, the power to detect differences between groups in the primary disease group was limited due to a small sample size ($n = 18$).

In addition to the clinical neurological evaluations, a standardized neuropsychological testing battery was administered to all patients at study entry and then annually for 2 years. A significant treatment effect favoring MTX was seen on measures of information processing speed ($p < 0.05$), and prose recall ($p < 0.05$) (17). Additionally, 35 consecutively enrolled patients were scheduled for gadolinium enhanced magnetic resonance imaging (MRI) scans at 6-week intervals for the first 6 months of treatment. The results of exploratory analyses demonstrated a treatment effect favoring MTX on absolute change in T2-weighted total lesion area (18). The change in T2-weighted total lesion area was significantly related to sustained progression of disability as measured by tests of manual dexterity but not EDSS.

This study demonstrated a statistically significant treatment effect favoring MTX that was most evident on validated tests of upper extremity function (16). The difference in outcome between treatment groups was apparent within 6 months of initiating therapy and was sustained for 2 years without evidence of significant toxicity. No patient discontinued therapy because of drug toxicity. The therapeutic benefit, however, was not sufficiently robust to be statistically significant when measured solely by the EDSS. This has often been misinterpreted to mean that methotrexate demonstrates only an effect on delaying progression of upper extremity dysfunction. Instead, it is likely that in this population, the EDSS score was not sensitive to change in the time frame of the study and that only with tests of upper extremity function was the benefit of treatment uncovered. It is possible that the therapeutic benefits observed with MTX in the context of this phase II study may be restricted to patients with secondary rather than primary progressive MS, although this conclusion is supported only by preliminary data and may be premature.

Although no major toxicity has yet been observed in patients with multiple sclerosis treated with methotrexate, instances of major toxicity may be expected with more widespread use of this drug. The RA population has provided reliable information regarding tolerability of oral MTX at the same dosage (19). Major toxicity observed in patients with rheumatoid arthritis consists principally of interstitial pulmonary fibrosis, liver fibrosis or cirrhosis, and bone marrow suppression. The American College of Rheumatology guidelines for monitoring methotrexate therapy in rhematoid arthritis suggest following complete blood count with platelet count, albumin creatinine and AST levels every 4 to 8 weeks (20).

Low-dose weekly oral methotrexate is not approved for use in patients with multiple sclerosis. Nonetheless, the observed treatment effect, modest toxicity, ready availability, and limited cost make it an attractive therapeutic option for some patients with progressive forms of MS.

III. CYCLICAL PULSES OF INTRAVENOUS METHYLPREDNISOLONE

Intravenous pulse glucocorticoids remain the treatment of choice for acute relapses in MS (21,22). The use of steroids as disease-modifying agents in progressive MS has also been studied. Two previous studies (23,24) examining the use of glucocorticoids in chronic progressive MS have suggested treatment effect, but because of design limitations the results were difficult to interpret. In 1998, results from the phase II dose comparison trial of cyclical pulses of intravenous methylprednisolone in SPMS patients demonstrated a modest treatment effect in favor of the high-dose treatment option (25).

In this phase II study, 108 patients with secondary progressive MS met the following entry criteria: (a) age 21 to 60 years, (b) disease duration longer than 1 year, and (c) baseline EDSS 4.0 to 6.5. SPMS was defined as progression of ≥ 0.5 EDSS points over 5 months in patients who had experienced one or more exacerbations with or without recovery to baseline EDSS during the 2 years preceding entry. Participants were randomized to receive either high-dose (500 mg, $n = 54$) or low-dose (10 mg, $n = 54$) methylprednisolone every 8 weeks for 2 years. Each bimonthly pulse was administered intravenously once each day for 3 days followed by a tapering course of oral methylprednisolone starting on day 4 and concluding on day 14. High-dose recipients initiated their tapering dose at 64 mg and took the following doses on days 2 to 11: 64, 48, 48, 32, 32, 24, 24, 8, 8, and 8 mg. Low-dose recipients initiated their tapering dose at 10 mg and took the following doses on days 2 to 11: 10, 8, 8, 6, 6, 4, 4, 2, 2, and 2 mg.

The primary outcome measure was a comparison of the proportion of patients experiencing treatment failure in each treatment arm. Treatment failure was defined by sustained worsening for 5 or more months on any component of a composite outcome measure or by relapse rate (three exacerbations treated with unscheduled methylprednisolone during 12 successive months). Components of the composite outcome measure included changes in EDSS (≥ 1.0 point increase for baseline EDSS 4.0 to 5.0, or ≥ 0.5 point increase for baseline EDSS 5.5 to 6.5), time ambulation (≥ 1.0 point increase from baseline), and standardized tests of manual dexterity (20% or more increase from baseline time on the best of two consecutive performances of BBT or 9HPT in either hand).

At the end of the 2 years, 53.7% of the low-dose group and 38.9% of the high-dose group met criteria for treatment failure. This difference was not statistically significant ($p = 0.18$). However, a significant treatment effect was seen with the preplanned secondary outcome, a long rank comparison of the survival curves of the low- and high-dose groups. The time to onset of sustained treatment failure was found to be delayed in the high-dose group ($p = 0.04$). Because the high-dose treatment failure rate did not reach 50%, an estimated median time to onset of sustained treatment failure could not be compared across treatment groups. More high-dose than low-dose recipients experienced drug-related adverse events, but serious drug-related adverse events were uncommon. Cessation of high-dose treatment was discontinued in only one patient, who experienced a transient psychotic reaction.

The results of this study demonstrate that cyclical pulses of steroids are safe, well-tolerated, suggest efficacy in delaying progression of disability in SPMS patients, and may provide an additional alternative disease-modifying treatment of SPMS patients with or without superimposed relapses. While it is widely used off label, the optimal dose, route of administration, and frequency of administration of this promising treatment remains unknown.

IV. CYCLOPHOSPHAMIDE (CYTOXAN)

Cyclophosphamide is an alkylating agent with potent cytotoxic and immunosuppressive effects that is widely used in the treatment of neoplastic and autoimmune disorders. Several unblinded trials of cyclophosphamide in chronic progressive MS have suggested a positive treatment effect (15a,26,27). However, these benefits were not confirmed in one single-blind placebo-controlled trial (28) or the double-blinded placebo-controlled Canadian Cooperative Multiple Sclerosis Study (29), in which patients were randomly assigned to treatment with intravenous cyclophosphamide and oral prednisone, daily oral cyclophosphamide, alternate-day prednisone, and weekly plasma exchange versus placebos with sham plasma exchange for up to 3 years. Reasons for the differing results have been attributed to differences in patient selection, drug doses, and criteria used to define clinical progression (30,31).

A comparison of induction versus induction and maintenance with cytoxan was reported by the Northeast Cooperative Multiple Sclerosis Treatment Group in 1993. In this trial, 256 progressive patients were randomized to four groups to receive two different (established and modified) induction regimens of IV cyclophosphamide/ACTH either with or without 24 monthly boosters (32). The study was designed to detect 15% stabilization or improvement on the nonbooster arms at 3 years compared to 40 to 45% stabilization on the booster arms. The EDSS and AI were used to assess neurological status. At 24 months, 24% of the no-booster group had stable or improved EDSS scores compared to 38% of the booster group ($p = 0.004$). At 30 months, 17% of the no-booster group and 27% of the booster group ($p = 0.004$) were stable or improved as assessed by EDSS. Time to treatment failure after 1 year was also prolonged in the booster-treated group ($p = 0.003$). Post hoc analysis suggested that patients under the age of 40 were more likely to respond to therapy.

The toxicities of cyclophosphamide include alopecia, hemorrhagic cystitis, leukopenia, myocarditis, pulmonary interstitial fibrosis, infertility, and malignancy. In light of these toxicities and conflicting evidence for efficacy, the role of cyclophosphamide as a disease-modifying therapy in MS remains unclear. Cyclophosphamide is most frequently used for selected patients with SPMS who have not responded to other, less toxic alternatives. The results of the NSCMSTG suggest treatment with cytoxan may be most effective when administered as induction followed by maintenance therapy.

V. MITOXANTRONE (NOVANTRONE)

Mitoxantrone is a cytotoxic anthracenedione that is currently approved as a first-line agent in the combination of therapy of acute nonlymphocytic leukemia and as initial; chemotherapy in conjunction with corticosteroids for pain related to advanced hormone-refractory prostate cancer. It has also been used to treat breast cancer, non-Hodgkin's lymphoma, and hepatoma. Its mechanism of action has not been fully elucidated, but it has cytocidal activity on both proliferating and nonproliferating cultured human cells and has been shown to have potent immunosuppressive actions on B- and T-lymphocyte activity (33–35). Because of these immunosuppressive actions, mitoxantrone has been studied in animal models of MS as well as in phase II and III trials for the treatment of RRMS and SPMS.

In 1998, the results of the European multicenter placebo-controlled phase III trial of mitoxantrone in progressive MS demonstrated a beneficial effect favoring treatment (36). In this study, 194 patients with SPMS with or without relapses, ages 18 to 55 years, with EDSS scores of 3.0 to 6.0 were randomized to receive mitoxantrone every 3 months for up to 24 months at a dose of 5 mg/m^2 ($n = 66$) or 12 mg/m^2 ($n = 63$) or placebo ($n = 65$). Participants underwent neurological evaluations every 3 months. In a subgroup of 110 patients, brain MRI sessions were performed annually for 2 years. The primary outcome measure was mean change in EDSS. Additional clinical outcomes included mean change in ambulation index, number of relapses requiring steroid therapy, time to first relapse requiring steroid therapy, proportion of patients experiencing sustained worsening of EDSS, percentage of patients without relapses requiring treatment, mean number of relapses, and time to first relapse.

There were significant treatment effects measured by the primary outcome measure ($p = 0.038$) and most of the secondary clinical outcomes. In general, high-dose recipients experienced a more robust treatment effect. In the subgroup who completed annual MRI scanning sessions, there was a significant reduction in the number of new T2-weighted lesions in both low-and high-dose groups ($p < 0.05$) compared to placebo at the end of 2 years. A significant decrease in the number of new gadolinium enhancing T1-weighted lesions was seen in the high-dose group only at the end of 1 year ($p = 0.016$), and this effect was sustained at the end of 2 years ($p = 0.004$).

Overall, mitoxantrone was well-tolerated during this study. Common side effects included a predictable and reversible leukopenia, mild alopecia, nausea, and menstrual disorders. Left ventricular ejection fraction decreased by 10% in 19 patients on mitoxantrone (19.2%) and in 9 patients on placebo (13.8%). An irreversible cardiomyopathy is reported to occur at cumulative doses of mitoxantrone over 140 mg/m^2 in cancer patients, but no evidence of clinically significant cardiac dysfunction was observed in this or other studies involving MS patients. Mitoxantrone is not currently widely used for the treatment of patients with MS, but its use will increase if approved by the FDA for use in SPMS. Concern remains regarding cardiac toxicity with long-term usage of mitoxantrone. Careful attention should be directed at monitoring cardiac status with serial transthoracic echoes, particularly as patients approach or exceed cumulative doses of 100 mg/m^2

VI. AZATHIOPRINE (IMMURAN)

Azathioprine is a nitroimidazole-substituted form of 6-mercaptopurine with broad-spectrum immunosuppressive effects. Azathioprine has been tested extensively in progressive and relapsing MS patients. In 1991, Yudkin et al. (37) conducted a metanalysis of 7 clinical trials of azathioprine in MS patients. Two of these studies were single-blind (38,39) and five were double-blinded, placebo controlled clinical trials (40–44). A summary of these trials is provided in Table 1. A total of 793 patients were enrolled in the seven trials. Entry criteria for each trial varied and trials included patients with all forms of multiple sclerosis: relapsing remitting, progressive after relapsing and remitting, and progressive from onset. Of the 793 patients, 719 were followed for at least 1 year; 563 patients in five trials were followed for 2 years; and 459 patients in three trials were followed for at least 3 years. Outcomes measures included mean change in Kurtzke disability status scores and probability of freedom from relapse.

Results of the metanalysis showed no clear benefit of treatment in terms of change in Kurtzke scores at 1 year, but a trend for favorable effect at 2 years. In the three trials that looked at treatment over at least 3 years, two showed a slightly greater benefit at 3 compared to 2 years. The difference between mean Kurtzke scores, however, was not robust. Difference in mean change at 3 years was only 0.24 points, and it is debatable whether this represents a clinically significant effect. However, effect on relapse rate was more convincing with treatment reducing risk of relapse even in the first year. Over 2 years, there was an even greater benefit reducing relapses—an effect which was maintained but not further reduced at 3 years.

More recently, Cavazutti et al. published results of a retrospective study comparing MRI lesion burden in 19 patients treated with azathioprine plus steroids versus 17 patients treated with steroids alone (45). Change in total lesion load was compared in two serial proton-density weighted scans at a mean interval of 2.5 years. A significant difference of

Table 1 Summary of Studies of Azathioprine in MS

Swinburn and Liversedge (38)	1973	50 RRMS 44 treated	AZA 2.5 mg/kg/day vs. PLC	2-year follow-up
Mertin et al. (41)	1982	45 RRMS 43 treated	Antilympyhocyte globulin + prednisolone + AZA for 1 month then AZA 3 mg/kg/day for 14 months vs. PLC	1-year follow-up
British and Dutch (56)	1988	354 RR and CPMS 25 treated	AZA 2.5 mg/kg/day vs. placebo	3-year follow-up
Milanese et al. (42)	1988	40 RR and CPMS 25 treated	AZA 2–2.5 mg/kg/day vs. PLC	3-year follow-up
Ghezzi et al. (39)	1989	185 RR and CPMS 135 treated	AZA 2.5 mg/kg/day vs. PLC	1-year follow-up
Ellison et al. (42)	1989	65 CPMS 61 treated	AZA + MP vs. AZA + PLC vs. PLC + PLC Dose titrated to desired WBC effect	3-year follow-up
Goodkin et al. (44)	1991	54 RRMS 43 treated	AZA 3 mg/kg/day vs. PLC	2-year follow-up

Key: RRMS, relapsing-remitting MS; CPMS, chronic progressive MS; AZA, azathioprine; PLC, placebo, MP, methylprednisolone; WBC, white blood cell.

total lesion area between the first and second scans was noted, favoring the azathioprine-treated group ($+15.6\%$ in control, -43.7% in azathioprine recipients). Further prospective studies are necessary to confirm a positive treatment effect of azathioprine on MRI lesion burden.

Although it is generally well tolerated, common side effects of azathioprine include leukopenia, anorexia, diarrhea and vomiting, abdominal pain, abnormal liver function, and skin rashes. To assess the long-term risk of development of cancer, Confavreux et al. conducted a case-control study in 1191 MS patients in the Lyon Multiple Sclerosis Database (46), in which 23 MS patients with cancer were identified: adenocarcinomas of the breast (7), cervix (3), uterine corpus (2), lung (2), kidney (1), and maxilla (1); basal cell epithelioma (1), squamous cell carcinoma (1), chronic myeloid leukemia (1), non-Hodgkin's lymphoma (1), solitary plasmacytoma (1), essential thrombocytopenia (1), and metastatic adenocarcinoma to the liver with unknown primary (1). Of these individuals, 14 had been treated with azathioprine. Each cancer case was matched to three cancer-free MS controls. In comparing risk associated with duration of therapy with azathioprine versus no treatment, MS patients had an increase in cancer risk of 1.3 (95% CI, 0.4 to 4.0) when treated less than 5 years, 2.0 (95% CI, 0.4 to 9.1) when treated 5 to 10 years, and 4.4 (95% CI, 0.9 to 20.9) when treated for more than 10 years. The authors concluded that there is little risk of development of cancer in the early years of treatment. The risk of development of malignancies in long term-treatment must be weighed with the potential benefit of treatment on an individual basis.

VII. 2-CHLORODEOXYADENOSINE (CLADRIBINE)

Cladribine is a purine nucleoside that selectively targets lymphoid cells (47,48). It has been approved for the treatment of hairy-cell leukemia but has also been shown to be effective in the treatment of autoimmune hemolytic anemia and immune thrombocytopenia (49).

In 1990, Sipe et al. conducted a phase II pilot study in four patients with chronic progressive MS treating with a 7-day infusion of six doses of 0.087 mg/kg IV per day. The results of this pilot study suggested a positive treatment effect as measured by sustained improvement on the Scripps Neurologic Rating Scale (SNRS) (50). In 1994, the results of a 2-year double-blind placebo-controlled crossover study of cladribine in 51 chronic progressive MS patients were published (51), again suggesting a positive treatment effect on the SNRS.

In 1999 the results of the phase III study of Cladribine in 159 patients which chronic progressive MS were reported (52). In that study, 48 of the 159 patients had PPMS and 111 patients had SPMS; their EDSS scores ranged from 3.0 to 6.5. Participants were randomly assigned to receive 2-chlorodeoxyadenosine 0.07 mg/kg/day for 5 consecutive days every 4 weeks for either two ($n = 53$, low-dose) or six ($n = 52$, high-dose) cycles or placebo ($n = 54$). All participants completed eight treatment cycles. Those completing active therapy cycles were switched to placebo for their remaining cycles for a total of eight treatment cycles and placebo recipients recieved eight treatment cycles. Patients underwent neurological evaluations (EDSS) bimonthly and MRI scanning sessions every 6 months for 12 months.

No clinical treatment effects were seen across groups as measured by mean changes in disability scores (EDSS and Scripps Neurological Rating Scale), proportion of patients experiencing a sustained increase on the EDSS scale (≥ 1.0 points on EDSS scale for baseline EDSS 3.0 to 5.0, or ≥ 0.5 point for baseline EDSS 5.5 to 6.5), or time to onset of confimed progression of disability. However, the placebo-controlled phase of this study lasted only 12 months, a time frame that may have been too brief to detect a significant effect on sustained progression of disability. Subgroup analysis demonstrated no significant difference in treatment effect between PPMS and SPMS patients.

Analysis of MRI data, however, demonstrated a positive treatment effect favoring Cladribine. Both low- and high-dose recipients with SPMS experienced fewer numbers of gadolinium enhancing T1-weighted lesions ($p = 0.007$, $p = 0.001$ respectively), and the proportion of SPMS patients having gadolinium enhanced T1-weighted lesions was significantly lower in Cladribine recipients (low dose, $p = 0.013$; high-dose, $p = 0.002$). None of these treatment effects were observed in the PPMS recipients.

Cladribine was well tolerated with the exception of a dose-dependent lymphocytopenia and thrombocytopenia. There is significant potential for long-term marrow suppression and possible complications of bleeding, anemia, or opportunistic infection. In the absence of a convincing effect on sustained progression of disability, it is unlikely that Cladribine will be widely used as an alternative disease-modifying therapy for patients with MS, although select patients with highly active disease on MRI may be potential candidates for treatment. Longer-term studies of Cladribine appear warranted.

VIII. CYCLOSPORINE

Cyclosporine is a cyclic undecapeptide immunosuppressant that was initially isolated from two soil fungi and recognized as an antifungal metabolite. Cyclosporine has been found to inhibit the production of a number of lymphokines, including interleukin-2, interleukin-3, migration inhibitory factor, and gamma interferon (53). However, cyclosporine appears to spare T lymphocytes that secrete a soluble factor critical for the expansion of nonspecific suppressor T cells. It appears possible that this T-cell subpopulation belongs to the CD4+CD45R+ subset of T cells known as suppressor inducer (54). Three major studies have assessed the efficacy of cyclosporine in MS, but overall, clinical benefits appear to be outweighed by toxicity and poor tolerability (55–57).

The first of these studies (55) was a double-blinded, controlled trial of 194 patients with clinically definite active relapsing MS: 98 were randomized to treatment with cyclosporine (5 mg/kg/day), and 96 to treatment with azathioprine (2.5 mg/kg/day). A total of 85 patients in the cyclosporine group and 82 in the azathioprine group completed a treatment period of 24 to 32 months, as stipulated by the study protocol. No significant changes were detected in EDSS, frequency of relapse, or overall treatment efficacy as assessed by patients and investigators at the end of the trial. Overall, only minor deterioration occurred in both groups during the trial. Side effects included the following: hypertrichosis, gingival hyperplasia, paresthesias, elevated serum creatinine, and elevated blood pressure. These side effects were seen more than twice as often in the cyclosporine group as in the azathioprine group. The authors concluded that cyclosporine as a single agent was not acceptable as the drug of final choice for the long-term immunosuppressive treatment of relapsing MS.

The second study was a double-blinded, placebo-controlled trial with patients who had either relapsing or chronic progressive clinically definite MS. A total of 82 patients were enrolled at centers in London ($n = 44$) and Amsterdam ($n = 38$) (56). The patients were begun on daily cyclosporine 10 mg/kg for 2 months, which was subsequently adjusted to minimize toxicity for the final 22 months of observation. The mean daily maintenance dose differed at the two sites (London 7.2 mg/kg, and Amsterdam, 5.0 mg/kg). While investigators in Amsterdam concluded that no beneficial clinical effects were seen and that side effects from cyclosporine presented a major problem, the investigators at the London site reported separately that patients had fewer relapses and a longer interval to first relapse on treatment over the 2-year study and better overall functional assessments for the first 6 months of treatment (56).

The most recent study was a multicenter effort undertaken in the United States (57). In this study, 273 clinically definite MS patients with a progessive course were randomized to receive cyclosporine for at least 2 years. Patients were moderately disabled, with EDSS scores ranging from 3.0 to 7.0. The dosage of cyclosporine was adjusted for toxicity, resulting in trough whole-blood levels from 310 to 430 mg/mL. Clinical outcome measures included (a) time to becoming wheelchair-bound, (b) time to dependency in activities of daily living, (c) time to sustained progression of neurological disability and (d) change in EDSS score from baseline. Cyclosporine treatment delayed time to confinement to wheelchair ($p = 0.038$) and the mean worsening in EDSS score for cyclosporine-treated patients (0.39 ± 1.07 points) was significantly less ($p = 0.002$) than for placebo-treated patients (0.65 ± 1.08), but statistically significant effects were not observed for the other criteria. A large and differential withdrawal rate (cyclosporine 44%; PLC 32%) complicted the analysis but did not appear to explain the observed effect of cyclosporine in delaying time to wheelchair confinement. Nephrotoxicity and hypertension were common and accounted for most of the excess loss of patients in the cyclosporine arm of the study.

The authors concluded that cyclosporine was associated with a modest benefit in the patients with chronic progressive MS in the study, but these benefits were not evident until 18 to 24 months after initiating therapy. Because of this delay in measurable benefit and the high incidence of toxicity, cyclosporine is not routinely used in the management of MS patients.

IX. CONCLUSION

Clinical and radiological evidence indicates that immunosuppressive therapies have a modest therapeutic effect on modifying the disease course in relapsing and progressive forms of MS. In the absence of head-to-head comparisons of therapeutic options, treatment decisions are generally driven by personal experience and clinical judgment. We favor monotherapy with weekly oral methotrexate, cyclical pulses of methylprednisolone, or 3-monthly mitoxantrone in MS patients with progression of disability. Mitoxantrone would be preferred in patients with rapidly progressive disease unresponsive to immunomodulators (interferon beta-la, interferone beta-lb, glatiramer acetate), whereas methotrexate or steroids might be preferred in frail patients or those with a more slowly progressive course. All three share the benefits of good tolerability and ease of administration, but there are also clear disadvantages. Methotrexate has interactions with commonly used medications such as aspirin and patients must abstain from alcohol. There are potential long-term consequences of steroid use, including osteoporosis, cataracts, cushingoid appearance, etc. Mitoxantrone has potential for cardiotoxicity at doses exceeding 120 mg/m^2, and there is a risk of infertility. Others favor cytoxan for patients who are suboptimally responsive to approved therapies and off-label treatment options. We consider cytoxan to be less appealing because of poor tolerability and absence of convincing effects in placebo-controlled trials.

REFERENCES

1. Grosflam J, Weinblatt ME. Methotrexate: Mechanism of action, pharmacokinetics, clinical indications, and toxicity. Curr Opin Rheumatol 1991; 3:363–368.
2. Weinblatt ME, Weissman BN, Holdsworth DE, et al. Long-term prospective study of methotrexate in the treatment of rheumatoid arthritis: 84-month update. Arthritis Rheum 1992; 35: 129–137.
3. Cronstein BN. The mechanism of action of methotrexate. *Rheum Dis Clin* North Am 1997; 23:739–755.
4. Alarcon GS, Schrohenloher RE, Bartolucci AA, et al. Suppression of rheumatoid factor production by methotrexate in patients with rheumatoid arthritis: Evidence for differential influences of therapy and clinical status on IgM and IgA rheumatoid factor expression. Arthritis Rheum 1990; 33:1156–1161.
5. Calabrese LH, Taylor JV, Wilke WS, et al. Methotrexate (MTX) immunoregulatory T-cell subsets and rhematoid arthritis: Is MTX an immunomodulator? Arthritis Rheum 1988; 31(suppl 1):C20.
6. Hine RJ, Everson MP, Hardon JM, et al. Methotrexate therapy in rheumatroid arthritis patients diminishes lectin-induced mono-nuclear cell proliferation. Rheumatol Int 1990; 10:165–169.
7. Weinblatt ME, Coblyn JS, Fox DA, et al. Efficacy of low-dose methotrexate in rheumatoid arthritis. N Engl J Med 1985; 312: 818–822.
8. Sperling RI, Benincaso AI, Anderson RJ, et al. Acute and chronic suppression of leukotriene B$_4$ synthesis ex vivo in neutrophils from patients with rheumatoid arthritis beginning treatment with methotrexate. Arthritis Rheum 1992; 35: 376–384.
9. Segal R, Yaron M, Tartakovsky B. Methotrexate: Mechanism of action in rheumatoid arthritis. Semin Arthritis Rheum 1990; 20:190–200.
10. Tak PP, Smeets TJM, Daha MR, et al. Analysis of the synovial cell infiltrate in early rheumatoid synovial tissue in relation to local disease activity. Arthritis Rheum 1997; 40:217–225.
11. Dolhain RJEM, Tak PP, Dijkmans BAC, et al. Methotrexat reduces inflammatory cell numbers, expression of monokines and of adhesion molecules in synovial tissue of patients with rheumatoid arthritis. Br J Rheum 1998; 37:502–508.

12. Nielsen HJ, Nielsen H, Georgsen J. Ranitidine for improvement of treatment resistant psoriasis. Arch Dermatol 1991; 127:270.

13. Nielsen JH, Hammer JH. Possible role of histamine in pathogenesis of autoimmune diseases: Implications for immunotherapy with histamine-2 receptor antagonists. Med Hypoth 1992; 39:349–355.

14. Goodkin DE, Rudick RA, VanderBrug Medendorp S, et al. Low-dose (7.5 mg) oral methotrexate reduces the rate of progression in chronic progressive multiple sclerosis. Ann Neurol 1995; 37:30–40.

15. Kurtzke JF. Rating neurologic impairment in multiple sclerosis: An expanded disability scale (EDSS). Neurology 1983; 33:1444–1452.

15a. Hauser SL, Dawson DM, Lehrich JR, et al. Intensive immunosuppression with high dose cyclophosphamide, plasma exchange, and ACTH. N Engl J Med 1983; 308:173–180.

16. Goodkin DE, Hertzgaard D, Seminary J. Upper extremity function in multiple sclerosis: Improving assessment sensitivity with box-and-block and nine-hole-peg-tests. Arch Phys Med Rehabil 1988; 69:850–854.

17. Fischer JS, Goodkin DE, Rudick RA, et al. Low-dose (7.5 mg) oral MTX improves neuropsychological function in patients with chronic progressive multiple sclerosis. Ann Neurol 1994; 36:289.

18. Goodkin DE, Rudick RA, VanderBrug Medendorp S, et al. Low dose oral methotrexate in chronic progressive multiple sclerosis: Analyses of serial MRIs. Neurology 1996; 47:1153–1157.

19. Goodman TA, Polisson RP. Methotrexate: Adverse reactions and major toxicities. Rheum Dis Clin North Am 1994; 20:513–528.

20. ACR; American College of Rheumatoloy Ad Hoc Committee on Clinical Guidelines. Guidelines for monitoring drug therapy in rheumatoid arthritis. Arthritis Rheum 1996; 39(5):723–731.

21. Kupersmith MJ, Kaufman D, Paty D, et al. Megadose corticosteroids in MS. Neurology 1994; 44:1–4.

22. Olivieri RL, Valentino P, Russo C, et al. Randomized trial comparing two different high doses of methylprednisolone in MS. A clinical and MRI study. Neurology 1998; 50:1833–1836.

23. Rinne UK, Sonninen V, Tuovinen T, Corticotrophin treatment in multiple sclerosis. Acta Neurol Scand. 1968; 44:207–218.

24. Milligan NM, Newcombe R, Compston DAS. A double-blind controlled trial of high dose methylprednisolone in patients with multiple sclerosis. 1. Clinical effects. J Neurol Neurosurg Psychiatry 1987; 50:511–516.

25. Goodkin DE, Kinkel RP, Weinstock-Guttman B, et al. A phase II study of IV methylprednisolone in secondary-progressive multiple sclerosis. Neurology 1998; 51:239–245.

26. Hommes OR, Lamers KJB, Reekers P. Effect of intensive immunosuppression on the course of chronic progressive multiple sclerosis. J Neurol 1980; 223:177–190.

27. Goodkin DE, Plencner S, Palmer-Saxerud K, et al. Cyclophosphamide in chronic progressive multiple sclerosis: Maintenance vs nonmaintenance therapy. Arch Neurol 1987; 44:823–832.

28. Likosky WH, Fireman B, Elmore R, et al. Intense immunosuppression in chronic progressive multiple sclerosis: the Kaiser study. J Neurol Neurosurg Psychiatry 1991; 54:1055–1060.

29. TCCMSG, The Canadian Cooperative Multiple Sclerosis Group. The Canadian cooperative trial of cyclophosphamide and plasma exchange in progressive multiple sclerosis. Lancet 1991; 337:441–446.

30. Noseworthy JA, Vandervoort MK, Penman M, et al. CTX and plasma exchange in multiple sclerosis (letter). Lancet 1991; 337:1540–1541.

31. Weiner HL, Hauser SL, Dawson DM, et al. CTX and plasma exchange in multiple sclerosis (letter). Lancet 1991; 337:1033–1034.

32. Weiner HL, Mackin GA, Orav EJ, et al. Intermittent cyclophosphamide pulse therapy in pro-

gressive multiple sclerosis: Final report of the Northeast Cooperative Multiple Sclerosis Treatment Group. Neurology 1993; 43:910–918.

33. Wang BS, Lumanglas AL, Ruszala-Mallon VM, Wallace RE, Durr FE. Induction of alloreactive immunosuppression by 1,4-bis[(2-aminoethyl)amino]-5,8-dihydroxy-9,10-anthracenedione dihydrochloride. Int J Immunopharmacol 1984; 6:475.

34. Wang BS, Lumanglas AL, Silva J, Ruszala-Mallon VM, Durr FE. Inhibition of induction of alloreactivity with MTXN. Int J Immunopharmacol 1986; 8:967–973.

35. Fidler JM, DeJoy SQ, Smith FR III, Gibbon JJ. Selective immunomodulation by the antineoplastic agent MTXN: Suppression of B lymphocyte function. J Immunol 1986; 137:727–732.

36. Hartung HP, Gonsette R. MTXN in progressive multiple sclerosis (MS): a PLC-controlled, randomized observer-blind European phase III multi-center study-clinical results. Mul Scler 1998; 4:325.

37. Yudkin PL, Ellison GW, Ghezzi A, Goodkin DE, et al. Overview of azathioprine treatment in multiple sclerosis. Lancet 1991; 338:1051–1055.

38. Swinburn WB, Liversedge LA. Long-term treatment of multiple sclerosis with azathioprine. J Neurol Neurosurg Psychiatry 1973; 36:124–126.

39. Ghezzi A, DiFalco M, Locatelli C, et al. Clinical controlled randomized trial of azathioprine in multiple sclerosis. In: Gonsette RE, Delmotte P, eds. Recent Advances in Multiple Sclerosis Therapy. Amsterdam: Elsevier, 1989.

40. BDMSATG. British and Dutch Multiple Sclerosis Azathioprine Trial Group. Double-masked trial of azathioprine in multiple sclerosis. Lancet 1988, 8604:179–183.

41. Mertin J, Rudge P, Kremer M, et al. Double-blind controlled trial of immunosuppression in the treatment of multiple sclerosis: final report. Lancet 1982; 8294:351–354.

42. Milanese C, La Mantia L, Salmaggi A, et al. Double blind controlled randomized study on azathioprine efficacy in multiple sclerosis: Preliminary results. Ital J Neurol Sci 1988; 9(1): 53–57.

43. Ellison GW, Myers LW, Mickey MR, et al. A placebo-controlled, randomized, double-masked, variable dosage, clinical trial of azathioprine with and without methylprednisolone in multiple sclerosis. Neurology 1989; 39:1018–1026.

44. Goodkin DE, Bailly RC, Teetzen ML. The efficacy of azathioprine in relapsin-remitting multiple sclerosis. Neurology 1991; 41:20–25.

45. Cavazzutti M, Merelli E, Tassone G, Mavilla L. Lesion load quantification in serial MR of early relapsing multiple sclerosis patients in azathioprine treatment. Eur Neurol 1997; 38:284–290.

46. Confavreux C, Saddier P, Grimaud J, et al. Risk of cancer from azathioprine therapy in multiple sclerosis: A case control study. Neurology 1996; 46:1607–1612.

47. Carson DA, Wasson DB, Taetle R, Yu A. Specific toxicity of 2-chlorodeoxyadenosine towards resting and proliferating human lymphocytes. Blood 1983; 62:737–743.

48. Carson DA, Wasson DB, Beutler E. Antileukemic and immunosuppressive activity of 2-chloro-2'-deoxyadenosine. Proc Natl Acad Sci USA 1984; 81:2232–2236.

49. Beutler E. Cladribine (2-chlorodeoxyadenosine). Lancet 1992; 340:952–956.

50. Sipe JC, Knobler RL, Braheny SL, et al. A neurologic rating scale (NRS) for use in multiple sclerosis. Neurology 1984; 34:1368–1372.

51. Sipe JC, Romine JS, Koziol JA, et al. Cladribine in the treatment of chronic progressive multiple sclerosis. Lancet 1994; 334:9–13.

52. Rice GPA, Filippi M, Comi G, et al. Therapeutic effect of MYLINAX (Cladribine) on disease activity and burden in progressive multiple sclerosis: clinical and MRI outcomes of a multicenter, randomized double-blind, placebo-controlled trial. Submitted.

53. Reem GH, Cook LA, Vilck J. Gamma interferon synthesis by human thymocytes and T lymphocytes by cyclosporine A. Science 1983; 22:63–65.

54. Rich S, Caprina MR, and Arthelger C. Suppressor T cell growth and differentiation: Identifica-

tion of a cofactor required from suppressor T cell function and distinct from interleukin 2. J Exp Med 1987; 159:1473–1490.

55. Kappos L, Patzold U, Poser S, et al. Cyclosporine versus azathioprine in the long-term treatment of multiple sclerosis: results of the German Multicenter Study. Ann Neurol 1988; 23: 56–63.

56. Rudge P, Koetsier JC, Mertin J, et al. Randomized double blind controlled trial of cyclosporine in multiple sclerosis. J Neurol Neurosurg Psychiatry 1989; 52:559–565.

57. TMSSG. The Multiple Sclerosis Study Group. Efficacy and toxicity of cyclosporine in chronic progressive multiple sclerosis: A randomized, double-blind, placebo-controlled clinical trial. Ann Neurol 1990; 27:591–605.

26

Treatment of Multiple Sclerosis: Bone Marrow Reconstitution, Total Lymphoid Irradiation, and Plasma Exchange

GEORGE P. A. RICE

The Multiple Sclerosis Clinic, London, Ontario, Canada

I. INTRODUCTION

The relative inadequacy of the treatments currently available for multiple sclerosis (MS) reflects, in large measure, our naïve understanding of the pathogenesis of the disease and the nature of its progression (1). Despite the vast amount of research (reviewed in Chap. 7) and the strong circumstantial evidence that MS is an autoimmune disease, it must be conceded that the study of immunological abnormalities in vitro has yielded little insight into the pathogenesis of the disease. There has been a penchant to interpret the disease process in the context of the latest immunological assays, be they for a new cytokine, adhesion molecule, or lymphocyte subset. Often interesting at the moment of publication, remarkably few of these observations have left insightful legacies. Few observations appear to be reproducible.

Lymphocytes are present in the nervous system of MS patients (2). Attempts to identify something unique about autoreactive lymphocytes in MS have failed. Preliminary studies that suggested linkage of susceptibility to T cell–receptor genes in patients with MS have not been confirmed (3). Neither has it been confirmed that T-cell expression is unique in perpheral blood lymphocytes. This is not surprising, given that the pattern of expression of T cell–receptor genes has not characterized any human autoimmune disease. Tantalizing reports of restricted T-cell gene utilization within plaques await confirmation

(4). Lymphocyte reactivity to brain antigens such as myelin basic protein and proteolipid has been described in MS patients but also in controls (5).

These lymphocytes appear to be activated and can release a variety of cytokines, possibly contributing to inflammation and demyelination (6), although a role for lymphocytes in repair and regulation should not be discounted. Most MS treatment strategies have been targeted at lymphocytes or the consequences of their activation.

We do not understand the fundamental immunological abnormality in MS, why the disease can start over a wide range of years, exactly how it is triggered, or how the disease can progress insidiously after one or more inaugural attacks. The events that determine the evolution of relapsing MS to progressive MS remain particularly mysterious. The inflammatory process itself, demyelination, and axonal transection are likely all important players (7).

Heroic treatment is justified only if the risk of treatment is less than the mortality of the disease. Survival is shortened moderately by MS and mortality rates increase with advancing disability. Wheelchair-confined patients face 10-year mortality rates of >50%. In desperation, there has been a tendency to embark on heroic treatments in such patients. Disability, to the point of requiring walking assistance (cane, walker, or wheelchair), develops in approximately 50% of patients within 15 years of disease onset (8) and in the majority of patients by 25 years. The course of the disease is variable. The determinants that identify a poor outcome are only partially understood. A more aggressive disease course is suggested by the occurrence of frequent attacks in the first 2 years of the disease and by early accumulation of disability (8). A large burden of disease on the magnetic resonance scan at the time of diagnosis bodes for a more ominous disease course (9). Identification of benign cases is suggested by an early age of onset, a low attack frequency in the first few years, and a minimal burden of disease on magnetic resonance imaging (MRI). Paradigms are being developed to identify less disabled patients who are at high risk for disease progression and who might have greater benefit from heroic intervention.

II. BONE MARROW ABLATION AND RECONSTITUTION

A. Rationale

Based on the supposition that MS is an immune-mediated disorder, there has been substantial interest in purging the immune system of its autoreactive lymphocytes by bone marrow ablation followed by reconstitution with allogeneic bone marrow transplantation (BMT) or autologous stem cell transplantation (ASCT) (10,11). This enthusiasm derives from the theoretical attraction of the procedure, an encouraging pilot experience in patients with MS (10–12) and other immune-mediated disorders, such as rheumatoid arthritis, systemic lupus erythematosus, immune-mediated thrombocytopenia, psoriasis, and inflammatory bowel disease (for review, see Ref. 13) and the reduction in morbidity and mortality. Although animal models of MS and other autoimmune disorders have not been useful crucibles for testing new treatments in MS, the fact that both spontaneous and induced autoimmune diseases in rodents can be "cured" by BMT/ASCT (14–16) provides the limited rationale that can be derived from imperfect animal models.

Marrow ablation and reconstitution is intended to result in the regeneration of an immune system that is naïve to the mysterious brain autoantigen. It is assumed that putative MS triggers operative at the onset of the disease are absent at the time of the marrow reconstitution.

B. The Treatment

Allogeneic BMT vs. Autologous Stem Cell Transplantation

Grafting of allogeneic bone marrow stem cells has been associated with higher mortality as well as with lingering concerns about graft versus host disease and the need for chronic immunosuppression. The mortality of such procedures has been substantially higher, in the range of 20%—an unacceptable figure for patients with MS. ASCT is associated with less mortality (about 1 to 3% in breast cancer patients; 10 to 15% in patients with hematological malignancies) and largely obviates graft versus host disease. If there is an immunological abnormality in MS that is present in early precursor cells, grafts of autologous stem cells, mobilized from the peripihery, run the risk of reintroducing the guilty immunocytes that triggered the original disease. For this reason, autologous stem cells are purged of T cells, usually with a T cell–specific monoclonal antibody (CD34) (10,11) or other T-cell manipulations (antithymocyte globulin, either in vitro or in vivo) (12). Stem cells can be obtained from bone marrow, but the harvesting procedure requires considerably more manipulation and general anesthesia. Peripheral stem cells can be harvested more easily with only the minor inconveniences occasioned by placement of the central line for the cytopheresis. Cytokines such as granulocyte-colony stimulating factor (g-CSF) are administered to facilitate mobilization of peripheral stem cells. Such cytokines could potentially aggravate MS lesions. It is thought that this complication can be minimized by cyclophosphamide treatment during the process of stem cell mobilization (10,11).

Bone Marrow Ablation in the Recipient

A variety of techniques has been used to prepare the recipient. Some of the regimens have employed high dose cytotoxic agents such as busulphan, or BEAM (**B**CNU + **E**toposide + cytosine **A**rabinoside + **M**elphalan) (10,11). Total lymphoid radiation (TLI, 150 cGy bid for 4 days) has been favored by others (12) as possibly being more immunosuppressive and includes radiation of the spinal cord.

Complications

Patients require multidisciplinary treatment with antiemetics, blood product support, nutrition, prevention of venous occlusive disease, and insightful management of potential infections. Revaccination of marrow recipients is necessary. ASCT should not be undertaken outside of specialized facilities. The mortality for ASCT should be less than 5%. The rates are higher in patients above 50 years of age and those who have received prior cytotoxic chemotherapy.

The Experience to Date

Because adequately powered and controlled phase II trials have not yet been conducted and follow-up has not been long enough in unrandomized observational studies, it is difficult to draw firm conclusions about the potential utility of this treatment. Only a handful of pilot observations has been reported, and there has been substantial variation in the methods of patients selection, recipient marrow ablation, and graft preparation. There also have been a handful of encouraging reports in MS patients who received BMT as treatment for concomitant hematological malignancies (17). The existing data provide only a mandate for further evaluation of the procedure.

More than 70 patients have been transplanted in pilot studies (10,11). There have been fatalities from complications of immunosuppression. Barring one fatality from increased MS activity, possibly from g-CSF administration, there do not appear to be MS-specific hazards. Although there have been anecdotal reports of disease stability or improvement in transplanted patients, it has been difficult to differentiate the effect of marrow ablation from the transplant itself. In the largest experience (12), of 23 patients who survived the procedure, 18 were deemed to be stable or better and 5 (22%) were deemed to have progressed. It is of note, however, that this experience was neither blinded nor controlled. The natural history of patients with untreated progressive MS would predict that about 30% of patients would worsen in a similar time frame (18).

There have been well-documented cases of MS exacerbations occurring in patients who have been successfully engrafted (19). Imperfect marrow ablation in the recipient (radio-resistant, disease-causing lymphocytes), reinfusion of central nervous system (CNS)-reactive mature lymphocytes with the ASCT (missed by T-cell purging), regeneration of CNS-reactive lymphocytes from progenitor cells (i.e., the same problem) are all reasonable explanations.

Future Prospects

BMT remains an unproven treatment in MS, but there is enough encouraging information to justify a substantial research effort. A definitive phase II trial is clearly worthwhile. The utilization of controls will be important. Longer studies will be necessary to differentiate the effects of marrow conditioning from marrow transplantation. Such experimentation should be done by groups with proven expertise in BMT. It will be important for all the clinical experience to be published to avoid the bias for publication of favorable reports. A registry of all treated patients would be welcome. If transplantation does not work, the hypothesis that MS is purely an autoimmune disorder might be questioned further.

III. TOTAL LYMPHOID IRRADIATION

A. Rationale

Total lymphoid irradiation (TLI) is undeniably effective in securing long-standing suppression of cell-mediated immunity. TLI prolongs organ transplant survival and can induce long-term remission in both natural and experimental autoimmune disorders. This approach has been studied in human autoimmune disorders, such as rheumatoid arthritis and multiple sclerosis.

B. The Treatment

Patients with progressive MS were treated with an 8 MeV photon beam from a Philips SL 75-10 linear accelerator (20,21). The radiation was given by mantle and inverted-Y approach. Care was taken to limit parotid radiation, so as to avoid devastating xerostomia, and radiation of the spleen field was restricted to protect the left kidney. The radiation dose was adjusted to deliver <1000 rads to the spinal cord. A total dose of 1980 cGy was given over 11 fractions.

C. The Experience to Date

In the largest placebo-controlled, double-blind study (40 patients total) (20,21), a significant effect was demonstrable at 6 months, and this effect persisted "significantly" for 18 months. The trend continued until 48 months, the end of the study. Subset analysis identified that the treatment response was confined to patients who had a radiation-induced lymphopenia of <900 lymphocytes per cubic millimeter. The same investigators reported, in an unblinded, open-label study, that low-dose prednisone (approximately 30 mg/day) enhanced the response (22).

Not all patients benefited from the treatment. Over the course of this study, more than 50% TLI-treated patients continued to progress. It is also worth emphasizing that the benefit in favor of TLI was significant statistically only for the first 18 months. Late recurrence of disease activity has also been reported in rheumatoid arthritis patients treated with TLI (23).

These favorable clinical results were not reproduced in a smaller (24 patient) and likely underpowered study that followed a similar protocol (24). Although a clinical benefit was not identified, a small but significant improvement of the MRI segregated with the TLI-treated group (24). An uncontrolled study of TLI was not encouraging (25).

Nausea, anorexia, weight loss, skin irritation, fatigue, dysphagia, vomiting, diarrhea, and hair loss are predictable in TLI-treated patients. There have been mortalities secondary to sepsis. Amenorrhea as well as axillary and inguinal hair loss are ubiquitous, and these factors pose significant challenges for the neurologists who performed blinded assessments in these studies. The late development of malignancy, which has some precedent from a previous study of TLI in Hodgkin's disease, remains a concern (26).

Among the 54 patients who participated in the New Jersey pilot and a subsequent open-label study, there have been six deaths (20). These occurred between 42 and 54 months after therapy.

D. Future Prospects

Although of theoretical interest, the marginal clinical and radiological benefits appear to be outweighed by an excess of morbidity and mortality. TLI cannot be recommended as a treatment for MS in routine practice.

IV. THERAPEUTIC PLASMA EXCHANGE

A. Rationale

Therapeutic plasma exchange (TPE) involves the removal of plasma and its replacement, generally with saline and albumin. In some earlier studies, plasma was replaced with intravenous immunoglobulin. Dissecting which manipulation was effective in combination treatment would be difficult. TPE has a well-established place in the treatment of neurological disorders such as acute exacerbations of myasthenia gravis and chronic inflammatory demyelinating polyneuropathy (for review, see Refs. 27 and 28). In diseases such as myasthenia gravis, the removal of the offending immunoglobulin is compatible with our understanding of the pathology of the disease. In MS, the potential mechanisms of action are unknown. Removal of demyelinating immunoglobulins, immune complexes, complement, and proinflammatory cytokines might be desirable from a theoretical perspective. Neuroelectric blocking factors have been identified in MS sera and their removal has some logic (29).

B. The Treatment

Replacement of plasma with saline/albumin is generally thought to be safe and well tolerated. The treatment is expensive, requires insertion of central lines, and carries with it some risk of discomfort and infection (30). The use of heparin during the procedure poses some risk of thrombocytopenia.

C. The Experience to Date

Progressive MS

Vamvakas (31) undertook a metaanalysis of six prospective, controlled studies of TPE in patients with progressive MS. A very modest but statistically significant effect in favor of treatment was identified. The metaanalysis might be questioned because of the substantial variability in TPE protocols, the use of concomitant immunosuppressive treatments, and the definition of control groups—not to mention any publication bias.

TPE for Rescue from Steroid-Refractory Acute Exacerbations

Long-term benefit in the first controlled trials in relapsing MS were not compelling and difficult to dissociate from concomitant immunosuppression (32). However, some observers had noted that patients with devastating exacerbations could be rescued by TPE (33–35). These observations prompted a recent study by Dr. Weinshenker and his colleagues (36) at the Mayo clinic. The study included patients with acute devastating exacerbations that were refractory to corticosteroid treatment. Patients with MS, acute disseminated encephalomyelitis, Devic's disease, Marburg disease, and acute regional demyelinating disorders were evaluated. The neurological deficits had been at their nadir for a minimum of 3 weeks, with trivial or no improvement after high-dose intravenous methylprednisolone. The patients were selected intensively. Patients with a flare-up that was superimposed on chronic progression were excluded, as were patients with chronic stable fixed deficits. This rigorous screening procedure accounts for the small number patients who met the eligibility criteria.

The study was innovative in the application of a new outcome measure. Rather than use the conventional outcome scale defined on the basis of disability, a scale was tailored to the nature of the exacerbation for each (36).

TPE was given over a period of seven treatments on alternate days. Intravenous immune globulin (IVIG) was not given. To maximize patient recruitment, a crossover protocol was used. Carryover effects from the first treatment were not deemed to be a significant hazard.

Of the 19 of TPE-treated patients, 8 had a significant improvement, compared to 1 of 17 sham-treated patients. The results were significant with one-sided statistical tests. The treatment gains of TPE were short-lived. Half of the patients who improved went on to further exacerbations, one of which was fatal.

D. Future Prospects

The success of TPE as a rescue treatment for severe, steroid-refractory exacerbations will be met with enthusiasm by MS neurologists, and we will see more application of this treatment in such cases. Physicians who resort to this treatment are reminded that these favorable outcomes were shown in highly selected patients. The desperate cry for relief of chronic fixed deficits will not be answered by this treatment.

V. CONCLUSIONS

MS can be a devastating disorder, even in the short and intermediate terms for a minority of MS patients. In these individuals, treatments entailing major risks can be justified. **It** must be emphasized that gains in knowledge are unlikely to be realized by study of patients outside of experimental protocols.

ACKNOWLEDGMENTS

The author is grateful to Drs. George Ebers, Stuart Cook, and George Ellison for insightful comments on these treatments and the manuscript.

REFERENCES

1. Ebers GC. Treatment of multiple sclerosis. Lancet 1994; 343:275–279.
2. Bruck W, Bitsch A, Kolenda H, Bruck Y, Stiefel M, Lassmann H. Inflammatory central nervous system demyelination: Correlation of magnetic resonance imaging findings with lesion pathology. Ann Neurol 1997; 43:783–793.
3. Hashiimoto LL, Mak TW, Ebers GC. T cell receptor alpha chain polymorphisms in multiple sclerosis. J Neuroimmunol 1992; 40:41–48.
4. Oksenberg JR, Stuart S, Begovich AB, et al. Limited heterogeneity of rearranged t-cell receptor V beta transcripts in brain of multiple sclerosis patients. Nature 1990; 345:344–346.
5. Olsson T, Zhi WW, Hojeberg B, et al. Autoreactive T lymphocytes in multiple sclerosis determined by antigen-induced secretion of interferon-gamma. J Clin Invest 1990; 86:981–985.
6. Huang YM, Xiao BG, Ozenci V, Kouwenhoven M, Teleshova N, Fredrikson S, Link H. Multiple sclerosis is associated with high levels of circulating dendritic cells secreting pro-inflammatory cytokines. J Neuroimmunol 1999; 99:82–90.
7. Charcot JM. Lectures on Disease of the Nervous System. London: The New Sydenham Society, 1977, pp 171–172.
8. Weinshenker BG, Bass B, Rice GP, et al. The natural history of multiple sclerosis: A geographically based study: I. Clinical course and disability. Brain 1989; 12:133–146.
9. Filippi M, Horsfield MA, Morrissey S, et al. Quantitative brain MRI lesion load predicts the course of clinically isolated syndromes suggestive of multiple sclerosis. Neurology 1994; 44: 635–641.
10. Burt RK. BMT for severe autoimmune diseases: An idea whose time has come. Oncology 1997; 11:1001–1014.
11. Burt RK, Burns WH, Miller SD. Bone marrow transplantation for multiple sclerosis: Returning to Pandora's box. Immunol Today 1997; 18:559–561.
12. Fassas A, Anagnostopoulos A, Kazis A, et al. Peripheral blood stem cell transplantation in the treatment of progressive multiple sclerosis: First results of a pilot study. Bone Marrow Transplant 1997; 20:631–638.
13. Ikehara S. Bone marrow transplantation for autoimmune diseases. Acta Haematol 1998; 99: 116–132.
14. van Gelder M, van Bekkum DW. Effective treatment of relapsing experimental autoimmune encephalomyelitis with pseudoautologous bone marrow transplantation. Bone Marrow Transplant 1996; 18:1029–1034.
15. Karussis D, Vourka-Karussis U, Mizrachi-Koll R, Abramsky O. Acute/relapsing experimental autoimmune encephalomyelitis: Induction of long lasting, antigen-specific tolerance by syngeneic bone marrow transplantation. Mult Scler 1999; 5:17–21.
16. Burt RK, Burns W, Hess A. Bone marrow transplantation for multiple sclerosis. Bone Marrow Transplant 1995; 16:1–6.
17. McAllister LD, Beatty PG, Rose J. Allogeneic bone marrow transplant for chronic myelogenous leukemia in a patient with multiple sclerosis. Bone Marrow Transplant 1997; 19:395–397.
18. Weinshenker BG, Bass B, Rice GP, et al. The natural history of multiple sclerosis: A geographically based study: 2. Predictive value of the early clinical course. Brain 1989; 112:1419–1428.

19. Jeffery D, Alshami E. Allogenic bone marrow transplantation in multiple sclerosis. Neurology 1998; 50:A147.

20. Cook SD, Troiana R, Zito G, et al. Deaths after total lymphoid irradiation for multiple sclerosis. Lancet 1989; 29:277–278.

21. Devereux C, Troiano R, Zito G, et al. Effect of total lymphoid irradiation on functional status in chronic multiple sclerosis: Importance of lymphopenia early after treatment—the pros. Neurology 1988; 38:32–37.

22. Cook SD, Devereux C, Troiano R, Bansil S, Zito G, Sheffet A, Jotkowitz A, Rohowsky-Kochan C, Dowling PC. Combination total lymphoid irradiation and low-dose corticosteroid therapy for progressive multiple sclerosis. Acta Neurol Scand 1995; 91:22–27.

23. Trentham DE, Belli JA, Anderson RJ, Buckley JA, Goetzl EJ, David JR, Austen KF, Cook SD, et al. Clinical and immunologic effects of fractionated total lymphoid irradiation in refractory rheumatoid arthritis. N Engl J Med 1981; 305:976–982.

24. Wiles CM, Omar L, Swan AV, Sawle G, Frankel J, Grunewald R, Joannides T, Jones P, Laing H, Richardson PH, et al. Total lymphoid irradiation in multiple sclerosis. J Neurol Neurosurg Psychiatry 1994; 57:154–163.

25. Buffoli A, Micheletti E, Capra R, Mattioli F, Marciano N. Progressive multiple sclerosis: Evaluation of the effectiveness of total lymph node irradiation. Radiol Med 1991; 81:899–901.

26. Sverdlow AJ, Douglas AJ, Hudson GV, et al. Risk of second primary cancers after Hodgkin's disease by type of treatment: analysis of 2846 patients in the British lymphoma investigation. BMJ 1992; 304:1137–1143.

27. Khatri BO. Therapeutic apheresis in neurological disorders. Ther Apheresis 1999; 3:161–171.

28. Shumak KH, Rock GA. Therapeutic plasma exchange. N Engl J Med 1984; 310:762–771.

29. Stefoski D, Schauf CL, McLeod BC, Haywood CP, Davis FA. Plasmapheresis decreases neuroelectric blocking activity in multiple sclerosis. Neurology 1982; 32:904–907.

30. Henze T, Prange HW, Talarschik J, et al. Complications of plasma exchange in patients with neurological diseases. Klin Wochenschr 1990; 68:1183–1188.

31. Vamvakas EC, Pineda AA, Weinshenker BG. Meta-analysis of clinical studies of the efficacy of plasma exchange in the treatment chronic progressive multiple sclerosis. J Clin Apheresis 1995; 10:163–170.

32. Weiner HL, Dau PC, Khatri BP, et al. Double-blind study of true vs. sham plasma exchange in patients treated immunosuppression for acute attacks of multiple sclerosis. Neurology 1989; 39:1143–1149.

33. Warren KG, Gordon PA, McPherson TA. Plasma exchange of malignant multiple sclerosis. Can J Neurol Sci 1982; 9:27–30.

34. Trouillas P, Neuschwander P, Tremis JP. Rapid modification of the symptomatology of progressive forms of multiple sclerosis by plasma exchange. Rev Neurol (Paris) 1986; 142:689–695.

35. Rodriguez M, Karnes WE, Bartleson JD, Pineda AA. Plasmapheresis in acute episodes of fulminating CNS inflammatory demyelination. Neurology 1993; 43:1100–1104.

36. Weinshenker BG, O'Brien PC, Petterson TM, et al. A randomized trial of plasma exchange in acute CNS inflammatory demyelinating disease. Ann Neurol 1999; 46:878–886.

27

Symptomatic Therapy

RANDALL T. SCHAPIRO

Fairview MS Center and University of Minnesota, Minneapolis, Minnesota

I. INTRODUCTION

The advent of immunomodulating medications has markedly altered the way clinicians view multiple sclerosis (MS). The often expressed view was that there was little to do for those with MS until these disease-modifying agents came on the scene. That was never the case. The management of symptoms in MS was and remains the single most common and necessary role of the physician interested in developing a management plan for a person with MS. Symptom management can improve the quality of life so significantly that it can make the difference in a person being able to live in today's society or not. There are many symptoms that occur regularly in MS. There are often several ways to manage those symptoms. This chapter discusses the medical management of MS symptomatology. Chapter 28 discusses in depth the rehabilitation of MS. It is essential to understand that neither stands alone. The proper management of MS involves medication and rehabilitation done simultaneously on an ongoing basis. When these occur together, symptom management in multiple sclerosis becomes real and alive!

II. FATIGUE

The single most disturbing and disabling symptom in MS is fatigue (1). There are five different fatigues that contribute to the alarmed feeling that bothers most with MS. Obviously normal fatigue occurs in those with disease as it does in those without. This is especially the case if the person is trying to prove competence by doing more than expected. The management strategy is to understand the situation and recognize that fatigue of this sort is not damaging but simply tiring. People who have MS are not fragile, and while the idea is not to test the system to see how far one can go before permanent problems occur, one can go pretty far and still live to tell the tale. However it is good for all, including those with MS, to plan and carry out the day in an efficient manner.

MS can lead to depression and depression can lead to fatigue. This is especially important to understand because there are treatments for depression that are efficient and effective. Demyelination in the brain typically leads to changes in the neurochemistry in the brain (2). This may manifest as the signs of depression, with sleep disturbances, eating disturbances, and fatigue. The specific serotonin release–inhibiting medications, of which there are many, can be of significant value because they not only treat depression but can also energize in the process (3). Fluoxetine, paroxetine, sertraline, etc., should accompany counseling for this specific type of fatigue.

Neuromuscular fatigue follows the repetitive stimulation of a demyelinated nerve. This "short-circuiting" type of fatigue presents as muscle fatigue with ongoing use of a muscle. It is best treated by rest, allowing the nerve and muscle to recover function. This is the reason that progressive resistive exercise must be done with caution, allowing for time for the nerve-muscle combination to recover between repetitions.

Deconditioning may be a problem in MS. This leads to another type of fatigue. A conditioning program with the prudent use of aerobic exercise can be valuable in this circumstance.

Lassitude is the term reserved for the overwhelming tiredness that comes with auto-immune diseases. This occurs with MS and is a sleepiness that is prevalent despite the absence of activity. Neurochemicals such as amantadine and fluoxetine are of benefit for this (3). Sometimes stimulants such as pemoline may be helpful (4). Modafinil (provigil), an agent utilized for the management of narcolepsy, has also found a home in treating MS lassitude. Care must be taken not to provoke agitation with the combinations of medicines to help treat fatigue. Also care must be taken to prevent oversedation with the medications used to treat other symptoms seen in MS. Iatrogenic fatigue may be a necessary but not welcomed side effect of aggressive management.

III. SPASTICITY

Ambulation problems are the result of many different factors. These include weakness, ataxia, sensory disturbances, and cognitive disturbances. Most of these are treated with rehabilitative techniques. Spasticity may disturb ambulation and also cause significant discomfort and positioning problems. Spasticity is the result of an upper motor neuron dsyfunction in regulation of impulses and neurochemistry. Its presence is not necessarily negative, as it may be present without significant weakness and it may be helpful in transferring techniques. However if it is causing discomfort, aggressive treatment is not only appropriate but necessary.

Exercise and removal of noxious stimuli are the first line of treatment. Baclofen (Lioresal) is usually the first medication utilized. It is effective at low to high dosing and the exact dose is determined by response. Usually it is begun at 5 mg tid, but doses of 40 mg qid may be necessary for some. The side effects of weakness, sedation, and cognitive problems are the limiting factors. The dose is titrated according to function. If baclofen is found to be ineffective on its own, tizanidine may be added to the baclofen for synergistic potential. These medications act differently and thus may be additive (5). Tizanidine is limited by side effects of fatigue and dry mouth but tends not to be associated with as much weakness as baclofen (6). Thus its use as a primary antispasticity agent becomes apparent if weakness is a prevalent symptom. Doses of 2 mg qd to 36 mg in divided doses may be necessary.

Spasms are common in MS and often occur during the nighttime hours or just before sleep. While baclofen and especially tizanidine are helpful for spasms, both clonazepam (Klonopin) and diazepam (Valium) are also indicated, taking advantage of their antispasticity and significant sedating potential. Gabapentin (Neurontin) is also very helpful for problematic spasms, with doses of up to 3 to 4 g but usually of 2000 mg or less (7). Occasionally L-dopa or dopaminergic agonists can help spasms at fairly low doses (8) and the serotinergic antagonist cyproheptadine (Periactin) (9) may treat spasticity with a high level of sedation.

Dantrolene (Dantrium) is often too weakening for most patients with MS, but it may be helpful at low doses for the spinal form of the disease.

The baclofen pump has been phenomenal for intractable spasticity unmanageable by oral medications. The Synchromed programmable pump has allowed for relief of severe spasticity with minimal side effects, but involves a surgical procedure and poses the problems of any mechanical device with catheter and occasionally pump difficulties (10). It requires an experienced physician to implant and control the dosage of the medication (usually different physicians).

Botulinum toxin (Botox) can be helpful for less severe, localized muscle spasm as seen occasionally in the face or the adductor muscles of the legs (11). Unfortunately, most spasms are in large muscles, the treatment of which requires too much toxin to be practical. Motor-point blocks and surgical procedures are done less often today.

IV. WEAKNESS

The weakness seen in MS is usually due to decreased central conduction secondary to demyelination. Occasionally weakness is caused by deconditioning. When that is the case, a strengthening program will potentially bring the muscle back to normality. However, there is usually a degree of decreased conduction, and progressive resistive exercises lead to fatigue, as described above.

The old adage "Use it or lose it" does apply to weakness in MS. Thus even if the muscle is neurologically weakened, it should be stimulated to prevent atrophy. Thus the therapist must carefully ferret out the muscles that can and should be strengthened by exercise. Medication can boost nerve condition. The aminopyridines are potassium blockers, which allow for faster and more efficient transmission in demyelinated nerves (12). They are chemicals available in compounding pharmacies. However the quality control is not universal and the incidence of seizures is unacceptable. Until better control of the blood levels can be obtained, their use is not recommended. Nonetheless, several reports indicated increased strength and endurance and decreased fatigue with the aminopyridines.

V. URINARY DYSFUNCTION

Urinary discomfort in MS is very common. The "MS bladder" can be big and boggy or small and muscular. In both cases the symptoms may be similar, including urgency, frequency, hesitancy, and incontinence. In the big bladder that fails to empty, the symptoms are secondary to overflow incontinence. In the small failure-to-store bladder, they are due to the hyperactivity of the bladder muscle. Diagnosis is key to treatment. Residual urine can be obtained via a catheter or ultrasound machine. If the residuals are high, catheterization techniques may be essential. Stimulants such as urecholine are rarely helpful but may be worth a try in selected individuals. Ataxia, numbness, weakness, and cognitive prob-

lems often make self-catheterization less desirable despite the appropriateness of the bladder for that technique.

Anticholinergic medication (oxybutynin, tolterodine, propantheline) can be titrated
to slow the hyperactive bladder (13). Care must be taken with these, especially in the
summer, as they can decrease the sweating response and inadvertently lead to hyperthermia and severe weakness.

Dyssynergia of the bladder and bladder sphincter is also common in MS. Urodynamic studies may be necessary to make this diagnosis. Alpha-blocking agents (terazosin,
phenoxygenzamine) may aid in better emptying if this condition is present (14).

VI. BOWEL DYSFUNCTION

Bowel problems in MS are reasonably frequent, although not as typical as bladder dysfunction. The most common problem is constipation. Often this is due to decreased fluid intake,
which takes place in order to control the bladder. Lack of physical activity can also contribute to the problem. Both of these can be solved if the right attitude is instilled and the
bladder can be regulated.

However, often a bowel program is helpful. This begins by the understanding that
the best time for a bowel movement is after a meal. This takes advantage of the gastrocolic
reflex. The addition of a bulk-forming substance (e.g., Metamucil, Fibercon, Per Diem)
can be important. If that fails, the addition of a gentle mechnical stimulant such as a
glycerine suppository or a TheraVac mini-enema on the third day of constipation often
works. The idea is to have a bowel movement about every 3 days or less. If that fails
stimulants in the form of Dulcolax suppositories may be necessary. Stimulation from
above with milk of magnesia or lactulose is sometimes the way to treat especially refractory constipation. Typically that is not necessary.

Sometimes the problem is the opposite, with urgency and incontinence. The goal
in this situation is to bulk up the stool to allow more time for the bowel movement sensation. Often transferring and undressing techniques become important here. The use of
Metamucil as a bowel regulator is the most frequent management suggestion. In this situation, more Metamucil with less fluid is utilized in order to allow the Metamucil to absorb
excess bowel fluid, making the stool bulkier. Bowel movements on a schedule in the
morning allow for more freedom during the day.

VII. SEXUAL DYSFUNCTION

The management of sexual dysfunction has evolved dramatically in the past decade. There
was a time when little could be done for the man or woman with MS who had sexual
difficulties. For the man with erectile dysfunction, treatment in the 1980s meant a penile
prosthesis. While these evolved into very functional and useful pieces of equipment, their
use in MS diminished because of the advent of injectable vasodilating medications. The
administration of papaverine and more recently prostaglandin (aprostadil) intracorporeally
made for a very firm and usable erection (15). The inconvenience and lack of spontaneity
is a problem. Vacuum tubes that drew blood into the penis, which was held by a rubber
band, became popular for a short time. Their clumsiness and perceived lack of effectiveness made them less popular. A prostaglandin (Alprostadil) that required injection was
put into a suppository form and given via the urethra (MUSE) (16). This is still used as is
the injection method. However, the most popular form of treatment has become sildenafil

(Viagra) (17). This pill, when taken 30 min prior to sexual activity, allows for a very natural, usable erection in many men with MS who previously could not achieve one. It requires lovemaking to work but has become the drug of choice in this circumstance. The dose is 50 to 100 mg 30 min prior to intercourse.

Women who have decreased lubrication have their choice of very natural vaginal lubricants. Vibrators can produce stimulation in numb areas and a frozen bag of peas can substitute as a vaginal/clitoral stimulant if necessary (18). The use of sildenafil in women has been discussed but data are lacking.

The key to beginning the management of sexual dysfunction is to ask about it. Too often the topic is avoided and thus the problem is not treated. Insurance companies have often chosen to see this as a condition that does not require treatment. This goes against the majority of opinion among people who want to be sexually active but cannot be as they were in the past. Today the methodology to make this possible exists.

VIII. PAIN

Pain in MS is very common. Over half of those with MS will have some pain (19). In some of these patients, the problem is quite obvious, with pain due to orthopedic, joint, or back problems, that may have occurred because of gait deviations, altering the normal joint relationships. These need to be treated by correction of the problem.

However, often the pain is a burning, irritative pain, a dysesthesia. This "nerve" pain may occur anywhere on the body. It likely is due to demyelination within the sensory tracts in the brain and spinal cord. Some antiseizure medications have been helpful in controlling the pain of MS (20). Carbamazepine has been used for many years for the nerve pain of neuralgia, especially the trigeminal neuralgia sometimes seen in MS. Doses of 800 mg or more are sometimes required, and this often leads to significant fatigue. Gabapentin has become more helpful, as it often decreases MS pain without the fatigue seen with carbamazepine. Doses of gabapentin must often reach 2000 mg or more for optimal effect.

Occasionally other anticonvulsant medications can be helpful for neuralgia, and other neurochemical agents including misoprostol (Cytotec) may serve as adjuvant medication (21).

The tricyclic antidepressants, including amitriptyline, are utilized, but again, they are quite sedating. They may allow for help in sleeping in the case of pain.

IX. TREMOR

Tremor can be especially disabling. It is not unusual to see tremor in a person who otherwise has retained good strength. It is also not unusual to see it in the more cognitively impaired, giving meaning to the descriptive term *cerebellar-cerebral MS*. The tremor is typically of the action variety. No real help is afforded by exercise; thus medical management is particularly important. There are no drugs that work universally in tremor management but many that have the potential to help sometimes. None of these pharmaceuticals were introduced specifically for tremor management and most have been poorly studied for this. Nonetheless, by experience, a variety have proved to be helpful.

Propranolol (Inderal) is a beta blocker that clearly helps patients with essential tremor and is often of some help with the cerebellar tremor of MS (22). Doses of over 160 mg are often necessary to get an effect. Primidone (Mysoline) will occasionally tone down the tremor with less than anticonvulstant dosages of 150 to 300 mg per day (23). Clonazepam (Klonopin) will provide a calming effect, which can diminish the tremor, as well its relative diazepam (Valium). The tuberculosis medication isoniazid (INH) in high dosage (300 mg three times per day) will, in some, decrease the gross tremor often described as "rubro" (24). Liver and blood toxicity must be guarded against. Ondansetron (Zofran) in dosages of 8 mg three times a day has had a better effect than most medications but its cost is especially prohibitive (25). Buspirone (Buspar) in dosages of 10 to 15 mg four times per day will occasionally help diminish tremor (26).

Often various combinations of these medications are necessary to get an effect, and trial and error is the rule.

Surgical procedures involving lesions in the extrapyramidal system proved more dangerous than helpful in the late 1960s. Now the question of stimulatory electrodes is raised, but unfortunately, to date, no good data are available on which to base this potential treatment for MS. It has been shown to be of value in the very different tremor of Parkinson's.

X. VISUAL DYSFUNCTION

Visual problems in MS are very common. Decreased vision due to disease of the optic nerve or tracts is particularly frequent due to their highly concentrated myelination. High-dose IV corticosteroids (methylprednisolone, 1000 mg per day for 3 to 5 days) often will shorten the course of acute visual loss secondary to optic nerve inflammation (27). There are no good data to indicate that low-dose steroid (usually given orally) makes a difference (27). Some have interpreted study data as showing a negative effect to the oral treatment, but that interpretation was made without a study designed to look at this specific question and must therefore be held in doubt.

Diplopia secondary to internuclear ophthalmoplegia or isolated brainstem involvement of the extraocular muscles and nerves is very annoying. Steroids can speed recovery in this situation as well, but often the healing is slow and incomplete. The brain is usually capable of fusing the images even in the face of muscle imbalance if patching of an eye is not too aggressively done early on in the course of the problem.

XI. PAROXYSMAL SPASMS

A unique symptom that occasionally occurs in MS is that of surrounding electrical short circuiting in the spinal cord. This results in a paroxysmal episode of spasm on sensory disturbance. These are called tonic spasms and can be frightening, especially if misunderstood. The spasm usually begins in the upper extremity but may spread to the legs or even the face. It lasts for seconds and may recur very frequently and then settle down without rhyme or reason. It is treated with anticonvulsants, particularly carbamazepine. Fairly low doses usually control the problem and, after it is settled, the medication can usually be withdrawn.

XII. PATHOLOGICAL LAUGHING/CRYING

Pathological laughing and crying is another symptom linked to diffuse brain damage. While it may occur with small strokes, it is not unusual with the more cortically involved MS pathology. It is a symptom of pseudobulbar palsy. The individual cries or less commonly laughs inappropriately and uncontrollably. Tricylic antidepressants (amitriptyline) have been helpful in gaining control of this embarrassing symptom.

XIII. CONCLUSION

The management of MS has changed dramaticaly in the past 10 years. Nonetheless, the backbone to managing MS properly remains the symptom management of the disease. Today we can truly begin to manage the disease itself, the symptoms of the disease, and the person with the disease. This truly improves the quality of life for those with MS.

REFERENCES

1. Krupp LB, Alvarez LA, La Rocca NG, Scheinberg LC. Fatigue in multiple sclerosis. Arch Phys Med Rehabil 1988; 45:435–437.
2. Wolinsky JS, Narayana PA, Fenstermacher MJ. Proton magnetic spectroscopy in multiple sclerosis. Neurology 1990; 40:1764–1769.
3. Schapiro RS. Symptom Management in Multiple Sclerosis. 3rd ed. New York: Demos Publications, 1998, p 27.
4. Weinshenker BG, Penman M, Bass B, Ebers GC, Rice GPA. A double-blind, randomized crossover trial of pemoline in fatigue associated with multiple sclerosis. Neurology 1992; 42: 1468–1471.
5. United Kingdom Tizanidine Trial Group. A double-blind, placebo-controlled trial of tizanidine in the treatment of spasticity caused by multiple sclerosis. Neurology 1994; 44(suppl 9):S70–S78.
6. Bass B, Weinshenker B, Rice GPA. Tizanidine versus baclofen in the treamtent of spasticity in patients with multiple sclerosis. Can J Neurol Sci 1988; 15:15–19.
7. Dunevsky A, Berel AB. Gabapentin for relief of spasticity associated with multiple sclerosis. Am J Phys Med Rehabil 1998; 77:451–454.
8. Calne DB. Drug treatment of spasticity and rigidity. Mod Trends Neurol 1975; 6:25–27.
9. Schapiro, RT. Symptom Management in Multiple Sclerosis, 3rd ed. New York: Demos Publications, 1998.
10. Penn RD, Savoy SM, Corcos D. Intrathecal baclofen for severe spinal spasticity. N Engl J Med 1989; 320:1517–1521.
11. Borg-Stein J, Fine Z, Mille RJ, Brin M. Botulinum toxin for the treatment of spasticity in multiple sclerosis. Am J Phys Med Rehabil 1993; 72:364–468.
12. Davis FA, Stefoski D, Rush J. Orally administered 4-aminopyridine improves clinical signs in multiple sclerosis. Ann Neurol 1990; 27:186–192.
13. Fowler CJ, van Kerrebroeck PE, Nordenbo A, Van Poppel H. Treatment of lower urinary tract dysfunction in patients with multiple sclerosis. Committee of the European Study Group of SUDIMS. J Neurol Neurosurg Psychiatry 1992; 55:986–989.
14. Betts CD, D'Mellow MT, Fowler CJ. Urinary symptoms and neurological features of bladder dysfunction in multiple sclerosis. J Neurol Neurosurg Psychiatry 1993; 56:245–250.
15. Chao R, Clowers DE. Experience with intracavernosal tri-mixture for the management of nellurogenic erectile dysfunction. Arch Phys Med Rehabil 1994; 75:276–278.
16. Schapiro RT. Symptom Management in Multiple Sclerosis, 3rd ed. New York: Demos Publications, 1998.
17. Viera AJ, Clenney TC, Shernerberger DW, Grea FF. Newer pharmacologic alternatives for erectile dysfunction. Am Fam Physician 1999; 60(4):1159–1166.
18. Schapiro RT. Symptom Management in Multiple Sclerosis, 3rd ed. New York: Demos Publications, 1998.

19. Stenager E, Knudsen I, Jensen K. Acute and chronic pain syndromes in multiple sclerosis. Acta Neurol Scand 1991; 84:197–200.
20. Schapiro RT. Symptom Management in Multiple Sclerosis, 3rd ed. New York: Demos Publications, 1998.
21. Reder AT, Arnason BG. Trigeminal neuralgia in multiple sclerosis relieved by a prostaglandin E analogue. Neurology 1995; 45:1097–1100.
22. Rudick R, Schiffer RB, and Herndon RM. Drug treatment of multiple sclerosis. Semin Neurol 1987; 7:150–159.
23. Wasielowski PG, Burns JM, Kolwer WC. Pharmacologic treatment of tremor. Mov Disord 1998; 13 suppl 3:90–100.
24. Bozek CB, Kastrukoff LF, Wright JM, Perry TL, Larsen TA. A controlled trial of isoniazid therapy for action tremor in multiple sclerosis. Neurology 1987; 234:36–39.
25. Rice GP, Lesaux, J, Vandenoort P, Maceuar L, Ebers GC. Ondansetron, a 5-HT3 antagonist, improves cerebellar tremor. J Neurol Neurosurg Psychiatry 1997; 62:282–284.
26. Trouillas P, Xie J, Adeleine P. Treatment of cerebellar ataxia with buspirone. Lancet 1996; 348:759.
27. Beck RW, Cleary PA, Angerson PAC Jr. A randomized, controlled trial of corticosteroids in the treatment of acute optic neuritis. N Engl J Med 1992; 326:581–588.

28

Symptomatic Treatment and Rehabilitation in Multiple Sclerosis

CHARLES R. SMITH

St. Agnes Hospital, White Plains, New York

LABE SCHEINBERG

Albert Einstein College of Medicine, New York, New York

I. INTRODUCTION

Multiple sclerosis (MS) is one of the more common diseases capable of producing severe disability in the young adult population. Since the total population of patients in the United States is estimated to be 350,000—that is, a prevalence of about 0.1%—and since a substantial number may suffer severe disability, MS is a disease of considerable social and economic impact.

The most frequent age of onset is between 20 and 45 years, with a mean age of onset of 33. As the female-to-male ratio is nearly 2:1 and the white-to-nonwhite ratio is also nearly 2:1, MS is primarily a disease of young adult white women.

The cause of MS is unknown. Available evidence suggests that autoimmune factors are important in the pathogenesis of lesions, but how these immunological aberrations are precipitated remains a mystery. Although epidemiological evidence implies that an environmental factor is important, no environmental agent has yet been identified that causes the disease.

The disease varies widely from individual to individual. Recently, four patterns of disease have been suggested for disease classification (1). Patients with the relapsing-remitting form have attacks that resolve completely or nearly so and disability is mild over the long term. Typically, attacks eventually decrease in frequency. For a few, the symptoms are only general sensory or visual, so-called benign MS. The progressive-relapsing type is similar to the relapsing-remitting form in that there are clear-cut attacks but recovery following episodes is incomplete and disability gradually mounts. Other patients never experience definite exacerbations but have slowly evolving neurological deficits, the primary progressive form. These patients typically manifest their disease later in life and primarily exhibit myelopathic signs and symptoms. Patients whose disease was initially relapsing-remitting and who later become chronic progressive are termed secondary progressive.

It is impossible to predict with accuracy which disease course a patient will follow. Approximately 85% of patients begin with relapsing-remitting disease. However, within 10 to 15 years of illness, about half of these patients will develop secondary progressive MS. Once a course has become progressive, spontaneous reversion to a remitting course is unlikely. However, many patients with progressive courses experience long periods of stability.

Some features of the disease may be of prognostic value. Female sex and onset of disease before age 40 years tends to have a better prognosis than male sex and disease of later onset. Relapsing-remitting disease is more favorable than slowly progressive disease. However, frequent attacks, especially in the first 2 years of illness, is an unfavorable prognostic sign. Symptoms primarily of a sensory nature, such as numbness or tingling or optic neuritis, are associated with a good prognosis. Early onset of motor signs—including ataxia, weakness, spasticity, or tremor—suggests a poor prognosis (2,3).

II. EVALUATING THE PATIENT

Because the course of MS can be difficult to predict, especially in the early years, attempts have been made to quantify impairment and disability to help in giving a prognosis, selecting patients for experimental protocols, monitoring the response, and determining future rehabilitative needs. The best-known and most widely used comprehensive scale for MS is the Minimal Record of Disability (MRD), developed by the International Federation of Multiple Sclerosis Societies (4).

The MRD was designed to adhere to the three-tier classification of dysfunction developed by the World Health Organization (WHO): impairment, the physical impact of the underlying organic disorder resulting in clinical signs and symptoms; disability, the personal limitations imposed on the activities of daily living; handicap, the environmental ramifications, which limits the disabled person from achieving an optimal social role.

The WHO impairment classification has been codified by the Kurtzke system, a two-part evaluation that assesses neurological impairment. The Extended Disability Status Scale (EDSS), a 20-step ordinal scale based on the neurological examination, measures overall function of the patient through the assignment of a numerical score selected from a 20-step ordinal scale (Table 1) (5). The derivation of the EDSS relies heavily on the Functional Systems (FS), a series of eight functional groupings based on objectively verifiable defects (Table 2) (5). These are mutually exclusive in terms of neuroanatomy and each is assigned a numerical rating indicative of the degree of involvement of that system.

Disability is measured by the Incapacity Status Scale and correlates with the Kurtzke, Pulses (6), Barthel (7), and Escrow (8) systems as standards. Handicap is measured by the Environmental Status Scale of Mellerup and Fog (9), which addresses the less tangible measures of an MS individual's social dysfunction as defined in different cultural settings. Regular and careful determinations of the MRD over the course of the disease may help to provide an estimation of the course to be expected. Another frequently used

Table 1 Kurtzke Expanded Disability Status Scale (EDSS) and Functional Systems (FS) Scores[a]

0.0	Normal neurological exam (all grade 0 in FS).
1.0	No disability, minimal signs in one FS (i.e., grade 1).
1.5	No disability, minimal signs in more than one FS (more than one grade 1).
2.0	Minimal disability in one FS (one FS grade 2, others 0 or 1).
2.5	Minimal disability in two FS (two FS grade 2, others 0 or 1).
3.0	Moderate disability if one FS (one FS grade 3, others 0 or 1) or mild disability in three or four FS (three or four FS grade 2 others 0 or 1) though fully ambulatory.
3.5	Fully ambulatory but with moderate disability in one FS (one grade 3) *and* one or two FS grade 2; *or* two grade 3 (others 0 or 1); or five grade 2 (others 0 or 1).
4.0	Fully ambulatory without aid, self-sufficient, up and about some 12 h a day despite relatively severe disability consisting of one FS grade 4 (others 0 or 1), *or* combination of lesser grades exceeding limits of previous steps and the patient can walk > 500 m without assist or rest.
4.5	Fully ambulatory without aid, up and about much of the day, may otherwise require minimal assistance; characterized by relatively severe disability usually consisting of one FS grade 4 (others or 1) *or* combinations of lesser grades exceeding limits of previous steps *and* the patient can walk >300 m without assist or rest.
5.0	Ambulatory without aid for at least 50 m; disability severe enough to impair full daily activities (e.g., to work a full day without special provision). (Usual FS equivalents are one grade 5 alone, others 0 or 1; combinations of lesser grades.) The patient should be able to walk ≥200 m without aid or rest.
5.5	Ambulatory without aid for at least 50 m; disability severe enough to preclude full daily activities. (Usual FS equivalents are one grade 5 alone, others 0 or 1; or combinations of lesser grades). Enough to preclude full daily activities. (Usual FS equivalents are one grade 5 alone, others 0 or 1; or combinations of lesser grades.) The patient should be able to walk ≥100 m without aid or rest.
6.0	Intermittent or unilateral constant assistance (cane, crutch, brace) required to walk at least 50 m. (Usual FS equivalents are combinations with more than one FS grade 3.)
6.5	Constant bilateral assistance (canes, crutches, braces) required to walk at least 50 m. (Usual FS equivalents are combinations with more than one FS grade 3.)
7.0	Unable to walk at least 50 m even with aid, essentially restricted to wheelchair; wheels self and transfers alone; up and about in wheelchair some 12 h a day. (Usual FS equivalents are combinations with more than one FS grade 4+; very rarely pyramidal grade 5 alone.)
7.5	Unable to take more than a few steps; restricted to wheelchair; may need aid in transfer; wheels self but cannot carry on in wheelchair a full day. (Usual FS equivalents are combinations with more than one FS grade 4+; very rarely pyramidal grade 5 alone.)
8.0	Essentially restricted to chair or perambulated in wheelchair, but out of bed most of day; retains many self-care functions; generally has effective use of arms. (Usual FS equivalents are combinations, generally grade 4+ in several systems.)
8.5	Essentially restricted to bed most of day; has some effective use of arm(s); retains some self-care functions. (Usual FS equivalents are combinations generally 4+ in several systems.)
9.0	Helpless bed patient; can communicate and eat. (Usual FS equivalents are combinations, mostly grade 4+.)
9.5	Totally helpless bed patient; unable to communicate effectively or eat or swallow. (Usual FS equivalents are combinations almost all grade 4+.)
10.0	Death due to MS.

Note: EDSS steps below 5 refer to patients who are fully ambulatory, and the precise step is defined by the Functional System (FS)score(s). EDSS steps from 5 up are defined by ability to ambulate, and *usual* equivalents in FS score are provided.

Table 2 Kurtzke Functional Systems (FS)

1 *Pyramidal Functions*
   0. Normal.
   1. Abnormal signs without disability.
   2. Minimal disability.
   3. Mild to moderate paraparesis or hemiparesis; or severe monoparesis
   4. Marked paraparesis or hemiparesis; moderate quadriparesis; or monoplegia.
   5. Paraplegia, hemiplegia, or marked quadriparesis.
   6. Quadriplegia.
   9. Unknown.
2 *Cerebellar Functions*
   0. Normal.
   1. Abnormal signs without disability.
   2. Mild ataxia.
   3. Moderate truncal or limb ataxia.
   4. Severe ataxia in all limbs.
   5. Unable to perform coordinated movements because of ataxia.
   9. Unknown.
3 *Brainstem Functions*
   0. Normal
   1. Signs only.
   2. Moderate nystagmus or some other mild disability.
   3. Severe nystagmus, marked extraocular weakness, or moderate disability of other cranial nerves.
   4. Marked dysarthria or other marked disability.
   5. Inability to swallow or speak.
   9. Unknown.
4 *Sensory Function*
   0. Normal.
   1. Vibration or figure-writing decrease only in one or two limbs.
   2. Mild decrease in touch or pain or position sense, and/or moderate decrease in vibration in one or two limbs; or vibratory decrease alone in three or four limbs.
   3. Moderate decrease in touch or pain or position sense, and/or essentially lost vibration in one or two limbs; or mild decrease in touch or pain and/or moderate decrease in all proprioceptive tests in three of four limbs
   4. Marked decrease in touch or pain or loss of proprioception, alone or combined, in one or two limbs; or moderate decrease in touch or pain and/or severe proprioceptive decrease in more than two limbs.
   5. Loss (essentially) of sensation in one or two limbs; or moderate decrease in touch or pain and/or loss of proprioception for most of the body below the head
   6. Sensation essentially lost below the head.
   9. Unknown.
5 *Bowel and Bladder Function* (rate on the basis of worse function, either bowel or bladder)
   0. Normal.
   1. Mild urinary hesitancy, urgency, or retention.
   2. Moderate hesitancy, urgency, retention of bowel or bladder or rare urinary incontinence (intermittent self-catheterization, manual compression to evacuate bladder, or finger evacuation of stool).
   3. Frequent urinary incontinence.
   4. In need of almost constant catheterization (and constant measures to evacuate stool).
   5. Loss of bladder function.
   6. Loss of bladder and bowel function
   9. Unknown: Not tested by oversight.

Table 2 Continued

6 *Visual (or Optic) Functions*
   0. Normal.
   1. Scotoma with visual acuity (corrected) better than or equal to 20/30.
   2. Worse eye with scotoma with maximal visual acuity (corrected) of 20/30 or 20/59.
   3. Worse eye with large scotoma, or moderate decrease in fields, but with maximal visual acuity (corrected) of 20/60 to 20/99.
   4. Worse eye with marked decrease of fields and maximal visual acuity (corrected) of 20/100 or 20/200; grade 3 plus maximal acuity of better eye of 20/60 or less.
   5. Worse eye with maximal visual acuity (corrected) less than 20/200; grade 4 plus maximal acuity of better eye of 20/60 or less.
   6. Grade 5 plus maximal visual acuity of better eye of 20/60 or less.
   9. Unknown.
7 *Cerebral (or Mental) Function*
   0. Normal.
   1. Mood alteration only (does not affect DSS score).
   2. Mild decrease in mentation.
   3. Moderate decrease in mentation.
   4. Marked decrease in mentation (chronic brain syndrome- moderate).
   5. Dementia or chronic brain syndrome—severe or incompetent.
   9. Unknown.
8 *Other functions* (any other neurological findings attributable to MS)
   a. *Spasticity*
       0. None.
       1. Mild (detectable only).
       2. Moderate (minor interference with function).
       3. Severe (major interference with function).
       9. Unknown.
   b. *Other*
       0. None.
       1. Any other neurological findings attributed to MS: Specify _____.
       9. Unknown.

assessment scale, the Ambulation Index, is a 10-point ordinal scale that, like the EDSS, is heavily weighted to gait (Table 3) (10).

Because of the inherent limitations imposed by these ordinal rating scales, a Clinical Outcomes Assessment Task Force was appointed by the National MS Advisory Committee on Clinical Trials of New Agents in MS in 1994 and charged with developing new clinical outcome measures for use in clinical trials. The Task Force recommended that the clinical outcome measures be multidimensional to reflect the varied clinical expression of MS across patients and over time, including cognitive function and should change relatively independently over time. The MS Functional Composite (MSFC) Measure was published in 1997 for use in evaluating new agents in clinical trials (11) and included a timed 25-ft walk (to test lower extremity function) (10), a nine-hole peg test (to test upper extremity function) (12) and a paced auditory serial addition test (PASAT-3'') (to test neuropsychological function) (13). The Task Force has yet to define measures for visual, sensory, bladder, bowel, and sexual functions.

Table 3   Ambulation Index (AI)

0	Asymptomatic; fully active; no gait abnormality reported or observed.
1	Walks normally but reports fatigue or difficulty running which interferes with athletic or other demanding activities.
2	Abnormal gait or episodic imbalance; gait disorder is noticeable to family and friends, and evident to examiner. Able to walk 25 ft in 10 s or less.
3	Walks independently; requires 10 s, but able to walk 25 ft in 20 s or less.
4	Requires unilateral support (cane, single crutch) to walk; uses support more than 80% of the time. Walks 25 ft in 20 s or less.
5	Requires bilateral support (canes, crutches, walker) and walks 25 ft in 20 s or less; or, requires unilateral support but walks 25 ft in greater than 20 s.
6	Requires bilateral support and walks 25 ft in greater than 20 s. May use wheelchair on occasion.
7	Walking limited to several steps with bilateral support; unable to walk 25 ft. May use wheelchair for most activities.
8	Restricted to wheelchair; able to transfer independently.
9	Restricted to wheelchair; unable to transfer independently.

III. PRIMARY SYMPTOMS

The symptoms or signs of MS may be categorized as primary, secondary, or tertiary. Primary symptoms are the physical manifestations on neurological function of a strategically located plaque of demyelination. Visual loss, weakness, incoordination, and urinary incontinence are examples. Secondary symptoms are the complications that ensue directly as a consequence of the primary ones and include pressure sores, urinary tract infection, and fibrous contractures of muscles. Tertiary symptoms are the emotional, social, and vocational ramifications of the disease on the patient, family, and community. This chapter focuses on evaluation and treatment of the most salient primary and the common secondary symptoms.

   In general terms, types of medical intervention could include prevention of the disease, modification of the expected course, restoration of function, and relief of symptoms. Currently, individual susceptibility to MS because of genetic type, ethnicity, heredity, or geography cannot be ascertained and immunization is unavailable. Although there have been recent advances in treatment that may favorably modify the course of the disease, there is as yet no cure for MS. Restoration of function depends to a large extent on regeneration of central nervous system tissue that is currently not possible. Fortunately, for many symptoms—including some of those that are the source of greatest disability, including spasticity, bladder and sexual dysfunction—there are effective medical and rehabilitative strategies. Both medical and rehabilitative interventions are discussed, since it is inappropriate to separate them. The goals of each are often identical. For example, treatment for urinary incontinence may also enable the patient to be vocationally and socially rehabilitated.

A. Gait

Many MS patients cite gait disturbance as their major primary symptom. Thorough evaluation will reveal whether spasticity, weakness, ataxia, or, as is frequently the case, a combination of these is responsible. Based on this analysis, the health care provider can design a treatment program that attempts to maximize the patient's existing ability.

Spasticity

Spasticity may be defined as a velocity-dependent increase in muscular tone associated with accelerated deep tendon reflexes and extensor plantar responses. Patients with spastic lower limbs walk stiffly, frequently exhibit foot drop and toe dragging during the swing phase of gait, and circumduct their lower limbs. In addition, many experience spasms, which are frequently painful, involving the thigh and calf muscles. Even though the mechanism of spasticity is not completely understood, there is effective medical therapy. When of spinal origin, spasticity is a symptom that frequently responds to medication.

Baclofen (Lioresal) is one of the most commonly used of the antispasticity medications. It is an analogue of gamma-aminobutyric acid, an inhibitory neurotransmitter. Stiffness and spasms, whether flexor or extensor, respond well to this drug. Reduced leg stiffness may result in more efficient gait and increased endurance. As response varies, a small initial dose, such as 5 mg three times a day, should be tried. The dosage should be gradually increased until the best response is achieved. Frequently, doses in excess of the manufacturer's recommendation are needed to obtain optimal results (14). Side effects include drowsiness, which usually disappears in a few days, and occasionally nausea, which can be avoided by taking the drug with meals. Patients with weakness may require lower extremity spasticity to maintain erect posture. The use of this medication to eliminate spasticity may then seem to aggravate weakness, resulting in worsened function. Careful self-titration is therefore necessary to achieve the best response and encourages the patient to participate actively in treatment.

In some patients, the response to oral baclofen or other oral antispasticity medications may be unsatisfactory, despite maximal doses. Side effects may limit the optimal dose in others. For these patients, intrathecally administered baclofen (ITB) may dramatically alleviate spasticity, increasing function and improving quality of life. If the patient responds to an intrathecal test dose, a battery-operated infusion pump is implanted into the abdominal wall; this is connected to a subcutaneous catheter delivering drug to the thecal space of the lumbar spine. The dose of ITB can easily be adjusted by a telemetry unit to tailor doses to the patient's optimal requirements. The pump's reservoir is easily refilled percutaneously at a frequency depending on the dose and concentration of the drug. Side effects are few, although some patients have had to have their pumps removed because of infection at the pump site or pump failure. Pumps must be replaced every 7 years, the life span of the battery. Although expensive and invasive, ITB has greatly improved the management of the severely spastic patient or the patient with significant spasticity who could not tolerate oral medication.

Tizanidine (Zanaflex), a drug recently approved by the FDA, is an alpha$_2$-noradrenergic receptor agonist, related to clonidine. It acts primarily on spinal polysynaptic reflexes. With this drug, unlike baclofen, weakness is not a frequent adverse effect. Frequent side effects include drowsiness and dry mouth. Some patients experience dizziness. Because of drowsiness, the drug is best started at low dosage, such as 2 mg at bedtime, and slowly increased until the desired effect is achieved. The recommended maximum dose is 36 mg in three divided daily doses. The drug should be used cautiously when combined with antihypertensive medications and never combined with clonidine, as the antihypertensive effect is enhanced (15).

Diazepam (Valium) is another effective oral antispastic drug but is less well tolerated than baclofen or tizanidine. It is best reserved for those who do not respond to or cannot tolerate baclofen or tizanidine. Sometimes, a combination of antispasticity drugs produces the best result, likely because they act on different receptors (16). A reasonable initial dose of diazepam is 2 mg three times a day. Because of its long half-life, diazepam seems to be particularly useful for sleep-disturbing nocturnal spasms. Side effects are similar to those with baclofen, but sedation is more prominent and abuse may occasionally be a problem.

Dantrolene sodium (Dantrium) acts to weaken spastic muscles by interfering with the myoneuronal contractile mechanism. Rarely, it can cause serious, life-threatening hepatotoxicity. Its use should be limited to those suffering from severe spasticity refractory to other treatments who are not ambulatory.

Clonidine may alleviate spasticity and is available as a convenient transdermal absorption system. It is worth trying in patients with troublesome nocturnal spasticity who have not responded to first-line drugs. The antiepileptic drug, gabapentin (Neurontin) has recently been described to relieve spasticity (17), but more studies are needed for confirmation.

Patients with spasticity should also be instructed in the technique of passive stretching of the spastic limbs several times daily through the full range of movement. Regular repetition relieves the stiffness of spasticity, which may last up to several hours, and prevents fibrous contracture and ankylosis of joints. Some patients may initially require the assistance of a physical therapist until they or their caregivers learn the techniques.

Other forms of exercise may also improve spasticity. Swimming is especially helpful. Not only does the cooling effect of the water ameliorate spasticity but the exercise increases endurance and a sense of well-being. Swimming is often the only nonfatiguing exercise option in hot, humid weather.

When spasticity is refractory to medical management, chemodenervation may be necessary. Phenol (5%) can be injected directly into motor nerves or into the site of motor point insertion (18). When lower extremity spasticity is the target in ambulatory patients, it is best to precede this with a trial of a short-acting local anesthetic to determine whether the treatment will significantly interfere with function.

Chemodenervation with botulinum toxin type A (BTA) is more recently added strategy to reduce spasticity (19). BTA is injected into the motor points of spastic muscles and produces relief of spasticity for up to 6 months. The precise mechanism of action is not known but includes the binding of BTA to the neuromuscular junction presynaptic nerve terminals. Somehow, this interferes with the fusion of the acetylcholine vesicles with the neuronal cell membrane. Unfortunately, the drug is expensive, must be given in relatively large amounts, and needs to be readministered at relatively frequent intervals. For these reasons, BTA is probably most useful for spasticity of the much smaller muscles of the upper limbs (20). With the introduction of new and effective strategies to relieve spasticity, destructive procedures such as selective dorsal rhizotomy and intrathecal instillation of alcohol are now rarely indicated.

Weakness

When weakness interferes with gait, management depends on its distribution, severity, and acuteness of onset. The most common involvement for the lower extremity conforms to the pattern of the upper motor neuron, that is, dorsiflexors and evertors of the foot, flexors of the hip, and abductors of the thigh. In the most subtle form, manual testing is normal but the patient may be unable to walk on the heel or hop on the affected leg. Others may complain of symptoms only after unusually strenuous exercise or under conditions of high ambient temperature.

Exercise

All patients should be maintained on an exercise program commensurate with their physical capabilities. Exercise will improve endurance and a sense of well-being. Recently, Petejan et al. (21) showed that aerobic exercise increased maximal oxygen consumption and maximal power output and significantly improved body composition and factors related to quality of life. Whether functional improvement occurs in strength or ambulation, for example, has yet to be shown. Specific exercises will also prevent complications associated with spasticity or weakness in those at risk.

Exercise can be either passive or active. Active exercises may include range-of-motion or resistive tasks. In active range-of-motion exercises, the patient actively moves the joint through as wide a range as possible, with gravity eliminated when weakness is severe, and then progresses as strength permits to moving the joint in the antigravity position. These exercises may require the aid of a therapist or the use of weights or pulleys to counterbalance the joint when the patient is too weak to move the joint actively.

In resistive exercises, the patient moves the joint through its full range of motion as resistance is applied in the opposite direction either by a therapist or by equipment. Many therapists believe that high-resistance, low-repetition exercises simultaneously develop strength and endurance.

Therapists currently use two types of active resistive exercises: isometric and isotonic. In isometric exercises, muscles contract around a joint without joint movement. In the preferred isotonic exercises, muscle contraction with joint movement is permitted and is performed against manually or mechanically applied resistance.

Progressive resistive exercise routines produce maximal strengthening of muscle by applying the greatest tolerable load to the muscles through the full range of motion for a given number of repetitions. Routines have been developed to best achieve the desired effect (22). If the patient cannot lift the part to be exercised, the effects of gravity can be minimized by use of a powder or skateboard or a partial counterbalance.

A comprehensive exercise program must also include exercise for cardiovascular fitness. Swimming, running, and cycling are typical activities. Swimming is preferred by many patients, especially those with significant lower limb motor impairments, and is often the only such exercise they can tolerate during the warmer months of the year.

Lower Extremity Orthotics

Assistive devices or orthotics are frequently necessary when weakness or spasticity interferes with gait. Proper prescription of an orthosis requires a thorough understanding of the pathophysiology of the gait abnormality. The patient must clearly understand the purpose and benefit of the device. It must be comfortable, relatively easy to don and doff (preferably without assistance), and reasonably acceptable in terms of cosmetics (23).

Patients with upper motor neuron lesions frequently exhibit foot drop during the swing phase of gait, mediolateral ankle instability, and insufficient push-off (24). This results from weakness of the foot dorsiflexors and evertors and may be aggravated by spasticity. Therefore an assistive device should provide resistance against plantar flexion during the swing phase, increase ankle stability at the time of heel strike, and be relatively rigid during push-offs lest the foot yield into dorsiflexion (25). The readily available posterior ankle-foot orthosis (PAFO) meets these requirements.

Several types of PAFO are available. All are worn within the patient's shoe and are secured by a strap around the calf. They differ in degree of rigidity and ankle support. For example, the so-called Seattle orthosis is stiff and provides maximal mediolateral ankle stability. It is best for patients with moderate to severe spasticity and/or weakness. The Teufel orthosis, on the other hand, resists plantar flexion but yields easily to dorsiflexion when stressed and affords limited mediolateral stability. This more flexible orthosis is best suited for patients with mild to moderate spasticity.

These devices are generally made to provide a slight degree of dorsiflexion of the sole plate, in the range of 5 to 10 degrees, to minimize toe drag. However, this may lessen knee stability (26). Instead of letting the foot down slowly from heel-strike to foot-flat by contracting the foot dorsiflexors, the patient rocks over the posterior portion of the heel, causing a bending movement at the knee that must be overcome by the knee extensors. Consequently, the degree of dorsiflexion should be only as much as is needed. Alternatively, part of the heel can be cut off at a 45-degree angle or a cushion wedge can be inserted into the heel of the orthotic (27). These tactics will move the groundreactive force forward.

Although advisable for some, the standard double-upright metal orthosis is not well tolerated by most MS patients because of the weight of the appliance. Studies in patients with hemiplegia have shown that functional ambulatory capacity is similar for the double-upright orthosis and the PAFO (28). Therefore, use of the more expensive and cumbersome double-upright should be reserved for special circumstances.

Once fitted, the orthosis should be checked to ensure that the calf band does not impinge on the peroneal nerve or place undue pressure on any a part of the skin, especially in patients with impaired sensation or spasticity; that the axis of any permitted ankle plantar or dorsiflexion closely approximates the location of the anatomic axis of the ankle joint; and that the patient demonstrates good function during ambulation (24). When the patient is standing, the sole and heel of the shoe should be flat on the floor. The entire gait cycle should be observed. Knee buckling during heel strike can arise from dorsiflexion of the orthosis exceeding that necessary for toe clearance. Hyperextension of the knee will occur if there is too much plantar flexion or if the sole plate extends too far forward (24).

Hyperextension of the knee joint, also termed *genu recurvatum* or "back knee," is a common alignment problem. This results from muscle imbalance in which the patient stabilizes the knee by extending it. Normally, this is limited by the posterior joint capsule and extension-limiting knee ligaments. However, these may gradually yield because of muscle weakness. Patients who have this problem and who wear a PAFO can limit the tendency by setting the ankle in some dorsiflexion, forcing the knee to bend during the first part of stance (25).

When more severe, genu recurvatum may be managed by a knee-ankle-foot orthosis (KAFO) designed to keep the knee in slight flexion. Alternatively, a "Swedish knee cage" may be used, but most orthotists feel that KAFOs apply force more effectively and will not slide down the leg. However, most MS patients find the KAFO too difficult to don and doff and too heavy.

Ataxia

When the cerebellum or its connections to the brainstem are affected, gait ataxia may result. Gait becomes broad-based and patients appear to weave from side to side or, with unilateral involvement, drift to one side. Because the cerebellum functions by comparing actual limb movement and position with that intended through proprioceptive mechanisms, it is not surprising that similar gait disturbances also follow dorsal column disease.

Findings on physical examination will distinguish whether ataxia arises from cerebellar or dorsal column disease or a combination of the two. Severe impairment of joint position sense, coupled with improved gait following increased use of visual cues, suggests dorsal column dysfunction, especially when other signs of cerebellar involvement (nystagmus, kinetic tremor of the extremities, dysarthria) are absent.

Ataxia from either cerebellar or dorsal column dysfunction does not respond to medication, but some patients may improve with specific physical therapy exercises. Sensory information can be enhanced by increased awareness of visual cues—for example, by watching the movement carefully with mirrors or by enhanced general sensory cues by placing light weights on the limbs. In this way, sensory feedback can be increased, improving performance (29). However, results are not as satisfying as for dorsal column causes for ataxia.

Frenkel's exercises have been suggested for the treatment of ataxia (Table 4) (30). This series of exercises of increasing difficulty improves lower extremity proprioceptive control. The exercises are done in each of four positions: lying sitting, standing, walking. By careful concentration and by slow repetition, some degree of coordination may be restored by the utilization of other senses. These exercises are physiologically sound insofar as they use total patterns, righting reflexes, and stabilization mechanisms while stressing prime movements. Some of Frenkel=s exercises also stress normal daily activities. However, their greatest value is in compensating for loss of proprioception by enhancing visual cues. Success is therefore limited when dysfunction arises from cerebellar lesions (29).

Canes, Crutches, and Walkers

When gait becomes hazardous, an assistive device should be considered. Gait aids should be carefully chosen to provide only as much assistance as is needed and no more. The more complicated the gait aid, the more cumbersome the gait and the less likely the patient will be to comply with the recommendation. Generally, patients will need to be trained to use the gait aid in a way that will closely mimic, to the extent physically possible, a normal gait pattern.

Canes provide the least support and walkers the most. A cane provides weight-bearing relief in the range of 20 to 25% of body weight (31). Because there is only a single point of contact with the body, support is limited. Generally, a cane is held in the hand opposite the involved side. This provides a more physiological gait as opposite arm and leg move together. When the dysfunction is unilateral, this also shifts weight away from the involved limb because contralateral arm support changes the center of gravity (32). The length of the cane should be adjusted so that the highest point is at the level of the greater trochanter, producing about 20–30 degrees flexion at the elbow (32). Four-legged or ''quad'' canes provide more stability at the expense of reducing speed (32).

Table 4 Frenkel's Exercises

Exercises While Supine

The patient lies on a bed or plinth with a smooth surface along which the heels may slide easily. A caster shoe rolling on a large board positioned under the lower extremities may be used to make the activities easier by reducing friction. The various motions to be practiced may be indicated by lines painted on the board. The head should be supported so that the patient can see the legs and feet.

   1. Flex the hip and knee of one extremity, sliding the heel along in contact with the bed. Return to the original position. Repeat with the opposite extremity.

   2. Flex as in exercise 1. Then abduct the flexed hip. return to the flexed position and then to the original position.

   3. Flex the hip and knee only halfway and then return to the extended position. Add abduction and adduction.

   4. Flex one limb at the hip and knee, stopping at any point in flexion or extension on command.

   5. Flex both lower extremities simultaneously and equally; add abduction, adduction, and extension.

   6. Flex both lower extremities simultaneously to the halfway position; add abduction and adduction to the half-flexed position. Extend. Stop in the pattern on command.

   7. Flex one extremity at the hip and knee with the heel held 2 in. above the bad. Return to the original position.

   8. Flex as in exercise 7. Bring the heel to rest on the opposite patella. Successively add patterns so that the heel is touched to the middle of the shin, to the ankle, to the toes of the opposite foot, to the bed on either side of the knee, and to the bed on either side of the leg.

   9. Flex as in exercise 7 and then touch the heel successively to the patella, shin, ankle, and toes. Reverse the pattern.

10. Flex as in exercise 7 and then on command touch the heel to the point indicated by the therapist.

11. Flex the hip and knee with the heel 2 in. above the bed. Place the heel on the opposite patella and slowly slide it down the crest of the tibia to the ankle. Reverse.

12. Use the pattern in exercise 11, but slide the heel down the crest of the opposite tibia, over the ankle and foot to the toes. If the heel is to reach the toes, the opposite knee must be flexed slightly during this exercise. Stop in the pattern of command.

13. With malleoli and knees in apposition, flex both lower extremities simultaneously with the heels 2 in. above the bed. Return to the original position. Stop in the pattern on command.

14. Perform reciprocal flexion and extension of the lower extremities with the heels touching the bed.

15. Perform reciprocal flexion and extension of the lower extremities with the heels 2 in. above the bed.

16. Perform bilateral simultaneous flexion, abduction, adduction, and extension with the heels 2 in. above the bed.

17. Place the heel precisely where the therapist indicates with the finger on the bed or the opposite extremity.

18. Follow with the toe the movement of the therapist's finger in any combination of lower extremity motion.

Exercises While Sitting

   1. Practice maintaining correct sitting posture for 2 min in an armchair with the back supported and the feet flat on the floor. Repeat in a chair without arms. Repeat without back support.

   2. Mark time to the counting of the therapist by raising only the heel from the floor. Progress to alternatively lifting the entire foot and replacing it precisely in a marked position on the floor.

Table 4 Continued

3. Make two cross marks on the floor with chalk. Alternately glide the foot over the marked cross; forward, backward, left and right.

4. Practice rising from and sitting on a chair to the therapist's counted cadence: (a) Flex the knees and draw the feet under the front edge of the seat. (b) Bend the trunk forward over the thighs. (c) Rise by extending the knees and hips and then straightening the trunk. (d) Bend the trunk forward slightly. (e) Flex the hips and knees to sit. (f) Straighten the trunk and sit back in the chair.

Exercises While Standing

1. Walking sideways. Balance is easier during sidewards walking because the patient does not have to pivot over the toes or heels, which decreases the base of support. The exercise is performed to a counted cadence: (a) Shift the weight to the left foot. (b) Place the right foot 12 in to the right. (c) Shift the weight to the right foot. (d) Bring the left foot over to the right foot. The size of the step taken to the right or left may be varied.

2. Walk forward between two parallel lines 14 in. apart, placing the right foot just inside the right line and the left foot just inside the left line. Emphasize correct placement. Rest after 10 steps.

3. Walk forward placing each foot on a footprint traced on the floor. Footprints should be parallel and 2 in. lateral to the midline. Practice with quarter steps, half steps, three-quarter steps, and full steps.

4. Turning. (a) Raise the right toe and rotate the right foot outward, pivoting on the heel. (b) Raise the left heel and pivot the left leg inward on the toes. Bring the left foot up beside the right.

Crutches are either axillary or nonaxillary. Two points of contact with the body provide more support. Axillary crutches can transfer as much as 80% of body weight away from the lower extremities; nonaxillary crutches, 40 to 50% (31). Nonaxillary crutches are the most commonly prescribed type for MS patients and paraparesis. Adequate axial balance is necessary and patients with significant ataxia should not, in general, be prescribed crutches.

The Lofstrand crutch has a padded hand bar and forearm cuff (32). The cuff helps to stabilize the arm and wrist, allowing for safer and easier gait. In addition, the patient is free to use the hand to grasp stair rails or open a door. The Canadian crutch can be used when there is triceps weakness (33); it has both a forearm and an arm cuff. The arm is supported with the elbow in extension. Both crutches can be provided with a four-legged base with a flexible point of attachment to the shaft providing for greater stability. The Lofstrand crutch should be adjusted so that the hand bars produce about 20 to 30 degrees of elbow flexion.

Walkers provide maximal support but at the cost of slow and awkward gait. They are particularly useful for patients with severe lower limb weakness or ataxia. A walker should be placed 10 to 12 in. in front of the patient. The patient should stand erect and have elbows flexed to 15 to 20 degrees (34). Walkers with wheels are excellent choices for patients with ataxia but are usually not suitable for patients with significant weakness. Because wheeled walkers introduce a measure of instability that can be dangerous, models with variable-resistance brakes, such as the Nova, make good choices. Any patient with significant lower limb weakness or ataxia being considered for a wheeled walker should first be evaluated for suitability by an experienced physical therapist.

Gait Training

As gait aides transfer some weight-bearing capacity from the lower to the upper extremities, adequate upper extremity strength and mobility are of prime importance in gait training. In addition, adequate truncal stability is necessary to maintain balance and correct posture. Walking should be undertaken only when the patient feels secure standing and has satisfactory posture (32).

Depending on the degree of difficulty, gait training may first require training on parallel bars, assuring the optimal development of upper body strength and general endurance in a safe and controlled situation. Gait training by an experienced physiotherapist is essential once the appropriate gait aid is prescribed. This is particularly true for crutches, the most difficult of the gait aids to use properly. Gait training is incomplete unless the patient demonstrates ability to negotiate stairs, inclines, and curbs. The safest stair-climbing technique is to advance the unaffected limb first when ascending and the affected limb first when descending.

Wheelchairs

When aid-assisted walking becomes unsafe or impossible, a wheelchair will be necessary. Frequently, a wheelchair serves as a supplementary means of transportation. For many, it provides a degree of independence that would otherwise be impossible. On the other hand, some patients may rely too heavily on a wheelchair. It should made clear to the patient that a wheelchair is an auxiliary means of transportation and that walking, even with an aid, is preferred (35).

When being fitted for a wheelchair, the patient should be fully clothed and wearing any braces normally used. If a patient is being fitted for a wheelchair while seated in an ordinary chair, the hips and knees should be at 90 degrees of flexion and the ankles in the neutral position (35). If necessary, the seat may be elevated or a wooden platform placed under the shoes to achieve this position. The following measurements should be taken:

1. The distance from the soles of the shoes to the upper horizontal level of the seat (add 2 in. to compensate for elevation of the footrests).
2. The distance between the outer borders of the thighs.
3. The distance from the back of the seat to within four finger breadths in back of the knee, taken along the midline.
4. The height of the armrest (the forearm should be at right angles to the arms with the palms down, plus 1 in.).
5. The distance between the chair and the lower angle of the scapula except in patients with quadriplegia, when the seat-to-occiput distance should be measured (35).

Normally, the footrest should be adjusted so that two finger breadths can be placed under the thigh at the forward end of the seat (35). This extra lift for the thighs, however, may not be advisable in patients predisposed to ischial pressure sores. The legs should not dangle over the end of the seat because of the danger of sciatic nerve compression.

The most common wheelchair in use today is the rear-wheel-drive folding chair. It weighs about 40 lb. For standard wheelchairs, the strength of upper extremities must be sufficient to self-propel. Hand rim projections are available for those with diminished hand grip.

Front-wheel-drive chairs are available but not frequently prescribed. They need less room for turning, but the occupants must lean forward to propel them. The trunk extensors must be strong enough to prevent the trunk from falling on the thighs (35). Sustaining this posture can be quite tiring.

Once provided with a wheelchair, the patient should be trained in backward and forward propulsion and turning as well as how and when to use the brakes. The patient must also be instructed in the proper methods of transferring from the wheelchair. The unassisted standing transfer requires adequate sitting balance, strong voluntary control of hip and knee extensors, or adequate extensor spasticity of the lower extremities, and reasonably strong upper extremities. Physical therapists can teach the necessary techniques for transferring into and out of bed or to other surfaces, into and out of the bathtub, and onto and off the toilet (36). Patients who cannot accomplish such transfers without extensive help may need a hydraulic lift.

Motorized chairs or scooters are available for patients with severe upper extremity disability or for those so weak that the effort of propelling a wheelchair precludes accomplishing daily activities. When needed, the use of motorized chairs or scooters should not be discouraged, as these modes of transportation can greatly increase mobility and quality of life. Patients must demonstrate sound judgment before they should be prescribed one of these.

B. Bladder

Pathophysiology

After gait, many MS patients cite bladder problems as the next most disabling symptom. Urinary symptoms have traditionally been divided into irritative and obstructive. Irritative symptoms include urinary urgency, frequency, nocturia, and urgency incontinence. Obstructive symptoms include hesitancy, diminished force of stream, "double voiding," involuntary interruption of stream, and postvoiding sense of fullness. Mere analysis of symptoms may be misleading (37,38). For example, symptoms suggestive of obstruction, such as hesitancy and diminished force of stream, may occur when bladder capacity is very small and no obstruction is present. Moreover, complicating infection may not only produce symptoms of cystitis but may also aggravate preexisting neurological complaints. A sudden change in bladder function that may be associated with other worsened neurological symptoms, especially increased lower extremity spasticity, should always suggest possible urinary tract infection (UTI).

It is most practical to classify neurourologic dysfunction in MS as failure to store urine, failure to fully empty the bladder, or a combination of the two, usually the result of detrusor-external sphincter dyssynergia (DESD) (37). The bladder that fails to store urine adequately has a smaller than normal capacity but empties completely. Patients will usually note urgency, frequency, and urgency incontinence because of uninhibited detrusor contractions. Responsible lesions may be located anywhere in the central nervous system above the sacral segments of the spinal cord. About half of MS patients with urinary complaints have this problem (37).

The bladder that fails to empty completely without DESD results from detrusor weakness or from the detrusor deafferentation. This is usually the result of a sacral cord lesion. An exception is the phase of "spinal shock" following, for example, acute transverse myelitis. Patients may complain of hesitancy, postvoiding sense of fullness (or no sense of fullness), weak urinary stream, infrequent voiding, or dribbling incontinence. Less than 10% of symptomatic patients have this problem (37).

In DESD, detrusor contractions occur but are usually weak and poorly sustained (39,40). They are associated with simultaneously occurring contractions of the somatically innervated external urethral sphincter (39,40). Patients may note involuntary interruption of the urinary stream, hesitancy, or complete inability to void. DESD results from lesions above the sacral spinal cord but below the pontine reticular formation. Lesions above the pons have not been shown to cause DESD. It appears that the "pontine micturition center" coordinates detrusor contraction and external urethral sphincter relaxation for the timely expulsion of urine via a long loop reflex extending from the second to fourth sacral cord segments to the pons. DESD is probably the most serious form of neurourologic dysfunction because detrusor contraction against a closed outlet facilitates ureteral reflux, which may jeopardize sterility of the upper urinary tracts.

Management

The goals of intervention are threefold: eradicate any infection; prevent subsequent infection; control the neurological symptoms (41). All patients presenting for the first time with bladder symptoms or those who experience a change in their usual symptoms should be evaluated for complicating UTI or other urological conditions (e.g., bladder calculus) with microscopic urinalysis and urine culture (41). Infection, if present, should be treated with appropriate antibiotics. If the urinalysis suggests another problem (as evidenced, for example, by persistent microscopic hematuria or crystalluria), bladder ultrasound, cystoscopy, or an intravenous pyelogram may be necessary.

Next, the amount of the postvoid residual (PVR) urine should be measured (41). The magnitude of the PVR directly correlates with the likelihood of complicating bladder infection. Normal bladder capacity is 350 to 500 mL. A significant PVR is one that exceeds 100 mL or an amount greater than 20% of the voided volume (42). All patients with a significant PVR should be placed on urinary antiseptics. Vitamin C, 1 g four times a day, acidifies the urine. With urinary pH maintained at ≤6, there is significant bacteriostasis. Some fruit juices, especially cranberry, decrease urinary pH; orange and other citrus juices tend to increase pH. Drugs such as methenamine hippurate (Hiprex) and methenamine mandelate (Mandelamine) reduce the incidence of UTI by generating formaldehyde salts in acid urine (43).

The PVR may be determined in several ways. Simple in-out catheterization following voiding is the easiest method. Both the voided and residual amount are recorded. Alternatively, the PVR can be determined by a radioisotope method using technetium 99–labeled hippurate (44) or by bladder ultrasonography.

Patients whose bladders fail to store urine usually respond to anticholinergic or smooth-muscle-relaxant drugs, including propantheline bromide (Pro-Banthine), oxybutynin chloride (Ditropan), and, for their anticholinergic side effects, the tricyclic antidepressants, such as imipramine HCl (Tofranil). Tolterodine (Detrol), a competitive muscarinic antagonist with high specificity for bladder muscarinic receptors, has significantly less systemic and central adverse effects than oxybutynin chloride (45). Long-acting preparations such as the sustained-release preparation of oxybutynin chloride (Ditropan XL) or the tricyclic antidepressants may allow overnight control. Vasopressin (DDAVP), insufflated at bedtime, has been shown to assist with nighttime control of irritative urinary symptoms in some patients (45). Recently an oral preparation of DDAVP has been released. Electrolyte imbalance is a possible complication. For those patients who wish treatment for irritative symptoms and who have PVRs near the significant range, the PVR should be rechecked following control of symptoms, because some may develop significant emptying problems.

The dose of medication given for control of symptoms should be determined by response. Occasionally, it may be necessary to exceed the manufacturer's recommendation. This is acceptable provided that no significant adverse reactions ensue (41). Some patients with hyperreflexic bladders can be taught to induce voiding by triggering detrusor contractions (42). Such triggers may include suprapubic tapping, stroking the glans penis, rubbing the thighs, or tugging on pubic hair. Other patients may be trained to void at specified intervals to ensure regular bladder emptying. It may take considerable practice to learn how to induce bladder contractions of sufficient duration and intensity. Frequently, simultaneous execution of a Valsalva maneuver will be needed. Voiding by reflex triggering should not be employed by patients with DESD because it may cause ureteral reflux.

Clean intermittent self-catheterization (ISC) is recommended for patients with high PVRs (41). This is a simple and safe technique that has been proven to reduce the frequency of UTI and to relieve symptoms (47). Semirigid clear plastic catheters, such as those manufactured by Mentor, are best for this purpose. The urethral meatus is cleansed with a towelette and the catheter introduced. Once the urine begins to flow, suprapubic pressure is applied to ensure complete evacuation. The catheter is then removed and washed with soap and water until next use. The frequency of catheterization varies depending on the magnitude of the PVR. Three to four times a day is frequently the initial prescription. This frequency may be reduced if the PVR decreases over time. Once emptying problems have been treated, medications for coincidental irritative symptoms can be prescribed.

Obviously, patients who are obese or who have impaired vision, sensation, manual coordination, or intellect or who suffer from spasticity of the thigh adductor muscles may not be able to perform ISC. Frequently, another person can be instructed in the technique or can at least assist the patient.

Some patients can reduce residual urine by Credé's method. The suprapubic area of the abdomen is compressed by the hand while at the same time a Valsalva maneuver is performed (42). This should not be done in patients with DESD, as the likelihood of ureteral reflux is enhanced.

An indwelling catheter may be necessary for those patients unable to perform ISC. This option should be a last resort. For some, a suprapubic vesicostomy is preferable to urethral catheterization because hygiene is easier to maintain (41). Also, the complication of acute epididymitis in men is avoided. Some men with refractory urinary incontinence can use condom catheters when needed, as while sleeping or on outings. These may be difficult to keep on, especially for older men, and continuous use can lead to penile ulceration.

C. Bowel

Not surprisingly, urinary, bowel, and sexual dysfunction tend to occur together, as these functions are believed to share similar central pathways and segmental levels of control. Most patients with bowel complaints cite constipation as the primary problem. The normal increment in colonic motility after eating is reduced in many MS patients (48). Other nonneurological factors may contribute to constipation, including lack of exercise because of immobility, inadequate dietary fiber and hydration (often because patients avoid ingesting adequate fluids to control irritative urinary symptoms), and the effects of medication (such as those used to control irritative urinary symptoms).

The patient should be encouraged to drink six to eight glasses of liquid daily and to eat high-fiber foods or, if needed, take unprocessed wheat bran, psyllium (Metamucil), or docusate sodium (Colace). These measures should ensure stool of soft consistency and may be enough to ensure bowel movements at least every 2 to 3 days. If constipation persists, mineral oil, suppositories, laxatives such as bisacodyl (Dulcolax) or enemas (e.g., Fleet, Theravac) may be required.

Fecal incontinence is much less frequent in MS patients than is constipation. If there is diarrhea, spurious diarrhea because of fecal impaction should be considered (49). A careful rectal examination should be the first step in assessing a complaint of persistent stool incontinence with diarrhea. Patients with fecal incontinence may respond to the regular use of suppositories, such as glycerine, or enemas to ensure bowel movements at a predictable time. Failing this, anticholinergic medications such as propantheline bromide or imipramine HCl may be used.

D. Sexual Symptoms

Sexual symptoms are a frequent source of disability in MS (50). Only one-fifth of males have adequate erections and at least one-third of females complain of anorgasmia or decreased libido. Symptoms may reflect the primary effect of MS plaques or psychological complications. Frequently both contribute. It is important to recognize that many medications can produce sexual dysfunction, including impotence and anhedonia, as an adverse effect.

Treatment depends on the cause. Psychological problems are best managed by individual, group, or couples counseling. For impotence, alprostadil, given either transurethrally (Muse) or intracavernously (Caverject), and sildenafil (Viagra) have been shown to be beneficial in neurogenic impotence and have largely obviated the need for penile implants. Most patients prefer sildenafil because of its convenience. For those not interested in medical treatments, vacuum devices are worth considering. For those with anorgasmia, directing the partner as to what is and what is not pleasurable may allow a lowering of the threshold for climax to occur. Sometimes the use of stimulants, such as vibrators, will help. When there is decreased vaginal lubrication, a water-soluble jelly, such as K-Y, is best.

E. Upper Extremities

Problems with the upper limbs include weakness, generally of the upper motor neuron type but occasionally mimicking a lower motor neuron pattern, dyssynergia because of cerebellar involvement with kinetic or postural tremor and dysdiadochokinesia, and sensory impairment with numbness, stereoanesthesia, ataxia, or pain. Occupational therapists are particularly interested in the assessment of upper extremity function and provide compensatory training and adaptive equipment. Upper extremity dysfunction can impair dressing, personal hygiene, eating, and writing. Numerous adaptive devices are available. They run the gamut from long straws to facilitate drinking to devices that spread pants, turn pages, hold playing cards, and extend the patient's reach for bathing, picking up objects, and clipping toenails. Imagination combined with a trial-and-error approach can often overcome a particular problem (51).

Some upper extremity orthotics tend to hinder rather than facilitate performance of activities impaired by MS. Static forearm splints, however, may be useful to prevent the formation of fibrous contractures due to spasticity of the finger flexors (52). Utensils for eating and food preparation can sometimes be affixed to the splint. Patients with fixed contractures or marked finger-flexor spasticity may need to use a hand roll to prevent their fingernails from gouging their palms.

Although some patients with tremor find that the use of weighted forearm cuffs improves performance (29), most find wearing them too tiring to be useful and weakness, if present, is aggravated. As in the case of the lower extremities, unremitting upper extremity spasticity may respond to motor point phenol blocks or BTA injection. The biceps brachii and flexor sublimis muscles respond well to chemodenervation. Unfortunately, the benefit is often short-lived and repeat blocks are required every 3 to 6 months. Oral antispastic medications do not consistently ameliorate upper limb spasticity nor does ITB.

F. Fatigue

Fatigue is one of the most disabling primary symptoms of MS. In fact, in one study, fatigue was the most likely of all primary symptoms to interfere with the activities of daily living (53).

The cause of fatigue in MS is unknown. For most, it seems to adopt a diurnal cycle, being greatest in the afternoon and least in the morning. It is worsened by physical activity and high ambient temperature. Interestingly, it does not correlate either with depression, with which it is frequently confused, or the degree of overall disability as measured by the Kurtzke EDSS (54).

Amantadine (Symmetrel) has been reported to be helpful (55), but frequently the benefit is not sustained. Pemoline (Cylert) has also been reported to ameliorate fatigue in MS, but this has not been confirmed in a recent trial (56). Anecdotal reports suggest that fluoxetine (Prozac) and modafinil (Provigil) may also be effective and are worth trying in patients refractory to other treatments.

In general, the patient should organize the day around the times when fatigue is worse to permit rest periods when needed. Homemaking may be particularly difficult. Highly fatiguing activities such as grocery shopping, laundry, and cooking should be scheduled for times of the day when fatigue is less likely. Housecleaning should be spread over several days and work space and utensils organized so that the patient can carry out tasks with the minimum of time and energy. In the kitchen or workplace, the patient should learn to sit, slide, and toss rather than stand, lift, and carry. On-site assessment of home or workplace by an occupational therapist may be necessary to devise optimal solutions.

G. Speech

Dysarthria, although frequent in MS, is an uncommon source of major disability. Severity of speech disturbance generally parallels the severity of neurological impairment. Impairment arises from lesions in the cerebral hemispheres, brainstem, or cerebellum. When communication is affected, a speech pathologist should be consulted, as most clinically significant disorders of motor speech are at least partly amenable to treatment. (Aphasia is rarely encountered in MS and is thus not discussed.)

Based on one of the few published reviews of dysarthria in MS (57), scanning speech marked by impaired emphasis and sudden articulatory breakdowns is not as frequent in patients with MS as is commonly believed. In this study, hypernasality and a breathy voice quality, the most common abnormalities, were each encountered in about 25% of patients. About 35% of patients had reduced vital capacity and 42% had inadequate ventilation.

Patients with defective articulation should first be taught to slow their rate of speech to make more time available for the tongue to compensate for the loss of control. Depending on the severity of the articulatory disturbance, phrases or even individual words may require a syllable-by-syllable attack (58) in which each syllable or word is pronounced separately and deliberately. Some consonants will require overarticulation to prevent their being slighted during speech (59).

With severe articulatory failure, exercises with specific speech muscles may be required. Examples include moving the tongue in and out of the mouth and from side to side. Frequently, such exercises are best performed in front of a mirror for visual feedback (58). Once tongue control has been mastered, progression to functional speech should follow.

When articulation is controlled, prosody can be regulated to reduce the resulting scanning quality of the speech. Normal syllabic stress and word emphasis can be reintroduced by varying the loudness, altering the pitch, and varying the duration of syllables to produce more nearly normal speech (60). Loudness control can be improved by using the loudness-level meter of a tape recorder for visual feedback (58).

Some patients have such severe motor speech disturbance that direct exercise of articulators and contextual speech therapy are of no substantial benefit. In this case, alternatives to speech—including picture, word, phrase, and alphabet boards—can be selected, depending on the patient's degree of motor, visual, and intellectual impairment. Also available are costly voice synthesizing computers.

H. Dysphagia

Dysphagia is not infrequent in MS patients (61). When it is a significant problem, however, it tends to be associated with more severe disease. Although potentially lethal, dysphagia has only recently received attention in MS.

Evaluation

The first step is to obtain an adequate history of the problem from the patient, family members, or nursing staff. Questions include onset, course, the effects of different food consistencies, the results of swallowing, and the presence of choking or coughing. Although a majority of patients who are aware of their problem can precisely identify where in the cycle and with what foods their symptoms appear, a patient with a severe swallowing disorder may be oblivious to it, especially if mentally compromised (62). When patients say that food seems to "stick" in the throat near the base of the tongue, the bolus is probably hesitating at the level of the valleculae. When the hesitation appears to be just below the larynx, the bolus is usually collecting in the piriform recesses (62).

Coughing and choking generally indicate aspiration into the airway. Difficulty with specific food consistencies often indicates the nature of the problem. Patients with prolonged oral transit times may find liquids easy to swallow but thicker materials and solids more difficult because of defective tongue manipulation. Conversely, when the swallowing reflex is reduced or absent, liquids may cause more problems than solids because they splash into the oropharynx before a swallowing reflex can be triggered (62).

Pertinent observations during the evaluation of dysphagia include range, rate and accuracy of lip, tongue, and soft palate movement during speech, reflex activity, and actual swallowing. It should be emphasized that many normal individuals exhibit a reduced or absence of the gag reflex and that the presence or absent gag reflex is not by itself an indication of the patient's ability to swallow (63).

The only reliable way to determine the cause of aspiration is with radiography (64). The "modified barium swallow" involves the video fluoroscopic analysis of swallowing employing small amounts of barium liquid, paste, and masticated material (62). During the study, the fluoroscope remains in the field of the oral cavity, pharynx, and cervical esophagus and at no time follows the bolus into the body of the esophagus. Otherwise aspiration following the swallow would be missed (62).

Analysis and Management

Aspiration during the lingual phase (when the tongue opposes on the hard palate to push the bolus toward the oropharynx) is secondary to disordered tongue control or a delayed or absent triggering of the swallowing reflex. Poor tongue control can result from cerebellar dysfunction or from pseudobulbar palsy. Consequently, the tongue loses control of the bolus, causing part or all of the bolus to roll back into the pharynx. When this happens, the pharyngeal response is not triggered because tongue action, and not just the presence of food in the pharynx, is important in triggering the swallowing reflex (65). Depending on the type and amount of food and the position of the patient, the food will deposit in the valleculae, the piriform recesses, or the airway.

When triggering of the swallowing reflex is delayed or absent, the bolus tumbles into the pharynx in an uncontrolled way. The amount and consistency of the food and the patient's position will determine where the bolus comes to rest. Treatment for poor tongue control includes compensatory positional changes, such as holding the head forward when preparing the bolus for swallowing, then throwing it back to allow the bolus to fall into the pharynx, or exercises to increase tongue range of motion, strength, and control to prevent the bolus from entering the pharynx prematurely (64,66).

There are several strategies to alleviate delayed or absent triggering of the swallowing reflex. The patient may hold the head flexed in preparation for the swallow, thus enlarging the vallecular space. This reduces the chance for aspiration by helping to trap the material in the valleculae during the reflex delay (64,66). The patient also can adopt a diet of thicker foods and liquids taken in smaller amounts per bolus. Thicker foods tend to remain in the valleculae longer, increasing the chance of reflex trigger. Commercially available thickeners, such as Thick-it, facilitate the swallowing of thin liquids in a palatable form.

The swallowing reflex can sometimes be facilitated by thermal stimulation of the anterior faucial arches, soft palate, or posterior tongue. For example, a chilled laryngeal mirror can be used to stroke the anterior faucial arch on each side with five or six stroking movements. The contact of the mirror does not trigger the swallow but allows the reflex to trigger more rapidly in a subsequent swallow (64,66). As many as 95% of patients treated this way exhibit improved reflex triggering for up to four swallows following stimulation (67).

If the larynx fails to close during the swallow, aspiration may ensue. If mild, this can be managed with the supraglottic swallow procedure. The patient inhales and holds the breath at the height of inspiration. The patient then swallows. Following the swallow, the patient coughs with exhalation, expectorating any residue that might be remaining in the pharynx or upper airway (64).

Aspiration following the swallow may result from reduced pharyngeal peristalsis, reduced laryngeal elevation, or oropharyngeal dysfunction, leaving residue in the pharynx. Inhalation when the swallow is completed leads to inhalation of these residues. Patients with this problem should cough and clear any residue remaining before inhaling after a swallow (64).

When dysphagia is severe enough, alternatives to oral intake may be necessary. The percutaneous gastrostomy is simple to perform and well accepted by both patient and caregivers, making it the option of choice.

IV. SECONDARY SYMPTOMS

The preceding sections have addressed most of the common secondary symptoms such as fibrous contractures, aspiration pneumonia, and UTI, which are a direct consequence of neurological dysfunction. Only pressure sores (decubitus ulcers) remain to be discussed.

About 15% of patients with MS develop pressure sores at some time during their illness, as many of the factors that enhance their development are present in patients with severe disease. This figure can be considerably reduced if the appropriate preventive measures are taken.

Several important factors contribute to the development of pressure sores. Applying to the skin and subcutaneous tissue pressure that exceeds capillary blood pressure diminishes the level of oxygenation needed to maintain cells. Ensuing venous stasis will preclude adequate removal of toxic metabolic by products, further compromising tissue survival. If these circulatory aberrations persist in a large enough area, a sore will develop (22). In addition, the tissue's susceptibility to destruction is increased if it is subjected to shearing forces, friction (as when patients are dragged across bedding), or moisture (from urinary incontinence) (68).

The paramount role of pressure as the initiator of sores is evidenced by the most common sites for their occurrence: the bony prominences of the buttocks (the ischial tuberositics and the sacrum), the lateral aspects of the hips (over the greater trochanter), the heels, and the malleoli of the ankles.

The first sign of tissue destruction, a reddened area that does not blanch when finger pressure is applied, should signal that continued pressure over the site may result in a frank sore. When tissue loss is confined solely to the epidermis, the lesion is referred to as a grade I sore and superficially resembles an abrasion. A grade II sore extends through the dermis to the subcutaneous fat and is a full-thickness skin defect. Both grade I and II sores can be completely reversed nonsurgically through use of antiseptic washes and saline dressings. A grade III sore extends through the subcutaneous fat, with extensive undermining. A grade IV sore extends down into underlying muscle and bone (69).

These sores may extend directly or by sinus tracts to result in osteomyelitis if bone is involved or pyarthrosis if they extend to joints. Grade III and IV sores usually require surgical treatment, including debridement devitalized tissue and myocutaneous flap surgery. When such surgery is necessary, the patient should be prepared by adopting a protein-rich diet to establish a positive nitrogen balance and promote wound healing. Any significant orthopedic complication such as fibrous contracture that will compromise positioning should be repaired prior to wound closure.

Physicians treating MS patients must identify those most at risk for pressure sores.

These include patients with weakness or spasticity of the lower limbs severe enough to preclude ambulation and those with significant loss of sensation, intellectual function, bladder or bowel incontinence, or poor nutrition and hypoalbuminemia (70).

After those at risk are identified, patients and their caregivers should be trained to examine the skin regularly for signs of tissue compromise, especially in the most commonly involved areas. Those who spend a great deal of time in a wheelchair must be taught to sit in a way that distributes pressure evenly over the buttocks and posterior thighs. They should also be taught to do pressure-relieving exercises such as pushing up from their wheelchairs and turning from side to side and forward every 15 min. They should be provided with wheelchair cushions designed to suit their body contours.

No one wheelchair cushion suits every patient. Ideally, the physician should confirm a cushion's suitability by using a pressure manometer to take readings over the bony prominences of the buttocks while the patient is seated. Although foam cushions are popular and can easily be modified to suit patient anatomy, they last only about 3 to 6 months.

Bedridden patients should learn how to turn themselves, if they are able, using side rails and overhead trapezes. Those who cannot turn themselves should be turned every 2 h. If these patients lie on a regular mattress, air mattresses or egg crates should be used to help distribute their weight. Specialized mattresses containing air, water, hydrophilic gels, or fluidized silicon beads (e.g., Clinitron), including some for home use, also are available.

Individuals with severe spasticity who develop fibrous contractures of the adductor or hamstring muscles or ankylosis of the hip and knee joints can lie only in restricted positions. Therefore, spasticity must be aggressively treated with medication and daily passive range-of-motion exercises. Care should be taken to prevent incontinence and excessive perspiration and maintain good personal hygiene.

V. CONCLUSION

The physician can do much to alleviate many of the most troubling symptoms of MS, including disorders of gait, bladder and bowel, upper extremities, speech, and deglutition. Such treatment entails careful assessment of the patient's neurological and other symptoms; knowledge of his or her intellectual, emotional, and social skills and demands; and an understanding of the patient's support network. Because the symptoms and needs of the patient with MS are so varied, the physician must also work closely with professionals in allied fields, including speech, physical, and occupational therapists; social workers; and rehabilitation specialists. Because there is no cure, one of the major functions of the physician is preempted. However, it should be kept in mind that although the challenges of treating the patient with MS are great, so too are the rewards: helping individuals continue, to the best of their ability, to contribute to the world around them.

ACKNOWLEDGMENT

This work was supported by National Institute on Disability and Rehabilitation Research Grant Number H133B30015–95.

REFERENCES

1. Lublin F, Reingold S; Defining the clinical course of multiple sclerosis: Results of an international survey. Neurology 1996; 46:907–911.

2.   Weinshenker BG, Bass B, Rice GPA, et al. The natural history of multiple sclerosis: A geographically based study. II: Predictive value of the early clinical course. Brain 1989; 112: 1419–1428.

3.   Weinshenker BG, Rice GPA, Noseworthy JH, et al. The natural history of multiple sclerosis: A geographically based study. III: Multivariate analysis of predictive factors and models of outcome. Brain 1991; 114:1045–1056.

4.   Minimal Record of Disability for Multiple Sclerosis. New York: International Federation of Multiple Sclerosis Societies, 1985.

5.   Kurtzke JF. Rating neurologic impairment in multiple sclerosis: An Expanded Dis- ability Status Scale (EDSS). Neurology 1983; 33:1114–1452.

6.   Moskowitz E, McCann C. Classification of disability in the chronically ill and aging. J Chronic Dis 1957; 5:342–346.

7.   Mahoney FL, Barthel DW. Functional evaluation: The Barthel index. Maryland State Med J 1965; 14:61–65.

8.   Granger CV. Assessment of functional status: A model for multiple sclerosis. Acta Neurol Scand 1981; 64(suppl 87):4047.

9.   Mellerup E, Fog T. The socioeconomic scale. Acta Neurol Scand 1981;64(suppl 87):130–138.

10.   Hauser SL, Dawson DM, Lehrich JR, et al. Intensive immunosuppression in progressive multiple sclerosis: A randomized three-armed study of high dose intravenous cyclophosphamide, plasma exchange, and ACTH. N Engl J Med 1983; 308:173–180.

11.   Rudick R, Antel J, Confavreux C, et al. Recommendations from the National Multiple Sclerosis Society Clinical Outcomes Assessment Task Force. Ann Neurol 1997; 42:379–382.

12.   Goodkin DE, Hertzgard D, Seminary J. Upper extremity function in multiple sclerosis: Improving assessment sensitivity with box-and-block and nine-hole-peg tests. Arch Phys Med Rehabil 1988; 69:850–854.

13.   Gronwall DMA. Paced auditory serial-addition task: A measure of recovery from concussion. Percept Mot Skills 1977; 44:367–373.

14.   Smith CR, LaRocca NG, Giesser BS, et al. High-dose oral baclofen: Experience in patients with multiple sclerosis. Neurology 1991; 41:1829–1831.

15.   The United Kingdom Tizanidine Study Group. A double-blind placebo-controlled trial of tizanidine in the treatment of spasticity caused by multiple sclerosis. Neurology 1994; 44(suppl 9):70–79.

16.   Davidoff RA. Antispasticity drugs: mechanisms of action. Ann Neurol 1985; 17:107–116.

17.   Dunevsky A, Perel A. gabapentin for relief of spasticity associated with multiple sclerosis. Am J Phys Med Rehabil 1998; 77:451–454.

18.   Moore CD. Regional block: A Handbook for Use in the Clinical Practice of Medicine and Surgery, 4th ed. Springfield, IL: Charles C Thomas, 1971.

19.   Borg-Stein J, et al. Botulinum toxin for the treatment of spasticity in multiple sclerosis: New observation. Am J Phys Med Rehabil 1993; 72:364–368.

20.   Borodic GE, Ferrante R, Weigner AW, et al. Treatment of spasticity with botulinum toxin. Ann Neurol 1992; 31:113.

21.   Petajan JH, Gappmaier E, White AT, et al. Impact of aerobic training on fitness and quality of life in multiple sclerosis. Ann Neurol 1996; 39:432–441.

22.   Penn RD, Savoy SM, Corcos D, et al. Intrathecal baclofen for severe spinal spasticity. N Engl J Med 1989; 320:1517–1521.

23.   Redford JB. Principles of orthotic devices. In: Redford JB, ed. Orthotics Etcetera. Baltimore: Williams & Wilkins, 1985, pp 1–20.

24.   Lehman JF. Lower limb orthotics. In: Redford JB, ed. Orthotics Etcetera. Baltimore: Williams & Wilkins, 1985, pp 278–351.

25.   Lehman JF, Esselman PC, Ko MJ, et al. Plastic ankle-foot orthoses: Evaluation of function. Arch Phys Med Rehabil 1983, 64:402–407.

26. Lehman JF, Warren CG, deLateur BJ. Biomechanical evaluation of knee stability in below knee braces. Arch Phys Med Rehabil 1970; 51:688–695.

27. Simons BC, Jebsen, RH, Wildman LE. Plastic short leg brace fabrication. Orthop Prosthet Appl J 1967; 21:215–218.

28. Fifth Workshop Panel on Lower Extremity Orthotics. Subcommittee on Design and Development, Committee on Prosthetics Research and Development. Division of Engineering. National Research Council, National Academy of Sciences-National Academy of Engineering. Atlanta, April 3–4, 1968, p 17.

29. Cailliet R. Exercise in multiple sclerosis. In: Basmajian IV, ed. Therapeutic Exercise. Baltimore: Williams & Wilkins, 1984, pp 407–420.

30. Frenkel HS. In: Granger FB, ed. Physical Therapeutic Technique. Philadelphia: Saunders, 1929.

31. Jebsan R. Use and abuse of ambulation aids. JAMA 1967; 199:63–68.

32. Varghese G. Crutches, canes and walkers. In: Redford JB, ed. Orthotics Etcetera, 3rd ed. Baltimore: Williams & Wilkins, 1986, pp 453–463.

33. Hoberman M, Basmajian JV. Crutch and cane exercises and use. In: Basmajian JV, ed. Therapeutic Exercise, 4th ed. Baltimore: Williams & Wilkins, 1984, pp 267–284.

34. Burgess E, Alexander A. Mobility aids. In: Atlas of Orthopedics. St. Louis: Mosby, 1975.

35. Kemenetz HL. Wheelchairs and other motor vehicles for the disabled. In: Redford JB. ed. Orthotics Etcetera, 3rd ed. Baltimore: Williams & Wilkins, 1986, pp 464–517.

36. Ellwood PM. Transfers: method equipment and preparation. In: Kottke FL, Stillwell GK, Lehman JF, eds. Krusen's Handbook of Physical Medicine and Rehabilitation. 3rd ed. Philadelphia: Saunders, 1982, pp 473–491.

37. Blaivas JG. Management of bladder dysfunction in multiple sclerosis. Neurology 1979; 30:12–18.

38. Goldstein 1, Siroky MB, Sax DS, et al. The urodynamic characteristics of multiple sclerosis. J Urol 1982; 128:541.

39. Blaivas JG, Sinha HP, Zayed AAH, et al. Detrusor external sphincter dyssynergia. J Urol 1981; 125:542–544.

40. Blaivas JG, Sinha HP. Zayed AAH, Labib KB. Detrusor external sphincter dyssynergia: A detailed electromyographic study. J Urol 1981; 125:545–548.

41. Blaivas JG, Holland NJ, Giesser B, et al. Multiple sclerosis bladder: Studies and care. Ann NY Acad Sci 1984; 436:328–345.

42. Khanna OP. Nonsurgical therapeutic modalities. In: Krane RJ, Siroky MB, eds. Clinical Neuro-urology. Boston: Little, Brown, 1979, pp 139–196.

43. Boyarsky S, Labay P, Nanick P, et al. Care of the Patient with Neurogenic Bladder. Boston: Little, Brown, 1979.

44. Strauss BS, Blaufox MD. Estimation of residual urine and urine flow rates without urethral catheterization. J Nucl Med 1970; 11:81–84.

45. Nilvebrant L, Hallen B, Larsson G. Tolterodine—A new bladder selective muscarinic receptor antagonist: Preclinical pharmacological and clinical data. Life Sci 1997; 60:1129–1136.

46. Valiquette G, Meade-D'Alisera P, Herbert J. Double-blind crossover trial of DDAVP for nocturia in MS. Neurology 1993; 43(suppl 2):A281.

47. Diokno AC, Childs SJ. Clean intermittent catheterization in urinary tract infection management. Infect Surg 1985; 4:185–190.

48. Glick ME, Meshkinpoor H, Haldeman S. Colonic dysfunction in multiple sclerosis. Gastroenterology 1982; 83:1002–1007.

49. Levine IS. Bowel dysfunction in multiple sclerosis. In: Maloney FP, Burks JS, Ringel SP. eds. Interdisciplinary Rehabilitation of Multiple Sclerosis and Neuromuscular Disorders. Philadelphia: Lippincott, 1985, pp 62–64.

50. Kalb R, LaRocca N, Kaplan S. Sexuality. In: Scheinberg L, Holland NJ, eds. Multiple Sclerosis, 2nd ed. 1987, pp 177–196.

51. Wolf BG. Occupational therapy for patients with multiple sclerosis. In: Maloney FP, Burks JS, Ringel SP, eds. Interdisciplinary Rehabilitation of Multiple Sclerosis and Neuromuscular disorders. Philadelphia: Lippincott, 1985, pp 103–128.

52. Long C, Schutt AH. Upper limbs orthotics. In: Redford IB, ed. Orthotics Etcetera. 3rd ed. Baltimore: Williams & Wilkins, 1986, pp 198–277.

53. Freal JE, Kraft GH, Coryell JK. Symptomatic fatigue in multiple sclerosis. Arch Phys Med Rehabil 1984; 65:135–138.

54. Krupp LB, Alvarez LA, LaRocca NG, et al. Fatigue in multiple sclerosis. Arch Neurol 1988; 45:435–437.

55. Murray TJ. Amantadine therapy for fatigue in multiple sclerosis. Can J Neurol Sci 1985; 12: 251–254.

56. Krupp LB, Coyle PK, Doscher C, et al. Fatigue therapy in multiple sclerosis: Results of a double-blind, randomized, parallel trial of amantadine, pemoline, and placebo. Neurology 1995; 45:1956–1961.

57. Darley FL, Brown JR, Goldstein NP. Dysarthria in multiple sclerosis. J Speech Hear Res 1972; 15:229–245.

58. Darley FL, Aronson AE, Brown JE. Motor Speech Disorders. Philadelphia: Saunders, 1975.

59. Farmakides MN, Boone DR. Speech problems of patients with multiple sclerosis. J Speech Hear Disord 1960; 25:385–390.

60. Robbins SD. Dysarthria and its treatment. J Speech Disord 1940; 5:113–120.

61. Abraham S, Samkoff L. Prevalence of dysphagia symptomatology in multiple sclerosis. Neurology 1992; 42(suppl 3):465.

62. Logemann JA. Evaluation of swallowing disorders. In: Evaluation and Treatment of Swallowing Disorders. San Diego, CA: College Hill Press, 1983, pp 89–125.

63. DeJong R. The Neurologic Examination. 4th ed. New York: Harper & Row, 1979. 15. DeLorme TL, Watkins AL. Technics of progressive resistance exercise. Arch Phys Med Rehab 1948; 29:263–273.

64. Logemann JA. Treatment for aspiration related to dysphagia: An overview. Dysphagia 1986; 1:34–38.

65. Larsen C. Neurophysiology of speech and swallowing. In: Logemann JA, ed. Relationship of Speech and Swallowing. New York: Thieme Stratton, 1985.

66. Logemann JA. Management of the patient with disordered oral feeding. In: Evaluation and Treatment of Swallowing Disorders. San Diego, CA: College Hill Press, 1983, pp 129–157.

67. Lazzara G, Lazarus C, Lojemann J. Impact of thermal stimulation on the triggering of the swallowing reflex. Presented at the American Speech Language Hearing Association Annual Meeting, San Francisco, 1984.

68. Reuler JBM, Cooney TG. The pressure sore: pathophysiology and principles of management. Ann Intern Med 1981, 94:661–666.

69. Shea JD. Pressure sores: Classification and management. Clin Orthop 1975; 112:89–100.

70. Narsete TA, Orgel MG, Smith D. Pressure sores. Am Fam Physician 1983; 28:135–139.

29

Experimental Therapies with T-Cell Vaccines, Oral Myelin, and Monoclonal Antibodies in Multiple Sclerosis

SUPRABHA BHAT AND JERRY S. WOLINSKY

The University of Texas—Houston, Health Science Center, Houston, Texas

I. INTRODUCTION

The development of specific immunotherapies that target potentially pathogenic cells in multiple sclerosis (MS) patients without compromising the immune system as a whole is an active quest. Nonspecific immunosuppression is associated with toxicity and only marginal therapeutic benefit. The ideal therapy for MS would selectively abolish the autoimmune response while leaving the host's responses to infectious agents intact. A more precise understanding of the pathogenic process of MS is necessary to achieve this goal.

Therapy could be directed at the trimolecular complex, inhibition of inflammatory events, enhancement of regulatory mechanisms, or enhancement of repair processes. In summary, the therapeutic strategies can be grouped into those that affect the initial events of antigen presentation to encephalitogenic T cells, the activation of these cells, or their migration into the target tissue.

II. T-CELL VACCINE

Accumulating evidence indicates that MS has an autoimmune component, mediated by autoreactive T-lymphocytes specific for myelin antigens. The putative T-cell autoantigen remains uncertain, but myelin basic protein (MBP) is considered a major candidate. Clonally expanded MBP-specific T cells persist for several years in the blood of MS patients and activated MBP and proteolipid peptide (PLP)–specific T cells migrate and accumulate in the CNS, where they have been identified in brain lesions of MS patients (1). It is not yet clear how these T cells are initially activated, but several studies suggest that viral antigens mimicking myelin epitopes or functioning as superantigens may be involved. Further, there is evidence that regulatory mechanisms that control autoreactive T cells in healthy subjects are potentially defective in MS patients. In addition to myelin-reactive T cells, B cells producing myelin specific antibodies and γδ T cells may also play important roles in the autoimmune cascade (2). As MBP-reactive T cells may be central in the initiation and perpetuation of the CNS inflammation in MS, specific immune therapies have been proposed to deplete them in attempts to improve the clinical course of the disease.

A. T-Cell Receptors

The T-cell receptor (TCR) is a subunit of the T cell that distinguishes it from other T cells. The TCR, like immunoglobulins, has both constant and variable complementary regions and is selected under the pressure of antigenic stimulation. The progeny of a given T-cell clone has a unique TCR and limited antigen specificity. While once felt to be entirely specific for a given epitope, some limited cross reactivity is now established in a manner analogous to some monoclonal antibodies.

The TCR approach in MS and other putative autoimmune diseases assumes that (a) the subpopulations of the putative autoaggressive effector T cells must utilize only a limited number of TCR genes, (b) the T-cell vaccine must provoke an immune response that recognizes the hypervariable regions of the naturally occurring TCR peptide present on the surface of disease causing T-cells, and (c) the resulting immune response must somehow inhibit or downregulate the activities of disease-causing T cells in a manner sufficient to provide a clinical benefit without toxicity.

An understanding of the immune response against TCR is a prerequisite for successful TCR vaccination therapy of MS and other antigen-specific autoimmune diseases.

B. T-Cell Receptor Studies

In the Lewis rat, the subpopulation of T-lymphocytes responsible for EAE utilizes the TCRβ chain 8.2 V region gene (3–6). Treatment with a vaccine consisting of a peptide fragment of Vβ8.2 reduced the level of central nervous system (CNS) infiltration and the severity of paralytic disease in the rat experimental allergic encephalomyelitis (EAE) model (7,8). Similarly, treatment of Lewis rats with a Vβ8.2–specific monoclonal antibody to deplete these cells before or after immnization with MBP significantly reduced the severity of the induced disease (9). The peptide studies in EAE raised the possibility that immunizing MS patients who express high cerebrospinal fluid (CSF) levels of Vβ6 T cells with a similar Vβ6 peptide might have a discernible biological effect on the levels of these cells and ultimately prove to have a clinical benefit. T cells of the γδ type are expected to participate in the cascade of organ-specific immune-mediated tissue destruction, not to orchestrate the process. In related experiments, Vγ6 T cells were shown to predominate in the CNS of mice during the early stages of EAE. Therefore a TCR peptide designed to immunize against Vγ6 T cells was explored. The TCR peptide immunization specific for Vγ6 chains did not protect against EAE but did alter the development of the disease. There was a delay in the onset of EAE and a reduction in disease severity in TCR peptide–treated animals (10). These and similar studies suggest that immunization to deplete a population of T cells that contain putative encephalitogenic autoreactive T cells can control EAE, whether mediated by anti-TCR antibodies or by regulating T cells. However, different TCR peptide vaccine approaches may vary in their effects based on their specificity of action in the immune cascade.

In the first study to assess the safety and immunogenicity of TCR peptide (11,12), MS patients with chronic progressive disease were treated with CDR2–based peptides of TCR Vβ5.2 or 6.1 (this sequence is expressed in MS plaques and on MBP-specific T cells). No toxicity was observed. Treatment did not cause broad immunosuppression and some treated subjects develop immune responses, including delayed-type skin reactivity and TCR peptide–specific antibodies. A phase I trial of a T-cell receptor (TCR) Vβ6 CDR2 region peptide vaccine was conducted in 10 MS patients with biased over representations of Vβ6 mRNA among the T cells isolated from their CSF (13). These patients were monitored for adverse events, immunogenicity of the peptide and changes in their CSF T-cell populations. The peptide was immunogenic in some patients, although none of the immunized patients produced detectable antipeptide antibodies. Five patients treated with 300 μg of vaccine displayed a slight decrease in CSF cellularity, and a lack of growth of CSF cells in cytokine-supplemented expansion cultures. This implied an absence of a subset of activated CD_4+ T cells and a reduction of Vβ6 mRNA levels among T cells in these cultures. In the five patients who received a lower vaccine dose of 100 μg, CSF cellularity was the same or slightly increased over prevaccination levels. CSF cells from one patient failed to grow in expansion cultures and cultured cells from two low dose patients underwent a change from an oligoclonal Vβ6 pattern to one that was more polyclonal. This clonal prevalence and overrepresentation of Vβ6+ TCR raises the possibility that immunization with a Vβ6 peptide vaccine may produce a regulatory immune response. A double-blind pilot trial with TCR peptide vaccine from the Vβ5.2 sequence was then conducted in patients with progressive MS. Vaccine responders had a reduced MBP response and remained clinically stable without adverse effects during 1 year of therapy, whereas the nonresponders had an increased MBP response and progressed clinically. Peptide-specific TH2 cells directly inhibited MBP-specific TH1 cells in vitro through the release of interleukin-10 (IL-10), implicating bystander suppression (14). A widely active vaccine for MS might involve a limited set of slightly modified CDR2 peptides from βV genes involved in T-cell recognition of MBP.

C. T Cell–Based Vaccine

The concept of T-cell vaccine in MS is similar to that of any other attenuated vaccine used against microbial agents in infectious diseases. T-cell vaccination is a procedure whereby MS patients are immunized with attenuated autologous MBP-reactive T cells. This procedure induces immune response to the vaccine cells and a depletion of MBP-reactive T cells (15). Since MBP-reactive T cells potentially hold an important position in initiation and perpetuation of brain inflammation, specific immune therapies designed to deplete them may improve the clinical course of the disease.

Six MS patients were inoculated three times with autologous attenuated MBP-specific T-cell clones at 2-month intervals. No toxicity was observed, and after the third inoculation, the precursor frequency of the MBP-specific T cells fell below detectable levels in all patients. Limited antiergotypic and pronounced anticlonotypic T-cell responses were seen. This clinical trial showed that antigen-specific T-cell vaccination is feasible in humans (16). Another study demonstrated that in the majority of T-cell vaccine recipients, MBP-reactive T cells remained undetectable in the circulation for 1 to 3 years after vaccination, but they reappeared in some individuals (3 of 9) coinciding with clinical exacerbations (17).

In a pilot trial, 8 MS patients were matched to control patients and received vaccination with irradiated T cells reactive to MBP. Excacerbations in the 2 years before and after vaccination were evaluated. The exacerbations decreased in 5 vaccinated patients with relapsing-remitting disease from 16 to 3, respectively, and from 12 to 10 in their matched controls. MRI showed a mean 8% increase in brain lesion load in vaccinated patients compared to 39.5% increase in controls (18). In the majority of vaccinated MS patients, γδ T-cells expand upon stimulation with the vaccine cells. This indicates that γδ T cells can be stimulated by activated αβ T cells, and that these γδ T-cell responses are upregulated after T-cell vaccination (21).

An extended phase I trial was done on 49 MS patients in Belgium and Houston to study the safety, immune responses and clinical effects of T-cell vaccination (19,20,22,23). Substantial long-term in vitro proliferative responses were observed in all treated patients. Reactive TCR αβ(+), CD8(+) and CD4(+) T cells and, to a lesser extent, γδ T cells and NK cells were observed to in vitro stimulation with vaccine cells. Upregulated antibody responses to the vaccine cells could not be detected in most patients. Thus, immunization with attenuated autoreactive T cells appears to induce a complex cellular response specifically targeted at vaccine cells, but no antibody responses. This type of vaccination induces an effective anticlonotypic T-cell response leading to a specific depletion of circulating MBP-reactive cells. While longitudinal clinical evaluation suggests a possible reduction of rate of clinical exacerbation, disability score, and brain lesions measured by MRI in vaccinated patients (22,23), these studies have lacked rigorous controls.

D. Conclusion

The TCR-peptide immunotherapy and T-cell vaccination are primarily designed to target the TCR of MBP-reactive T cells. Unfortunately, the TCR V gene repertoire of MBP autoreactive T cells varies considerably among patients with MS. No common TCR V gene pattern has emerged for the disease association. Thus, the heterogeneous expression of TCR V gene products among a general MS population complicates attempts to develop an immunotherapy directed at a ''common'' variable regions of the TCR. A treatment agent designed to target certain TCR V gene product may be useful in one patient but not in other, which hampers its clinical usefulness.

Attenuated T-cell vaccine induces a complex cellular response specifically targeted at vaccine cells, but no antibody responses. The T-cell responses induced by immunization are restricted to the immunizing clones and do not affect MBP-reactive clones not used for immunization, which may be a limiting factor in therapeutic efficacy. Investigation on the treatment efficacy of T-cell vaccination is ongoing at several centers.

III. ORAL MYELIN

Immune tolerance refers to a state of systemic unresponsiveness to a specific antigen. Oral administration of antigen is a long recognized method of inducing systemic immune tolerance. Ingested antigen processing in Peyer's patches is central in the induction of oral tolerance. This method of inducing immune nonresponsiveness has been applied to the prevention and treatment of experimental models of autoimmune disease, including

EAE and other organ-specific autoimmune diseases such as collagen-induced arthritis, adjuvant arthritis, uveoretinitis, thyroiditis, and graft rejection.

Extensive research has led to the conclusion that two mechanisms are operative in the mediation of oral tolerance–active suppression by transforming growth factor-beta (TGF-β)–secreting T cells and clonal anergy or deletion of antigen specific T cells (24). Several factors appear to determine which mechanism of tolerance is operative. These include antigen dose, the form of antigen presentation, and the timing of antigen administration. It is believed that low doses of antigen induce active suppression, intermediate antigen doses induce clonal T-cell anergy, and high doses induce clonal T-cell deletion. Repeated ingestion of low doses of antigen induces active suppression. Under this condition, the suppression of an autoimmune attack to target tissues is mediated by anti-inflammatory cytokines such as TGF-β, IL-10, and IL-4, which are released from regulatory T cells triggered in an antigen-specific manner. Suppression of ongoing inflammatory reaction in an antigen-nonspecific fashion by activated T cells at the target organ is termed "bystander suppression."

A. Studies in EAE

That oral administration of MBP could protect Lewis rats from the induction of EAE was demonstrated as early as 1988 (25,26,27). The oral administration of MBP to susceptible mice prevented the induction of EAE with MBP (28). In a chronic relapsing model of EAE, oral administration of MBP either prior to MBP challenge or on the first day of clinical signs decreased the number and severity of EAE relapses (24). A decrease in the severity and frequency of clinical attacks with reduced CNS inflammation and demyelination followed the administration of myelin after the first clinical attack of chronic, relapsing EAE in Lewis rats and strain 13 guinea pigs (29). Finally, when mice with confirmed neurological deficits from chronic relapsing EAE were fed whole bovine myelin for 6 months, inflammation and demyelination in the CNS was suppressed and there was no exacerbation of clinical disease status compared with the control group. After 6 months of treatment, there was no increased sensitization of myelin antigens seen, as measured by anti-MBP or anti-PLP antibodies (30). The administration of recombinant IL-2 reversed the tolerance induced by feeding low doses of MBP. However, it did not overcome the tolerance induced by high doses of MBP. This suggests that the relative balance between suppressor and effector mechanisms can be overcome in low-dose tolerance but that T-cell deletion occurs in the high-dose group. Moreover, the oral administration of MBP to MBP-specific TCR transgenic mice resulted in a profound reduction in proliferative response and decrease of transgenic T cells in the blood, mesenteric nodes, and spleen, indicating that the cells were deleted from these sites or silenced. These and other studies suggest that oral administration of myelin, MBP, or other potentially encephalitogenic peptides of myelin can block EAE induction and modify the course of established acute, chronic, or recurrent disease.

B. Studies in MS

Based on the above results, a 1-year phase II double-blind study was conducted in 30 patients with early relapsing-remitting MS. Half of the patients ingested capsules containing bovine myelin, the remainder received placebo. At the end of the year, 6 of 15 myelin-treated patients had one or more major attacks, compared with 12 of the 15 placebo-controlled patients who had one or more relapses ($p = 0.06$). There was no difference in the overall change in disability between the two groups. Subgroup analysis suggested that males and HLA-DR2-negative subjects might derive the greatest benefit from this treatment. No improvement was seen in the DR2-positive individuals and females. This result was particularly surprising, as females and those with the DR2 molecule are over-represented in this disease (31). When 17 patients with relapsing-remitting MS were fed bovine myelin (containing both MBP and PLP) daily for a minimum of 2 years, a marked increase in the relative frequencies of MBP- and PLP-specific TGF-β1 secreting T-cell lines was found when compared to 17 nontreated MS patients. In contrast, no change in the frequency of the MBP- or PLP-specific, interferon gamma (IFN-γ) or tetanus toxoid–specific secreting T cells were seen. These results suggest that the oral administration of antigens generates antigen-specific TGF-β1–secreting T cells, which may represent a distinct cytokine-secreting lineage of T cells (TH3) (32,33).

Given these observations, a 2-year phase III double-blind multicenter placebo-controlled trial of oral bovine myelin (Myloral) involving 500 subjects with well-defined relapsing-remitting MS was conducted. This was the first major attempt to determine if a protein that is also a self antigen, administered into the gut, could counterregulate a presumed ongoing CNS autoimmune process. Unfortunately, preliminary reports from the completed trial indicate no differences in the frequency of relapses or progression of disability between those taking the drug and those receiving placebo (34). Several major assumptions were made by this study. First, that encephalitogenic T lymphocytes are reacting to a specific identified self-antigen(s) intrinsic to myelin, such as MBP or PLP, that damage myelin directly or through activation of macrophages and other agents of inflammation. This may not be the case. The evidence for increased MBP T-cell reactivity relies on in vitro culture techniques that may not reflect in vivo reality. Myelin protein components may not be the primary sensitizing T-cell antigen or even the secondary neo-antigen after primary CNS damage in MS. Second, that bovine myelin was an appropriate source of myelin. This may have been inappropriate, as bovine myelin does not express the putative immunodominant epitope of human MBP. Similarly, the dose, formulation, or timing of administration of Myloral may have been inappropriate. Finally, that human gut epithelial cells or gut-associated lymphoid tissue (GALT) in Peyer's patches, lamina propria, or intraepithelial lymphocytes process intact bovine myelin into appropriate proteins or peptide fragments for presentation to and activation of counterregulatory T cells may be incorrect. MBP is relatively unique among proteins in that the intact molecule can bind directly to class II for presentation to T-cells. However, there is as yet limited evidence that MBP was efficiently presented in these patients.

C. Oral Tolerance with Glatiramer Acetate

Further studies show that the suppression of EAE by oral glatiramer acetate is probably mediated by glatiramer acetate–specific T-suppressor (T2) cells, which are of the T-helper (CD4+, TH2) type and secrete anti-inflammatory cytokine TGF-β. Glatiramer acetate–specific TH2/TH3 cells, isolated from mesentric lymph nodes of mice and rats fed with glatiramer acetate, demonstrated the ability to suppress whole spinal cord homogenate or MBP-induced EAE in naïve rats and mice. In various EAE models in mice and rats, a significant reduction in the incidence and severity of disease following oral administration of glatiramer acetate has recently been demonstrated (36).

This suggests that ongoing inflammation at the target organ is suppressed through bystander suppression. Similar regulatory cells were produced following parenteral administration of glatiramer acetate and are implicated in the beneficial clinical effect of parenteral glatiramer acetate in MS patients (35). A large multinational, multicenter phase III clinical trial with oral Copaxone is now under way.

IV. ALTERED PEPTIDE LIGANDS

Altered peptide ligands (APLs) are defined as analogues of immunogenic peptides modi-fied at their TCR contact sites in a way that results in antagonism, anergy, or partial activation of antigen-specific T cells. When developed for encephalitogenic T cells, they result in downregulation of EAE (37). While these peptides may not stimulate T-cell clonal proliferation, they nevertheless can retain the capacity to activate some TCR-mediated effector functions.

An immunodominant epitope of MBP, VHFFKNIVTPRTP (P87-99), is a major target of T cells isolated from lesions of MS patients and in EAE. T cells found in EAE lesions bear the same amino acids in the third complementary determining region of the TCR as those found in MS lesions. IFN-γ and tumor necrosis factor–alpha (TNF-α) are two cytokines that are critical in the pathogenesis of EAE and MS. TNF-α is a mediator of cell recruitment in inflammatory infiltrates (40) and is a critical cytokine in the patho-genesis of EAE and probably of MS (41). As an example, draining lymph node cells from rats immunized with the native encephalitogenic peptide induce EAE when transfered to naive recipients. When challenged together with each of the three TCR anatagonists, administration of P87-99 (91K > A), P87-99 amino acid sequence substituted with an alanine at MBP residue 91 for the native lysine), but not P87-99 (95T > A) or P87-99 (96P > A), reduced the production of TNF-α and IFN-γ. The peptides P87-99 (95T > A) and P87-99 (96P > A) could compete more effectively with P87-99 for binding to MHC and could antagonize the in vitro response of T cells to P87-99 more effectively than did P87-99 (91K > A). However, only P87-99 (91K > A) prevented and reversed EAE, indicating that the extent of MHC or TCR competition does not predict success in treating EAE. APL may induce T-cell populations that secrete regulatory cytokines upon stimulation by the native peptide (38) or may decrease the ratio of IFN-γ/IL-4 secreted by encephalitogenic THI cells (39).

Following induction of EAE with a T-cell clone that is specific for the MBP epitope P87-99, the inflammatory infiltrate in the CNS contained a diverse collection of T cells with heterogeneous receptors. When this clone was tolerized in vivo with an analogue of P87-99, established paralysis was reversed, inflammatory infiltrates regressed, and the heterogeneous T-cell infiltrate disappeared from the brain, with only the T-cell clones that incited disease remaining in the original lesions. Treatment with this APL appeared to selectively silence pathogenic T cells that would actively signal for the efflux of other T cells to be recruited to the site of disease as a result of their production of IL-4 and reduction of TNF-α within the lesion. This phenomenon is likely mediated by downregula-tion of the production of TNF-α and by the action of IL-4. IL-4 is associated with recovery from disease and is seen in MS lesions (42,43). Inflammation is a dynamic process, and T-cell tolerance with APL leads to regression and dissolution of an inflammatory infil-terate. By selectively targeting the initial trigger for inflammation, the secondary infiltrate can be controlled. This may be relevant for highly selective immune therapy of autoim-mune disease in the face of determinant spreading (44) and nonspecific amplification of the inflammatory response.

When certain neurotropic viruses trigger inflammation in the CNS, immune cells in the inflammatory infiltrate attack neighboring myelin antigens in the CNS (45). This immune response then spreads to various epitopes on various myelin antigens, a process known as *epitope spreading* (46). Certain APLs actually resemble the immunogenic portion of certain neurotropic viruses and can be used to subvert epitope spreading. Suppression of the spreading response may be possible by administering various APLs that mimic the structure of both certain microbes and a component of myelin. These APLs induce IL-4 and either prevent or reverse EAE. Administration of such APLs may clear an entire inflammatory infiltrate that contains a diverse collection of T and B cells from the brain (39,46).

A double-blind randomized placebo-controlled phase I clinical trial evaluated the safety and tolerability of CGP 77116 (APL) in MS patients. Twenty three patients were treated with CGP 77116. The total exposure to CGP 77116 ranged from 4 to 200 mg over a 4-week treatment period. Most adverse events were as expected for the MS population and were generally more frequent in the placebo group. Most frequent adverse events were transient mild to moderate injection-site reactions of pain, erythema, wheal, burning, and itching, which did not require treatment. Cranial MRI with gadolinium did not show drug-related worsening of disease. There was no significant change in the Kurtzke EDSS scale during the study period. Anti-CGP antibodies were not detected in the sera. The APLs now in phase II clinical trials in MS have a K→A substitution at position 91 and thus neither bind anti-MBP antibody nor trigger MBP-specific T-cells (46).

V. MONOCLONAL ANTIBODIES

Monoclonal antibodies (mAbs) recognize and bind to a single structural motif on a specific antigen with exquisite specificity. CD4+ T-cells, which recognize peptide fragments in the context of the major MHC II molecule binding pocket, orchestrate cellular and humoral immune reactions through the secretion of immunoregulatory cytokines and via cell-to-cell contact. Distinct types of helper CD4+ T cells are identified based on their cytokine production capacity. TH1-type cells secrete IFN-γ and TNF-α and are involved in cell-mediated immunity. TH2-type cells secrete IL-4 , IL-5 and TGF-β and exert their primary function in humoral immune reactions and in modulating TH1 T-cell responses. Experimental animal models have shown that autoantigen-reactive CD4+ TH1-type cells are central for disease induction and progression. These cells are considered to play a pivotal role in a number of human autoimmune diseases such as rheumatoid arthritis and MS. In animals, depletion of CD4+ T cells interferes with disease induction in EAE (47), adjuvant arthritis (48), and systemic lupus erythematosus models (49). Several trials have studied the effects of infusions of various mAbs in patients with chronic progressive MS in the hope of developing an immunologically specific, nontoxic form of therapy.

Murine mAbs, which specifically deplete or interfere with the function of discrete T-cell subsets, can prevent or delay the onset of EAE (47,50) and reverse signs of already established clinical disease (51). Murine mAb is a foreign protein, which elicits antimouse antibody responses (HAMA) in humans that could block its therapeutic action (59). Chimeric mAbs are genetically engineered by combining a human constant region to the variable region of a murine antibody. Humanized mAbs are further engineered to be even more similar to human antibodies.

Many different mAbs with specificity for CD4, TCR, cytokines, adhesion molecules, and costimulation receptors have been studied.

A. Anti-CD4 Antibody

CD4 is a cell-surface antigen found almost exclusively on the helper subset of T lymphocytes. Since the pathogenesis of EAE and presumably MS involves CD4+ TH1 T cells that control many aspects of immune function, CD4 it is a logical target for intervention. Experiments with animal models of autoimmune disease indicate that anti-CD4 antibodies are effective in reversing various spontaneous and induced diseases, even in advanced clinical stages, in nonhuman primates (52). Very early work with a murine anti-CD4 mAb showed that it prevented the development of EAE (47,51). Treatment with anti-CD4 reversed EAE even when given to paralyzed animals. Anti-CD4 mAb selectively depleted CD4 bearing T cells from lymph nodes and spleen in mice (51) but did not appreciably deplete CD4 T cells in the rat EAE model (47). However, treatment with both CD4+ cell-depleting or CD4+ blocking/nondepleting mAb inhibited disease progression in mice with chronic relapsing EAE (53). In Lewis rats, anti-CD4 mAb does not ablate the encephalitogenic CD4+ cells or prevent the development of resistance to EAE, but it may inhibit EAE by preventing the function of already activated effector cells (54). EAE in primates is often quite severe compared to that seen in the rodent models. Treatment of rhesus monkeys with OKT4+4A an (anti-CD4 mAb) can reverse clinical signs of EAE (55). Outbred long-tailed macaques on anti-CD4 mAb treatment showed prolonged survival and in some cases complete reversal of clinical EAE (56). However, of caution, mice with chronic CNS toxoplasmosis develop fatal disease when treated with anti-CD4 mAb. This therapy, while targeted to a very specific T-cell subpopulation, induces substantial immunodeficiency. Pretreatment with a nondepleting anti-CD4 mAb (H129.19), which produces long-lasting receptor saturation, fully protected PL/J mice from EAE (57). These results further illustrate the varied mechanisms through which mAbs directed at the same molecule may exert their effects.

Phase I trials were conducted in chronic progressive MS patients using anti-T12, anti-T4, and anti-T11 mAbs. Anti-T11 mAb decreased T-cell activation by phytohemagglutination and anti-T4 mAb infusions abolished pokeweed mitogen-induced immunoglobulin synthesis without lysis of the CD4+ T-cell subpopulation (59). Early trials with anti-CD4 antibodies in chronic progressive MS patients were carried out with infusions of murine anti-CD4 mAb. Patients received five daily infusions (0.2 mg/kg/day) of either murine anti-CD2 (an antigen more widely expressed on T cells) or anti-CD4 mAb. These were reported to be tolerated without side effects (58). The infusions suppressed several in vitro measures of the immune response. Eighteen hours after the first anti-CD4 mAb infusion, there was an approximately 50% decrease in circulating CD4+ lymphocytes accompanied by a twofold increase in the percentage of circulating CD8+ cells. However, as is typical when murine mAbs are given across species, most subjects developed antimouse antibody responses that were almost exclusively IgG isotype. These may block the therapeutic action of the mAbs (59).

A phase I open label trial with murine anti-T CD4/BF5 mAb was done in 35 patients with active MS (18 progressive and 17 relapsing-remitting). Therapy induced a marked CD4+ lymphocyte depletion. Only minor general side effects were noted in 22 patients and only upon the first mAb infusion. These side effects may be related to release of cytokines from T cells directly stimulated by the mAb infusions. Functional disability was stabilized at 1 year in only 6 of the 35 patients and after 2 years in only 2 of 21 patients. No changes in the lesions were noted on magnetic resonance imaging (MRI) scans performed after treatment (60).

Single and repeated infusions of a chimeric murine/human anti-CD4 mAb, CM-T412, resulted in a profound selective depletion of CD4+ cells in a phase I study in MS patients (61,62). This led to a randomized double-blind placebo controlled MRI-monitored phase II trial in 71 patients with active relapsing remitting and secondary progressive MS. As expected, infusion of the mAbs resulted in a long-lasting reduction of circulating

CD4+ T cells. However, there was no significant effect on the primary measure of efficacy, the number of enhanced lesions on monthly gadolinium-enhanced MRI over 9 months. There was a significant 41% decrease in the number of clinical relapses (secondary efficacy parameter) after 9 months ($p = 0.02$) (63). An analysis on the phenotypes and function of circulating T cells in treated MS patients correlated the absence of therapeutic success with failure of the mAb to delete primed IFN-γ–producing T cells, cells strongly implicated in the pathogenesis of autoimmune disease (64).

CD52 is a surface antigen found on both T cells and macrophages. In a pilot study, seven MS patients treated with Campath-IH (humanized anti-CD52 mAb) had a substantial reduction in disease activity as measured by gadolinium-enhancing lesions on MRI (65). Five-day pulse treatment of 27 MS patients with Campath-IH in a randomized controlled clinical trial depleted 95% of their circulating lymphocytes. Counts of CD4 and CD8 remained at 30 to 40% of pretreatment values 18 months later. A third of these patients developed antibodies against the thyrotropin receptor and carbimazole-responsive autoimmune hyperthyroidism. Altogether 12 out of 37 Campath-IH–treated MS patients developed Graves disease, while none of 600 patients treated for various other disorders with Campath-IH have done so. This suggests that patients with MS are uniquely susceptible to this complication (66). The earlier report showed that a single pulse of Campath-IH suppressed MRI markers of MS disease activity for at least 6 months. An extended follow-up in 27 additional patients showed that MRI markers of disease activity were significantly suppressed for at least 18 months in all patients. However, half of these patients experienced progressive disability, assumed to be due to axonal degeneration conditioned by high pretreatment disease activity. Treatment with Campath-IH causes the immune response to shift away from the TH1 phenotype, suppressing MS disease activity but permitting the generation of antibody-mediated thyroid autoimmunity (67). In a crossover treatment trial in 25 secondary progressive MS patients, treatment was associated with a reduction in the number and volume of enhancing lesions ($p < 0.01$), but decrease in brain volume was seen in 13 patients during the 18 months posttreatment period (68).

An open-label trail of Muromonab (Orthoclone OKT3) was conducted by Weinshenker et al. (78). OKT3 is an IgG2a mAb that is pan-T-cell–reactive. Sixteen MS patients with rapidly progressive disease were treated daily with 5-mg infusions of OKT3 on 10 consecutive days. Side effects were severe and common and included hypotension, skin rash, nausea, fever, and diarrhea. One patient had an acute anaphylactic reaction. Four patients deteriorated > 1.0 points on their EDSS. There was a 73% stabilization rate, and two patients had clinical improvement at 1-year follow-up. The investigators concluded that the severe and potentially life-threatening toxicity precluded the use of Muromonab-CD3 in the treatment of MS.

B. Anti-TCR Antibodies

Immunoglobulins and their close relatives, the antigen-specific T-cell receptors, are recognition proteins that express structures which can serve as self-immunogens. Healthy humans produce antibodies against variable region–defined recognition structures termed *idiotypes*, as well as against constant-region structures, and the level of these can increase markedly in autoimmune disease. Most recent analyses employing synthetic peptide technologies and construction of recombinant TCR document that autoantibodies directed against both variable- and constant-region markers of the TCR $\alpha\beta$ occur in healthy individuals. Two of the major autoimmunogeneic regions of the TCR $\alpha\beta$ are ''constitutive'' markers. All individuals tested have natural antibodies against these regions. Alterations in the levels of antibody, usage of IgM or IgG isotypes, and specificity for a particular peptide-defined region vary with natural physiological processes (aging, pregnancy), artificial allografting, retroviral infection, and the inception and progression of autoimmune diseases. The most frequently observed autoantibodies are against TCR Vβ CDR1 and Fr3 markers. It is hypothesized that these are normally involved in immunoregulation.

The natural tendency in T cell–mediated autoimmune conditions to develop focused antigen-specific responses that overutilize certain TCR V region segments prompted the induction of anti-TCR–specific T cells and antibodies that can inhibit the pathogenic T cells and promote recovery from disease. In some strains, such as the Lewis rat and the PL/J mouse, the encephalitogenic MBP-specific T cells overexpress a particular V region gene (Vβ 8.2) of the TCR (69,70). Administration of a combination of anti-Vβ8.2 and anti-Vβ13 mAbs resulted in a long-term elimination of T cells involved in the response to MBP in B10.PL mice. When given before MBP immunization, anti-TCR antibody treatment leads to nearly complete protection against EAE and also results in a dramatic reversal of paralysis in diseased mice (71). When SJL/J mice with relapsing EAE induced by a PLP 139-151–specific T-cell line expressing 88% Vβ2 were treated with anti-Vβ2 mAb, clinical and histological disease severity was markedly reduced, both when given at the time of cell transfer or when given at clinical disease onset (72).

R 73 is a mAb specific for rat TCR αβ. Administration of a low dose of R 73 protects rats from EAE. When treatment was started shortly before the onset of clinical signs, R 73 completely suppressed the induction of EAE, and when treatment was started on the day of onset of clinical signs, recovery was hastened (73).

Specific TCR mAbs have not been directly administered to MS patients, but the induction of polyvalent anti-TCR antibodies by TCR peptides might contribute to the responses seen in MS patients treated in several peptide pilot studies. This subject is reviewed in Sec. II of this chapter.

C. Anticytokine Antibodies

Cytokines play important signaling roles in cellular immune mechanisms. These soluble glycoproteins are nonimmunoglobulin in nature. They act nonenzymatically to regulate immune cell function. As a potent mediator of inflammation, the cytopathic cytokine TNF appears to be important in the pathogenesis of EAE and MS. A myriad of other cytokines undoubtedly influence the immune system and are potential targets of immune modulators with mAbs or soluble ligands. Monoclonal antibody to TNF can prevent either active or transferred EAE in mice (74,75). Anti-TNF antibody effectively inhibits the development of EAE in SJL/J mice by interfering with the effector rather than the induction phase of the disease (77).

Intravenous infusions of murine-human chimeric anti-TNF mAb (CA2) were administered twice in an interval of 2 weeks to two rapidly progressive MS patients. Clinical status, contrast-enhanced MRI, and peripheral blood and CSF immunologic status were monitored. Although clinically significant neurological changes were not noted in either patient, the number of gadolinium-enhancing lesions increased, as did CSF lymphocyte counts and the IgG index after each infusion in both patients. This suggests that CA2 treatment caused immune activation and an increase in disease activity (79).

EAE in rats was prevented by administration of a P55-TNF-IgG fusion protein (TNFR-IgG). TNFR-IgG, when administered before disease onset, appears to act by inhibiting an effector function of activated T cells and possibly other inflammatory leukocytes (76). The hypothesis that neutralization of TNF by a recombinant TNF receptor P55 immunoglobulin fusion protein (Lenercept) might reduce or halt MS progression was evaluated in a large phase II randomized, multicenter placebo-controlled study of 168 patients, most with relapsing-remitting MS. Patients received infusions of 10, 50, or 100 mg of Lenercept or placebo every 4 weeks for up to 48 weeks. The number of treated patients experiencing exacerbations was increased compared to the placebo group ($p = 0.007$), and their exacerbations occurred earlier ($p = 0.006$). There was no significant difference between the groups on any MRI study measured. Anti–fusion protein antibodies were present in a substantial number of treated patients (80). The recombinant TNF receptor P55 immunoglobulin fusion protein had repeatedly shown potent preventive and therapeutic effects in various EAE protocols. However, as has frequently occurred, the EAE results were not predictive of the drugs effect in MS.

IL-10 is a TH2 immunomodulatory cytokine with known downregulatory effects upon TH1 responses and macrophages. In murine EAE, the administration of anti-IL-10 mAb before the onset of signs had no effect when given early postsensitization. It caused marked worsening when given immediately before onset of signs (81). Anti-IL-2 mAbs have a beneficial effect on passive EAE but not on active disease (82,83). IFN-γ is regarded as an inflammatory cytokine, and hence an antibody to this cytokine is expected to lessen the severity of EAE. Parodoxically, four independent groups have shown that such a treatment exacerbates active or passive disease (84–87). Because of the intricate balance of cytokines in maintaining immune regulation, partial redundancy in the effects of many cytokines, fluctuations in the balance during beneficial as well as autodestructive immune responses, and the differential effects that reduction or elimination of the effects of a cytokine systemically or within the CNS might have in the cascade of organ-specific immune damage, cytokine-specific immune therapy may be less predictable and useful than originally anticipated.

D. Anti–Adhesion Molecule Antibodies

Alpha$_4$ beta$_1$ integrin (VLA-4) expressed on T cells is crucial for their adhesion to human vascular cell adhesion molecule-1 (VCAM-1) expressed on luminal surface of inflamed endothelium. Autoreactive lymphocytes activated in the periphery must migrate to the CNS before they can orchestrate tissue damage. Cell adhesion is an early step in leukocyte extravasation across the blood-brain barrier (BBB) in inflammatory CNS disease. Antibodies against VLA-4 that block interaction with VCAM-1 should prevent cell infiltration. Murine anti-VLA-4 mAbs suppress clinical and pathological features of EAE in mice and guinea pigs (88).

Humanized mAb AN 100226 is equivalent to the murine mAb AN 100226m in binding to α4β1 integrin and in blocking cell adhesion. In a phase I, placebo-controlled, five-level dose-escalation study of a single intravenous dose of humanized mAb anti-alpha$_4$ integrin (Natalizumab, Antegren), 0.03 to3.0 mg/kg of the drug or placebo was studied in 28 stable relapsing-remitting or secondary progressive MS patients. All doses were safe and well tolerated (89). Seventy two similar patients were then evaluated in a randomized, double-blind, placebo-controlled trial to determine the acute effects of Natalizumab on MRI lesion activity. Each subject received two intravenous infusions of mAb or placebo 4 weeks apart and was then followed for 24 weeks with serial MRI and clinical assesments. The treated group exhibited significantly fewer new enhancing lesions than did the placebo group over the first 12 weeks. No significant difference was seen between the two groups in the second 12 weeks of the study. The number of acute exacerbations was not different between the two groups during the first 12 weeks but was higher in the treatment group in the second 12 weeks ($p = 0.005$). The investigators concluded that short-term treatment with Antegren results in a significant reduction in number of new active lesions on MRI (90).

From a phase I uncontrolled dose-escalation study with humanized anti-CD11/CD18 mAB (Hu23F2G) in 24 MS patients, it was concluded that HU23F2G was tolerated at doses that achieved high degrees of leukocyte CD11/CD18 saturation with in vivo inhibition of leukocyte migration (91). A phase II, multicenter, randomized, double-blind, placebo-controlled trial of Hu23F2G was conducted in 169 patients with acute MS exacerbations. Subjects were enrolled within 7 days of symptom onset to one of four treatment groups: placebo ($n = 43$), methylprednisolone (MP) 1g IV qd for 3 days ($n = 41$), Hu23F2G 1 mg/kg IV ($n = 44$), or Hu23F2G 2 mg/kg IV ($n = 41$). Efficacy endpoints were the neurological rating scale and the EDSS change from day 0 to day 90 and brain MRI abnormality change from day 0 to day 5. Hu23F2G was ineffective in improving neurological status at a single dose of 1 or 2 mg/kg. MP treatment was associated with a greater decrease in areas of contrast enhancements on brain MRI than placebo or Hu23F2G (Fred Lublin, Philadelphia, PA, and the Hu23F2G MS study group).

E. Antibodies to Costimulation Receptors

Antigen bound to MHC alone is not sufficient to activate T cells. The TCR must not only contact the antigen in the MHC antigen binding groove but also requires a concurrent second signal or costimulation from the APC. When T cells are activated, they express cell surface molecules that are not present on naïve cells. In autoimmune disease, the autoreactive cells will express activation antigens, whereas normal cells do not. Autoreactive cells would be selectively eliminated by cytotoxic mAb to the activation antigen given at this time.

Several studies have shown that direct interference with the interaction of B7 (macrophage membrane–enclosed surface antigen) and CD28, a T-cell surface antigen, disrupts a costimulatory pathway and leads to antigen-specific unresponsiveness. Interference with B7/CD28 is an effective means of preventing induction of relapsing EAE (92,93) and of treating ongoing disease (94,95).

CD40, although originally identified as a constitutive B-cell antigen, is expressed by many cells, including dendritic cells, macrophages, and astrocytes. CD154 (CD40L), the ligand for CD40, is transiently expressed primarily by activated CD4 T cells. Recently CD154 has been identified on a subpopulation of activated B cells. CD40 ligation leads to upregulation of costimulatory molecules B7–1 and B7–2 on the antigen-presenting cells (APCs), enhancing their ability to activate naïve T cells. CD40-CD154 interactions are crucial for B-cell activation and differentiation and for production of IL-12 by APCs, which biases CD4 T-cell responses toward TH1. CD40–CD154 interactions may be involved in directing CNS migration of encephalitogenic cells and/or in their ability to activate CNS macrophages/microglia. When anti-CD154 mAbs was administered to SJL mice at either the peak of acute disease or during remission, clinical disease progression and CNS inflammation were effectively blocked. The proportion of anti-CD154 mAb treated mice with relapses (37%) was significantly reduced compared with that for control mice (81%). In vitro T-cell proliferation assays showed that anti-CD154–treated animals with ongoing R-EAE had inhibited TH1 responsiveness and epitope spreading (96).

VI. CONCLUSION

A possible advantage of using mAbs is the potential for specific depletion or modulation of an individual subset of cells, such as helper or suppressor T-lymphocyte populations. This is a clear advantage only when a specific subpopulation of cells is linked with disease pathogenesis. In MS, a specific immunological target for mAb therapy has not been identified yet.

REFERENCES

1. Zhang J, Stinissen P, Medaer R, et al. T-cell vaccination: clinical application in autoimmune diseases. J Mol Med 1996; 74:653–662.
2. Stinissen P, Raus J, Zhang J. Autoimmune pathogenesis of multiple sclerosis: role of autoreactive T-lymphocytes and new immunothereupetic strategies. Crit Rev Immunol 1997; 17:33–75.
3. Burns FR, Li X, Shen N, et al. Both rat and mouse T-cell receptors specific for the encephalitogenic determinant of myelin basic protien use similar Vα and Vβ chain genes even through the major histocompatibility complex and encephalitogenic determinants being recognized are different. J Exp Med 1998; 169:27–39.
4. Chluba J, Steeg C, Becker A, et al. T-cell receptor β chain usage in myelin basic protien-specific rat T-lymphocytes. Eur J Immunol 1989; 19:279–284.
5. Gold DP, Offner H, Sun D, et al. Analysis of T-cell receptor β chains in Lewis rats with experimental allergic encephalomyelitis: Conserved CDR3 regions. J Exp Med 1991; 174: 1467–1476.
6. Wilson DB, Steinman L, Gold DP. The V-region disease hypothesis: New evidence suggests it is probably wrong. Immunol Today 1993; 14:376–380.
7. Vandenbark AA, Hashim, G, Offner H. Immunization with a synthetic T-cell receptor V region protects against EAE. Nature 1989; 341:541–544.
8. Howell MD, Winters ST, Olee T, et al. Vaccination against experimental allergic encephalomyelitis with T-cell receptor peptides. Science 1989; 246:668–669.
9. Imrich H, Kugler C, Torres-Nagel N, et al. Prevention and treatment of Lewis rat experimental allergic encephalomyelitis with a monoclonal antibody to the T-cell receptor Vβ8.2 segment (abstr). Eur J Immunol 1995; 25:1960–1964.
10. Olive C. Modulation of experimental allergic encephalomyelitis in mice by immunization with a peptide specific for gamma delta T-cell receptor. Immunol Cell Biol 1997; 75:102–106.
11. Bourdette DN, Whitham RH, Chou YK, et al. Immunity to TCR peptides in multiple sclerosis: I. Successful immunization of patients with synthetic V beta 5.2 and V beta 6.1 CDR2 peptides. J Immunol 1994; 152:2510–2519.
12. Chou YK, Morrison WJ, Weinberg AD, et al. Immunity to TCR peptides in multiple sclerosis: II. T-cell recognition of Vβ5.2 and Vβ6.1 CDR2 peptides (abstr). J Immunol 1984; 152:2520–2529.
13. Gold DP, Smith RA, Golding AB, et al. Results of a phase I clinical trial of a T-cell receptor vaccine in patients with multiple sclerosis. II. Comparitive analysis of TCR utilization in CSF T-cell populations before and after vaccination with a TCRVβ6 CDR2 peptide. J Neuroimmunol 1997; 76:29–38.
14. Vandenbark AA, Chou YK, Whitham R, et al. Treatment of multiple sclerosis with T-cell receptor peptides: Results of a double-blind pilot trial. Nature Med 1996; 10:1109–1115.
15. Hermans G, Denzer U, Lohse A, et al. Cellular and humoral immune responses against autore-

active T-cells in multiple sclerosis patients after T-cell vaccination. J Autoimmun 1999; 13: 233–246.

16. Zhang J, Raus J. T-cell vaccination in multiple sclerosis: Hopes and facts. Acta Neurol Belg 1994; 94:112–115.

17. Zhang J, Vandevyver C, Stinissen P, et al. In vivo clonotypic regulation of human myelin basic protien-reactive T-cells by T-cell vaccination. J Immunol 1995; 155:5868–5877.

18. Medaer R, Stinissen P, Truyen L, et al. Depletion of myelin-basic-protein autoreactive T-cells by T-cell vaccination: Pilot trial in multiple sclerosis. Lancet 1995; 346:807–808.

19. Hermans G, Denzer U, Lohse, A, et al. Cellular and humoral immune responses against autoreactive T-cells in multiple sclerosis patients after T-cell vaccination. J Autoimmun 1999; 13: 233–246.

20. Zhang J, Stinissen P, Medaer R, et al. T-cell vaccination: Clinical application in autoimmune diseases. J Mol Med 1996; 74:653–662.

21. Stinissen P. Zhang J, Vandevyver C, et al. Gamma delta T-cell responses to activated T-cells in multiple sclerosis patients induced by T-cell vaccination. J Neuroimmunol 1998; 87:94–104.

22. Zhang J, Raus J. T-cell vaccination in multiple sclerosis. Mult Scler 1996; 1:353–356.

23. Stinissen P, Zhang J, Medaer R, et al. Vaccination with autoreactive T-cell clones in multiple sclerosis: Overview of immunological and clinical data. J Neurosci Res 1996; 45:500–511.

24. Whitacre CC, Gienapp IE, Meyer A, et al. Treatment of autoimmune disease by oral tolerance to autoantigens. Clin Immunol Immunopathol 1996; 80:S31–S39.

25. Higgins P, Weiner HL. Suppression of experimental autoimmune encephalomyelitis by oral administration of myelin basic protein and its fragments. J Immunol 1988; 140:440.

26. Bitar DM, Whitacre CC. Suppression of experimental autoimmune encephalomyelitis by oral administration of myelin basic protein. Cell Immunol 1988; 112:364.

27. Lider O, Santos LMB, Lee CSY, et al. Suppression of experimental autoimmune encephalomyelitis by oral administration of myelin basic protein: II. Suppression of disease and in vitro immune responses is mediated by antigen-specific CD8+ T lymphocytes. J Immunol 1989; 142:748.

28. Jewell SD, Gienapp IE, Cox KL, et al. Oral tolerance as therapy for experimental autoimmune encephalomyelitis and multiple sclerosis: Demonstration of T-cell anergy. Immunol Cell Biol 1998; 76:74–82.

29. Brod SA, Al-Sabbagh A, Sobel RA, et al. Suppression of experimental autoimmune encephalomyelitis by oral administration of myelin antigens: IV. Suppression of chronic relapsing disease in the Lewis rat and strain 13 guinea pig. Ann Neurol 1991; 29:615.

30. Al-Sabbagh AM, Goad EP, Weiner HL, et al. Decreased CNS inflammation and absence of clinical exacerbation of disease after six months oral administration of bovine myelin in diseased SJL/J mice with chronic relapsing experimental autoimmune encephalomyelitis. J Neurosci Res 1996; 45:424–429.

31. Weiner HL, Friedman A, Miller A, et al. Double blind pilot trial of oral tolerization with myelin antigens in multiple sclerosis. Science 1993; 259:1321–1324.

32. Fukaura H, Kent SC, Pietrusewicz MJ, et al. Induction of circulating myelin basic protein and proteolipid protein-specific transforming growth factor-beta$_1$-secreting Th3 T-cells by oral administration of myelin in multiple sclerosis patients. J Clin Invest 1996; 98:70–77.

33. Hafler DA, Kent SC, Pietrusewicz MJ, et al. Oral administration of myelin induces antigen-specific TGF-beta$_1$-secreting T cells in patients with multiple sclerosis. Ann NY Acad Sci 1997; 835:120–131.

34. Brod SA. Gut response: Therapy with ingested immunomodulatory proteins. Arch Neurol 1997; 54:1300–1302.

35. Miller A, Shapiro S, Gershtein R, et al. Treatment of multiple sclerosis with copolymer-1(Copaxone): Implicating mechanisms of Th1 to Th2/Th3 immune-deviation. J Neuroimmunol 1998; 92:113–121.

36. Teitelbaum D, Arnon R, Sela M. Immunomodulation of experimental autoimmune encephalomyelitis by oral administration of copolymer 1. Proc Natl Acad Sci USA 1999; 96:3842–3847.

37. Sloan-Lancaster J, Allen PM. Altered peptide ligand-induced partial T-cell activation: Molecular mechanism and role in T-cell biology. Annu Rev Immunol 1996; 14:1–27.

38. Karin N, Mitchell D, Ling N, et al. Reversal of experimental autoimmune encephalomyelitis by a soluble variant of a myelin basic protien epitope: T-cell receptor antogonism and reduction of interferon γ and tumour necrosis factor α production. J Exp Med 1998; 180:2227–2237.

39. Brocke S, Gijbels K, Allegretta M, et al. Treatment of experimental encephalitis with a peptide analogue of myelin basic protein. Nature 1996; 379:343–346.

40. Selmaj K, Raine CS, Cannela B, et al. Identification of lymphotoxin and tumour necrosis factor in multiple sclerosis lesions. J Clin Invest 1991; 87:949–954.

41. Raine CS. Tumour necrosis factor revisited, with promise. Nature Med 1995; 1:211–214.

42. Racke M, Bonomo A, Scott D, et al. Cytokine-induced immune deviation as a therapy for inflammatory autoimmune disease. J Exp Med 1994; 180:1961–1966.

43. Cannela B, Raine CS. The adhesion molecule and cytokine profile of multiple sclerosis lesions. Ann Neurol 1995; 37:424–435.

44. Lehmann PV, Forsthuber T, Miller A, et al. Spreading of T-cell immunity to cryptic determinants of an antigen. Nature 1992; 358:155–157.

45. Ufret-Vincenty R, Quigley N, Tresser N, et al. In vivo survival of antigen-specific T-cells that induce experimental autoimmune encephalomyelitis. J Exp Med 1998; 188:1725–1738.

46. Steinman L, Conlon P. Viral damage and the breakdown of self-tolerance. Nature Med 1997; 3:1085–1087.

47. Brostoff SW, Mason DW. Experimental allergic encephalomyelitis: Successful treatment in vivo with a monoclonal antibody that recognizes T-helper cells. J Immunol 1984; 133:1938.

48. Pelegri C, Morante MP, Castellote C, et al. Treatment with an anti-CD4 monoclonal antibody strongly ameliorates established rat adjuvant arthritis. Clin Exp Immunol 1996; 103:273–278.

49. Tomer Y, Blank M, Shoenfeld Y. Suppression of experimental antiphospholipid syndrome and systemic lupus erythematosus in mice by anti-CD4 monoclonal antibodies. Arthritis Rheum 1994; 37:1236–1244.

50. Waldor MK, Hardy RR, Hayakawa K, et al. Disappearance and reappearance of B-cells after in vivo treatment with a monoclonal anti-I-A antibodies. Proc Natl Acad Sci USA 1984; 81:2855–2858.

51. Waldor MK, Sriram S, Hardy R, et al. Reversal of experimental allergic encephalomyelitis with monoclonal antibody to a T-cell subset marker. Science 1985; 227:415–417.

52. Van Lambalgen R, Jonker M. EAE in Rhesus monkeys: II. Treatment of EAE with anti-T lymphocyte subset monoclonal antibodies. Clin Exp Immunol 1987; 67:305.

53. O'Neill JK, Baker D, Davison AN, et al. Control of immune-mediated disease of the central nervous system with monoclonal (CD4-specific) antibodies. J Neuroimmunol 1993; 45:1–14.

54. Sedgwick JD, Mason DW. The mechanism of inhibition of experimental allergic encephalomyelitis in the rat by monoclonal antibody against CD4. J Neuroimmunol 1986; 13:217–232.

55. Van Lambalgen R, Jonker M. Experimental allergic encephalomyelitis in rhesus monkeys: II. Treatment of EAE with anti-T lymphocyte subset monoclonal antibodies. Clin Exp Immunol 1987; 68:305–312.

56. Rose LM, Alvord EC Jr, Hruby S, et al. In vivo administration of anti-CD4 monoclonal antibody prolongs survival in longtailed Macaques with experimental allergic encephalomyelitis. Clin Immunol Immunopathol 1987; 45:405–423.

57. Biasi G, Facchinetti A, Monastra G, et al. Protection from EAE: Non-depleting anti-CD4 mAb treatment induces peripheral T-cell tolerance to MBP in PL/J mice. J Neuroimmunol 1997; 73:117–123.

58. Hafler DA, Ritz J, Stuart F, et al. Anti-CD4 and Anti-CD2 monoclonal antibody infusions in

subjects with multiple sclerosis. Immunosupprressive effects and human anti-mouse responses. J Immunol 1988; 141:131–138.

59. Hafler DA, Weiner HL. Immunosuppression with monoclonal antibodies in multiple sclerosis. Neurology 1988; 38:42–47.

60. Rumbach L, Racadot E, Armspach JP, et al. Biological assesment and MRI monitoring of the therapeutic efficacy of a monoclonal anti-CD4 antibody in multiple sclerosis. Mult Scler 1996; 1:207–212.

61. Lindsey JW, Hodgkinson S, Mehta R, et al. Phase I clinical trial of chimeric monoclonal antibody in multiple sclerosis. Neurology 1994; 44:413–419.

62. Lindsey JW, Hodgkinson S, Mehta R, et al. Repeated treatment with chimeric anti-CD4 antibody in multiple sclerosis. Ann Neurol 1994; 36:183–189.

63. Van Oosten BW, Lai M, Hodgkinson S, et al. Treatment of multiple sclerosis with the monoclonal anti-CD4 antibody cM-T412 : Results of a randomized, double-blind, placebo-controlled, MR-monitored phase II trial. Neurology 1997; 49:351–357.

64. Rep MH, Van Oosten BW, Roos MT, et al. Treatment with depleting CD4 monoclonal antibody results in a preferential loss of circulating naïve T-cells but does not affect IFN-gamma secreting TH1 cells in humans. J Clin Invest 1997; 99:2225–2231.

65. Moreau T, Coles A, Wing M, et al. Campath-IH in multiple sclerosis. Mult Scler 1996; 1: 357–365.

66. Coles AJ, Wing M, Smith S, et al. Pulsed monoclonal antibody treatment and autoimmune thyroid disease in multiple sclerosis. Lancet 1999; 354:1691–1695.

67. Coles AJ, Wing MG, Moleneux P, et al. Monoclonal antibody treatment exposes three mechanisms underlying the clinical course of multiple sclerosis. Ann Neurol 1999; 46:296–304.

68. Paolillo A, Coles AJ, Moleneux, et al. Quantitive MRI in patients with secondary progressive MS treated with monoclonal antibody Campath IH. Neurology 1999; 53:751–757.

69. Vandenbark AA, Chou YK, Bourdette DN, et al. T-cell receptor peptide therapy for autoimmune disease. J Autoimmun 1992; 5(suppl A): 83–92.

70. Vandenbark AA, Hashim GA, Offner H. T-cell receptor peptides in treatment of autoimmune disease: rationale and potential. J Neurosci 1996; 43:391–402.

71. Zaller DM, Osman G, Kanagawa O, et al. Prevention and treatment of murine allergic encephalomyelitis with T-cell receptor V beta-specific antibodies. J Exp Med 1990; 171:1943–1955.

72. Whitham R. H, Wingett D, Wineman J, et al. Treatment of relapsing autoimmune encephalomyelitis with T-cell receptor V beta-specific antibodies when proteolipid protein is the autoantigen. J Neurosci 1996; 45: 104–116.

73. Matsumoto Y, Tsuchida M, Hanawa H, et al. Successful prevention and treatment of autoimmune encephalomyelitis by short-term administration of anti-T-cell receptor alpha beta antibody. Immunology 1994; 81:1–7.

74. Ruddle NH, Bergman CM, McGrath KM, et al. An antibody to lymphotoxin and tumour necrosis factor prevents transfer of experimental allergic encephalomyelitis. J Exp Med 1990; 172: 1193–1200.

75. Baker D, Butler D, Scallon BJ, et al. Control of established allergic encephalomyelitis by inhibition of TNF activity within the CNS using monoclonal antibodies and TNF receptor immunoglobulin fusion proteins. Eur J Immunol 1994; 24:2040–2048.

76. Korner H, Lemckert FA, Chaudhri G, et al. Tumour necrosis factor blockade in actively induced experimental autoimmune encephalomyelitis prevents clinical disease despite activated T-cell infiltration to the central nervous system. Eur J Immunol 1997; 27:1973–1981.

77. Selmaj K, Raine CS, Cross AH. Anti-tumour necrosis factor therapy abrogates autoimmune demyelination. Ann Neurol 1991; 30:694–700.

78. Weinshenker BG, Bass B, Karlik S, et al. An open trial of OKT3 in patients with multiple sclerosis. Neurology 1991; 41:1047–1052.

79. Van Oosten BW, Barkhof F, Truyen L, et al. Increased MRI activity and immune activation

in two multiple sclerosis patients treated with the monoclonal anti-tumor necrosis factor antibody CA2. Neurology 1996; 47:1531–1534.

80. The Lenercept multiple sclerosis study group and the university of British Columbia MS/MRI analysis group. TNF neutralisation in MS. Neurology 1999; 53:457–465.

81. Cannella B, Gao YL, Brosnan C, et al. IL-10 fails to abrogate experimental autoimmune encephalomyelitis. J Neurosci Res 1996; 45:735–746.

82. Engelhardt B, Diamantstein T, Wekerle H. Immunotherapy of experimental autoimmune encephalomyelitis: Differential effect of anti-IL-2 receptor antibody therapy on actively induced and T-line mediated EAE of the Lewis rat. J Autoimmunol 1989; 2:61–73.

83. Duong TT, St. Louis J, Gilbert JJ, et al. Effect of anti-interferon-gamma and anti-interleukin-2 monoclonal antibody treatment on the development of actively and passively induced EAE in the SJL/J mouse. J Neuroimmunol 1992; 36:105–115.

84. Willenborg DO, Fordham SA, Cowden WB, et al. Cytokines and murine autoimmune encephalomyelitis: Inhibition of enhancement of disease with antibodies to select cytokines, or by delivery of exogenous cytokines using a recombinant vaccinia virus system. Scand J Immunol 1995; 41:31–41.

85. Billiau A, Heremans H, Vandekerckhove F, et al. Enhancement of EAE in mice by antibodies against IFN-gamma. J Immunol 1988; 140:1506–1510.

86. Lublin FD, Knobler RL, Kalman B, et al. Monoclonal anti-gamma interferon antibodies enhance EAE. Autoimmunity 1993; 16:267–274.

87. Duong TT, Finkelman FD, Singh B, et al. Effect of anti-interferon-gamma monoclonal antibody treatment on the development of EAE in resistant mouse strains. J Neurolimmunol 1994; 53:101–107.

88. Leger OJ, Yednock TA, Tanner L, et al. Humanization of a mouse antibody against human alpha-4 integrin: A potential therapeutic for the treatment of multiple sclerosis. Hum Antibodies 1997; 8:3–16.

89. Sheremata WA, Vollmer TL, Stone LA, et al. A safety and pharmacokinetic study of intravenous Natalizumab in patients with MS. Neurology 1999; 52:1072–1074.

90. Tubridy N, Behan PO, Capildeo R, et al. The effect of anti-alpha4 integrin antibody on brain lesion activity in MS. The UK Antegren study group. Neurology 1999; 53:466–472.

91. Bowen JD, Petersdorf SH, Richards TL, et al. Phase I study of a humanized anti-CD11/CD18 monoclonal antibody in multiple sclerosis. Clin Pharmacol 1998; 64:339–346.

92. Kuchroo VK, Das MP, Brown JA, et al. B7–1 and B7–2 costimulatory molecules differentially activate the TH1/TH2 development pathways: Application to autoimmune disease therapy. Cell 1995; 80:707–718.

93. Perrin PL, Scott D, June CH, et al. Role of B7/CD28/CTLA-4 in the induction of chronic relapsing EAE. J Immunol 1995; 154:1481–1490.

94. Miller SD, Vanderlugt CL, Lenshow DJ, et al. Blockade of CD28/B7–1 interaction prevents epitope spreading and clinical relapses of murine EAE. Immunity 1995; 3:739–745.

95. Vanderlugt CL, Neville KL, Nikcevich KM, et al. Pathologic role and temporal appearance of newly emerging autoepitopes in relapsing autoimmune encephalomyelitis. J Immunol 2000; 169:670–678.

96. Howard LM, Miga AJ, Vanderlugt CL, et al. Mechanisms of immunotherapeutic intervention by anti-CD40L (CD154) antibody in an animal model of multiple sclerosis. J Clin Invest 1999; 103:281–290.

30

Future Immunotherapies

CHRISTINE ROHOWSKY-KOCHAN

University of Medicine and Dentistry of New Jersey and New Jersey Medical School, Newark, New Jersey

I. INTRODUCTION

Multiple sclerosis (MS), a chronic demyelinating disease of the human central nervous system (CNS), is believed to have an autoimmune pathogenesis involving cell-mediated and humoral immune responses to myelin antigens. The hallmark of diseased MS brain tissue is the white matter plaque, which represents regions of myelin loss and gliosis with relative sparing of axons. The mechanism of oligodendroglial cell death and myelin sheath destruction remains undefined. It has been proposed that perhaps due to a failure of self-tolerance or by a process involving molecular mimicry and bystander activation, activated T cells specific for an infectious agent penetrate the blood-brain barrier and cross-react with myelin proteins. Production of immune mediators such as cytokines and chemokines by these activated T cells and by resident macrophages, microglia, and astrocytes may initiate the inflammatory process leading to the destruction of the myelin sheath. Evidence suggests that the myelin-producing oligodendrocyte may die via an apoptotic mechanism. This scenario for the pathogenesis of MS consists of numerous integrated pathways amenable to possible therapeutic immune intervention. This chapter explores some of the avenues for future therapeutic strategies and provides supporting evidence from studies in MS as well as from experimental autoimmune encephalomyelitis (EAE), the prototypic animal model of MS.

II. CYTOKINES

There is a considerable amount of evidence that cytokines, produced by autoantigen-reactive T cells and by other cells, are involved in the pathogenesis of MS. Although the

Th1/Th2 paradigm may be too simplistic for MS and other human diseases presumed to be autoimmune-mediated, one cannot dispute that proinflammatory cytokines contribute to the demyelinating process whereas anti-inflammatory cytokines suppress the inflammation. Interferon-γ (IFN-γ), the prototypic Th1 cytokine, appears to play a critical role in the pathogenesis of MS, and the regulation of this cytokine is an extremely important step in the overall scheme of an inflammatory response. Several cytokines are capable of inducing IFN-γ expression. IL-12, a heterodimeric cytokine, is a potent inducer of IFN-γ production in resting and activated T and NK cells (1–3); in vitro and in vivo studies have demonstrated that IL-12 is a powerful inducer of Th1 responses and suppresses Th2 responses (4). IL-12 signaling is mediated through the heterodimeric IL-12 receptor (IL-12R) (5,6). Expression of the β2 subunit of the receptor is more restricted than that of β1 and control of IL-12Rβ2 expression may constitute a mechanism for regulating IL-12 responsiveness (7–9). Cross-linking of the IL-12 receptor activates the Janus kinases, Jak-2 and Tyk-2 (10), which leads to the tyrosine phosphorylation of STAT3 and STAT4 transcription factors (11,12) and induction of IFN-γ mRNA synthesis.

In the second edition of this handbook, we detailed the studies performed on IL-12 in EAE. Additional evidence for the critical role that IL-12 plays in the pathogenesis of EAE is indicated by the resistance to EAE induction of IL-12 knockout animals (13). EAE studies suggest that immunotherapies that interfere with the biological function of IL-12 may be useful in MS. The role of IL-12 in MS is unclear, since the reports on IL-12 production in MS are conflicting. Increased mRNA expression of CD80 and IL-12 p40 were also observed in acute MS plaques but not in strokes (14). Increased IL-12 p70 production was reported by some groups (15,16), whereas others have reported normal levels of the heterodimer but decreased levels of the IL-12 p40 chain (17,18). The IL-12 p40 has been shown to act as a natural antagonist of the IL-12 heterodimer and down regulates its activity (19,20). Systemic administration of the IL-12 (p40)$_2$ homodimer significantly diminished the clinical severity and lesions in chronic relapsing EAE (21). Thus, the IL-12 p40 homodimer may be an attractive therapeutic agent in MS. Alternatively, agents that down regulate expression of the β2 chain of the IL-12 receptor or that block the signaling pathways may also be attractive therapeutic candidates. A defect in the capacity to upregulate the IL-12Rβ2 subunit has been identified in an EAE-resistant strain of mice (22). If IL-12 production is confirmed to be elevated in MS, administration of humanized anti-IL-12 monoclonal antibodies may be an alternative form of therapy. Anti-IL-12 was effective in treating a Th1-mediated disease in mice by inducing Fas-mediated apoptosis of the Th1 cells (23). Agents that inhibit the signaling cascade may also be potential therapeutic agents.

IL-18, or IFN-γ–inducing factor, is a recently described cytokine that shares structural features with the IL-1 family of proteins and functional properties with IL-12. The activation of IL-18 is mediated by interleukin-1β–converting enzyme (24). The role of IL-18 in inducing IFN-γ production is unclear. IL-18 has been shown to induce IFN-γ production either alone (24) or synergistically with IL-12 (25–27). The signal transduction pathways utilized by IL-18 have not been clearly elucidated, although they appear to be different than those used by IL-12. IL-18 may be involved in the upregulation of the central mediators instigating apoptotic cell death, since IL-18 upregulates FasL expression on CD4$^+$ T cells and NK cells (28,29), whereas IFN-γ upregulates Fas antigen expression. Neutralizing antibodies to IL-18 block EAE induction by shifting the Th1/Th2 balance toward autoantigen-specific Th2 cells (30). Thus, it appears that perturbation of the

Th1/Th2 balance among autoreactive T cells may be an effective mode of restraining the pathogenic effect of these lymphocytes.

III. Costimulatory Molecules

Activation of T cells requires two distinct signals, an antigen-specific one mediated by recognition of the peptide-MHC complex by the T cell receptor (TCR) and an antigen-nonspecific signal delivered by costimulatory molecules expressed on antigen-presenting cells (APCs). The interaction of CD80/CD86 with CD28 on T cells promotes T-cell activation and proliferation, whereas ligation with CTLA-4 provides an inhibitory or regulatory signal. Since the CD80/CD86:CD28/CTLA-4 costimulatory pathway plays an important role in the activation and regulation of the immune response, it represents a promising therapeutic avenue for manipulating autoimmune diseases. Evidence exists implicating the CD80/CD86-CD28/CTLA-4 pathway in the pathogenesis of EAE and MS. Blocking the CD80/CD86-CD28/CTLA-4 costimulatory pathway had profound effects on the initiation of EAE. Treatment with anti-CD80 antibodies reduced the incidence of EAE, whereas anti-CD86 antibodies increased the severity of EAE (31). Likewise, anti-CD80 antibody therapy prevented intramolecular epitope spreading and resolved relapses of chronic EAE (32). Administration of CTLA-4Ig protected against active induction of EAE (33–35); whereas in another study, CTLA-4 therapy exacerbated the disease (36,37). Blockade of CTLA-4 in vivo resulted in exacerbated disease, and in vitro studies demonstrated enhancement of T-cell responses to the immunizing peptide as well as epitope spreading (37). Another study showed that blockade of the CD28 molecule attenuated established EAE (38), suggesting that this therapy may be a more effective means of inhibiting existing autoimmune responses.

Manipulation of the CD80/CD86-CD28/CTLA-4 costimulatory pathway may be of therapeutic benefit in the treatment of MS. However, autoreactive T cells from MS patients have been found to be less dependent on costimulation signals, perhaps as a consequence of chronic activation by autoantigen in the CNS (39,40). Although it remains to be determined whether blockade of this costimulatory pathway inhibits reactivation of memory autoreactive T cells, it appears that it may be beneficial in preventing the activation and expansion of newly activated autoreactive T cells and bystander cells. The results of a phase I study using CTLA-4Ig to treat psoriasis patients, a presumed T cell–mediated human disease, showed clinical improvement in at least 50% of treated patients (41). Consideration has to be given to the mode of delivery, since some of these costimulatory molecules may not be able to enter the CNS efficiently. Gene delivery of CTLA-4Ig into the CNS using a nonreplicating adenoviral vector significantly ameliorated the development of EAE, whereas systemic administration of CTLA-4Ig had very little effect on the course of the disease (42).

Another costimulatory interaction important in T-cell regulation is that between CD40 and CD154. CD40 is expressed by a variety of cells such as B cells, macrophages, dendritic cells, and endothelial cells, whereas CD154 (CD40L) is expressed primarily on activated T cells and B cells. The role of CD40-CD154 in T-cell differentiation has not been completely established. CD40-CD154 interactions are involved in regulating IL-12 production by dendritic cells and macrophages. Anti-CD154 antibodies have been reported to prevent a Th1-mediated autoimmune disease, inflammatory colitis, by blocking IL-12 secretion (43). It has also been reported that direct triggering of CD154 activates T cells and induces Th2-type cytokine production, such as IL-4 but not Th1 cytokines (44,45). Moreover, CD154-deficient mice expressing a MBP-specific TCR transgene did not develop EAE (46). Treatment using anti-CD154 antibodies has been found to be effective in inhibiting actively induced and established EAE (47,48). Data indicate that inhibition of EAE induction is probably due to a block in T-cell activation as a result of decreased CD80 expression and not to migration of the activated T cells to the CNS. On the other hand, inhibition of established EAE may result from both blocking migration of autoreactive T cells into the CNS as well as blocking priming of T cells to other autoantigenic epitopes.

Evidence supporting the role of CD40-CD154 interactions in MS is provided by the finding of activated T helper cells expressing CD154 colocalizing with CD40-bearing cells in active lesions of MS patients (48). Since CD40-CD154 interactions regulate diverse pathways of the immune response, therapeutic strategies designed to modulate this interaction may be a treatment modality for autoimmune diseases. Such strategies may include the use of anti-CD40 or anti-CD154 humanized antibodies, antagonists, or chimeric molecules that bind to either CD40 or CD154. Alternatively, therapies could be aimed at targeting the intracellular signaling pathways and inactivating such molecules as CRAF-1, CAP-1, TRAF1, or TRAF2, which are associated with CD40 signaling.

IV. APOPTOSIS

In recent years, convincing evidence has accumulated that apoptosis, a physiological mechanism of cell death in the immune system, may also be involved in the pathogenesis of autoimmune diseases such as MS and diabetes. Fas (CD95), a member of the TNF/ nerve growth factor receptor superfamily, is expressed by various cell types, whereas its natural ligand, FasL (CD95L, which also belongs to the TNF protein superfamily), is expressed predominantly on cells found in lymphoid organs. Neither Fas nor its ligand are constitutively expressed by CNS cells. Interactions between the FasL-expressing cell and the receptor result in the apoptotic death of the Fas-expressing cells. In MS, the Fas/ FasL–mediated apoptotic pathway may be critical in promoting the death of FasL-expressing autoreactive T cells in the periphery and/or in the CNS as well as death of susceptible non-T-cell CNS target cells. The death-receptor ligand pair, FasL and Fas, appear to contribute both to the pathological process leading to demyelination and oligodendrocyte destruction as well as to the recovery phase of the disease.

With respect to the periphery, apoptosis is an essential mechanism for clonal deletion and tolerance, for downregulating the immune response, and for eliminating autoreactive T cells. Activation-induced apoptosis of autoreactive T cells may be altered in MS. Consequently, reactivation of these T cells may result in their migration into the CNS and initiation of the inflammatory process. Elevated soluble CD95L levels in the sera of relapsing-remitting MS patients implied that T-cell apoptosis mediated by the CD95-CD95L interaction was impaired (49,50). Impaired apoptotic deletion of myelin basic protein–reactive T cells in MS patients has been reported (51,52). Additional evidence for a failure of the CD95-mediated apoptotic process is provided from EAE studies. Interventions that would specifically enhance the susceptibility to apoptosis of autoreactive T lymphocytes may be beneficial in MS. The protein kinase inhibitor bisindolylmaleimide has been found to be useful in modulating the apoptosis of human autoreactive T cells in vitro (53) as well as to be an effective treatment in EAE (54). Perhaps potent apoptosis-enhancing substances affecting exclusively autoreactive T cells may be developed. It is conceivable that targeting of antisense *bcl-2* oligonucleotides to autoreactive T cells either in the periphery or in the CNS may be a therapeutic option.

Several lines of evidence support the role of Fas/FasL in MS brain tissues. CD95 expression was reported to be enhanced in oligodendroglial cells in the MS lesion (55). Macrophages that had phagocytosed Fas$^+$ cells were also detected. The nature of the FasL-expressing cell is not conclusive, since FasL was expressed by oligodendrocytes and astrocytes in one study (55) and by microglial cells and T cells in another report (56). Apoptosis, as detected by TUNEL positivity, colocalized with CD95 ligand expression, suggesting that a FasL-mediated suicide of the oligodendrocytes may occur in MS (55). Therapeutic strategies designed to protect oligodendrocytes from cell death may promote remyelination in MS lesions. Agents that upregulate expression specifically in oligodendrocytes of anti-apoptotic molecules such as *bcl-2 (bcl-xl)* or of the caspase-inhibitory protein p35 may inhibit apoptosis and confer protection to the myelin-producing cells. Transgenic mice that expressed the p35 anti-apoptotic protein were resistant to EAE induction, and the number of apoptotic oligodendrocytes were significantly reduced in these animals (57). Caspase inhibitory peptides that block the apoptosis-inducing proteolytic activity may also be utilized to promote oligodendrocyte survival. Administration of a caspase inhibitory peptide substantially decreased infarct injury and brain swelling in an animal model of acute stroke (58). Likewise, treatment with a peptide inhibitor suppressed fatal liver destruction in mice (59).

As mentioned, IFN-γ is believed to be a critical factor in the pathogenesis of MS. One mechanism by which IFN-γ may contribute to the pathogenesis of MS is by induction of Fas receptor expression on oligodendrocytes, rendering them susceptible to apoptosis. Therapies aimed at inhibiting IFN-γ production may suppress oligodendrocyte apoptosis. Studies have demonstrated that IFN-β can block T-cell apoptosis (60), and it is conceivable that it may have a similar effect on this death pathway of other cell types.

Downregulation of CD95/CD95L expression in the CNS may result in less oligodendrocyte cell death and destruction of the myelin sheath. In contrast, increased induction of CD95/CD95L-mediated apoptosis of autoreactive T cells in the periphery may be beneficial as well. Intervention in apoptotic processes might serve as a potential therapeutic strategy in MS, but interference in these processes is a two-edged sword. A critical consideration is to target proposed apoptosis inhibitors to oligodendrocytes and apoptosis enhancers to autoreactive T cells.

V. CHEMOKINES

Chemokines are a superfamily of small proinflammatory chemotactic cytokines that function in mediating the trafficking of leukocytes in physiological surveillance as well as in recruiting inflammatory cells to sites of tissue damage. Some chemokines selectively attract neutrophils and eosinophils and others act specifically toward monocytes, dendritic cells, and T cells. Although it is known that activated T cells can cross the blood-brain barrier, the mechanisms by which these T cells remain in the CNS and recruit other cells is not clear. Chemokines are now recognized as participants in the regulation of inflammatory cell invasion to the CNS through modulation of adhesion molecules as well as by other pathways.

Numerous studies have analyzed chemokine expression and production in EAE. High levels of CNS chemokine mRNA expression of macrophage inflammatory protein (MIP)-1α (61,62); MIP-1β (61); regulated upon activation, normal T cell–expressed and secreted (RANTES) (63); IFN-γ–inducible protein of 10 kDa (IP-10) (64); and monocyte chemoattractant protein-1 (MCP-1) (64) have been detected before the onset of clinical EAE and throughout the acute disease phase. Astrocytes near the inflammatory lesion were the cellular source of IP-10 and MCP-1 (64). Additional studies showed that CNS-specific chemokine expression never preceded histological signs of EAE (65), suggesting that chemokines amplify CNS lesion formation by recruiting nonspecific inflammatory cells rather than initiating the inflammatory lesion.

A role for chemokines in the pathogenesis of EAE was demonstrated by the finding that anti-MIP-1α antibodies inhibited the development of passive transfer of EAE, reduced the inflammatory CNS response, and ameliorated ongoing disease (66). Anti-MCP-1 antibodies did not protect animals from EAE but were able to block relapses (62).

Analysis of the chemokines expressed in MS lesions demonstrated that RANTES appears to be the first chemokine associated with lesion formation (67). Enhanced expression of RANTES, MCP-1 and MIP-1β in blood vessel endothelium, astrocytes and macrophages was associated with lesions that had a small degree of inflammation (67). In active lesions, MCP-1 and MIP-1α was expressed predominantly by macrophages and MIP-1β by macrophages, whereas RANTES was expressed by blood vessel endothelium, perivascular cells, and astrocytes within plaques. MCP-1–reactive astrocytes were also detected in chronic MS lesions (67).

Elevated levels of MIP-1α were found in the cerebrospinal fluid (CSF) of MS patients but not in noninflammatory neurological disease controls (68). During MS attacks, elevated levels of IP-10, monokine induced by interferon-γ (Mig), and RANTES were found in the CSF (69). Moreover, CXCR3, an IP-10/Mig chemokine receptor, was expressed on lymphocytes in active MS lesions, whereas CCR5, a RANTES receptor, was detected on lymphocytes, macrophages, and microglia (69). CXCR3-reactive T cells were reported to be increased in the blood of relapsing-remitting MS patients, while both CCR5$^+$ and CXCR3$^+$ T cells were increased in progressive MS patients (70). Thus, these studies provide evidence that chemokines are associated with MS pathogenesis and suggest that blocking of CCR5 and/or CXCR3 using antibodies or antagonists may be another therapeutic approach. Mice injected with chemokine DNA vaccines were protected from EAE induction (71). Protection was dependent on targeting the chemokine present at the inflammatory site and was believed to be mediated by antichemokine antibodies. This strategy of naked DNA vaccination has numerous advantages. Therapeutic approaches utilizing chemokine receptor antagonists may also be beneficial. A series of 4-hydroxy-pipieridines which potently inhibit binding of MIP-1α and RANTES to the human CCR1 chemokine receptor have been described (72).

VI. HORMONES

MS and other autoimmune diseases are more common in women than in men. In MS, the female-to-male ratio is between 2:1 and 3:1. Although the mechanisms for gender dimorphism in MS are not known, increasing evidence suggests that sex hormones may play an important role. The initial clinical signs of MS usually appear after sexual maturation (73). Exacerbation rates have been reported to decrease during pregnancy, with disease amelioration occurring (73–76). Disease activity as assessed by magnetic resonance imaging (MRI) declined during pregnancy, with a rebound to prepregnancy levels during the postpartum period (76). In contrast, increases in the number of MS attacks were observed postpartum (73–76). Fluctuations of MS symptoms were shown to occur during the normal menstrual cycle, with worsening of symptoms just prior the onset of menses (77,78).

Gender dimorphism has been studied in the EAE model. PLP-peptide-reactive cells from female animals were more effective at transferring EAE and induced more severe disease than male cells (79). The frequency of autoantigen-specific T cells was not affected by gender. Female mice receiving adoptively transferred female MBP-specific T cells had a more rapid onset of disease with increased mean clinical scores than male recipients (80). Likewise, female animals were more severely affected upon adoptive transfer of male MBP-specific T cells. Thus, gender-related differences appear to influence both induction and effector phases of EAE. A possible mechanism responsible for this gender-related difference in encephalitogenicity may be deficient IL-12 production by male antigen-stimulated lymph node cells (81). Studies on the effects of hormones in EAE have also been conducted. Treatment of animals with oral contraceptives containing a high ratio of estrogen to progesterone or with estradiol alone inhibited EAE, whereas progesterone treatment potentiated the disease (82,83). A recent study showed that estriol treatment (using doses comparable to levels during late pregnancy) reduced the severity of EAE, while progesterone treatment had no effect (84). Moreover, IL-10 production was shown to be increased in MBP-specific T cells from estriol-treated animals. Testosterone was found to decrease severity of EAE, and this effect may be mediated partly by enhanced production of IL-10 by autoantigen-specific T cells (85). Androgen-selected T cells were found to secrete less IFN-γ and more IL-10 than untreated cells (86).

There have been a limited number of reports on the effect of estrogen and progesterone on the development of human Th1 and Th2 cytokine responses. Progesterone was shown to favor the development of cells producing Th2-type cytokines in response to PPD and to transiently induce IL-4 production in established Th1 clones (87,88). Estrogen enhanced both IL-10 and IFN-γ secretion of PLP-specific T-cell clones but had no effect on IL-4 or transforming growth factor-β (TGF-β) production (89). The estrogen effects were biphasic. High estrogen doses, similar to physiological concentrations circulating during pregnancy, enhanced IL-10 secretion, whereas low doses (similar to nonpregnancy levels) triggered IFN-γ. These studies provide preliminary evidence that sex hormones may modulate the cytokine secreted by T cells. Moreover, it was recently reported that female MS patients with high estradiol and low progesterone levels had evidence of greater disease activity (assessed by the number of gadolinium-enhancing lesions on brain MRI) than patients with low estrogen and progesterone levels (90). Although additional studies are warranted to confirm these findings, they provide evidence that estradiol and progesterone may influence disease activity in MS and may be effective therapeutically in MS.

VII. STEM CELL TRANSPLANTATION

Most current MS therapies as well as the modalities detailed above are aimed at decreasing the exacerbation rate and degree of myelin injury. Successful therapy should also include agents or means by which to replace the lost myelin and damaged axon. An exciting and recently developed therapeutic approach entails the utilization of either embryonic or adult stem cells to promote remyelination. By definition, a stem cell possesses the ability of self-renewal and multilineage differentiation. Human embryonic pluripotent stem cells have been successfully cultured and studies have shown that adult stem cells can differentiate into developmentally unrelated cell types (91,92). Experimental evidence in support of the potential of stem cell or progenitor transplantion has been shown (91–93).

Human neural progenitor cells have been expanded in vitro and transplanted into adult rat brains (94). These precursors migrated specifically along the routes normally taken by the endogenous neuronal precursors and differentiated into neural and glial phenotypes. Neural stem cells transplanted at birth into the brain of a dysmyelinated shiverer mouse showed widespread engraftment and an overabundance of MBP (95). Perhaps in MS, allogeneic hematopoietic stem cell transplants may be used with the hope that the ongoing autoantigen T-cell reactivity might be inhibited. Transplantation of hematopoietic stem cells from normal mice into diabetogenic animals abrogated the diabetogenic T-cell response (91). Alternatively, transplantation of neural stem cells or their progenitors or of glial cells may result in remyelination and regeneration of function (92).

More primitive than neural stem cells, embryonic stem cells were shown to be induced to differentiate into a population of cells enriched for oligodendrocyte precursors (96). Transplantation of these cells into the spinal cords of myelin-deficient rats resulted in migration and ensheathment of the demyelinated axon (96).

Although many issues need to be addressed, clinical stem cell transplantation may be of great benefit in the near future in the treatment of MS as well as other neural degenerative diseases.

VIII. GENE THERAPY APPROACHES

Various gene therapy approaches may also be of benefit in MS. In principle, gene therapy should permit the efficient delivery of therapeutic agents, allowing for their long-term production from a single treatment. Genetically modified autoreactive T cells may serve as a vector for delivering therapeutic factors to the site of tissue injury. Autoantigen-specific T cells modified with the IL-10 (97), IL-4 (98), or TGF-β (99,100) transgene were shown to be effective in ameliorating ongoing EAE. Proteolipid protein–reactive T cells expressing a transgene for platelet-derived growth factor (PDGF) produced active PDGF upon stimulation with the autoantigen and were capable of triggering proliferation of oligodendrocyte progenitor cells (101). Delivery of cytokines such as IL-4 using non-replicative viral vectors was also effective in ameliorating ongoing EAE (102,103). A cell-based gene vector approach has also been utilized (104). Injection of fibroblasts infected with a retrovirus expressing soluble TNF receptors were found to significantly ameliorate both acute and relapsing EAE (104). Alternatively, CNS stem cells may be used as vehicles for the delivery of immunomodulatory agents into the CNS. Such an approach has been successfully tried for the treatment of brain tumors (105). Another gene therapy approach involves using modified B cells expressing an encephalitogenic determinant of a myelin antigen to downregulate the autoreactive T cells (Y. Ron, personal communication). Adoptive transfer of such genetically modified B cells protected the genetically susceptible animals from EAE induction. Thus, experimental evidence suggests that therapeutic delivery systems could be developed that either inhibit autoreactive T cells in the CNS or repair the damaged myelin sheaths in MS.

IX. CONCLUSIONS

There are many issues that need to be addressed before many of the therapeutic agents that have been shown to be efficacious in preventing or treating an experimental model of autoimmunity can be tested in humans. It is possible that therapies combining several of these immunomodulatory agents may be most effective in treating MS. Further advancement in immunology and molecular biology will increase our understanding of the complex and intertwined processes involved in maintaining immune homeostasis and will enable us to unravel the pathogenic mechanisms involved in MS and to treat this disease using the immune system's own strategies.

REFERENCES

1. D'Andrea A, Rengaraju M, Valiante NM, et al. Production of natural killer cell stimulatory factor (interleukin-12) by peripheral blood mononuclear cells. J Exp Med 1992; 176:1387–1398.
2. Gately MK, Wolitzky AG, Quinn PM, Chizzonite R. Regulation of human cytolytic lymphocyte responses by interleukin-12. Cell Immunol 1992; 143:127–142.
3. Kobayashi M, Fitz L, Ryan M, et al. Identification and purification of natural killer cell stimulatory factor (NKSF), a cytokine with multiple biologic effects on human lymphocytes. J Exp Med 1989; 170:827–845.
4. Trinchieri G. Interleukin-12: A cytokine produced by antigen-presenting cells with immunoregulatory functions in the generation of T-helper cells type 1 and cytotoxic lymphocytes. Blood 1994; 84:4008–4027.
5. Chua AO, Chizzonite R, Desai BB, et al. Expression cloning of a human IL-12 receptor component: A new member of the cytokine receptor superfamily with strong homology to gp130. J Immunol 1994; 153:128–136.
6. Presky DH, Yang H, Minetti LJ, et al. A functional interleukin 12 receptor complex is composed of two β-type cytokine receptor subunits. Proc Natl Acad Sci USA 1996; 93:14002–14007.
7. Wu C-Y, Warrier RR, Wang X, Presky DH, Gately MK. Regulation of interleukin-12 receptor β1 chain expression and interleukin-12 binding by human peripheral blood mononuclear cells. Eur J Immunol 1997; 27:147–154.
8. Szabo SJ, Dighe AS, Gubler U, Murphy KM. Regulation of the interleukin (IL)-12R β2 subunit expression in developing T helper 1 (Th1) and Th2 cells. J Exp Med 1997; 185:817–824.
9. Rogge L, Barberis-Maino L, Biffi M, et al. Selective expression of an interleukin-12 receptor component by human T helper 1 cells. J Exp Med 1997; 185:825–831.
10. Bacon CM, McVicar DW, Ortaldo JR, Rees RC, O'Shea JJ, Johnston JA. Interleukin 12 (IL-12) induces tyrosine phosphorylation of JAK2 and TYK2: Differential us of Janus family tyrosine kinases by IL-2 and IL-12. J Exp Med 1995; 181:399–404.
11. Jacobson NG, Szabo SJ, Weber-Nordt RM, et al. Interleukin 12 signaling in T helper type 1 (Th1) cells involves tyrosine phosphorylation of signal transducer and activator of transcription (Stat)3 and Stat4. J Exp Med 1995; 181:1755–1762.
12. Bacon CM, Petricoin EF, Ortaldo JR, et al. Interleukin 12 induces tyrosine phosphorylation and activation of STAT4 in human lymphocytes. Proc Natl Acad Sci USA 1995; 92:7307–7311.
13. Segal BM, Dwyer BK, Shevach EM. An interleukin (IL)-10/IL-12 immunoregulatory circuit controls susceptibility to autoimmune disease. J Exp Med 1998; 187:537–546.
14. Windhagen A, Newcombe J, Dangond F, et al. Expression of costimulatory molecules B7-1 (CD80), B7-2 (CD86) and interleukin-12 cytokine in multiple sclerosis lesions. J Exp Med 1995; 182:1985–1996.
15. Balashov KE, Smith DR, Khoury SJ, Hafler DA, Weiner HL. Increased interleukin 12 production in progressive multiple sclerosis: Induction by activated CD4+ T cells via CD40 ligand. Proc Natl Acad Sci USA 1997; 94:599–603.
16. Comabella M, Balashov KE, Issazadeh S, Smith DR, Weiner HL, Khoury SJ. Elevated interleukin-12 in progressive multiple sclerosis correlates with disease activity and is normalized by pulse cyclophosphamide therapy. J Clin Invest 1998; 102:671–678.

17. Rohowsky-Kochan C, Molinaro D, Choudhry A, Kahn M, Cook SD. Impaired interleukin-12 production in multiple sclerosis patients. Mult Scler 1999; 5:327–334.

18. Ferrante P, Fusi ML, Saresella M, et al. Cytokine production and surface marker expression in acute and stable multiple sclerosis: Altered IL-12 production and augmented signaling lymphocytic activation molecule (SLAM)-expressing lymphocytes in acute multiple sclerosis. J Immunol 1998; 160:1514–1521.

19. Ling P, Gately MK, Gubler U, et al. Human IL-12 p40 homodimer binds to the IL-12 receptor but does not mediate biologic activity . J Immunol 1995; 154:116–127.

20. Gillessen S, Carvajal DM, Ling P, et al. Mouse interleukin-12 (IL-12) p40 homodimer: A potent IL-12 antagonist. Eur J Immunol 1995; 25:200–206.

21. Lad N. Interleukin-12: A new target for immunosuppressive therapy in multiple sclerosis (abstr). IBC Proc 1997.

22. Chang JT, Shevach EM, Segal BM. Regulation of interleukin (IL)-12 receptor β2 subunit expression by endogenous IL-12: A critical step in the differentiation of pathogenic autoreactive T cells. J Exp Med 1999; 189:969–978.

23. Fuss IJ, Marth T, Neurath MF, Pearlstein GR, Jain A, Strober W. Anti-interleukin 12 treatment regulates apoptosis of Th1 T cells in experimental colitis in mice. Gastroenterology 1999; 117:1078–1088.

24. Okamura H, Tsutsui H, Komatsu T, et al. Cloning of a new cytokine that induces IFN-γ production by T cells. Nature 1995; 378:88–91.

25. Ahn H-J, Maruo S, Tomura M, et al. A mechanism underlying synergy between IL-12 and IFN-γ-inducing factor in enhanced production of IFN-γ. J Immunol 1997; 159:2125–2131.

26. Robinson D, Shibuya K, Mui A, et al. IGIF does not drive Th1 development but synergizes with IL-12 for inteferon-γ production and activates IRAK and NFκB. Immunity 1997; 7:571–581.

27. Yoshimoto T, Takeda K, Tanaka T, et al. IL-12 up-regulates IL-18 receptor expression on T cells, Th1 cells, and B cells: Synergism with IL-18 for IFN-γ production. J Immunol 1998; 161:3400–3407.

28. Dao T, Ohashi K, Kayano T, Kurimoto M, Okamura H. Interferon-γ-inducing factor, a novel cytokine, enhances Fas ligand-mediated cytotoxicity of murine T helper 1 cells. Cell Immunol 1996; 173:230–235.

29. Tsutsui H, Nakanishi K, Matsui M, et al. IFN-γ-inducing factor upregulates Fas ligand-mediated cytotoxic activity of murine natural killer cell clones. J Immunol 1996; 157:3967–3973.

30. Wildbaum G, Youssef S, Grabie N, Karin N. Neutralizing antibodies to IFN-γ-inducing factor prevent experimental autoimmune encephalomyelitis. J Immunol 1998; 161:6368–6374.

31. Kuchroo VK, Prabhu Das MR, Brown JA, et al. B7–1 and B7–2 costimulatory molecules activate differentially the Th1/Th2 developmental pathways: Application to autoimmune disease therapy. Cell 1995; 80:707–718.

32. Miller SD, Vanderlugt CL, Lenschow DJ, et al. Blockade of CD28.B7–1 interaction prevents epitope spreading and clinical relapses of murine EAE. Immunity 1995; 3:739–745.

33. Perrin PJ, Scott DE, Quigley L, et al. Role of B7:CD28/CTLA-4 in the induction of chronic relapsing experimental allergic encephalomyelitis. J Immunol 1995; 154:1481–1490.

34. Khoury SJ, Akalin E, Chandraker A, et al. CD28-B7 costimulatory blockade by CTLA4Ig prevents actively induced experimental autoimmune encephalomyelitis and inhibits Th1 but spares Th2 cytokines in the central nervous system. J Immunol 1995; 155:4521–4524.

35. Arima T, Rehman A, Hickey WF, Flye MW. Inhibition by CTLA4Ig of experimental allergic encephalomyelitis . J Immunol 1996; 156:4916–4924.

36. Perrin PJ, Maldonado JH, Davis TA, June CH, Racke MK. CTLA-4 blockade enhances clinical disease and cytokine production during experimental allergic encephalomyelitis. J Immunol 1996; 157:1333–1336.

37. Karandikar NJ, Vanderlugt CL, Bluestone JA, Miller SD. Targeting the B7/CD28:CTLA-4 costimulatory system in CNS autoimmune disease. J Neuroimmunol 1998; 89:10–18.

38. Perrin PJ, June CH, Maldonado JH, Ratts RB, Racke MK. Blockade of CD28 during in vitro activation of encephalitogenic T cells or after disease onset ameliorates experimental autoimmune encephalomyelitis. J Immunol 1999; 163:1704–1710.

39. Scholz C, Patton KT, Anderson DE, Freeman GJ, Hafler DA. Expansion of autoreactive T cells in multiple sclerosis is independent of exogenous B7 costimulation. J Immunol 1998; 160:1532–1538.

40. Lovett-Racke AE, Trotter JL, Lauber J, Perrin PJ, June CH, Racke MK. Decreased dependence of myelin basic protein-reactive T cells on CD28-mediated costimulation in multiple sclerosis patients. J Clin Invest 1998; 101:725–730.

41. Abrams JR, Lebwohl MG, Guzzo CA, et al. CTLA4Ig-mediated blockade of T-cell costimulation in patients with psoriasis vulgaris. J Clin Invest 1999; 103:1243–1252.

42. Croxford JL, O'Neill JK, Ali RR, et al. Local gene therapy with CTLA4-immunoglobulin fusion protein in experimental allergic encephalomyelitis. Eur J Immunol 1998; 28:3904–3916.

43. Stuber E, Strober W, Neurath M. Blocking the CD40L-CD40 interaction in vivo specifically prevents the priming of T helper 1 cells through the inhibition of interleukin-12 secretion. J Exp Med 1996; 183:693–698.

44. Blotta MH, Marshall JD, DeKruyff RH, Umetsu DT. Cross-linking of the CD40 ligand on human CD4+ T lymphocytes generates a costimulatory signal that up-regulates IL-4 synthesis. J Immunol 1996; 156:3133-3140.

45. van Essen D, Kikutani H, Gray D. CD40 ligand-transduced co-stimulation of T cells in the development of helper function. Nature 1995; 378:620–623.

46. Grewal IS, Foellmer HG, Grewal KD, et al. Requirement for CD40 ligand in costimulation induction, T cell activation, and experimental allergic encephalomyelitis. Science 1996; 273: 1864–1867.

47. Weinberg AD, Wegmann KW, Funatake C, Whitham RH. Blocking OX-40/OX-40 ligand interaction in vitro and in vivo leads to decreased T cell function and amelioration of experimental allergic encephalomyelitis. J Immunol 1999; 162:1818–1826.

48. Gerritse K, Laman JD, Noelle RJ, et al. CD40-CD40 ligand interactions in experimental allergic encephalomyelitis and multiple sclerosis. Proc Natl Acad Sci USA 1996; 93:2499–2504.

49. Zipp F, Otzelberger K, Dichgans J, Martin R, Weller M. Serum CD95 of relapsing remitting multiple sclerosis patients protects from CD95-mediated apoptosis. J Neuroimmunol 1998; 86:151–154.

50. Zipp F, Weller M, Calabresi PA, et al. Increased serum levels of soluble CD95 (APO-1/Fas) in relapsing-remitting multiple sclerosis. Ann Neurol 1998; 43:116-120.

51. Zang YCQ, Kozovska MM, Hong J, et al. Impaired apoptotic deletion of myelin basic protein-reactive T cells in patients with multiple sclerosis. Eur J Immunol 1999; 29:1692–1700.

52. Macchi B, Matteucci C, Nocentini U, Caltagirone C, Mastino A. Impaired apoptosis in mitogen-stimulated lymphocytes of patients with multiple sclerosis. Neuroreport 1999; 10:399–402.

53. Wendling U, Aktas O, Schmierer K, Zschenderlein R, Zipp F. Partial synergy of bisindolylmaleimide with apoptotic stimulus in antigen-specific T cells—Implications for multiple sclerosis. J Neuroimmunol 2000; 103:69–75.

54. Zhou T, Song L, Yang P, Wang Z, Liu D, Jope RS. Bisindoloyleimide VIII facilitates Fas-mediated apoptosis and inhibits T cell-mediated autoimmune diseases. Nature Med 1999; 5: 42–48.

55. Dowling PC, Shang G, Raval S, Menonna J, Cook SD, Husar W. Involvement of the CD95 (APO-1/Fas) receptor/ligand system in multiple sclerosis brain. J Exp Med 1996; 184:1513–1518.

56. D'Souza SD, Bonetti B, Balasingam V, et al. Multiple sclerosis: Fas signaling in oligodendrocyte cell death. J Exp Med 1996; 184:2361–2370.

57. Hisahara S, Araki T, Sugiyama F, et al. Targeted expression of baculovirus p35 caspase inhibitor in oligodendrocytes protects mice against autoimmune-mediated demyelination. EMBO J 2000; 19:341–348.

58. Hara H, Friedlander RM, Gagliardini V, et al. Inhibition of interleukin-1b converting enzyme family proteases reduces ischemic and excitotoxic damage. Proc Natl Acad Sci USA 1997; 94:2007–2012.

59. Rodriquez I, Matsuura K, Ody C, Nagata S, Vassalli P. Systemic injection of a tripeptide inhibits the intracellular activation of CPP32-like proteases in vivo and fully protects mice against Fas-mediated fulminant liver destruction and death. J Exp Med 1996; 184:2067–2072.

60. Pilling D, Akbar AN, Girdlestone J, et al. Interferon-β mediates stromal cell rescue of T cells from apoptosis. Eur J Immunol 1999; 29:1041–1050.

61. Ransohoff RM. Mechanisms of inflammation in MS tissue: Adhesion molecules and chemokines. J Neuroimmunol 1999; 98:57–68.

62. Karpus WJ, Lukacs NW, McRae BL, Strieter RM, Kunkel SL, Miller SD. An important role for the chemokine macrophage inflammatory protein-1α in the pathogenesis of the T cell–mediated autoimmune disease, experimental autoimmune encephalomyelitis. J Immunol 1995; 155:5003–5010.

63. Godiska R, Chantry D, Dietsch G, Gray P. Chemokine expression in murine experimental autoimmune encephalomyelitis. J Neuroimmunol 1995; 58:167–176.

64. Ransohoff RM, Hamilton TA, Tani M, et al. Astrocyte expression of mRNA encoding cytokines IP-10 and JE/MCP-1 in experimental autoimmune encephalomyelitis. FASEB J 1993; 7:592–600.

65. Glabinski A, Tani M, Tuohy VK, Tuthill RJ, Ransohoff RM. Central nervous system chemokine mRNA accumulation follows leukocyte entry at the onset of murine acute experimental autoimmune encephalomyelitis. Brain Behav Immun 1996; 9:315–330.

66. Karpus WJ, Ransohoff RM. Cutting edge commentary: Chemokine regulation of experimental autoimmune encephalomyelitis: Temporal and spatial expression patterns govern disease pathogenesis. J Immunol 1998; 161:2667–2671.

67. Simpson JE, Newcombe J, Cuzner ML, Woodroofe MN. Expression of monocyte chemoattractant protein-1 and other β-chemokines by resident glia and inflammatory cells in multiple sclerosis lesions. J Neuroimmunol 1998; 84:238–249.

68. Miyagishi R, Kikuchi S, Fukazawa T, Tashiro K. Macrophage inflammatory protein-1α in the cerebrospinal fluid of patients with multiple sclerosis and other inflammatory neurological diseases. J Neurol Sci 1995; 129:223–227.

69. Sørensen TL, Tani M, Jensen J, et al. Expression of specific chemokines and chemokine receptors in the central nervous system of multiple sclerosis patients. J Clin Invest 1999; 103:807–815.

70. Balashov KE, Rottman JB, Weiner HL, Hancock WW. CCR5+ and CXCR3+ T cells are increased in multiple sclerosis and their ligands MIP-1α and IP-10 are expressed in demyelinating brain lesions. Proc Natl Acad Sci USA 1999; 96:6873–6878.

71. Youssef S, Wildbaum G, Maor G, et al. Long-lasting protective immunity to experimental autoimmune encephalomyelitis following vaccination with naked DNA encoding C-C chemokines. J Immunol 1998; 161:3870–3879.

72. Ng HP, May K, Bauman JG, et al. Discovery of novel non-peptide CCR1 receptor antagonists. J Med Chem 1999; 42:4680–4694.

73. Birk K, Ford C, Smeltzer S, Ryan D, Miller R, Rudick RA. The clinical course of multiple sclerosis during pregnancy and the puerperium. Arch Neurol 1990; 47:738–742.

74. Korn-Lubetzki I, Kahana E, Cooper G, Abramsky O. Activity of multiple sclerosis during pregnancy and puerperium. Ann Neurol 1984; 16:229–231.

75. Thompson DS, Nelson LM, Burns A, Burks JS, Franklin GM. The effects of pregnancy in multiple sclerosis: A retrospective study. Neurology 1986; 36:1097–1099.

76. van Walderveen MA, Tas MW, Barkhof F, et al. Magnetic resonance evaluation of disease activity during pregnancy in multiple sclerosis. Neurology 1994; 44:327–329.

77. Smith R, Studd JW. A pilot study of the effect upon multiple sclerosis of the menopause, hormone replacement therapy and the menstrual cycle. J R Soc Med 1992; 85:612–613.

78. Zorgdrager A, De Keyser J. Premenstrual exacerbations of multiple sclerosis. J Neurol Neurosurg Psychiatry 1998; 65:279–280.

79. Bebo BF Jr, Schuster JC, Vandenbark AA, Offner H. Gender differences in experimental autoimmune encephalomyelitis develop during the induction of the immune response to encephalitogenic peptides. J Neurosci Res 1998; 52:420–426.

80. Voskuhl RR, Pitchekian-Halabi H, MacKenzie-Graham A, McFarland HF, Raine CS. Gender differences in autoimmune demyelination in the mouse: Implications for multiple sclerosis. Ann Neurol 1996; 39:724–733.

81. Kim S, Voskuhl RR. Decreased IL-12 production underlies the decreased ability of male lymph node cells to induce experimental autoimmune encephalomyelitis. J Immunol 1999; 162:5561–5568.

82. Arnason BG, Richman DP. Effect of oral contraceptives on experimental demyelinating disease. Arch Neurol 1969; 21:103–108.

83. Jansson L, Olsson T, Holmdahl R. Estrogen induces a potent suppression of experimental autoimmune encephalomyelitis and collagen-induced arthritis in mice. J Neuroimmunol 1994; 53:203–207.

84. Kim S, Liva SM, Dalal MA, Verity MA, Voskuhl RR. Estriol ameliorates autoimmune demyelinating disease: Implications for multiple sclerosis. Neurology 1999; 52:1230–1238.

85. Dalal M, Kim S, Voskuhl RR. Testosterone therapy ameliorates experimental autoimmune encephalomyelitis and induces a T helper 2 bias in the autoantigen-specific T lymphocyte response. J Immunol 1997; 159:3–6.

86. Bebo BF Jr, Schuster JC, Vandenbark AA, Offner H. Androgens alter the cytokine profile and reduce encephalitogenicity of myelin-reactive T cells. J Immunol 1999; 162:35–40.

87. Piccinni MP, Giudizi MG, Biagiotti R, et al. Progesterone favors the development of human T helper cells producing Th2-type cytokines and promotes both IL-4 production and membrane CD30 expression in established Th1 cell clones. J Immunol 1995; 155:128–133.

88. Correale J, Arias M, Gilmore W. Steroid hormone regulation of cytokine secretion by proteolipid protein-specific CD4+ T cell clones isolated from multiple sclerosis patients and normal control subjects. J Immunol 1998; 161:3365–3374.

89. Gilmore W, Weiner LP, Correale J. Effect of estradiol on cytokine secretion by proteolipid protein-specific T cell clones isolated from multiple sclerosis patients and normal control subjects. J Immunol 1997; 158:446–451.

90. Bansil S, Lee HJ, Jindal S, Cook SD. Correlation between sex hormones and magnetic resonance imaging lesions in multiple sclerosis. Acta Neurol Scand 1998; 98:1–4.

91. Weissman IL. Translating stem and progenitor cell biology to the clinic: Barriers and opportunities. Science 2000; 287:1442–1446.

92. Gage FH. Mammalian neural stem cells. Science 2000; 287:1433–1438.

93. Antel JP, Nalbantoglu J, Olivier A. Neuronal progenitors-learning from the hippocampus. Nature Med. 2000; 6:249–250.

94. Fricker RA, Carpenter N, Winkler C, Greco C, Gates MA, Bjorklund A. Site-specific migration and neuronal differentiation of human neural progenitor cells after transplantation in the adult rat brain. J Neurosci 1999; 19:5990–6005.

95. Yandava B.D., Billinghurst L.L., Snyder E.Y. Global cell replacement is feasible via neural stem cell transplantation: Evidence from the dysmyelinated shiverer mouse brain. Proc Natl Acad Sci USA 1999; 96:7029–7034.

96. Brüstle O, Jones KN, Learish RD, et al. Embryonic stem cell-derived glial precursors: A source of myelinating transplants. Science 1999; 285:754–756.

97. Tuohy VK, Mathisen PM. T-cell design: Optimizing the therapeutic potential of autoreactive T cells by genetic modification. Res Immunol 1998; 149:82–90.

98. Shaw MK, Lorens JB, Dhawan A, et al. Local delivery of interleukin 4 by retrovirus-transduced T lymphocytes ameliorates experimental autoimmune encephalomyelitis. J Exp Med 1997; 185:1711–1714.

99. Chen LZ, Hochwald GM, Huang C, et al. Gene therapy in allergic encephalomyelitis using myelin basic protein-specific T cells engineered to express latent transforming growth factor-beta 1. Proc Natl Acad Sci USA 1998; 95:12516–12521.

100. Thorbecke GJ, Umetsu DT, DeKruyff RH, Hansen GS, Chen LZ, Hochwald GM. When engineered to produce latent TGF-beta 1, antigen specific T cells down regulate Th1 cell-mediated autoimmune and Th2 cell-mediated allergic inflammatory processes. Cytokine Growth Factor Rev 2000; 11:89–96.

101. Mathisen PM, Yu M, Yin L, et al. Th2 T cells expressing transgene PDGF-A serve as vectors for gene therapy in autoimmune demyelinating disease. J Autoimmun 1999; 13:31–38.

102. Furlan R, Poliani PL, Galbiati F, et al. Central nervous system delivery of interleukin 4 by a nonreplicative herpes simplex type 1 viral vector ameliorates autoimmune demyelination. Hum Gene Ther 1998; 9:2605–2617.

103. Martino G, Furlan R, Galbiati F, et al. A gene therapy approach to treat demyelinating diseases using non-replicative herpetic vectors engineered to produce cytokines. Mult Scler 1998; 4:222–227.

104. Croxford JL, Triantaphyllopoulos KA, Neve RN, Feldmann M, Chernajovsky Y, Baker D. Gene therapy for chronic relapsing experimental allergic encephalomyelitis using cells expressing a novel soluble p75 dimeric TNF receptor. J Immunol 2000; 164:2776–2781.

105. Benedetti S, Pirola B, Pollo B, et al. Gene therapy of experimental brain tumors using neural progenitor cells. Nature Med 2000; 6:447–450.

Index

About the Editor

STUART D. COOK is President of the University of Medicine and Dentistry of New Jersey (UMDNJ), and R. D. Kushner and M. J. Serwitz Professor in the Department of Neurosciences, UMDNJ-New Jersey Medical School, Newark. Additionally, he is an Attending Physician at University Hospital, Newark, and serves as Consultant to the Veterans Administration Medical Center, East Orange, and Hackensack Hospital, New Jersey. The coauthor of numerous medical publications and a Fellow of the American Academy of Neurology, Dr. Cook serves on the International Medical Advisory Board of the National Multiple Sclerosis Society. He received the A.B. degree (1957) in chemistry from Brandeis University, Waltham, Massachusetts, and the M.S. (1959) and M.D. (1962) degrees from the University of Vermont, Burlington.

ISBN 0-8247-0485-1